Disorders of Brain and Mind 2

'This is without doubt the best introduction to neuroscience for psychiatrists.'
British Journal of Psychiatry, reviewing the previous volume of *Disorders of Brain and Mind*

In recent years there have been major advances in areas of clinical neuroscience including neurogenetics, neuroimaging and the scientific study of consciousness. *Disorders of Brain and Mind 2* brings together the most salient advances in the field since the previous volume was published in 1998.

In this entirely new collection of articles, the scope is again wide. Imaging of the normal and abnormal mind figures prominently, and there is also coverage of genes and behaviour, brain development, consciousness and aggression. New disease-orientated chapters detail recent advances in dementia, affective illness and drug use and abuse. Clinical chapters are paired with those describing neuropathology or experimental models of the disease in question.

The distinguished editors have assembled an authoritative team of contributors from the fields of psychiatry, clinical and cognitive neuroscience, and psychology. This book will appeal to anyone who has a clinical or scientific interest in the mind and its disorders.

Maria A. Ron is Professor of Neuropsychiatry at the Institute of Neurology, University College London.

Trevor W. Robbins is Professor of Experimental Psychology and Head of the Department of Experimental Psychology, University of Cambridge.

Disorders of Brain and Mind 2

Edited by

Maria A. Ron and
Trevor W. Robbins

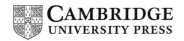

CAMBRIDGE
UNIVERSITY PRESS

PUBLISHED BY THE PRESS SYNDICATE OF THE UNIVERSITY OF CAMBRIDGE

The Pitt Building, Trumpington Street, Cambridge, United Kingdom

CAMBRIDGE UNIVERSITY PRESS

The Edinburgh Building, Cambridge CB2 2RU, UK

40 West 20th Street, New York, NY 10011-4211, USA

477 Williamstown Road, Port Melbourne, VIC 3207, Australia

Ruiz de Alarcón 13, 28014 Madrid, Spain

Dock House, The Waterfront, Cape Town 8001, South Africa

http://www.cambridge.org

First published 2003

Printed in the United Kingdom at the University Press, Cambridge

Typefaces Minion 10.5/14 pt, Formata and Formata BQ   *System* LaTeX 2$_\varepsilon$ [TB]

A catalogue record for this book is available from the British Library

Library of Congress Cataloguing in Publication data

ISBN 0 521 00456 X paperback

Every effort has been made in preparing this book to provide accurate and up-to-date
information which is in accord with accepted standards and practice at the time of publication. Nevertheless, the authors, editors and publisher can make no warranties that
the information contained herein is totally free from error, not least because clinical
standards are constantly changing through research and regulation. The authors, editors and publisher therefore disclaim all liability for direct or consequential damages
resulting from the use of material contained in this book. Readers are strongly advised
to pay careful attention to information provided by the manufacturer of any drugs or
equipment that they plan to use.

Contents

Contributors

Kate D Baker
Behavioural and Brain Sciences Unit,
Institute of Child Health, 30 Guilford
Street, London WC1N 1EH, UK

Clare Beasley
Research Worker, Section of Experimental
Neuropathology and Psychiatry, Institute of
Psychiatry, De Crespigny Park, Denmark
Hill, London SE5 8AF, UK

R J R Blair
Senior Lecturer, Institute of Cognitive
Neuroscience and Department of
Psychology, University College London,
Alexandra House, 17 Queen Square,
London WC1N 3AR, UK

Ed Bullmore
Professor of Psychiatry, University of
Cambridge, Department of Psychiatry,
Addenbrooke's Hospital, Cambridge
CB2 2QQ, UK

Don R Cherek
Professor, Human Psychopharmacology
Laboratory, Department of Psychiatry and
Behavioral Sciences, Mental Sciences
Institute, University of Texas Health Science
Center – Houston, 1300 Moursund Street,
Houston, Texas 77030, USA

Xavier Chitnis
Research Worker, Neuroimaging Research
Group, Department of Neurology, Institute
of Psychiatry, De Crespigny Park, Denmark
Hill, London SE5 8AF, UK

R J Dolan
Kinross Professor of Neuropsychiatry,
Wellcome Department of Cognitive
Neurology, Functional Imaging
Laboratory, Institute of Neurology,
12 Queen Square, London
WC1N 3BG, UK

Ian Ellison-Wright
Consultant Psychiatrist, Avon and
Wiltshire Mental Health Partnership
NHS Trust, The Old Manor Hospital,
Wilton Road, Salisbury SP2 7EP, and
Honorary Senior Lecturer, Department
of Psychological Medicine, Institute of
Psychiatry, De Crespigny Park, Denmark
Hill, London SE5 8AF, UK

Ian Everall
Professor of Experimental
Neuropathology and Psychiatry,
Section of Experimental Neuropathology
and Psychiatry, Institute of Psychiatry,
De Crespigny Park, Denmark Hill,
London SE5 8AF, UK

Jacqueline Foong
Consultant Psychiatrist, National Hospital for Neurology and Neurosurgery, Queen Square, London WC1N 3BG, and Honorary Senior Lecturer, Institute of Neurology, Queen Square, London WC1N 3BG, UK

Chris Frith
Professor in Neuropsychology, Wellcome Department of Cognitive Neurology, Institute of Neurology, University College London, 12 Queen Square, London WC1N 3BG, UK

Rebecca Gittins
MRC DPhil Student, University Department of Clinical Neurology (Neuropathology), Radcliffe Infirmary, Oxford OX2 6HE, UK

Michel Goedert
Member of the Scientific Staff, Medical Research Council Laboratory of Molecular Biology, Hills Road, Cambridge CB2 2QH, UK

Magdalena Götz
Max-Planck Institute of Neurobiology, Am Klopferspitz 18A, 82152 Planegg-Martinsried, Germany

P M Grasby
Cyclotron Unit, Clinical Sciences Centre, Hammersmith Hospital, Du Cane Road, London W12 0NN, UK

Paul J Harrison
Professor, University Department of Psychiatry, Warneford Hospital, Oxford OX3 7JX, UK

John R Hodges
MRC Professor of Behavioural Neurology, University Neurology Unit, Addenbrooke's Hospital, Cambridge; and MRC Cognition and Brain Sciences Unit, 15 Chaucer Road, Cambridge CB2 2EF, UK

Simon Killcross
Senior Research Fellow, School of Psychology, Cardiff University, PO Box 901, Tower Building, Park Place, Cardiff CF10 3YG, UK

Keith Matthews
Professor of Psychiatry, Department of Psychiatry, Dundee University, Ninewells Hospital and Medical School, Dundee DD1 9SY, UK

Andy N Mead
Research Fellow, Laboratory of Experimental Psychology, University of Sussex, Falmer, Brighton BN1 9QG, UK

Peter J Nestor
Research Associate, University Neurology Unit, Addenbrooke's Hospital, Hills Road, Cambridge CB2 2QQ, UK

Cynthia J Pietras
Postdoctoral Fellow, Human Psychopharmacology Laboratory, Department of Psychiatry and Behavioral Sciences, Mental Sciences Institute, University of Texas Health Science Center – Houston, 1300 Moursund Street, Houston, Texas 77030, USA

Robert Plomin
MRC Research Professor and Deputy Director of the SGDP Research Centre, Social, Genetic and Developmental Psychiatry Research Centre, Institute of Psychiatry, King's College London, De Crespigny Park, Denmark Hill, London SE5 8AF, UK

Tamzin L Ripley
Research Fellow, Laboratory of
Experimental Psychology, University
of Sussex, Falmer, Brighton
BN1 9QG, UK

Trevor W Robbins
Professor of Cognitive Neuroscience,
Department of Cognitive Neuroscience,
Downing Street, Cambridge CB2 3EB, UK

Robert D Rogers
University Lecturer in (Non-clinical)
Psychology, Department of Psychiatry,
University of Oxford, Warneford Hospital,
Oxford, OX3 7JX, UK

Maria A Ron
Professor of Neuropsychiatry, Institute
of Neurology, Queen Square, London
WC1N 3BG, UK

David H Skuse
Professor of Behavioural and Brain
Sciences, Behavioural and Brain Sciences
Unit, Institute of Child Health, 30 Guilford
Street, London WC1N 1EH, UK

Sean A Spence
University of Sheffield, Academic
Department of Psychiatry, The Longley
Centre, Sheffield S5 7JT, UK

Maria Grazia Spillantini
William Scholl Lecturer in Neurology, Brain
Repair Centre and Department of
Neurology, University of Cambridge,
Robinson Way, Cambridge CB2 2PY, UK

David N Stephens
Professor of Experimental Psychology,
Laboratory of Experimental Psychology,
University of Sussex, Falmer, Brighton
BN1 9QG, UK

Siân A Thompson
Research Fellow, University Neurology
Unit, Addenbrooke's Hospital, Hills Road,
Cambridge CB2 2QQ, UK

Brenda Williams
Senior Lecturer, Section of Experimental
Neuropathology and Psychiatry, Institute of
Psychiatry, De Crespigny Park, Denmark
Hill, London SE5 8AF, UK

Part I

Genes and behaviour

Genes and behaviour: cognitive abilities and disabilities in normal populations

Robert Plomin

Institute of Psychiatry, King's College, London, UK

Introduction

During the past three decades, the behavioural sciences have emerged from an era of strict environmental explanations for differences in behaviour to a more balanced view that recognizes the importance of nature (genetics) as well as nurture (environment). This shift occurred first for behavioural disorders, including rare disorders such as autism (0.001 incidence), more common disorders such as schizophrenia (0.01), and very common disorders such as reading disability (0.05). More recently it has become increasingly accepted that genetic variation contributes importantly to differences among individuals in the normal range of variability as well as for abnormal behaviour. Moreover, many behavioural disorders, especially common ones, may represent the quantitative extreme of the same genetic and environmental factors responsible for variation in the normal range. That is, genetic influence on disorders such as reading disability may not be due to genes specific to the disorder but rather to genes that contribute to the normal range of individual differences in reading ability. This view, known as the quantitative trait locus (QTL) perspective, has important conceptual implications because it implies that some common disorders may not be disorders at all but rather the extremes of normal distributions. This QTL perspective has far-reaching implications for molecular genetics and for neuroscience. If many genes of small effect are involved, it will be much more difficult to find them. It will also be much more difficult to explore the brain mechanisms that mediate genetic effects on behaviour.

These issues are the topic of this chapter, which focuses on cognitive abilities and disabilities. Basic introductions to quantitative genetics (such as twin and adoption designs), molecular genetics and research that uses these genetic methods to investigate behaviour are available elsewhere (Plomin et al. 2001a), as are more detailed discussions of genetic research in neuroscience (Crusio and Gerlai 1999; Pfaff et al. 2000).

The very standard deviation

It is important to begin with a discussion of the different perspectives or levels of analysis used to investigate behaviour because so much follows conceptually as well as methodologically from these differences in perspective (Figure 1.1). Research on cognitive abilities and disabilities focuses on within-species interindividual differences – for example, why some children are reading disabled and others are not. In contrast, textbooks in cognitive neuroscience seldom mention individual differences and concentrate instead on species-universal or species-typical (normative) aspects of cognitive functioning (Gazzaniga 2000; Thompson 2000). Neuroscience has focused on understanding how the brain works on average – for example, which bits of the brain light up under neuroimaging for particular tasks. Until now, genetics has entered neuroscience largely in relation to gene targeting in mice in which mutations are induced that break down normal brain processes. In humans, rare single-gene mutations are the centre of attention. This approach tends to treat all members of the species as if they were genetically the same except for a few rogue mutations that disrupt normal processes. In this sense, the species-typical perspective of neuroscience assumes that mental illness is a broken brain. In contrast, the individual-differences perspective considers variation as normal – the very standard deviation. Common mental illness is thought to be the quantitative extreme of the normal distribution.

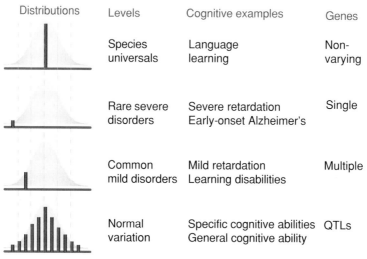

Figure 1.1   Levels of analysis.

Although perspectives are not right or wrong – just more or less useful for particular purposes – the species-typical perspective and the individual-differences perspective can arrive at different answers because they ask different questions. The distinction between the two perspectives is in essence the difference between means and variances. There is no necessary connection between means and variances, either descriptively or aetiologically. Despite its name, analysis of variance, the most widely used statistical analysis in the life sciences, is actually an analysis of mean effects in which individual differences are literally called the *error term*. Instead of treating differences between individuals as error, and averaging individuals across groups as in analysis of variance, individual-differences research focuses on these interindividual differences. Variation is distributed continuously, often in the shape of the familiar bell curve, and is indexed by variance (the sum of squared deviations from the mean), or the square of variance, which is called the standard deviation.

The two perspectives also differ methodologically. Most species-typical research is experimental in the sense that subjects are randomly assigned to conditions which consist of manipulating something such as genes, lesions, drugs and tasks. The dependent variable is the average effect of the manipulation on outcome measures such as single-cell recordings of synaptic plasticity, activation of brain regions assessed by neuroimaging, or performance on cognitive tests. Such experiments ask whether such manipulations *can* have an effect on average in a species. For example, a gene knock-out study investigates whether an experimental group of mice who inherit a gene that has been made dysfunctional differs, for example in learning or memory, from a control group with a normal copy of the gene. A less obvious example can be seen in recent experimental research that manipulated tasks and found that average blood flow assessed by positron emission tomography (PET) in the human species is greater in the prefrontal cortex for high-intelligence tasks than for low-intelligence tasks (Duncan et al. 2000).

In contrast, rather than creating differences between experimental and control groups through manipulations, the individual-differences perspective focuses on naturally occurring differences between individuals. One of the factors that makes individuals different is genetics. The individual-differences perspective is the foundation for quantitative genetics, which focuses on naturally occurring genetic variation, the stuff of heredity. Although 99.9% of the human DNA sequence is identical for all human beings, the 0.1% that differs – 3 million base pairs (enough for every gene for each of us to be different) – is ultimately responsible for the ubiquitous genetic influence found for all individual-differences traits including cognitive abilities and disabilities (Plomin et al. 2001*a*). Individual-differences research is correlational in the sense that it investigates factors that *do* have an effect in the world outside the laboratory. Continuing with the previous examples, an individual-differences approach would ask whether naturally occurring genetic variation in mice is associated with individual differences in mouse learning and memory. Genes can be knocked out and shown to have major effects on learning and memory but this does not imply that the gene has anything to do with the naturally occurring genetic variation that is responsible for hereditary transmission of individual differences in performance on learning and memory tasks. The PET experiment that compared average performance on high- and low-intelligence tasks could be addressed from an individual-differences perspective by comparing cortical blood flow in high- and low-intelligence individuals rather than comparing average performance on tasks (Duncan et al. 2000).

Other perspectives or levels of analysis lie in between these two extremes of species universals and normal variation. The effects of rare severe disorders caused by a single gene are dramatic. For example, mutations in the gene that codes for the enzyme phenylalanine hydroxylase, if untreated, cause phenylketonuria (PKU) that is associated with a severe form of mental retardation. This inherited condition occurs in 1 in 10 000 births. At least 100 other rare single-gene disorders include mental retardation as part of the syndrome (Wahlström 1990). Such rare single-gene disorders can be viewed as aberrations from the species type, exceptions to the species rule. In contrast, common disorders – such as mild mental retardation and learning disabilities – seldom show any sign of single-gene effects and appear to be caused by multiple genes as well as by multiple environmental factors. Indeed, quantitative genetic research suggests that such common disorders are usually the quantitative extreme of the same genes responsible for variation throughout the distribution. Genes in such multiple-gene (polygenic) systems are called quantitative trait loci (QTL) because they are likely to result in dimensions (quantitative continua) rather than disorders (qualitative dichotomies). For example, as discussed later, reading disability has been linked to the short arm of chromosome 6 (6p21) in several QTL analyses (Willcutt et al., in press). When the gene responsible for this linkage is isolated, the QTL prediction is that it will not reveal a gene for reading disability per se. Rather, the gene is one of many that are expected to contribute quantitatively to reading performance throughout the distribution. In other words, in terms of the genetic aetiology of common disorders, there may be no disorders, just dimensions. Other than simple and rare single-gene or chromosomal disorders, mental illness may represent the extreme of normal variation.

In summary, the individual-differences perspective views variation as normal and distributed continuously; common disorders are viewed as the extremes of these continuous distributions. As indicated at the outset, perspectives are not right or wrong. But they are different, and the proper interpretation of genetic research depends on understanding these differences. The perspectives are complementary in the sense that a full understanding of behaviour requires integration across all levels of analysis.

Quantitative genetics

Although much human genetic research focuses on rare single-gene disorders (see Chapter 2 by Skuse and Baker) and much genetic research using animal models focuses on gene knockouts (see Chapter 19 by Stephens et al.), the present chapter concentrates on the genetics of individual differences, both quantitative genetics and molecular genetics. Quantitative genetic research such as twin and adoption studies is hardly needed any longer merely to ask whether and how much genetic factors influence behavioural traits, because the answers are 'yes', and 'a lot' for nearly all dimensions and disorders that have been studied (Plomin et al. 2001a). However, new quantitative genetic techniques make it possible to go beyond these rudimentary questions to investigate how genes and environment affect developmental change and continuity, comorbidity and heterogeneity, and the links between disorders and normal variation. Using these techniques, quantitative genetic research can lead to better diagnoses based in part on aetiology rather than solely on symptomatology. They can also chart the course for molecular genetic studies by identifying the most heritable components and constellations of disorders as they develop and as genetic vulnerabilities correlate and interact with the environment. The future of genetic research on cognitive abilities and disabilities lies with molecular genetic research that attempts to identify specific genes responsible for heritability. Although progress in identifying genes for complex traits such as cognitive abilities and disabilities has been slow, when such genes are found the next step will be to understand the brain mechanisms that mediate genetic effects on behaviour.

This chapter focuses on genetics but it should be mentioned at the outset that quantitative genetic research is at least as informative about nurture as it is about nature. In the first instance, it provides the best available evidence for the importance of the environment, in that the heritability of complex traits is seldom greater than 50%. In other words, about half of the variance cannot be explained by genetic factors. In addition, two of the most important findings about environmental influences on behaviour have come from genetic research. The first finding is that, contrary to socialization theories from Freud onwards, environmental influences operate to make children growing up in the same family as different as children growing up in different families, which is called nonshared environment (reviewed by Plomin et al. 2001b). The second finding, called the nature of nurture, is that genetic factors influence the way we experience our environments (reviewed by Plomin 1994). For this reason, most measures of the environment used in behavioural research show genetic influence. For the same reason, associations between environmental measures and behavioural outcome measures are often substantially mediated genetically. The way forward in research is to bring together genetic and environmental strategies, for example, using environmental measures in genetically sensitive designs to investigate interactions and correlations between nature and nurture. The present chapter's focus on genetics is not intended to denigrate the importance of environmental influences or to imply biological determinism.

General cognitive ability

General cognitive ability (g) is a highly heritable quantitative trait that varies from a low end of mild mental retardation to a high end of gifted individuals (Plomin 1999a). One of the most consistent findings from individual-differences research on human cognitive abilities and disabilities during the past century is that diverse cognitive processes intercorrelate. Despite the diversity of cognitive tests, individuals who perform well on one test tend to do well on other tests. In a meta-analysis of 322 studies that included hundreds of different kinds of cognitive tests, the average correlation among the tests was about 0.30 (Carroll 1993). A technique called factor analysis, in which a composite score is created that represents what is shared in common among the measures, indicates that g accounts for about 40% of the total variance of cognitive tests (Jensen 1998). However, g is not just a statistical abstraction – one can simply look at a matrix of correlations among such measures and see that there is a positive manifold among all tests and that some measures (such as spatial and verbal ability) intercorrelate more highly on average than do other measures (such as nonverbal memory tests). Because all of these measures intercorrelate to some extent, g is also indexed reasonably well by a simple total score on a diverse set of cognitive measures, as is done in IQ tests. This overlap emerges not only for traditional measures of reasoning, spatial, verbal and memory abilities such as those mentioned above but also for information-processing tasks that rely on reaction time and other cognitive tasks used to assess, for example, working memory (Anderson 1992; Stauffer et al. 1996; Baddeley and Gathercole 1999; Deary 2000).

General cognitive ability was recognized nearly a century ago by Charles Spearman (1904, 1927), who used g as a neutral signifier that avoided the many connotations of the word *intelligence*. g is one of the most reliable and valid traits in the behavioural domain (Jensen 1998). Its long-term stability after childhood is greater than for any other behavioural trait (Deary et al. 2000), it predicts important social outcomes such as educational and occupational levels far better than any other trait (Gottfredson 1997), and it is a key factor in cognitive ageing (Salthouse and Czaja 2000). There are of course many other important noncognitive abilities, such as athletic ability, but there seems to be nothing to be gained by lumping all such abilities together as is done with the popular notion of 'multiple intelligences' (Gardner 1983). Also, g by no means guarantees success either in school or in the workplace – achievement also requires personality, motivation and social skills, currently referred to as 'emotional intelligence' (Goleman 1995).

Although the concept of *g* is widely accepted (Neisser et al. 1996; Carroll 1997; Snyderman and Rothman 1987), acceptance is not universal. The arguments against *g* have been reviewed (Jensen 1998). They include ideological issues such as political concerns and the notion that *g* merely reflects knowledge and skills that happen to be valued by the dominant culture (Gould 1996). Objections of a more scientific nature include theories that focus on specific abilities (Gardner 1983; Sternberg 1985). However, when these theories are examined empirically, *g* shines through. For example, one of the major advocates of a 'componential' view to cognitive processing conceded that 'We interpret the preponderance of evidence as overwhelmingly supporting the existence of some kind of general factor in human intelligence. Indeed, we are unable to find any convincing evidence at all that militates against this view' (Sternberg and Gardner 1983). *g* is not the whole story – group factors representing specific abilities are also important levels of analysis – but trying to tell the story of cognitive abilities without *g* loses the plot entirely.

The existence of *g* appears to go against the tide of current cognitive neuroscience which considers cognitive processes as 'modular' – specific and independent (Fodor 1983; Pinker 1994). However, as mentioned earlier, research in cognitive neuroscience focuses on species-typical processes. *g* is not about average performance – it is about individual differences in performance, and the fact that individuals who perform well on some tasks tend to perform well on most tasks. The investigation of individual differences represents a different level of analysis where the data clearly point to *g*. The existence of *g* does not imply that the source of *g* must be a single general physical (dendritic complexity, myelinization), physiological (synaptic plasticity, speed of nerve conduction) or psychological (working memory, executive function) process (Deary 2000). It seems more reasonable to suppose that *g* represents a concatenation of such physical, physiological and psychological processes that are all enlisted to solve functional problems. As an analogy, athletic ability depends on psychological (motivation), physiological (oxygen transport) and physical (bone structure) processes. Athletic ability is not one of these things, it is all of these things.

There is more research addressing the genetics of *g* than any other human characteristic. Dozens of studies including more than 8000 parent–offspring pairs, 25 000 pairs of siblings, 10 000 twin pairs and hundreds of adoptive families all converge on the conclusion that genetic factors contribute substantially to *g* (Plomin et al. 2001*a*). Estimates of the effect size, called heritability, vary from 40–80% but estimates based on the entire body of data are about 50%, indicating that genes account for about half of the variance in *g*. Sorting the results by age indicates that heritability increases from about 0.20 in infancy to about 0.40 in childhood and to 0.60 or higher later in life (McGue et al. 1993), even for individuals 80+ years old (McClearn et al. 1997). This increase in heritability throughout the lifespan is interesting, because it is counterintuitive in relation to Shakespeare's 'slings and arrows of outrageous fortune' accumulating over time. This finding suggests that people actively select, modify and even create environments conducive to the development of their genetic proclivities. For this reason, it may be more appropriate to think about *g* as an appetite rather than an aptitude.

The most important finding comes from multivariate genetic analysis, which is used to examine covariance among specific cognitive abilities, rather than the variance of each trait considered separately. It yields a statistic called the *genetic correlation*, which is an estimate of the extent to which genetic effects on one trait correlate with genetic effects on another trait independent of the heritability of the two traits. That is, although all cognitive abilities are moderately heritable, the genetic correlations between them could be anywhere from 0.0, indicating complete independence, to 1.0, indicating that the same genes influence different cognitive abilities. In the case of cognitive abilities, multivariate genetic analyses have consistently found that genetic correlations among cognitive abilities are very high – close to 1.0 (Petrill 1997). In other words, if a gene were found that is associated with a particular cognitive ability, the same gene would be expected to be associated with all other cognitive abilities as well. As noted earlier, *g* accounts for about 40% of the total variance of cognitive tests. In contrast, multivariate genetic research indicates that *g* accounts for nearly *all* of the genetic variance of cognitive tests. That is, what is in common among cognitive abilities is almost completely genetic in origin. This finding has the interesting converse implication that what is specific to each cognitive test is largely environmental – what makes us good at all tests is largely genetic but what makes us better at some tests than others is largely environmental.

This finding from multivariate genetic research provides clues for understanding how the brain works from an individual-differences perspective. Spearman, who first described *g* in 1904, noted that ultimate understanding of *g* 'must needs come from the most profound and detailed study of the human brain in its purely physical and chemical aspects' (Spearman 1927, p. 403). The simplest brain model of genetic *g* is that there is a single fundamental brain process that permeates all other brain processing such as neural speed (e.g. myelinization), power (e.g. number of neurons) or fidelity (e.g. density of dendritic spines). The opposite model is that there are many brain processes that are uncorrelated phenotypically and genetically, but lead to a genetic correlation in performance on cognitive tasks because all of these brain processes are enlisted by the cognitive tasks. A middle position is that multiple brain processes underlie *g* in cognitive tasks but these processes are correlated phenotypically and genetically. That is, genetic *g* might exist in the brain as well as the mind. To test these different models about brain mechanisms responsible for *g*, it is necessary to identify reliable individual differences in brain processes and investigate the phenotypic and genetic relationships among these processes.

Human research on *g* can make progress towards understanding brain mechanisms using neuroimaging techniques (Kosslyn and Plomin 2001). However, mouse models of *g* would facilitate the precise analysis of basic brain mechanisms using techniques such as single cell recordings, micro-stimulation, targeted gene mutations, antisense DNA that disrupts gene transcription and DNA expression studies. Clearly, there are major differences in brain and mind between the human species and other animals, most notably in the use of language and the highly developed prefrontal cortex in the human species. However, *g* in humans does not depend on the use of language – a strong *g* factor emerges from a battery of completely nonverbal tests (Jensen 1998) – and low-level tasks such as information-processing tasks assessed by reaction time contribute to *g* (Deary 2000). Indeed, *g* can be used as a criterion to identify animal models of individual differences in cognitive processes. If *g* represents the way in which genetically driven components of the brain work together to solve problems, it would not be unreasonable to hypothesize that *g* exists in all animals (Anderson 2000). Although much less well documented than *g* in humans, increasing evidence exists for a *g* factor in mice across diverse tasks of learning, memory and problem solving (Plomin 2001).

Specific cognitive abilities

Although *g* is important, there is much more to cognitive functioning. Cognitive abilities are usually considered in a hierarchical model (Figure 1.2). General cognitive ability is at the top of the hierarchy, representing what all tests of cognitive ability have in common. Below general cognitive ability in the hierarchy are broad factors of specific cognitive abilities, such as verbal ability, spatial ability, memory and speed of processing. These broad factors are indexed by several tests, shown at the bottom of the hierarchy in Figure 1.2. In addition to specific tests, the bottom of the hierarchy can also be considered in terms of elementary processes thought to be involved in information processing.

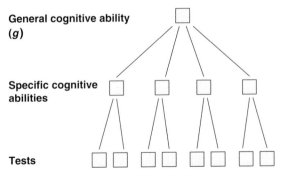

General cognitive ability
(*g*)

Specific cognitive abilities

Tests

Figure 1.2　Hierarchical model of cognitive abilities.

Many specific cognitive abilities show genetic influence in twin studies, although the magnitude of the genetic effect is generally lower than that for general cognitive ability (Plomin and DeFries 1998). Family and twin studies suggest that the genetic contribution may be stronger for some cognitive abilities such as verbal and spatial than for other abilities, especially nonverbal memory. Recent studies of twins reared apart generally confirm these findings. Developmental genetic analyses indicate that genetically distinct specific cognitive abilities can be found as early as 3 years of age and show increasing genetic differentiation from early to middle childhood. Twin studies also indicate genetic influence on information-processing measures and brain-wave measures of EEG and event-related potentials (Plomin et al. 2001*a*).

Mental retardation

If genetics substantially influences general cognitive ability, one might expect that low IQ scores are also due to genetic factors. However, this conclusion does not necessarily follow. For example, mental retardation can be caused by environmental trauma, such as birth problems, nutritional deficiencies and head injuries. Given the importance of mental retardation, it is surprising that no twin or adoption studies of diagnosed mental retardation have been reported. Nonetheless, one sibling study suggests that moderate and severe mental retardation may be due largely to nonheritable factors. In a study of over 17 000 white children, 0.5% were moderately to severely retarded (Nichols 1984). The siblings of these retarded children were not retarded – the siblings' average IQ was 103 and ranged from 85–125. In other words, moderate to severe mental retardation showed no familial resemblance, which implies that mental retardation is not heritable. Although most moderate and severe mental retardation may not be inherited from generation to generation, it is often caused by noninherited DNA events, such as new gene mutations and new chromosomal abnormalities such as Down's syndrome (see Chapter 2 by Skuse and Baker). This suggestion of low overall heritability for moderate to severe mental retardation does not contradict the finding that mental retardation is a symptom for some rare single-gene syndromes such as phenylketonuria (1 in 10 000 births).

In contrast, in this same study, siblings of mildly retarded children (1.2% of the sample) showed lower than average IQ scores. The average IQ for these siblings of mildly retarded children was only 85. These important findings – that mild mental retardation is familial whereas moderate and severe retardation is not familial – also emerged from the largest family study of mild mental retardation, which considered 80 000 relatives of 289 mentally retarded individuals (Reed and Reed 1965). This parent–offspring family study showed that mild mental retardation is very strongly familial. If one parent is mildly retarded, the risk for retardation in their children is about 20%. If both parents are retarded, the risk is nearly 50%.

Although mild mental retardation runs in families, it could do so for reasons of nurture rather than nature. Twin and adoption studies of mild mental retardation are needed to disentangle the relative roles of nature and nurture. Although no proper twin or adoption studies of diagnosed mild mental retardation have been reported, three small twin studies suggest that low IQ is at least as heritable as IQ in the normal range (Plomin 1999*a*). These studies also suggest that mild mental retardation may be the lower end of the distribution of the same genetic and environmental factors that are responsible for general cognitive ability.

Reading disability

Reading is the primary problem in about 80% of children with a diagnosed learning disorder. As many as 10% of children have difficulty learning to read. For some, specific causes can be identified, such as mental retardation, brain damage, sensory problems and deprivation. However, many children without such problems find it difficult to read. Children with a specific reading disorder (also known as *dyslexia*) read slowly, and often with poor comprehension. When reading aloud, they perform poorly.

Family studies have shown that reading disability runs in families. The largest family study included 1044 individuals in 125 families with a reading-disabled child and 125 matched control families (DeFries et al. 1986). Siblings and parents of the reading-disabled children performed significantly worse on reading tests than did siblings and parents of control children. Earlier twin studies suggested that familial resemblance for reading disability involves genetic factors (Bakwin 1973; Decker and Vandenberg 1985). Although one twin study showed little evidence of genetic influence (Stevenson et al. 1987), the largest twin study confirmed genetic influence on reading disability (DeFries et al. 1999). For more than 250 twin pairs in which at least one member of the pair was reading disabled, twin concordances were 66% for identical twins and 36% for fraternal twins, a result suggesting moderate genetic influence.

As part of this twin study, a new method was developed to estimate the genetic contribution to the mean difference between the reading-disabled probands and the mean reading ability of the population. DF extremes analysis (DeFries and Fulker 1985, 1988) takes advantage of quantitative scores of the relatives of probands rather than just assigning a dichotomous diagnosis to the relatives and comparing twin concordances for the disorder. To the extent that reading deficits of probands are heritable, the quantitative reading scores of identical co-twins will be more similar to that of the probands than will the scores of fraternal twins. In other words, the mean reading score of identical co-twins will regress less far back toward the population mean than will that of fraternal co-twins, which is the case for reading disability (DeFries and Gillis 1993). Half of the mean difference between the probands and the population is heritable. This is called 'group heritability' to distinguish it from the usual heritability estimate, which refers to differences between individuals rather than to mean differences between groups. Results of DF extremes analysis indicates that group heritability for reading disability is moderate and similar to individual heritability estimates for reading, suggesting that reading disability is quantitatively rather than qualitatively different from the normal range of reading ability (DeFries and Gillis 1993).

Various modes of transmission have been proposed for reading disability. The autosomal dominant hypothesis takes into account the high rate of familial resemblance but fails to account for the fact that about a fifth of reading-disabled individuals do not have affected relatives. An X-linked recessive hypothesis is suggested when a disorder occurs more often for males than females, as is the case for reading disability. However, the X-linked recessive hypothesis does not work well as an explanation of reading disability. One of the hallmarks of X-linked recessive transmission is the absence of father-to-son transmission, because sons inherit their X chromosome only from their mother. Contrary to the X-linked recessive hypothesis, reading disability is transmitted from father to son as often as from mother to son. It is now generally accepted that, like most complex disorders, reading disability is caused by multiple genes as well as by multiple environmental factors.

Communication disorders

Despite the strong trend of much linguistic theorizing to invoke an innate basis for language (Pinker 1994), genetic research has been slow in coming to the field of language, but the field is making up for lost time (Gilger 1997; Plomin and Dale 2000; Rice 1996). DSM–IV (American Psychiatric Association 1994) includes four types of communication disorders: expressive language (putting thoughts into words) disorder, mixed receptive (understanding the language of others) and expressive language disorder, phonological (articulation) disorder and stuttering (speech interrupted by prolonged or repeated words, syllables or sounds). Hearing loss, mental retardation and neurological disorders are excluded.

Several family studies, examining communication disorders broadly, indicate that communication disorders are familial (Stromswold 2001). For children with communication disorders, about a quarter of their first-degree relatives report similar disorders, compared with about 5% for the relatives of controls (Felsenfeld 1994). Three twin studies of communication disorders found evidence for extremely high heritability, with average concordances of about 90% for identical twins and 50% for fraternal twins (Lewis and Thompson 1992; Bishop et al. 1995; Tomblin and Buckwalter 1998). The only adoption study of communication disorders confirms the twin results (Felsenfeld and Plomin 1997).

These disorders are frequently comorbid but little is known about the genetic and environmental links between them as they emerge in infancy and early childhood.

Multivariate genetic analysis suggests that DSM–IV diagnostic categories may not reflect the genetic origins of these disorders (Plomin and Dale 2000). For example, expressive and receptive language disorders overlap genetically, whereas genetic factors appear to be different for individuals who have articulation problems and those who do not (Bishop et al. 1995).

A large-scale study of twins in infancy and early childhood is under way in the UK to investigate the genetics of early-onset language problems and their relationship to other cognitive and behaviour problems (Plomin and Dale 2000). The study shows that vocabulary delay is highly heritable (73% group heritability using DF extremes analysis) as early as 2 years of age (Dale et al. 1998). Examples of multivariate genetic findings include a high genetic correlation between lexical (vocabulary) and grammatical (sentence complexity) development (Dale et al. 2000) and a strong genetic correlation between language and nonverbal cognitive development (Price et al. 2000).

Family studies of stuttering over the past 50 years have shown that about a third of stutterers have other stutterers in their families. The Yale Family Study of Stuttering includes nearly 600 stutterers and more than 2000 of their first-degree relatives (Kidd 1983). About 15% of the first-degree relatives reported that they had stuttered at some point in their life, about five times greater than the base rate of approximately 3% in the general population. Moreover, about half of the affected first-degree relatives were considered to be chronic stutterers. One small twin study of stuttering suggests that familial resemblance is heritable, with concordances of 77% for identical twins (17 pairs) and 32% for fraternal twins (13 pairs) (Howie 1981). A large twin study that included a single item about stuttering in a question-naire study also found evidence for substantial genetic influence (Andrews et al. 1991). Although much remains to be learned about the genetics of stuttering, the evidence as it stands suggests substantial genetic influence (Yairi et al. 1996).

Molecular genetics

The twentieth century began with the rediscovery of Mendel's laws of heredity. The word *genetics* was only invented in 1903. Fifty years later it was understood that DNA was the mechanism of heredity. The genetic code was cracked in 1966; the 4-letter alphabet (G, A, T, C) of DNA is read as 3-letter words that code for the 20 amino acids that are the building blocks of proteins. The crowning glory of the century and a tremendous start to the new century is the Human Genome Project which has provided a working draft of the sequence of the 3 billion letters of DNA in the human genome.

When the working draft of the human genome sequence was published in February 2001, much publicity was given to the finding that there are fewer than half as many genes (30 000) in the human genome as expected – about the same number of genes as in mice and worms. A bizarre spin in the media was that having only 30 000 genes implies that nurture must be more important than we thought. The idea that fewer genes means more free will is silly. Do flies have more free will than us because they have fewer genes? However, the finding that the human species does not have more genes than other species is important in suggesting that the number of genes is not responsible for the greater complexity of the human species. In part, the greater complexity of the human species occurs because during the process of decoding genes into proteins, human genes, more than the genes of other species, are spliced in alternative ways to create a greater variety of proteins. The greater complexity of the human species may be due to quality rather than quantity: other subtle variations in genes rather than the number of genes may be responsible for differences between mice and men. If subtle DNA differences are responsible for the differences between mice and men, even more subtle differences are likely to be responsible for individual differences within the species.

Another interesting finding from the Human Genome Project is that only 2% of the 3 billion letters in our DNA code involves genes in the traditional sense, that is, genes that code for amino-acid sequences. This 2% figure is similar in other mammals. On an evolutionary time scale, mutations are quickly weeded out from these bits of DNA that are so crucial for development. When mutations are not weeded out, they can cause one of the thousands of severe but rare single-gene disorders. However, it seems unlikely that the other 98% of DNA is just along for the ride. For example, variations in this other 98% of the DNA are known to regulate the activity of the classical genes. For this reason, the other 98% of DNA might be the place to look for genes associated with quantitative rather than qualitative effects on behavioural traits.

The most exciting development for behavioural genetics is the identification of the DNA sequences that make us different from each other. There is no human genome sequence – we each have a unique genome. Indeed, about one in every thousand DNA letters differs, about 3 million variations in total. Many of these DNA differences have already been identified. The Human Genome Project has spawned new technologies that will make it possible to investigate simultaneously thousands of DNA variants as they relate to behavioural traits. These DNA differences are responsible for the widespread heritability of psychological disorders and dimensions. That is, when we say that a trait is heritable, we mean that variations in DNA exist that cause differences in behaviour.

DNA variation has a unique causal status in explaining behaviour. When behaviour is correlated with anything else, the old adage applies that correlation does not imply causation. For example, when parenting is shown to be correlated with children's behavioural outcomes, this does not imply that the parenting caused the outcome environmentally. Indeed, it has been shown that parental behaviour to some extent reflects genetic effects on children's behaviour (Plomin 1994). When it comes to interpreting correlations between biology and behaviour, such correlations are often mistakenly interpreted as if biology causes behaviour. For example, correlations between neurotransmitter physiology and behaviour, or between neuroimaging indices of brain activation and behaviour, are often interpreted as if brain differences cause behavioural differences. However, these correlations do not necessarily imply causation. Behavioural differences can cause brain differences. In contrast, in the case of correlations between DNA variants and behaviour, the behaviour of individuals does not change their genome. Expression of genes can be altered but the DNA sequence itself does not change. For this reason, correlations between DNA differences and behavioural differences can be interpreted causally: DNA differences cause the behavioural differences and not the other way around.

Integration of quantitative genetics and molecular genetics

Since its origins early in the twentieth century, quantitative genetics has focused on commercially valuable traits in plants and animals and socially important traits in the human species, especially behavioural dimensions and disorders. Techniques were developed such as twin and adoption designs for humans, and inbred strain and selection studies for animals, in order to investigate the extent to which genetic factors contribute to the observed differences in such complex traits. Such studies consistently pointed to an important role for genetics even for the most complex of all traits, behaviour. However, the evidence pointed to the involvement of many genes as well as many environmental factors, so that it seemed hopeless to identify specific genes responsible for the genetic contribution to most behavioural traits. In contrast to the focus of quantitative genetics on important phenotypes and on naturally occurring genetic variation responsible for phenotypic differences, molecular genetics focused on genes and techniques to create new mutations in model organisms such as the fruit fly, in order to investigate how genes work. Because of their differences in perspectives and methods, these two approaches to genetics diverged steadily during the twentieth century.

In the 1980s the development of a new generation of polymorphisms in DNA itself began to make it possible to identify genes responsible for the heritability of complex traits influenced by many genes as well as by many environmental factors. As mentioned earlier, the pace of this integration has been accelerated dramatically as a result of the Human Genome Project which has brought us to the threshold of a postgenomic world in which the genome sequence of our species and others is known. Most importantly for the analysis of complex traits, several million DNA variations (polymorphisms) in the genome sequence are being identified which are the ultimate causes of the ubiquitous heritability of complex traits.

If many genes influence a trait, the trait is likely to be distributed quantitatively in a continuous distribution. For this reason, such genes are often referred to as quantitative trait loci (QTLs). The name implies that complex traits influenced by multiple genes are thought to be distributed as continuous, quantitative dimensions rather than as discontinuous, qualitative disorders. Unlike single-gene effects that are necessary and sufficient for the development of a disorder, QTLs act like probabilistic risk factors. Although QTLs are inherited in the same mendelian manner as single-gene effects, if many genes affect a trait then each gene is likely to have a relatively small effect. This makes it much more difficult to detect QTLs than single-gene effects but the potential availability of millions of DNA markers makes this daunting prospect possible. A revolutionary implication of the QTL perspective is that there may be no disorders from a genetic perspective. Disorders may merely be the quantitative extreme of the same genetic factors that contribute to heritability throughout the dimension (Plomin et al. 1994). That is, there may be no genes specific to a disorder – genes associated with a disorder might have the same effect throughout the distribution. In other words, a QTL associated with reading disability may actually be associated with the entire continuum of reading ability, that is, with the high end and middle of the distribution as well as the low end.

In the case of single-gene effects such as phenylketonuria that cause severe mental retardation, the gene is necessary and sufficient for the development of the disorder. In contrast, cognitive disorders in childhood such as reading disability are much more common than any known single-gene disorders, with risks often reported to be as high as 1 in 10. Traditional methods for identifying single-gene effects such as the use of large family pedigrees are unlikely to succeed in identifying QTLs because the effect size of individual QTLs will be relatively small. The earliest attempts to find genes for behavioural disorders focused on schizophrenia and manic-depressive psychosis at a time when gene-hunting techniques were limited to identifying a single gene necessary and sufficient to cause the disorder. Although there has never been any solid evidence that these disorders are caused by a single gene, this single-gene approach was all that was available at that time for finding genes. Although there are several promising leads, no clear-cut associations with schizophrenia and bipolar affective disorder have been identified (Baron 2001). We now realize that such designs are only able to detect genes of major effect size.

Identifying QTLs

Molecular genetic studies in the cognitive domain were begun relatively recently and have used QTL approaches from the start, which may contribute to the quicker successes in this domain. An example of a behavioural QTL is the association between apolipoprotein-E and late-onset dementia (Corder et al. 1993), an association that has been replicated in scores of studies and remains the only known predictor of this common disorder in later life. Although a particular allele in this gene leads to a five-fold increased risk for dementia, it is a QTL in the sense that many people with this allele do not have dementia and most people with dementia do not have this genetic risk factor. As described in the following section, a replicated QTL linkage has been found for another cognitive disorder, reading disability.

The advantage of linkage approaches, including QTL linkage approaches, is that they can systematically scan the genome for linkages using just a few hundred DNA markers. QTL linkage designs use many small families (usually siblings) rather than a few large families. The disadvantage is that they can only detect QTLs that account for a substantial amount (perhaps 10%) of the genetic variance. In contrast, allelic association can detect QTLs that account for 1% of the variance but thousands of DNA markers are needed to screen the genome systematically for association because association can only be detected if a DNA marker is very close to a QTL. In other words, linkage is systematic but not powerful and allelic association is powerful but not systematic (Risch and Merikangas 1996). For this reason, allelic association approaches have largely been limited to studies of 'candidate' genes. If, as is usually the case, a DNA marker in or near a candidate gene is not itself functional (that is, it does not produce a coding difference), the marker may be close enough to a functional QTL to be in linkage disequilibrium with it and thus yield an indirect association with the disorder. One problem with a candidate gene approach is that, for behavioural disorders, any of the thousands of genes expressed in the brain could be viewed as candidate genes. The way out of this conundrum is to conduct a systematic scan of the genome for allelic association using many thousands of DNA markers, although tens of thousands or even hundreds of thousands of DNA markers would be needed to identify or exclude all QTL associations (Kruglyak 1999). Such systematic large-scale genome scans or scans of all known candidate gene polymorphisms are becoming possible with new technologies that can quickly genotype thousands of DNA markers (Watson and Akil 1999).

Progress in identifying genes associated with behaviour and other complex traits has been slower than expected, in part because research to date has been under-powered for finding QTLs of small-effect size, especially in linkage studies. Very large studies are needed in order to identify QTLs of small-effect size (Cardon and Bell 2001). A daunting target for molecular genetic research on complex traits such as behaviour is to design research powerful enough to detect QTLs that account for 1% of the variance, while providing protection against false positive results in genome scans of thousands of genes. In order to break the 1% QTL barrier, samples of many thousands of individuals are needed for research on disorders (comparing cases and controls) and on dimensions (assessing individual differences in a representative sample). Another factor in the slow progress to date is that only a few candidate gene markers have been examined rather than systematic scans of gene systems or of the entire genome. The Human Genome Project will accelerate progress towards identifying all functional DNA variants expressed in the brain, especially those for entire neurotransmitter pathways.

QTLs and cognitive abilities and disabilities

Mild mental retardation and general cognitive ability

QTL linkage or association studies of mild mental retardation have not yet been reported even though quantitative genetic research mentioned earlier suggests that mild mental retardation represents the lower extreme of the same multiple genetic and environmental factors that affect cognitive functioning in the normal range. Although systematic QTL studies of mild mental retardation have not been reported, a QTL perspective suggests that QTL studies of normal IQ or even high IQ could identify QTLs that are also associated with mild mental retardation. This is part of the rationale for an allelic association study comparing high-IQ and control individuals called the IQ QTL Project (Plomin 2002). The first phase of the project employed an allelic association strategy using DNA markers in or near candidate genes likely to be relevant to neurological functioning, such as genes for neuroreceptors. Allelic association results were reported for 100 DNA markers for such candidate genes (Plomin et al. 1995). Although several significant associations were found in an original sample, only one association was replicated in an independent sample. However, a recent attempt to replicate this finding was not successful (Hill et al., in press).

As mentioned earlier, attempts to find QTL associations with complex traits have begun to go beyond candidate genes to conduct systematic genome scans using dense maps of DNA markers. As part of the IQ QTL Project, a first attempt to use this approach to identify QTLs associated with IQ focused on the long arm of chromosome 6, and found replicated associations for a DNA marker that happened to be in the gene for insulin-like growth factor-2 receptor (*IGF2R*) (Chorney et al. 1998), which has been shown to be especially active in brain regions most involved in learning and memory (Wickelgren 1998). Another polymorphism in the *IGF2R* gene has been genotyped and similar results were found for the new polymorphism in a new sample (Hill et al., in press).

The problem with using a dense map of markers for a genome scan is the amount of genotyping required. In order to scan the entire genome at 1 million DNA basepair intervals (1 Mb), about 3500 DNA markers would need to be genotyped. This would require 700 000 genotypings in a study of 100 high 'g' individuals and 100 controls. With markers at 1 Mb intervals, no QTL would be farther than 500 000 base pairs from a marker. Moreover, it is generally accepted that 10 to even 100 times as many markers would be needed in order to detect all QTLs (Kruglyak 1999;

Abecasis et al. 2001; Reich et al. 2001). Despite the daunting amount of genotyping required for a systematic genome scan, this approach has been fuelled by the promise of 'SNPs on chips' which can quickly genotype thousands of DNA markers of the single nucleotide polymorphism (SNP) variety.

DNA pooling, developed for use in the IQ QTL Project, provides a low-cost and flexible alternative to SNPs on chips for screening the genome for QTL associations (Daniels et al. 1998). DNA pooling greatly reduces the need for genotyping by pooling DNA from all individuals in each group and comparing the pooled groups so that only 14 000 genotypings are required to scan the genome in the previous example involving 3500 DNA markers. A scan of 1842 DNA markers using DNA pooling and a multiple-stage design found two markers that yielded significant results in two independent case–control studies but neither reached significance in a third within-family study (Plomin et al. 2001*c*). Rather than genotyping additional anonymous DNA markers, the IQ QTL Project is now focusing on functional polymorphisms such as SNPs in coding regions (cSNPs) and SNPs in regulatory regions in which the marker can be presumed to be the QTL.

Reading disability

The first QTL linked to a human behavioural disorder by a QTL linkage approach has been reported and replicated for reading disability (Cardon et al. 1994). The method used was sib-pair QTL linkage, which is conceptually similar to DF extremes analysis. Instead of comparing identical and fraternal twins, siblings are compared who share 0, 1 or 2 alleles for a particular DNA marker. If siblings who share more alleles are also more similar for a quantitative trait such as reading ability, then QTL linkage is implied. QTL linkage analysis is much more powerful when one sibling is selected on the basis of an extreme score on the quantitative trait. When one sibling was selected for reading disability, the reading ability score of the co-sibling was also lower when the two siblings shared alleles for markers in a certain region on the short arm of chromosome 6 (6p21). Significant linkage was also found for markers in this region in an independent sample of fraternal twins and in three replication studies (Grigorenko et al. 1997; Fisher et al. 1998; Gayán et al. 1999). The linkage to chromosome 6 appears for both phonological and orthographic reading measures. In 1983, linkage to chromosome 15 was reported using traditional analyses of pedigrees (Smith et al. 1983). Chromosome 15 linkage (15q21) for reading disability has also been replicated in several studies (Smith et al. 1991; Grigorenko et al. 1997; Schulte-Körne et al. 1997).

The next step is to pin down the specific genes responsible for these QTL regions (Smith et al. 1998). When the specific genes are identified (so far, the QTL linkage has only been tracked to its neighbourhood of several million base pairs of DNA rather than to a specific location), it will be of great interest to investigate the extent to which the gene's effects are specific to reading, or affect language or other cognitive processes more broadly.

Communication disorders

A single-gene disorder with its primary effect on language has been reported, albeit for a single family (Fisher et al. 1998). This family included 15 linguistically impaired relatives whose speech has low intelligibility and who have deficits in nearly all aspects of language but especially grammar. The family showed a simple dominant mode of inheritance that could be traced to one grandmother. A region on the long arm of chromosome 7 (7q31) was found that is linked to the disorder in this family (Lai et al. 2001). The same region has also been linked with autism (International Molecular Genetics Study of Autism Consortium 1998).

QTL linkage studies of specific language impairment are under way in Oxford and Edinburgh. Quantitative genetic results can help to chart the course for molecular genetic research in this area. At the most rudimentary level, the Twins Early Development Study (TEDS), described earlier, has shown that language problems even at 2 years of age are highly heritable, suggesting that language impairment is a good target for molecular genetic research. Although it is not unreasonable to focus on specific language impairment, quantitative genetic research suggests that genetic effects on persistent language problems may be general to cognitive development rather than specific to language (Plomin and Dale 2000). For this reason, TEDS has launched an allelic-association genome scan using DNA pooling in an attempt to identify some QTLs responsible for general language impairment and general cognitive impairment and comorbidity between them.

Once QTLs are found for language disability, hypotheses derived from quantitative genetic research can be tested empirically, for example, to assess the extent to which QTLs are specific to language (or to some specific component of language) or general to cognitive impairment. Indeed, all the questions raised by quantitative genetics – about developmental change and continuity, about multivariate issues of heterogeneity and comorbidity and the links between the normal and abnormal, and about the interplay between nature and nurture – can be addressed much more precisely and profitably once specific genes are identified (Plomin and Rutter 1998).

Conclusions

Despite the slow progress to date in finding genes associated with cognitive abilities and disabilities, their substantial heritability means that DNA polymorphisms exist that affect these traits. I am confident that we will find some of them. Although attention is now focused on finding specific genes associated with complex traits, the greatest impact for the neurobehavioural sciences will come after genes have been identified. Few behavioural scientists are likely to join the hunt for genes because it is difficult and expensive, but once genes are found, it is relatively easy and inexpensive to use them (Plomin and Rutter 1998). DNA can be obtained painlessly and inexpensively from cheek swabs – blood is not necessary. Cheek swabs yield enough DNA to genotype thousands of genes, and the cost of genotyping can be surprisingly inexpensive.

It is critical for the future of the behavioural sciences that we be prepared to use DNA in our research and eventually in our clinics. What has happened in the area of dementia in the elderly will be played out in many areas of the behavioural sciences. As mentioned earlier, the only known risk factor for late-onset Alzheimer's dementia (LOAD) is a gene, apolipoprotein E, involved in cholesterol transport. A form of the gene called allele 4 quadruples the risk for LOAD but is neither necessary nor sufficient to produce the disorder; hence, it is a QTL. Although the association between allele 4 and LOAD was reported less than a decade ago (Corder et al. 1993), it has already become de rigueur in research on dementia to genotype subjects for apolipoprotein E in order to ascertain whether the results differ for individuals with and without this genetic risk factor. Genotyping apolipoprotein E will become clinically routine if a genetic risk factor is found to predict differential response to interventions or treatments.

In terms of clinical work, DNA may eventually lead to gene-based diagnoses and treatment programmes. The most exciting potential for DNA research is to be able to predict genetic risk for an individual and to intervene to prevent problems before full-blown disorders emerge and create cascades of complications that are difficult to counteract. Interventions for behavioural disorders, and even for single-gene disorders, are likely to involve environmental rather than genetic engineering. For example, as mentioned earlier, phenylketonuria (PKU), a metabolic disorder that can cause severe mental retardation, is caused by a single gene on chromosome 12. A particular form of the gene, found in 1 per 10 000 babies, damages the developing brain postnatally. This form of mental retardation has been largely prevented, not by high-tech solutions such as correcting the mutant DNA or by eugenic programmes or by drugs, but rather by a change in diet that prevents the mutant DNA from having its damaging effects. For this reason, newborns have for decades been screened for PKU in order to identify those with the disorder so their diet can be changed. The example of PKU serves as an antidote to the mistaken notion that genetics implies therapeutic nihilism, even for a single-gene disorder. This point is even more important in relation to complex disorders that are influenced by many genes and by many environmental factors as well.

The search for genes involved in behaviour has led to a number of ethical concerns (Plomin 1999b). For example, there are fears that the results will be used to justify social inequality, to select individuals for education or employment, or to enable parents to pick and choose among their fetuses. These concerns are largely based on misunderstandings about how genes affect complex traits (Rutter and Plomin 1997), but it is important that behavioural scientists knowledgeable about DNA continue to be involved in this debate. Students in the behavioural sciences must be taught about genetics in order to prepare them for this future.

As the recent advances from the Human Genome Project begin to be absorbed in behavioural genetic research, optimism is warranted about finding more QTLs associated with behavioural dimensions and disorders. The future of genetic research lies in moving from finding genes (genomics) to finding out how genes work (functional genomics). Functional genomics is usually considered in terms of bottom-up molecular biology at the cellular level of analysis. As an antidote to the tendency to define functional genomics at the cellular level of analysis, the phrase *behavioural genomics* has been proposed (Plomin and Crabbe 2000). Indeed, behavioural genomics may pay off more quickly than other levels of analysis in terms of prediction, diagnosis, therapy and intervention in relation to behavioural disorders and normal behavioural variation. In addition to producing indisputable evidence of genetic influence, the identification of specific genes associated with learning and language delays and disorders will revolutionize genetic research by providing measured genotypes for investigating genetic links between behaviours, for tracking the developmental course of genetic effects, and for identifying interactions and correlations between genotype and environment (Plomin and Rutter 1998). Identification of specific genes might also provide greater precision in diagnoses and individually tailored educational programmes and therapies. For example, gene-based classification of disorders may bear little resemblance to our current symptom-based diagnostic systems. Indeed, from a QTL perspective, common disorders may be the quantitative extreme of normal genetic variation rather than qualitatively different, as mentioned earlier. Most importantly, gene-based prediction of early-onset disorders offers the hope for preventive intervention rather than waiting to intervene when language and learning problems begin to cast a long and wide shadow over children's development.

Bottom-up and top-down levels of analysis of gene–behaviour pathways will eventually meet in the brain (Andreasen 2001). The grandest implication for science is that DNA will serve as an integrating force across diverse disciplines.

REFERENCES

Abecasis GR, Noguchi E, Heinzmann A et al. (2001). Extent and distribution of linkage disequilibrium in three genomic regions. *Am J Hum Genet*, 68, 191–7.

American Psychiatric Association (1994). *Diagnostic and Statistical Manual of Mental Disorders*, 4th edn (DSM–IV). Washington, DC: APA.

Anderson B (2000). The *g* factor in non-human animals. In *The Nature of Intelligence*, ed. GR Bock, JA Goode and K Webb, pp. 79–95. Chichester: John Wiley and Sons (Novartis Foundation Symposium 233).

Anderson M (1992). *The Development of Intelligence: Studies in Developmental Psychology*. Hove: Psychology Press.

Andreasen NC (2001). *Brave New Brain: Conquering Mental Illness in the Era of the Genome*. Oxford: Oxford University Press.

Andrews G, Morris-Yates A, Howie P and Martin N (1991). Genetic factors in stuttering confirmed. *Arch Gen Psychiatry*, 48, 1034–5.

Baddeley A and Gathercole S (1999). Individual differences in learning and memory: psychometrics and the single case. In *Learning and Individual Differences: Process, Trait, and Content Determinants*, ed. PL Ackerman, PC Kyllonen and RD Roberts, pp. 31–55. Washington, DC: American Psychological Association.

Bakwin H (1973). Reading disability in twins. *Dev Med Child Neurol*, 15, 184–7.

Baron M (2001). Genetics of schizophrenia and the new millennium: progress and pitfalls. *Am J Hum Genet*, 68, 299–312.

Bishop DVM, North T and Donlan C (1995). Genetic basis of specific language impairment: evidence from a twin study. *Dev Med Child Neurol*, 37, 56–71.

Cardon LR and Bell J (2001). Association study designs for complex diseases. *Nat Genet*, 2, 91–9.

Cardon LR, Smith SD, Fulker DW, Kimberling WJ, Pennington BF and DeFries JC (1994). Quantitative trait locus for reading disability on chromosome 6. *Science*, 266, 276–9.

Carroll JB (1993). *Human Cognitive Abilities*. New York: Cambridge University Press.

Carroll JB (1997). Psychometrics, intelligence, and public policy. *Intelligence*, 24, 25–52.

Chorney MJ, Chorney K, Seese N et al. (1998). A quantitative trait locus (QTL) associated with cognitive ability in children. *Psychol Sci*, 9, 1–8.

Corder EH, Saunders AM, Strittmatter WJ et al. (1993). Gene dose of apolipoprotein E type 4 allele and the risk of Alzheimer's disease in late onset families. *Science*, 261, 921–3.

Crusio WE and Gerlai RT (1999). *Handbook of Molecular-Genetic Techniques for Brain and Behavior Research*. Amsterdam: Elsevier.

Dale PS, Simonoff E, Bishop DVM et al. (1998). Genetic influence on language delay in 2-year-old children. *Nat Neurosci*, 1, 324–8.

Dale PS, Dionne G, Eley TC and Plomin R (2000). Lexical and grammatical development: a behavioral genetic perspective. *J Child Lang*, 27, 619–42.

Daniels J, Holmans P, Plomin R, McGuffin P and Owen MJ (1998). A simple method for analyzing microsatellite allele image patterns generated from DNA pools and its application to allelic association studies. *Am J Hum Genet*, 62, 1189–97.

Deary I (2000). *Looking Down on Human Intelligence: From Psychometrics to the Brain*. Oxford: Oxford University Press.

Deary IJ, Whalley LJ, Lemmon H, Crawford JR and Starr JM (2000). The stability of individual differences in mental ability from childhood to old age: follow-up of the 1932 Scottish Mental Survey. *Intelligence*, 28, 49–55.

Decker SN and Vandenberg SG (1985). Colorado twin study of reading disability. In *Biobehavioral Measures of Dyslexia*, ed. DB Gray and JF Kavanagh, pp. 123–35. Parkton, MD: York Press.

DeFries JC and Fulker DW (1985). Multiple regression analysis of twin data. *Behav Genet*, 15, 467–73.

DeFries JC and Fulker DW (1988). Multiple regression analysis of twin data: etiology of deviant scores versus individual differences. *Acta Genet Med Gemellol*, 37, 205–16.

DeFries JC and Gillis JJ (1993). Genetics and reading disability. In *Nature, Nurture and Psychology*, ed. R Plomin and GE McClearn, pp. 121–45. Washington, DC: American Psychological Association.

DeFries JC, Vogler GP and LaBuda MC (1986). Colorado Family Reading Study: an overview. In *Perspectives in Behavior Genetics*, ed. JL Fuller and EC Simmel, pp. 29–56. Hillsdale, NJ: Lawrence Erlbaum.

DeFries JC, Knopik VS and Wadsworth SJ (1999). Colorado Twin Study of reading disability. In *Reading and Attention Disorders: Neurobiological Correlates*, ed. DD Duane, pp. 17–41. Baltimore, MD: York Press.

Duncan J, Seitz RJ, Kolodny J et al. (2000). A neural basis for general intelligence. *Science*, 289, 457–60.

Felsenfeld S (1994). Developmental speech and language disorders. In *Nature and Nurture During Middle Childhood*, ed. JC DeFries, R Plomin and DW Fulker, pp. 102–19. Oxford: Blackwell.

Felsenfeld S and Plomin R (1997). Epidemiological and offspring analyses of developmental speech disorders using data from the Colorado Adoption Project. *J Speech Lang Hear Res*, 40, 778–91.

Fisher SE, Vargha-Khadem F, Watkins KE, Monaco AP and Pembrey ME (1998). Localisation of a gene implicated in a severe speech and language disorder. *Nat Genet*, 18, 168–70.

Fodor JA (1983). *The Modularity of Mind*. Cambridge, MA: MIT Press.

Gardner H (1983). *Frames of Mind: The Theory of Multiple Intelligences*. New York: Basic Books.

Gayán J, Smith SD, Cherny SS et al. (1999). Quantitative-trait locus for specific language and reading deficits on chromosome 6p. *Am J Hum Genet*, 64, 157–64.

Gazzaniga MSE (2000). *Cognitive Neuroscience: A Reader*. Oxford: Blackwell.

Gilger JW (1997). How can behavioral genetic research help us understand language development and disorders? In *Towards A Genetics of Language*, ed. ML Rice, pp. 77–110. Hillsdale, NJ: Lawrence Erlbaum.

Goleman D (1995). *Emotional Intelligence*. New York: Bantam Books.

Gottfredson LS (1997). Why g matters: the complexity of everyday life. *Intelligence*, 24, 79–132.

Gould SJ (1996). *The Mismeasure of Man*, 2nd edn. New York: W W Norton.

Grigorenko EL, Wood FB, Meyer MS et al. (1997). Susceptibility loci for distinct components of developmental dyslexia on chromosomes 6 and 15. *Am J Hum Genet*, 60, 27–39.

Hill L, Chorney MJ, Chorney K et al. (in press). A quantitative trait locus not associated with cognitive ability in children: a failure to replicate. *Psychol Sci*.

Howie P (1981) Concordance for stuttering in monozygotic and dizygotic twin pairs. *J Speech Hear Res*, 5, 343–8.

International Molecular Genetics Study of Autism Consortium (1998). A full genome screen for autism with evidence for linkage to a region on chromosome 7q. *Hum Mol Genet*, 7, 571–8.

Jensen, AR (1998). *The g Factor: The Science of Mental Ability*. Wesport: Praeger.

Kidd K (1983). Recent progress on the genetics of stuttering. In *Genetic Aspects of Speech and Language Disorders*, ed. C Ludlow and J Cooper, pp. 197–213. New York: Academic Press.

Kosslyn S and Plomin R (2001). Towards a neuro-cognitive genetics: goals and issues. In *Psychiatric Neuroimaging Research: Contemporary Strategies*, ed. D Dougherty, SL Rauch and JF Rosenbaum, pp. 491–515. Washington, DC: American Psychiatric Press.

Kruglyak L (1999). Prospects for whole-genome linkage disequilibrium mapping of common disease genes. *Nat Genet*, 22, 139–44.

Lai CS, Fisher SE, Hurst JA, Vargha-Khadem F and Monaco AP (2001). A forkhead-domain gene is mutated in a severe speech and language disorder. *Nature*, 413, 519–23.

Lewis BA and Thompson LA (1992). A study of developmental speech and language disorders in twins. *J Speech Hear Res*, 35, 1086–94.

McClearn GE, Johansson B, Berg S et al. (1997). Substantial genetic influence on cognitive abilities in twins 80+ years old. *Science*, 276, 1560–63.

McGue M, Bouchard TJ Jr, Iacono WG and Lykken DT (1993). Behavioral genetics of cognitive ability: a life-span perspective. In *Nature, Nurture, and Psychology*, ed. R Plomin and GE McClearn, pp. 59–76. Washington, DC: American Psychological Association.

Neisser U, Boodoo G, Bouchard TJ Jr et al. (1996). Intelligence: knowns and unknowns. *Am Psychol*, 51, 77–101.

Nichols PL (1984). Familial mental retardation. *Behav Genet*, 14, 161–70.

Petrill SA (1997). Molarity versus modularity of cognitive functioning? A behavioral genetic perspective. *Curr Directions Psychol Sci*, 6, 96–9.

Pfaff DW, Berrettini WH, Joh TH and Maxson SC (2000). Genetic influences on neural and behavioral functions. Boca Raton, FL: CRC Press.

Pinker S (1994). *The Language Instinct.* New York, NY: William Morrow and Co.

Plomin R (1994). *Genetics and Experience: The Interplay Between Nature and Nurture.* Thousand Oaks, CA: Sage Publications.

Plomin R (1999*a*). Genetic research on general cognitive ability as a model for mild mental retardation. *Int Rev Psychiatry*, 11, 34–6.

Plomin R (1999*b*). Genetics and general cognitive ability. *Nature*, 402, C25–9.

Plomin R (2001). The genetics of g in human and mouse. *Nat Rev Neurosci*, 2, 136–41.

Plomin R (2002). Quantitative trait loci (QTLs) and general cognitive ability. In *Molecular Genetics of Human Personality*, ed. J Benjamin, R Ebstein and RH Belmaker, pp. 211–30. Washington, DC: American Psychiatric Press.

Plomin R and Crabbe JC (2000). DNA. *Psychol Bull*, 126, 806–28.

Plomin R and Dale PS (2000). Genetics and early language development: a UK study of twins. In *Speech and Language Impairments In Children: Causes, Characteristics, Intervention and Outcome*, ed. DVM Bishop and BE Leonard, pp. 35–51. Hove: Psychology Press.

Plomin R and DeFries JC (1998). Genetics of cognitive abilities and disabilities. *Sci Am*, May, 62–9.

Plomin R and Rutter M (1998). Child development, molecular genetics, and what to do with genes once they are found. *Child Dev*, 69, 1223–42.

Plomin R, Owen MJ and McGuffin P (1994). The genetic basis of complex human behaviors. *Science*, 264, 1733–9.

Plomin R, McClearn GE, Smith DL et al. (1995). Allelic associations between 100 DNA markers and high versus low IQ. *Intelligence*, 21, 31–48.

Plomin R, DeFries JC, McClearn GE and McGuffin P (2001*a*). *Behavioral Genetics*, 4th edn. New York: Worth Publishers.

Plomin R, Asbury K and Dunn J (2001*b*). Why are children in the same family so different? Nonshared environment a decade later. *Can J Psychiatry*, 46, 225–33.

Plomin R, Hill L, Craig I, McGuffin P et al. (2001*c*). A genome-wide scan of 1842 DNA markers for allelic associations with general cognitive ability: a five-stage design using DNA pooling. *Behav Genet*, 31, 497–509.

Price TS, Eley TC, Dale PS, Stevenson J and Plomin R (2000). Genetic and environmental covariation between verbal and non-verbal cognitive development in infancy. *Child Dev*, 71, 948–59.

Reed EW and Reed SC (1965). *Mental Retardation: A Family Study*. Philadelphia: Saunders.

Reich DE, Cargill M, Bolk S et al. (2001). Linkage disequilibrium in the human genome. *Nature*, 411, 199–204.

Rice ML (1996). *Toward a Genetics of Language*. Hillsdale, NJ: Lawrence Erlbaum.

Risch N and Merikangas KR (1996). The future of genetic studies of complex human diseases. *Science*, 273, 1516–17.

Rutter M and Plomin R (1997). Opportunities for psychiatry from genetic findings. *Br J Psychiatry*, 171, 209–19.

Salthouse TA and Czaja SJ (2000). Structural constraints on process explanations in cognitive aging. *Psychol Aging*, 15, 44–55.

Schulte-Körne G, Grimm T, Nöthen MM, Müller-Myhsok B, Propping P and Remschmidt H (1997). Evidence for linkage of spelling disability to chromosome 15. *Am J Med Genet (Neuropsychiatric Genet)*, 74, 661 (abstract).

Smith SD, Kimberling WJ, Pennington BF and Lubs HA (1983). Specific reading disability: identification of an inherited form through linkage analysis. *Science*, 219, 1345–47.

Smith SD, Kimberling WJ and Pennington BF (1991). Screening for multiple genes influencing dyslexia. *Read Writ*, 3, 285–98.

Smith SD, Kelley PM and Brower AM (1998). Molecular approaches to the genetic analysis of specific reading disability. *Hum Biol*, 70, 239–56.

Snyderman M and Rothman S (1987). Survey of expert opinion on intelligence and aptitude testing. *Am Psychol*, 42, 137–44.

Spearman C (1904). General intelligence, objectively determined and measured. *Am J Psychol*, 15, 201–93.

Spearman C (1927). *The Abilities of Man: Their Nature and Measurement*. New York: Macmillan.

Stauffer JM, Ree MJ and Carretta TR (1996). Cognitive-components tests are not much more than *g*: an extension of Kyllonen's analyses. *J Gen Psychol* 193–205.

Sternberg RJ (1985). *Beyond IQ: A Triarchic Theory of Human Intelligence*. Cambridge: Cambridge University Press.

Sternberg RJ and Gardner MK (1983). A componential interpretation of the general factor in human intelligence. In *A Model for Intelligence*, ed. HJ Eysenck, pp. 231–54. Berlin: Springer Verlag.

Stevenson J, Graham P, Fredman G and McLoughlin V (1987). A twin study of genetic influences on reading and spelling ability and disability. *J Child Psychol Psychiatry*, 28, 229–47.

Stromswold K (2001). The heritability of language: a review and meta-analysis of twin, adoption and linkage studies. *Language*, 77, 647–723.

Thompson RF (2000). *The Brain: a Neuroscience Primer*, 3rd edn. New York: Worth.

Tomblin JB and Buckwalter PR (1998). Heritability of poor language achievement among twins. *J Speech Lang Hear Res*, 41, 188–99.

Wahlström J (1990). Gene map of mental retardation. *J Ment Deficiency Res*, 34, 11–27.

Watson SJ and Akil H (1999). Gene chips and arrays revealed: a primer on their power and their uses. *Biol Psychiatry*, 45, 533–43.

Wickelgren I (1998). Tracking insulin to the mind. *Science*, 280, 517–19.

Willcutt EG, DeFries JC, Pennington BF, Smith SD, Cardon LR and Olson RK (2002). Genetic etiology of comorbid reading difficulties and ADHD. In *Behavioral Genetics in the Postgenomic Era*, ed. R Plomin, J DeFries, IC Craig and P McGuffin, pp. 227–46. Washington, DC: APA Books.

Yairi E, Ambrose N and Cox N (1996). Genetics of stuttering: a critical review. *J Speech Lang Hear Res*, 39, 771–84.

Genes and behaviour: finding a genetic substrate for cognitive neuropsychiatry

David H Skuse and Kate D Baker

Institute of Child Health, London, UK

Introduction

Cognitive neuropsychiatry was recently defined (Halligan and David 2001) as a 'systematic and theoretically driven approach to explain clinical psychopathologies in terms of deficits to normal cognitive mechanisms'. The aim of cognitive neuropsychiatry is to identify the neural substrates of cognitive mechanisms that, when impaired, may underlie the phenomenology of psychiatric disorder. Consequently, it is a quintessentially multidisciplinary endeavour, founded in both basic neuroscience and clinical psychiatry. The progress being made in identifying circumscribed brain circuits that are involved in specific cognitive tasks, with the aid of functional neuro-imaging techniques, is remarkable, yet relatively little discussion has been addressed to the issue of the genetic mechanisms that direct the development of these neurocognitive systems. There is increasing convergence between the identification of specific neural substrates and subjective experience, such as the recognition of certain emotions. The addition of genetics and developmental science to the research agenda will increase the power of the discipline to dissect aetiologies and pathological mechanisms.

Approaches to gene-finding in psychiatric research

Most psychiatric genetic research has focused on the hunt for genes that predispose to complex and heterogeneous clinical conditions, such as schizophrenia or manic depression (McGuffin et al. 2001). Additionally, human behavioural genetics has to date focused largely on the identification of genes that contribute to individual phenotypic variance in a trait (see Chapter 1 by Plomin). This is a desperately difficult undertaking, beyond demonstrating – for instance, through the investigation of twins – that a certain characteristic is likely to be more or less strongly influenced by (as yet unidentified) genetic factors in combination with experience during development, and by chance events. If we wish to discover 'how genes build brains' (Jennings 1999), we might start from the realization that single genes, or gene systems, may play a crucial role in the development or regulation of brain structures (Skuse and Baker, in press). Such genes might be so crucial to normal development that they are not polymorphic; there are no 'individual differences' for behavioural geneticists to study. Altmuller et al. (2001) recently commented on the 'considerable effort and expense' that have been expended in whole-genome screens aimed at detection of genetic loci contributing to the susceptibility to complex human disorders. They conclude the success of positional cloning attempts based on whole-genome screens has been limited, and many of the fundamental questions relating to the genetic epidemiology of complex human disease remain unanswered.

Classical approaches to the investigation of psychiatric genetics could usefully be complemented by a search for genes of major effect in the formation of neural systems that serve cognitive or emotional functions, and which therefore play an important role in the regulation of mental life. This approach would be analogous and complementary to that of cognitive neuropsychiatry, with its emphasis on the identification of cognitive processes that, if disturbed, lead to symptoms that are common to a variety of conventionally specified psychiatric disorders. The aim of *genetic cognitive neuropsychiatry* is to find genes that are major players in regulating aspects of brain development that are of relevance to cognitive processes. Many of these genes are unlikely to be subject to individual variation in functional terms – they are too highly conserved – so should not be expected alone to contribute towards individual differences in cognitive abilities. Their identification may nevertheless allow us to gain insights into the processes by which a normal brain is assembled, and the manner in which these processes are regulated by both genetic and environmental means.

Naturally occurring human genetic anomalies, in which candidate genes are either deleted or mutated, can be associated with quite specific neurocognitive consequences, which are reflected in symptom patterns. Such symptoms may in some cases be similar to those of idiopathic mental disorders such as autism or schizophrenia, although it should not be assumed that the genes in question necessarily play a role in predisposing to the idiopathic variants of those conditions. What can be stated, according to the framework outlined above, is that a genetic anomaly leading to a neurocognitive impairment can illuminate molecular and neurobiological processes which, when disrupted by any of a variety of means, can give rise to an equivalent biological or behavioural outcome. We should take note of the fact that genetic mechanisms are unlikely to code for domain-specific modules, but for the predisposition of selected brain regions to undertake certain tasks.

The regional specialization of cognitive processes found in adults is the result, not of unfettered genetic activity through the life span, but of a subtle interplay during development between genetic predisposition and experience. By studying the structural and functional consequences for brain development of abnormalities in the genome, insights might also be gained concerning the evolution of important neural systems.

There is remarkable conservation of genetic material through evolution and of genetically mediated processes in development (Allman 2000) and this conservation can be harnessed experimentally. The impact of manipulation of candidate genes on brain structure and behavioural function can be investigated with animal models, a well-established approach to learning about gene function in vivo. By elucidating key genes of importance for human brain development and utilizing experimental techniques of developmental biology (see Chapter 4 by Beasley et al., Chapter 15 by Killcross and Chapter 16 by Matthews), we can begin not only to identify genomic processes that could influence predisposition to mental illness, but also to understand how they do so. It is possible a significant proportion of such genes will be transcription factors (Gilbert 2000), which regulate the expression of other genes – often by means of a cascade of events. For example, the transcription factor AP-2, which plays a critical role in the regulation of neural gene expression and neural development throughout the brain, may regulate the expression of monoaminergic neurons or candidate genes within the monoamine system, according to Damberg et al. (2001). Polymorphisms that lead to variable expression of these key regulatory genes could have profound downstream effects on brain structural and functional development.

We cannot deliberately target and disrupt genes in humans in order to see what effects there will be on brain and behaviour. We can nevertheless learn about the consequences of sporadic or inherited genetic anomalies upon brain structure and function in humans. This can be achieved by studying chromosomal aneuploidies, microdeletions and single gene mutations that have cognitive or behavioural phenotypes. When a naturally occurring genetic anomaly is strongly associated with an aberrant cognitive or behavioural outcome we are given the opportunity to explore key developmental processes and to isolate genetic pathways which influence these processes. Discovering such genetic regulators alone will not allow us to explain why some people are cleverer than others, or are more prone to depression, or are liable to become psychotic under stress. However, their discovery may allow us to begin to understand how the brain normally works as a coherent whole, because we can identify the structural and functional consequences of a developmental abnormality. We can use our knowledge about which structures are affected to infer their function, which can be confirmed from functional imaging data in normal individuals. Accordingly, piece by piece, we can begin to link together knowledge about how some genes are vital to the development and maintenance of brain-based abilities such as attention, face recognition, even 'theory of mind'.

Ideally, we need to model proposed gene–biology–behaviour associations in a model system (for instance a mouse mutant). Naturally, we could not expect to find high-level cognitive deficits in an animal-model system. Therefore, it may prove more fruitful to forget, for now, about high-level deficits (as characterized by phenotyping of complex behavioural or cognitive traits) and to focus upon what Gottesman termed 'endophenotypes' (Gottesman 1997). Endophenotypes are genetically influenced latent traits, which may be only indirectly related to the classical disease symptoms as defined in ICD–10 or DSM–IV (World Health Organization 1992; American Psychiatric Association 1996). They reflect an underlying susceptibility to the disease phenotype (or some *forme fruste* of it). In psychiatry we are likely to be interested in endophenotypes that are measurable by neurophysiological or neuropsychological means, for reasons of specificity that will be discussed further. However, characteristic behavioural traits may also be found in carriers of susceptibility loci, as discussed in Skuse (2001). Crucial characteristics of any endophenotype include the fact that it can be measured before the explicit onset of the illness, and that it represents the genetic liability of nonaffected relatives of probands with the disorder. For example, there seems little doubt that the range of learning and social difficulties reported in the families of autistic probands, a quintessentially highly heritable condition (albeit a genetically complex one), reflect vulnerability traits (Pickles et al. 2000).

If the same susceptibility loci contribute to specific aspects of phenotypes in a variety of apparently nosologically distinct conditions, this could illuminate some currently puzzling aspects of comorbidity. In the search for genes that predispose to the development of child psychiatric disorders, it may prove unproductive to seek the genetic components of relatively amorphous syndromes, or 'comorbid' disorders. Broad heritability can of course be established with the aid of twin studies, which give us useful but often nonspecific information about the nature of the genetic components of complex disorders. For a deeper understanding of the genetic predisposition to psychiatric conditions, it may be more profitable to seek the genetic basis of endophenotypes that are common to a number of diseases or disorders and which reflect the neural substrate underlying symptoms rather than syndromes. Hence, if a clinical disorder is genetically and phenotypically complex, we might ask, could each genetic locus contribute to distinct aspects of the illness phenotype? It is possible for example that there may be separate susceptibility genes for the language impairments in autism and for the social deficits associated with the condition.

Neurodevelopmental disorders that result in psychiatric phenotypes represent the end points of aberrant pathways of brain development. Genetically influenced dysfunction could have originated as early as during fetal life. In such cases it seems reasonable to assume we should find evidence of endophenotypes in the early childhood of individuals with a given genetic susceptibility. The identification and definition of such characteristics would be of value for several reasons. First, in family-genetic investigations, one may be less likely falsely to identify as unaffected, individuals who are at genetic risk but who do not manifest the full illness phenotype. Second, the characteristics of the endophenotype may shed light on fundamental processes that are disrupted as a consequence of the inherited genetic susceptibility. Of course, we should bear in mind that susceptibility to an endophenotype does not necessarily imply the genetic locus responsible for that endophenotype is involved in the disease process. The gene could be in linkage disequilibrium with the locus of interest. Such proximity would be useful for linkage or association studies, but is useless for gaining an understanding of the biological processes that lead to the disease phenotype.

The characteristics of potentially valuable endophenotypes, whether physiological or psychological, functional or structural in nature, are clear. First, they should be measurable reliably, both over time and by different observers. Good reliability in the measurement of psychiatric symptomatology has been the touchstone sought by psychiatric researchers for decades, arguably at the expense of validity. Second, they should be sensitive to genetic susceptibility, in that all those with the susceptibility locus should manifest the endophenotype. Third, endophenotypes should be specific to the disorder in question. These are demanding criteria, for without measuring the genetic locus itself, and knowing just what its characteristics are, one has to assume that those 'at risk' individuals without an endophenotype are not genetically vulnerable. Perhaps the closest we have yet come to such a measure concerns individuals at risk of Huntington's disease, an autosomal dominant condition with virtually 100% penetrance, in which the single susceptibility locus has been identified. Gray et al. (1997) studied a sample of individuals who were at genetic risk, but who did not yet show any signs of the disease clinically. They were compared to people who presented for genetic testing, but who turned out not to carry the gene for Huntington's disease. A highly selective deficit in the recognition of disgust was confirmed in those whom genetic testing proved to be Huntington's gene carriers. These people were free from clinical symptoms. They did not perform significantly more poorly than noncarriers on any of the background tests, or on any other face-processing tasks, including the recognition of other basic emotions. Gray et al. (1997) concluded their finding strongly indicated the importance of the basal ganglia, whose development is compromised by the disease, in the neural system underlying the emotion of disgust.

In multiple-feature psychiatric conditions the search for reliable endophenotypes has so far been only moderately successful. For example, deficits in smooth-pursuit eye movements, and a failure to inhibit the P50 auditory event-evoked EEG response, appear to cosegregate with the genetic risk of schizophrenia (Adler et al. 1999). It is arguable that information processing and attentional and inhibitory deficits are central to this condition's psychopathology, therefore such measures could point towards a neural substrate which fulfils the aims of cognitive neuropsychiatry. However, it is important to note that the reliability of these measures is often not high enough to discriminate risk status at the individual level. Additionally, the proposed features may be nonspecific expressions of attentional deficits, which are found in association with many psychiatric disorders (Ross et al. 2000). As detailed above, taking a symptom-based rather than a diagnostic approach, and moving away from family studies towards study of genetically similar (with respect to specific loci) unrelated individuals, may reduce some of these uncertainties.

Examples are given of three approaches. First, the investigation of mutated genes, with cognitive consequences for the phenotype, which are inherited in classic mendelian fashion (Box 2.1). In this section the potential relevance of imprinted genetic loci is also considered. Second, the investigation of microdeletion syndromes, in which a piece of chromosome is missing with its associated genetic material (Box 2.2). Third, the study of chromosomal aneuploidies, in which an entire chromosome is missing or duplicated – a sporadic event, in which dosage of a whole variety of genes is upset.

Mutated genes and mental retardation: the case of Fragile X syndrome

Fragile X syndrome is often quoted as being the single most common form of inherited mental handicap after Down's syndrome, but it is probably far less common than was once thought. In the general population its prevalence is between 1.5 and 2.5 per 10 000 males (De Vries et al. 1997; Turner et al. 1997). In a large population of children at schools for the mentally retarded, the prevalence could be as high as 1.3% (De Vries et al. 1997), with no difference in prevalence between those with mild and those with moderate to severe mental retardation. The mutation underlying the disease is a CGG triplet repeat expansion occurring within an untranslated portion of the *FMR1* gene. The clinical severity of the disorder, which is far greater in males than females, is substantially more marked if there are more than 200 CGG repeats, for this is associated with transcriptional silencing of the gene. Expansions in the number of CGG repeats occur exclusively during female transmission of *FMR1*.

The full mutation (fM) is associated with deficits in short-term visual memory, in visuospatial skills, in visuomotor coordination, in the processing of sequential information and in executive function skills. Attention deficits and hyperactivity are found in most cases of both referred and nonreferred subjects

Box 2.1 Genetic mechanisms associated with disease and disorder

Genetic mutations and polymorphisms

A certain amount of confusion has arisen in the use of the terms 'mutation' and 'polymorphism' (Skuse 1997). A germ-line *mutation* occurs in the DNA of cells that will produce gametes and will be inherited by the cells of subsequent generations. From the point of view of molecular biology, any change in a DNA sequence is a mutation, but most are neutral, with no effect on the phenotype. This is because most of the human genome is not transcribed, much is not translated, and even within the coding regions a base change could lead to the substitution of one synonymous codon for another. There are many synonyms in the genetic code, and the protein product is not necessarily affected at all. These neutral mutations will nevertheless lead to DNA *polymorphisms*, which are alternative forms of DNA sequence within a population. Such polymorphisms are of great importance in all forms of medical genetic research, because they can serve as distinctive inheritable markers at specific positions on chromosomes. Polymorphisms involving microsatellite DNA produce variable number tandem repeats (VNTRs) which are proving especially useful for mapping purposes.

The term 'mutation' has come to imply an alteration in gene product that is detectable by some change in the phenotype of the organism. That is an unsatisfactory convention because the evidence for such change will depend on the sensitivity of the measures used to detect the difference in the phenotype. The term 'mutation' should not be taken to imply disease, as such. In complex disorders, the phenotype will be influenced by the interaction of a variety of polymorphisms (each of which is a 'mutation') in different genes, on different chromosomes. Each of these 'mutations' is insufficient to produce a disordered phenotype in its own right, but they act in combination to increase susceptibility to disease. One such mutation would be necessary, but not sufficient, to bring about a detectable phenotype. The others would be neither necessary nor sufficient, in their own right, to produce the phenotype. In other words, the genotype at any given locus can affect the probability of a detectable phenotype, but does not fully determine its outcome. We should remember that environmental factors have a crucial part to play too, as will be shown.

Sometimes dominant conditions result in phenotypes that become more severe in successive generations. A mechanism associated with this phenomenon is known as anticipation (McInnis 1996), and is exemplified by the Fragile X syndrome (Turner et al. 1997) and by Huntington's disease (Huntington's Disease Collaborative Research Group 1993). Trinucleotide repeat expansions have been proposed as its biological basis (Margolis et al. 1999). Trinucleotide repeats are triplets of nucleotides, usually cytosine, guanine and arginine. These are designated CGG, CAG and so on. The repeats may occur within genes, or they may be found in regions of DNA that lie between genes. If they lie actually within genes they may be in transcribed sequences (so-called exons), or within DNA sequences that are excised by the RNA-making machinery (so-called introns). Expansions occur in the course of DNA replication (Margolis et al. 1999) and the repeats grow in length as they are passed from one generation to the next. For reasons that we do not understand, there are proportionately more neurological than other diseases caused by expansion of CTG, CGG, CAG or GAA repeats (Weatherall 1999). The conditions caused by the expansion are associated with considerable phenotypic heterogeneity. There is inevitably variability in the length of the repeat sequences, and in the degree to which they disrupt transcription and function of the genes with which they are associated. Conditions associated with this phenomenon, which have a characteristic cognitive or behavioural phenotype, include Fragile X syndrome (CGG repeats), Huntington's chorea and other conditions such as dentatorubral-pallidoluysian atrophy (CAG repeats) and myotonic dystrophy (CTG repeats).

Imprinted genes

A small proportion of genes is systematically different in their activity, depending on whether they have been inherited from mother or from father. This phenomenon is known as genomic imprinting (Tilghman 1999). There is consequently monoallelic expression; that is to say, the gene is expressed from only one of the pair of alleles, but it is important to note this may only be detected in certain tissues, or at certain periods of development. There is no alteration in the underlying DNA sequence. The existence of imprinted genes in a region may be revealed when the only active copy is mutated or lost due to a structural abnormality of the chromosome containing it. Alternatively, that chromosome, or region of a chromosome, may show uniparental disomy, both copies of the gene in question (and part of the surrounding genome) having been inherited from just one parent. In general, the clinical phenotypes that result from abnormalities involving imprinted loci tend to be severe. One of the best-known examples is Prader–Willi syndrome, which is due to nonexpression of a critical genetic locus on the long arm of chromosome 15, at 15q11-13. The phenotype is due to loss of a cluster of paternally expressed alleles, the equivalent maternal alleles having been silenced by imprinting. The candidate gene(s) accounting for the syndrome have not yet been identified (Hanel and Wevrick 2001). Intriguingly, loss of a maternally expressed allele in the same region (UBE3) leads to a phenotypically different condition, Angelman syndrome.

Box 2.2 Chromosomal mechanisms associated with disease and disorder

Structural chromosomal anomalies

Structural abnormalities can arise in a variety of ways. Structural abnormalities include deletions of part of the long or short arms, which may be terminal or interstitial – meaning they occur within the arm. It is rather remarkable that we can develop at all with gross numerical abnormalities. Gene dosage is usually a delicate affair, and if it is interfered with in a major way (by monosomy or triploidy for example) a phenotype results.

Spontaneous breaks in chromosomal material can occur during the formation of the germ cells, during recombination, which occurs normally only during meiosis. The germ cells contain just 23 chromosomes, and if any of these are broken they can be repaired. However, sometimes if two breaks have occurred the joins may mismatch, resulting in a 'translocation' of material from one chromosome to another. If such breaks have damaged genetic material, phenotypes may result even though there is no net loss of genetic material. If there is a net gain or loss of genetic material, chromosomal structural abnormalities are known as 'unbalanced'. Other forms of break include loss of material from within the q or p arm (interstitial), or from the end of the arm (terminal). Material may be turned around within the arm (paracentric inversion), or between arms (pericentric). Rarely, there is a normal complement of chromosomes but one pair derives from maternal or paternal origin. Obviously, cells that contained all three copies have been lost, in such instances. Rather more frequently, a small area of one chromosome within the long or the short arm derives from maternal or paternal origins on both copies. This may not cause any problems provided the region does not contain an imprinted locus, containing a gene that is expressed systematically from either a maternal or a paternal allele.

Two conditions caused by microdeletions (loss of a few Mb of DNA) that have attracted considerable interest among developmental psychologists and psychiatrists respectively are Williams syndrome (Korenberg et al. 2000) and velo-cardio-facial syndrome, also known as 22q11.2 syndrome (Shprintzen et al. 1978). The former is of interest because of its peculiar neurocognitive profile of verbal and social strengths, despite serious learning difficulties (Bellugi et al. 2000). The latter has attracted recent considerable attention because of the suggestion that the psychopathological features of the syndrome could share a neurocognitive basis with schizophrenia (Murphy et al. 1999).

Numerical chromosomal anomalies

Numerical chromosomal abnormalities include too few and too many chromosomes. Complete duplication or erasure of a chromosome is only possible with the sex chromosomes, and chromosome 21, much beyond birth. So, for instance there are duplications of the sex chromosomes (e.g. XXX, XYY, XXY), and there is monosomy (45,X, but never 45,Y). The best-known examples are Down's syndrome (trisomy 21; Chapman and Hesketh 2000) and sex chromosome aneuploidies such as Turner syndrome (45,X; Lippe 1996) and Klinefelter syndrome (47,XXY; Geschwind et al. 2000). Other sex chromosome aneuploidies have been relatively little studied from the point of view of their cognitive or behavioural characteristics.

(Baumgardner et al. 1995). The notion current some years ago that Fragile X syndrome is commonly associated with autism has not been supported by more recent rigorous analyses. The most comprehensive review on this issue is by Dykens and Volkmar (1997). The consensus seems to be that a minority of Fragile X males do have classical autism (from 15–25%; McCabe et al. 1999) but the majority show behavioural characteristics that could be regarded as 'autistic-like' in character. These include gaze avoidance, shyness, social anxiety and withdrawal. Some of them could be regarded as having an autistic spectrum disorder, or the broader autistic phenotype (LeCouteur et al. 1996). A proportion are found to have stereotypies, impulsivity and to be oversensitive to certain perceptual experiences. In contrast to males with classical autism, they are able to recognize facial expressions and emotions in others (Turk and Cornish 1998). Females with Fragile X syndrome have a more variable clinical picture than affected males. They are said to show similar difficulties in social interaction, including shyness, gaze avoidance and poor modulation of interpersonal communication (Lachiewicz and Dawson 1994; Sobesky et al. 1996). They may also be more prone to sadness, and even depression (Thompson et al. 1994). They also have poor attention skills (Franke et al. 1999). It has been suggested that many such problems with activity and sensory stimuli may relate to anomalies in the posterior cerebellar vermis and caudate nucleus (Reiss et al. 1995*a*). However, the neuropsychological deficits are associated with rather nonspecific brain changes on MRI, especially within the temporal cortex and hippocampus.

There is no simple relationship between neuropsychological test performance, structural brain abnormalities and CGG triplet-repeat lengths (Merenstein et al. 1996). Therefore more subtle genetic mechanisms may be responsible for variation in the phenotype. In both males and females, the degree of cognitive and behavioural abnormality may be related to the extent to which the trinucleotide CGG repeat is methylated, and hence the amount of Fragile X protein that is produced (Tassone et al. 1999). If no *FMR1* protein is produced there will be moderate to severe mental disability; this situation is found virtually exclusively in males, for females have two copies of the *FMR1* gene, and even if one is mutated the other can compensate to a degree, in certain circumstances. If the male in question is a mosaic, so that it is only a proportion of his cells in which the mutation occurs, or if his full mutation is only partially methylated, the IQ deficit will be less marked. The phenotype in females depends on the inactivation pattern of the X chromosome. If the normal X is the active one, in any particular clone of cells, the functions of those cells will be relatively unimpaired and the corresponding phenotypic feature will not be found (Reiss et al. 1995*a*).

The mutation in the *FMR1* gene was detected, and the gene cloned, in 1991 (Verkerk et al. 1991) and was the first of the trinucleotide repeat expansions to be discovered. Unfortunately, in the decade since its discovery, and despite the fact that the condition has since been studied exhaustively, the role of this gene in normal development has yet to be established. We do know that the protein is associated with ribosomes, and it is believed to bind to specific RNAs and to regulate their expression in a manner that is necessary for correct neuronal development (Inoue et al. 2000). We also have a mouse model of Fragile X, and these mice have certain of the features of the human condition including macro-orchidism and impaired spatial learning abilities, although these features are dependent on the strain of mouse used in the investigation (Dobkin et al. 2000). In general, the degree of learning impairment in the mouse has not been as marked as is found in humans, and there could be various explanations for this. In humans other factors may interact with the gene to generate the full phenotype, so that the gene in fact performs different functions in different organisms. Alternatively, the gene may perform the same function in man as in mouse but disruption of this function has more widespread effects in animals with more complex brain structure and function.

Mutated genes, speech and language: the remarkable KE family

A decade or so ago, a family presented to a clinical genetics department in London, with a dominantly inherited disorder of speech which rendered many family members almost incomprehensible (Hurst et al. 1990). In subsequent work, based around this fascinating chance encounter, Vargha-Khadem et al. (1995) have studied the unique three-generation pedigree of the KE family. It is clear that they suffer from a severe speech and language disorder, which is indeed transmitted as an autosomal-dominant monogenic trait. The UK investigators were not the only researchers to take an interest in the KE family. Encountering the family whilst visiting this country, having seen a programme about them on television, Gopnik (1990) subsequently generated considerable excitement by claiming they had a fundamental disorder of grammar. She suggested the mutation was in a gene that affected a component of Universal Grammar (in the Chomskyian sense). In fact, the dominant characteristic of the phenotype is not language at all, but speech. Affected members have a severe impairment in the selection and sequencing of fine orofacial movements, which are necessary for articulation, in the form of a developmental verbal dyspraxia. However, there are also deficits in several facets of language processing, such as the ability to break up words into their constituent phonemes, and grammatical skills, including production and comprehension of word inflections and syntactical structure (Gopnik and Crago 1991). Although the mean nonverbal IQ of affected members is lower than that of unaffected members, there are affected individuals in the family who have nonverbal ability close to the population average. Despite having severe speech and language difficulties, therefore, nonverbal deficits are not thought to represent significant aspects of the disorder.

The importance of this study is two-fold. First, there is the way in which a combination of approaches was imaginatively used to try and locate the gene responsible for the cognitive and behavioural deficit. Second, there is the way in which the effects of the mutation on brain function and structure were investigated. Fortunately for the investigators, it was possible unambiguously to identify the core deficit in the genetic disorder, in the sense that they found measures that distinguished reliably between those who carried the mutation and those who did not. It is rather unusual for a behavioural phenotype to characterize carriers of the mutation so precisely, and yet, as we shall see later, failure to take account of variability in the genetically modified population can make interpretation of data for deletion mapping very difficult indeed. In this remarkable family, every one of the affected members studied was impaired relative to nonaffected members on just three tests. These were word repetition, nonword repetition and simultaneous and sequential orofacial movements (Vargha-Khadem et al. 1998). The investigators report that the scores of the affected members did not overlap at all with those of unaffected members / age-matched normal controls.

They then compared brain activation patterns with positron emission tomography (PET) in two affected family members and with four normal controls. Prior predictions were made about the areas of the brain that were likely to be affected by the genetic anomaly. Areas identified as being more active than normal included the left supplementary motor area (SMA), the subjacent cingulate cortex on the left and the left preSMA/cingulate cortex. On the other hand, decreases in activation were observed in the head and the tail of the left caudate nucleus, the left premotor cortex, a part of Broca's area, and a left ventral prefrontal area. To take the examination of the effects of the mutation on the development of the brain further, they employed a technique which is sensitive to subtle changes in grey matter density that are not detectable by conventional structural imaging analysis (voxel-based morphometry; Wright et al. 1995). Analysis of images is automatic, and nonoperator dependent. There were found to be regions in which the affected group, carrying the mutation, had either significantly more or significantly less grey matter than comparisons, who were unaffected members of the same family. Cases had less grey matter in the preSMA/cingulate cortex, Broca's area and the caudate nucleus. These regions were already known to be functionally abnormal from the PET scanning study. In particular, the head of the caudate nucleus was abnormal bilaterally, and this seemed likely to be causally related to the phenotype. Direct measures of the size of the caudate revealed affected individuals had smaller left and right volumes than the unaffected family members.

Previous work had mapped the locus responsible, *SPCH1*, to a 5.6-cM interval of region 7q31 on chromosome 7 (Fisher et al. 1998). The team also identified an unrelated individual, CS, in whom speech and language impairment is associated with a chromosomal translocation involving the *SPCH1* interval (Lai et al. 2000). CS presented with a severe orofacial dyspraxia, although there had been normal early feeding and gross motor development. Both the KE family and CS demonstrated substantial impairment of expressive and receptive language abilities. In both cases, general intelligence was relatively spared, although there was some lowering of IQ. Their deficits were more profound in the verbal domain. In a further set of investigations, Lai et al. (2001) identified *FOXP2*, which encodes a putative transcription factor, as the gene disrupted by the translocation breakpoint in CS. With remarkable prescience, they were also able to show that affected members of the KE family had a point mutation in the very same gene. Lai et al. (2001) propose that, in both cases, *FOXP2* haploinsufficiency in the brain at a key stage of embryogenesis leads to abnormal development of neural structures that are important for speech and language. The corollary of this finding is that *SPCH1* contributes to the development of a cognitive-motor brain system involved in speech/language functions, and is a necessary component of that system. The authors comment that this is the first gene to have been implicated in such pathways, 'and it promises to offer insights into the molecular processes mediating this uniquely human trait'.

Microdeletion syndromes: a predisposition to schizophrenia in 22q11 deletion syndromes

The 22q11 deletion syndromes comprise several clinical conditions described on the basis of the predominant congenital anomalies. They include velo-cardio-facial syndrome (VCFS), DiGeorge syndrome (DGS) and conotruncal facial anomaly (CFA). All three are caused by a microdeletion on the long arm of chromosome 22 at position q11.2 (Scambler et al. 1992). The deletion has a population frequency of approximately 1 in 4000 (Du Montcel et al. 1996) and most cases are sporadic, although approximately 25% are inherited (Ryan et al. 1997). Over 100 congenital anomalies have been described in association with this chromosomal anomaly.

Table 2.1. Evidence for psychiatric disorders in association with 22q11.2 microdeletions

Study	Year	Sample size	Ascertainment	Age (years)	SZ (%)[a]	Other diagnoses (%)
Shprintzen et al.	1992	90	VCFS[b] clinical referral	14 (mean onset of psychosis)	>10	—
Papolos et al.	1996	25	Psychiatric referral	12 (mean onset of psychosis)	—	64 bipolar also ADHD[c]
Murphy et al.	1999	50	Various	31 (mean)	24	42 psychiatric disorder, 30 psychotic
Ryan et al.	1997	252	Various	3–18	—	9 behavioural or psychotic disorder
Ryan et al.	1997	61	Various	18–51	—	18 psychiatric disorder
Arnold et al.	2001	20 vs. 11 siblings	Genetics clinic	11, 6–20 (mean, range)	15 schizotypal	60 psychiatric disorder 40 mood disorders also ADHD, ODD[d]

[a] SZ, schizophrenia; [b] VCFS, velo-cardio-facial syndrome;
[c] ADHD, attention-deficit hyperactivity disorder; [d] ODD, oppositional defiant disorder.

The commonest are cleft palate, cardiac anomalies, hypocalcaemia, hypernasal speech and typical craniofacial features comprising microcephaly, broad nasal root with deficient nasal alae, malar flattening and auricular anomalies. Because of the bewildering number of potential anomalies, and the overlapping syndromic descriptors, the term 22q11DS is often employed, and is the abbreviation we will use here.

The first report that patients with 22q11DS were experiencing a high rate of psychiatric disorder came in 1992 from Shprintzen et al. They reported that over 10% of patients attending their specialist outpatient service had psychiatric problems, with their onset in early adulthood; 'chronic schizophrenia with paranoid delusions' was the commonest diagnosis. Since then several other authors have reported high rates of schizophrenia and other disorders (see Table 2.1). Populations with schizophrenia but without a clinical diagnosis of a 22q11DS have also been screened for the presence of undetected deletions, and microdeletion rates are found to be significantly higher (2–3%) than one would find in the general population (Karayiorgou et al. 1995). This is especially marked in studies of childhood-onset schizophrenia (Usiskin et al. 1999). Where schizoaffective patients with other features of the deletion syndrome were included a phenomenally high rate of deletion was detected, albeit in a small sample (Bassett et al. 1998). Given that the lifetime risk of developing schizophrenia is estimated to be around 1%, these rates represent a very considerably increased risk in the 22q11DS population. No associations have been found between the presence of psychiatric disorder and other features of 22q11DS such as learning difficulty (which carries approximately a three-fold increased risk of schizophrenia relative to the general population) or cardiac anomalies. In studies of children and adolescents with the microdeletion, disorders of mood and attention have been highly prevalent (Papolos et al. 1996; Arnold et al. 2001). These included attention-deficit hyperactivity disorder (ADHD), oppositional defiant disorder, separation anxiety disorder, specific phobias, generalized anxiety disorder and depressive disorders.

The comorbidity of schizophrenia with bipolar and other affective disorders in this population lends weight to the idea that affective and schizophreniform disorders lie on the same psychopathological spectrum. Additionally such comorbidity could lend support to the hypothesis that all psychoses share some aetiological factors, including genetic predisposition. Alternatively, the findings in different age groups could indicate the progressive manifestations of the same underlying neurodevelopmental abnormality. Further study of psychiatric features in both children and adults with 22q11DS is necessary before any such claims can be substantiated. What is clear is that this microdeletion syndrome offers an unparalleled opportunity to explore the genetic and neurodevelopmental basis of complex psychiatric conditions. 22q11DS individuals who develop psychotic illness presumably have a shared aetiology to their disease and thus a common disrupted neurodevelopmental pathway, in contrast to the schizophrenic population as a whole in whom there may be multiple aberrant neurodevelopmental routes to the same clinical outcome. To reflect this aetiological homogeneity one might expect that the clinical picture of individuals with the microdeletion and schizophrenia would be rather similar. Gothelf et al. (1999) described four individuals with VCFS and schizophrenia who demonstrated early age of onset, chronic and disabling course of disease and poor response to classic neuroleptic drugs and electroconvulsive therapy. This contrasts with Murphy et al. (1999), who reported a somewhat mild phenotype. Individuals with VCFS and schizophrenia had fewer negative symptoms (SANS ratings) and a later age of onset when compared with a control group of non-VCFS schizophrenics. Hence, as yet there is no strong evidence for uniformity amongst 22q11DS individuals with psychiatric disorder.

Many of the developmental and neuropsychological features of 22q11DS are reminiscent of the premorbid features predicted to be antecedents to adult psychosis in nonsyndromal schizophrenia. These developmental features have been examined in several ways: studies of children in high-risk groups, e.g. the Copenhagen, New York and Jerusalem projects, follow-back studies of schizophrenic populations, e.g. the Maudsley project, and cohort studies (see Davies et al. 1998 for a review). A common finding is that high-risk children reach developmental milestones such as motor and speech skill maturity at a later age, and experience social difficulties during adolescence (Done et al. 1994; Jones et al. 1994). Comparisons have also been made between the premorbid functional status in schizophrenia and bipolar disorders (Cannon et al. 1997), and a spectrum of poor social adjustment has been proposed, with those children at the most severe end of the spectrum being most vulnerable to schizophrenia. Whether a similar relationship exists within the group of individuals with 22q11DS, and whether early social and emotional difficulties are reflective of underlying cognitive and neurodevelopmental variation within the group, has yet to be determined.

Individuals with 22q11DS demonstrate a greatly increased vulnerability to schizophrenia, other psychiatric disorders and learning difficulties, but there is marked variation in the type and severity of symptomatology. To explore this syndrome within the framework of genetic cognitive neuropsychiatry it is necessary to identify endophenotypic features that segregate with the microdeletion and which reflect aberrant neural structure and function, regardless of clinical status. There is preliminary evidence of a specific pattern of neuropsychological function in 22q11DS, comprising poor nonverbal skills, language impairment and executive dysfunction (Swillen et al. 1997; Moss et al. 1999). However, behavioural descriptions to date have been too broad, and results too variable, to be considered endophenotypic. Similarly, structural brain-imaging studies have so far contributed little to our understanding of the syndrome, with diverse and diffuse abnormalities reported (Chow et al. 1999; Eliez et al. 2000). A report in 1997 offered the first evidence of neurophysiological abnormality in 22q11DS, showing abnormal central auditory processing of novel sounds (Cheour et al. 1997). This work must be extended to determine whether there are indeed markers of aberrant neurodevelopment which are characteristic of the microdeletion. These endophenotypic features may point towards cognitive mechanisms accounting for increased vulnerability to schizophrenia in this group, and also indicate the developmental processes that are disrupted by loss of a gene or genes within the deleted region. The next step would be to analyse the developmental function of this gene so that other factors could be identified, both genetic and environmental, which impact on the same fundamental developmental processes.

Traditional genetic approaches, such as genetic linkage analysis (genome scanning with polymorphic genetic markers in multiply affected families) and association studies (comparing genotype in unrelated affected individuals) have suggested that a locus at 22q11 may be a minor risk factor for schizophrenia in the general population. Pulver et al. (1994) reported weak linkage (lod = 1.54) at 22q12 – q13.1 in a study of 38 families and follow-up studies in larger populations have replicated this (Wildenauer et al. 1996; Levinson and Coon 1998; Shaw et al. 1998). There appears to be significant overlap between the loci of genetic susceptibility to schizophrenia and bipolar disorder in this region and on chromosomes 10, 13 and 18 (see Wildenauer et al. 1999 for review). Kelsoe et al. (2001) reported significant linkage (maximum lod score 3.8) at D22S278, a marker within 22q11, in 20 families with bipolar disorder. However, the failure to demonstrate significant linkage reinforces the point that in complex disorders of polygenic origin, focusing on the identification of genetically influenced neurodevelopmental processes in atypical groups will be more fruitful.

The typically deleted region in 22q11DS spans about 3 Mb, involving a critical deletion overlap sequence of 750 kB, named the DiGeorge syndrome critical region (DGCR) (see Scambler 2000). The first biologically attractive molecule within the deletion, from the point of view of psychosis, was the COMT enzyme, a key regulator of catecholamine synthesis, which would provide a simple link between 22q11 and the dopamine and serotonin hypotheses. However, Karayiorgou et al. (1998) analysed four variants of the COMT allele and found no associations with schizophrenia. Additionally, Murphy et al. (1999) assessed low- and high-activity COMT alleles in their study of VCFS adults with schizophrenia and found no difference in allele frequency between those with and without psychosis. It therefore seems more likely that alleles of a different gene or genes are responsible for the phenotype. Haploinsufficiency of Tbx1, a transcription factor, has been shown to mimic accurately the cardiac phenotype of 22q11DS in mice (Lindsay et al. 2001). Whether the same gene is responsible for the cognitive and behavioural features of VCFS has yet to be determined. Interestingly, it has been shown that all mice with a heterozygous deletion that includes Tbx1 show abnormal aortic arch development early in embryogenesis, but only 32% of embryos still show abnormalities at birth (Lindsay and Baldini 2001). This indicates that developmental disruption caused by this genetic anomaly can be compensated for. Whether this is true of the psychiatric manifestations of the syndrome is, of course, an important and fascinating possibility.

Chromosomal aneuploidies: imprinting, sexual dimorphic social skills and the X chromosome

It seems at first improbable that any aspect of human behaviour that is as complex as one's awareness and response to social cues could be significantly influenced by a small number of genes. Evidence that there are X-linked genes whose effect is to heighten social perceptiveness came from another rare chromosomal disorder, Turner syndrome (Skuse et al. 1997). The genetic locus in question was imprinted, and represented the first evidence that there is at least one imprinted gene on the X chromosome.

Turner syndrome (TS) is associated with distinctive physical characteristics, the most reliable of which are short stature and low production of female sex hormones. It has been known for many years that it is associated with a distinctive intellectual profile (Rovet 1995). Verbal ability is in the normal range, but visuospatial skills are impaired. More recently, other characteristics have been described, including memory deficits, attentional problems, motor impairment and difficulties in social relationships. Structural brain correlates of TS have been investigated using neuro-imaging, and have revealed abnormalities in the parietal lobes (Murphy et al. 1993; Reiss et al. 1995*b*). One study (Murphy et al. 1993) also found that women with TS had reduced volume of the hippocampus, caudate, lenticular and thalamic nuclei, a finding that is consistent with reports of deficits in long-term memory (Pennington et al. 1985; Murphy et al. 1994).

At first glance it is surprising that loss of an X chromosome should have neuro-developmental consequences, because in normal females, the second X chromosome is inactivated very early in embryonic development (Willard 1995). This X-inactivation is random: in some cells the X inherited from the mother is in-activated, in others the X inherited from the father. The Y chromosome has few functions other than primary sex determination, so if X-inactivation did not occur, then normal males, with XY karyotype, would have only half as much gene product as females. X-inactivation ensures equal dosage of gene product for both sexes. Thus normal females, normal males, and females with TS, all have only one activated X chromosome. Why then should females with TS differ from those with two sex chromosomes? The conventional explanation is the haploinsufficiency hypothesis, which attributes the phenotype of TS to genes on the X chromosome that are the exception to the general rule of X-inactivation (Zinn and Ross 1998). Molecular studies have confirmed that there is a region of the X chromosome (the pseudo-autosomal region) that escapes inactivation, so genes from both X chromosomes are active in normal females. In this region, there is evidence that males have functionally equivalent genes on the Y chromosome, so both males and females have a double dose of gene product. More recently, other regions of the X chromosome that escape inactivation have been discovered (Carrel et al. 1999). According to the haploinsufficiency hypothesis, the phenotypic abnormalities in TS, including the cognitive profile, can be explained in terms of a deficiency of gene products from a region of the X chromosome that escapes inactivation. Adverse effects could be direct effects of genes on brain development, or more indirect consequences of the hormonal deficiencies that result from the genetic deficit.

Recently, we suggested that imprinted genes might play a role in determining the phenotype associated with TS. Genomic imprinting is another mechanism whereby one member of a pair of alleles is inactivated, but in this case, the inactivation is not random, but is determined by the parental origin of the chromosome. Imprinted

X-linked genes have recently been identified in humans (Naumova et al. 1998), as well as autosomal imprinted genes that are expressed in the brain (Keverne 1997; Reik and Walter 1998; Davies et al. 2001). We argued that if humans had imprinted genes affecting neurodevelopment on the X chromosome, then we would expect to see neurocognitive differences between females with a single X chromosome (i.e. monosomic TS), depending on the parental origin of the X chromosome (Skuse et al. 1997). Suppose there were an X-linked gene that was expressed only when inherited from the father. Girls with a single maternal X chromosome would lack the relevant gene product, whereas those with a single paternal X chromosome would show normal gene expression. Furthermore, because the single X in Turner syndrome is entirely normal, it is plausible that the actions of X-linked imprinted loci could be associated with sexual dimorphism of equivalent phenotypic features in normal ($46, X^m Y$) males and ($46, X^m X^p$) females (Skuse 1999). Thus, the imprinted locus hypothesis predicts (i) differences within TS, depending on parental origin of the X chromosome, and (ii) sex differences in the normal population, for phenotypes which depend on expression of a paternally derived X-linked gene. This was the pattern of results we reported in a study of social adjustment in TS. Although TS females in general had a somewhat elevated risk of impaired social adjustment, the risk of serious difficulties was substantially greater in those with a maternal X chromosome ($45, X^m$) than in those with a paternal X chromosome ($45, X^p$) (Skuse et al. 1997).

In further research into the potential neurocognitive mechanisms associated with these findings (Bishop et al. 2000) we anticipated that the $45, X^m$ group might have an impairment in verbal memory as the basis for abnormalities in their social interaction. However, although this group did show subtle abnormalities of verbal memory, as indicated by enhanced forgetting of previously well-encoded material, this was unrelated to social adjustment difficulties. Another surprising finding from this study was the relatively good performance on immediate recall, which was particularly striking in the $45, X^p$ group. This result could not be accounted for in terms of the greater age and verbal ability of this subgroup. Our study revealed a different pattern of results for initial perception and subsequent retention of visuospatial materials. In a copying task, where no memory is implicated, both groups of monosomic females did poorly, and those with $45, X^m$ genotype scored lowest. However, those with $45, X^p$ genotype forgot a disproportionate amount over a delay, and made errors similar to those of adults with right temporal-lobe lesions.

How can such results be explained? The contrasting patterns of forgetting for verbal and nonverbal material seen in relation to parental origin could indicate that there is a complementary set of imprinted genes on the X chromosome that affects the development of lateralized brain regions important for memory function.

There is increasing evidence for the role of imprinted genes in brain development (Keverne 1997) and functioning (Pilgrim and Reisert 1996). The apparent conjunction of oppositely imprinted domains is not surprising; allele-specific gene expression of this sort, with contrasting phenotypic consequences, has been increasingly frequently recognized in recent years (Reik and Walter 1998). However, our data could be accounted for by a more parsimonious explanation that postulated a single imprinted locus on the X chromosome that affected timing of early neurodevelopmental events. Suppose there were a maternally imprinted gene which had the effect of slowing down language development. Studies of the consequences of lateralized brain injuries in children suggest that verbal and nonverbal functions compete for hemispheric representation (Bishop 1988). Verbal functions develop early and usually become established in the left hemisphere, leaving the right hemisphere available for visuospatial functions. However, if the left hemisphere is damaged early in life, then verbal functions can become established in the right hemisphere, and visuospatial functions suffer as a consequence. It is possible that what we see in TS is a response to abnormal early development of the right temporoparietal region. In those with the $45,X^p$ genotype, language develops early and verbal memory functions become established in the left temporal lobe, leaving visuospatial functions to be carried out by the defective right hemisphere. However, in those with $45,X^m$ genotype, language development is slower to get started. Because of anomalies in the right temporal region, visuospatial functions do not develop normally but start instead to compete for representational space in the left temporal region. Consequently, verbal memory suffers.

This account is highly speculative, but is compatible with two facts. First, we know that in normal males (with $X^m Y^p$ genotype), language development is typically slower than in normal females (who may have either X^m or X^p activated). Second, several studies have suggested that in individuals with TS, the left hemisphere is less involved than normal in processing verbal information and more involved in processing nonverbal information. Since the majority of females with TS have $45,X^m$ genotype, we would expect to see this pattern of results. This account also has the advantage that it can explain why we fail to find any sex difference in verbal memory in our normal controls. To see disruptive effects on lateralized memory functions, one would need to have a slowing of language development *plus* pre-existing brain abnormality that led to more intense competition between verbal and visuospatial functions. Previous attempts to find evidence of imprinted genes have focused on the physical phenotype in TS, and not found any influence of parental origin on characteristics such as short stature, neck webbing or gonadal abnormalities (Mathur et al. 1991). The haploinsufficiency account has been widely accepted as an explanation for aspects of the physical phenotype of TS. However, our data suggest that a different explanation, in terms of genomic imprinting, might be needed to explain some of the neurocognitive consequences of X monosomy.

Conclusion

As we emerge from the 'Decade of the Brain', into what might be termed the 'Post-Genomic era', one of the major tasks facing those seeking a scientific basis for neuropsychiatry will be to conceptually link advances in genetic research with advances in brain research. Presumably, genes that contribute to neurodevelopmental dysfunction are affecting behaviour by altering brain function. We are still quite a way off identifying just which genes are important for cognitive development, although considerable progress has been made with regard to their role in developmental neurobiology of the brain (Skuse and Baker, in press). Quantitative genetic techniques are revealing replicable evidence for genetic predispositions to learning problems, such as dyslexia (see Chapter 1 by Plomin). However, so far progress in finding genetic loci that predispose to psychiatric disorders has been slow, with claims of progress countered almost simultaneously by contrary views and failures of replication (Altmuller et al. 2001). One possible explanation is that the conventional approach to phenotype definition (in terms of illness or disorder categories) is not the most efficient way to go about discovering the genetic mechanisms in question. We suggest we need to focus more carefully on the discrete cognitive characteristics that contribute to the clinical picture. These characteristics could be more closely linked to the genetic mechanisms that shape our personality, and our suspicion is that they act upon behaviour in indirect ways.

The study of chromosomal anomalies with cognitive or behavioural phenotypes should enable us to identify genes that contribute to the normal development of cognitive brain systems. The characterization of the consequences of even a single gene mutation, such as that causing the speech disorder of the KE family, could bring about insight into the development of neural systems that have general relevance to disorders of speech and language. Once we can establish the identity of just one gene that is linked to the development or function of a cognitive brain system, and we can demonstrate that gene has been conserved through evolution, its neurobiological role can be investigated. Using transgenic technology, we can even explore what that gene does if introduced, for example, into the genome of an experimental animal, such as a mouse. Identifying the gene is merely the first step, but a necessary one. In order to deletion-map our candidate successfully, we need to measure aspects of the phenotype that are most closely linked to the underlying genetic mechanisms. Such phenotypic characteristics may be both subtle and indirectly linked to the obvious clinical features of the disorder.

REFERENCES

Adler LE, Freedman R, Ross RG, Olincy A and Waldo MC (1999). Elementary phenotypes in the neurobiological and genetic study of schizophrenia. *Biol Psychiatry*, 46, 8–18.

Allman JM (2000). *Evolving Brains*. New York: Scientific American Library.

Altmuller J, Palmer LJ, Fischer G, Scherb H and Wjst M (2001). Genomewide scans of complex human diseases: true linkage is hard to find. *Am J Hum Genet*, 69, 936–50.

American Psychiatric Association (1996). *Diagnostic and Statistical Manual (Edition 4): Primary Care Version: International version with ICD-10 Codes*. Washington, DC: American Psychiatric Association Press.

Arnold PD, Siegel-Bartelt J, Cytrynbaum C, Teshima I and Schachar R (2001). Velo-cardio-facial syndrome: Implications of microdeletion 22q11 for schizophrenia and mood disorders. *Am J Med Genet*, 105, 354–62.

Bassett A, Hodgkinson K, Chow E, Correia S, Scutt L and Weksberg R (1998). 22q11 deletion syndrome in adults with schizophrenia. *Am J Med Genet*, 81, 328–37.

Baumgardner TL, Reiss A, Fruend LS and Abrams MT (1995). Specification of the neuro-behavioural phenotype in males with fragile X syndrome. *Pediatrics*, 95, 744–52.

Bellugi U, Lichtenberger L, Jones W, Lai Z and St George MI (2000). The neurocognitive profile of Williams Syndrome: a complex pattern of strengths and weaknesses. *J Cogn Neurosci*, 12 (Suppl. 1), 7–29.

Bishop DVM (1988). Language development after focal brain damage. In *Language Development in Exceptional Circumstances*, ed. DVM Bishop and K Mogford, pp. 203–19. Edinburgh: Churchill Livingstone.

Bishop DV, Canning E, Elgar K, Morris E, Jacobs PA and Skuse DH (2000). Distinctive patterns of memory function in subgroups of females with Turner syndrome: evidence for imprinted loci on the X-chromosome affecting neurodevelopment. *Neuropsychologia*, 38, 712–21.

Cannon M, Jones P, Gilvarry C et al. (1997). Premorbid social functioning in schizophrenia and bipolar disorder: similarities and differences. *Am J Psychiatry*, 154, 1544–50.

Carrel L, Cottle AA, Goglin KC and Willard HF (1999). A first-generation X-inactivation profile of the human X chromosome. *Proc Natl Acad Sci USA*, 96, 14440–4.

Chapman RS and Hesketh LJ (2000). Behavioral phenotype of individuals with Down syndrome. *Ment Retard Dev Disabil Res Rev*, 6, 84–95.

Cheour M, Haapanen ML, Hukki J et al. (1997). The first neurophysiological evidence for cognitive brain dysfunctions in children with CATCH. *Neuroreport*, 8, 1785–7.

Chow E, Mikulis D, Zipursky R, Scutt L, Weksberg R and Bassett A (1999). Qualitative MRI findings in adults with 22q11 deletion syndrome and schizophrenia. *Biol Psychiatry* 46, 1436–42.

Damberg M, Garpenstrand H, Hallman J and Oreland L (2001). Genetic mechanisms of behavior – don't forget about the transcription factors. *Mol Psychiatry*, 6, 503–10.

Davies N, Russell A, Jones P and Murray R (1998). Which characteristics of schizophrenia predate psychosis? *J Psychiatr Res*, 32, 121–31.

Davies W, Isles AR and Wilkinson LS (2001). Imprinted genes and mental dysfunction. *Ann Med*, 33, 428–36.

De Vries BB, van den Ouweland AM, Mohkamsing S et al. (1997). Screening and diagnosis for the fragile X syndrome among the mentally retarded: an epidemiological and psychological survey. Collaborative Fragile X Study Group. *Am J Hum Genet*, 61, 660–7.

Dobkin C, Rabe A, Dumas R, El Idrissi A, Haubenstock H and Brown WT (2000). Fmr1 knockout mouse has a distinctive strain-specific learning impairment. *Neuroscience*, 100, 423–9.

Done J, Crow T, Johnstone E and Sacker A (1994). Childhood antecedents of schizophrenia and affective illness: social adjustment at ages 7 and 11. *Br Med J*, 309, 699–703.

Du Montcel ST, Mendizabai H, Ayme S, Levy A and Philip N (1996). Prevalence of 22q11 microdeletion. *J Med Genet*, 33, 719.

Dykens EM and Volkmar FR (1997). Medical conditions associated with autism. In *Handbook of Autism and Developmental Disorders*, ed. DJ Cohen and FR Volkmar, pp. 388–410. New York: John Wiley and Sons.

Eliez S, Schmitt E, White C and Reiss A (2000). Children and adolescents with VCFS: a volumetric MRI study. *Am J Psychiatry*, 157, 409–15.

Fisher SE, Vargha-Khadem F, Watkins KE, Monaco AP and Pembrey ME (1998). Localisation of a gene implicated in a severe speech and language disorder. *Nat Genet*, 18, 168–70.

Franke P, Leboyer M, Hardt J et al. (1999). Neuropsychological profiles of FMR-1 premutation and full-mutation carrier females. *Psychiatry Res*, 87, 223–31.

Geschwind DH, Boone KB, Miller BL and Swerdloff RS (2000). Neurobehavioral phenotype of Klinefelter syndrome. *Ment Retard Dev Disabil Res Rev*, 6, 107–16.

Gilbert SF (2000). Transcription factors. In *Developmental Biology*, 6th edn. Sunderland, MA: Sinauer Associates, Inc.

Gopnik M (1990). Genetic basis of grammar defect. *Nature*, 347, 26.

Gopnik M and Crago MB (1991). Familial aggregation of a developmental language disorder. *Cognition*, 39, 1–50.

Gothelf D, Frisch A, Munitz H et al. (1999). Clinical characteristics of schizophrenia associated with VCFS. *Schizophr Res*, 35, 105–12.

Gottesman II (1997). Twins: en route to QTLs for cognition. *Science*, 276, 1522–3.

Gray JM, Young AW, Barker WA, Curtis A and Gibson D (1997). Impaired recognition of disgust in Huntington's disease carriers. *Brain*, 120, 2029–38.

Halligan PW and David AS (2001). Cognitive neuropsychiatry: towards a scientific psychopathology. *Nat Rev Neurosci*, 2, 209–15.

Hanel ML and Wevrick R (2001). The role of genomic imprinting in human developmental disorders: lessons from Prader–Willi syndrome. *Clin Genet*, 59, 156–64.

Huntington's Disease Collaborative Research Group (1993). A novel gene containing a trinucleotide repeat that is expanded and unstable on Huntington's disease chromosomes. *Cell*, 72, 971–83.

Hurst JA, Baraitser M, Auger E, Graham F and Norell S (1990). An extended family with a dominantly inherited speech disorder. *Dev Med Child Neurol*, 32, 352–5.

Inoue SB, Siomi MC and Siomi H (2000). Molecular mechanisms of fragile X syndrome. *J Med Invest*, 47, 101–7.

Jennings C (1999). Flies by night. *Nat Neurosci*, 2, 591.

Jones P, Rodgers B, Murray R and Marmot M (1994). Child developmental risk factors for adult schizophrenia in the British 1946 birth cohort. *Lancet*, 344, 1398–402.

Karayiorgou M, Morris MA, Morrow B et al. (1995). Schizophrenia susceptibility associated with interstitial deletions of chromosome 22q11. *Proc Natl Acad Sci USA*, 92, 7612–16.

Karayiorgou M, Gogos JA, Galke BL et al. (1998). Identification of sequence variants and analysis of the role of the catechol-O-methyl-transferase gene in schizophrenia susceptibility. *Biol Psychiatry*, 43, 425–31.

Kelsoe JR, Spence MA, Loetscher E et al. (2001). A genome survey indicates a possible susceptibility locus for bipolar disorder on chromosome 22. *Proc Natl Acad Sci USA*, 98, 585–90.

Keverne EB (1997). Genomic imprinting in the brain. *Curr Opin Neurobiol*, 7, 463–8.

Korenberg JR, Chen XN, Hirota H et al. (2000). VI. Genome structure and cognitive map of Williams syndrome. *J Cogn Neurosci*, 12 Suppl., 89–107.

Lachiewicz AM and Dawson DV (1994). Behavior problems of young girls with fragile X syndrome: factor scores on the Conners' Parents' Questionnaire. *Am J Med Genet*, 51, 364–9.

Lai CS, Fisher SE, Hurst JA et al. (2000). The SPCH1 region on human 7q31: genomic characterization of the critical interval and localization of translocations associated with speech and language disorder. *Am J Hum Genet*, 67, 357–68.

Lai CS, Fisher SE, Hurst JA, Vargha-Khadem F and Monaco AP (2001). A forkhead-domain gene is mutated in a severe speech and language disorder. *Nature*, 413, 519–23.

LeCouteur A, Bailey A, Goode S et al. (1996). A broader phenotype of autism: the clinical spectrum in twins. *J Child Psychol Psychiatry*, 37, 785–801.

Levinson DF and Coon H (1998). Chromosome 22 workshop. *Psychiatr Genet*, 8, 115–20.

Lindsay EA and Baldini A. (2001). Recovery from arterial growth delay reduces penetrance of cardiovascular defects in mice deleted for the DiGeorge syndrome region. *Hum Mol Genet*, 10, 997–1002.

Lindsay EA, Vitelli F, Su H et al. (2001). Tbx1 haploinsufficiency in the DiGeorge syndrome region causes aortic arch defects in mice. *Nature*, 410, 97–101.

Lippe BM (1996). Turner syndrome. In *Pediatric Endocrinology*, ed. MA Sperling, pp. 387–421. Philadelphia: WB Saunders.

Margolis RL, McInnis MG, Rosenblatt A and Ross CA (1999). Trinucleotide repeat expansion and neuropsychiatric disease. *Arch Gen Psychiatry*, 56, 1019–31.

Mathur A, Stekol L, Schatz D, McLaren NK, Scott ML and Lippe B (1991). The parental origin of the single X chromosome in Turner syndrome: Lack of correlation with parental age or clinical phenotype. *Am J Hum Genet*, 48, 682–6.

McCabe ER, de la Cruz F and Clapp K (1999). Workshop on fragile X: future research directions. *Am J Med Genet*, 85, 317–22.

McGuffin P, Riley B and Plomin R (2001). Genomics and behavior. Toward behavioral genomics. *Science*, 291, 1232–49.

McInnis MG (1996). Anticipation: an old idea in new genes. *Am J Hum Genet*, 59, 973–9.

Merenstein SA, Sobesky WE, Taylor AK, Riddle JE, Tran HX and Hagerman RJ (1996). Molecular-clinical correlations in males with an expanded FMR1 mutation. *Am J Med Genet*, 64, 388–94.

Moss E, Batshaw M, Solot C et al. (1999). Psychoeducational profile of the 22q11.2 microdeletion: a complex pattern. *J Pediatr*, 134, 193–8.

Murphy DGM, DeCarli C, Daly E et al. (1993). X-chromosome effects on female brain: a magnetic resonance imaging study of Turner's syndrome. *Lancet*, 342, 1197–200.

Murphy DGM, Allen G, Haxby JV et al. (1994). The effects of sex steroids, and the X chromosome on female brain function: a study of the neuropsychology of adult Turner syndrome. *Neuropsychologia*, 32, 1309–23.

Murphy K, Jones L and Owen M (1999). High rates of schizophrenia in adults with VCFS. *Arch Gen Psychiatry*, 56, 940–5.

Naumova A, Leppert M, Barker D, Morgan K and Sapienza C (1998). Parental origin-dependent, male offspring-specific transmission-ratio distortion at loci on the human X chromosome. *Am J Hum Genet*, 62, 1493–9.

Papolos DF, Faedda GL, Veit S et al. (1996). Bipolar spectrum disorders in patients diagnosed with VCFS: does a hemizygous deletion of chromosome 22q11 result in bipolar affective disorder? *Am J Psychiatry*, 153, 1541–7.

Pennington BF, Heaton RK, Karzmark P, Pendleton MG, Lehman R and Shucard DW (1985). The neuropsychological phenotype in Turner syndrome. *Cortex*, 21, 391–404.

Pickles A, Starr E, Kazak S et al. (2000). Variable expression of the autism broader phenotype: findings from extended pedigrees. *J Child Psychol Psychiatry*, 41, 491–502.

Pilgrim C and Reisert I (1996). Sex, hormones and the developing neuron. *Frontiers Endocrinol*, 20, 125–34.

Pulver AE, Karayiorgou M, Wolyniec PS et al. (1994). Sequential strategy to identify a susceptibility gene for schizophrenia: report of potential linkage on chromosome 22q12-q13.1: Part 1. *Am J Med Genet*, 54, 36–43.

Reik W and Walter J (1998). Imprinting mechanisms in mammals. *Curr Opin Genet Dev*, 8, 154–64.

Reiss AL, Abrams MT, Singer HS, Ross JL and Denckla MB (1995a). Neurodevelopmental effects of the FMR-1 full mutation in humans. *Nat Med*, 1, 159–67.

Reiss AL, Mazzocco MMM, Greenlaw R, Freund LS and Ross JL (1995b). Neurodevelopmental effects of X-monosomy: a volumetric imaging study. *Ann Neurol*, 38, 731–8.

Ross RG, Olincy A, Harris JG, Sullivan B and Radant A (2000). Smooth pursuit eye movements in schizophrenia and attentional dysfunction: adults with schizophrenia, ADHD, and a normal comparison group. *Biol Psychiatry*, 48, 197–203.

Rovet J (1995). Turner syndrome. In *Syndrome of Nonverbal Learning Disabilities: Neurodevelopmental Manifestations*, ed. BP Rourke, pp. 351–71. New York: Guilford Press.

Ryan AK, Goodship JA, Wilson DI et al. (1997). Spectrum of clinical features associated with interstitial chromosome 22q11 deletions: a European collaborative study. *J Med Genet*, 34, 798–804.

Scambler P (2000). The 22q11 deletion syndromes. *Hum Mol Genet*, 9, 2421–6.

Scambler PJ, Kelly D, Lindsay E et al. (1992). Velocardiofacial syndrome associated with chromosome 22 deletions encompassing the DiGeorge locus. *Lancet*, 339, 1138–9.

Shaw SH, Kelly M, Smith AB et al. (1998). A genome-wide search for schizophrenia susceptibility genes. *Am J Med Genet*, 81, 364–76.

Shprintzen RJ, Goldberg RB, Lewin ML et al. (1978). A new syndrome involving cleft palate, cardiac anomalies, typical facies, and learning disabilities: velo-cardio-facial syndrome. *Cleft Palate J*, 15, 56–62.

Shprintzen R, Goldberg R, Golding-Kushner K and Marion R (1992). Late-onset psychosis in the VCFS. *Am J Med Genet*, 42, 141–2.

Skuse D (1997). Genetic factors in the aetiology of child psychiatric disorders. *Curr Opin Pediatr*, 9, 354–60.

Skuse D (1999). Genomic imprinting of the X-chromosome: a novel mechanism for the evolution of sexual dimorphism. *J Lab Clin Med*, 133, 23–32.

Skuse DH (2001). Endophenotypes and child psychiatry. *Br J Psychiatry*, 178, 395–6.

Skuse DH and Baker K (in press). Neurodevelopmental genetics of brain. In *Encyclopaedia of the Human Genome*. London: Nature Publishing Group.

Skuse DH, James RS, Bishop DVM et al. (1997). Evidence from Turner's syndrome of an imprinted X-linked locus affecting cognitive function. *Nature*, 387, 705–8.

Sobesky WE, Taylor AK, Pennington BF et al. (1996). Molecular/clinical correlations in females with fragile X. *Am J Med Genet*, 64, 340–5.

Swillen A, Devriendt K, Legius E et al. (1997). Intelligence and psychosocial adjustment in VCFS: a study of 37 children and adolescents with VCFS. *J Med Genet*, 34, 453–8.

Tassone F, Hagerman RJ, Ikle DN et al. (1999). FMRP expression as a potential prognostic indicator in fragile X syndrome. *Am J Med Genet*, 84, 250–61.

Thompson NM, Gulley ML, Rogeness GA et al. (1994). Neurobehavioral characteristics of CGG amplification status in fragile X females. *Am J Med Genet*, 54, 378–83.

Tilghman SM (1999). The sins of the fathers and mothers: genomic imprinting in mammalian development. *Cell*, 96, 185–93.

Turk J and Cornish K (1998). Face recognition and emotion perception in boys with fragile-X syndrome. *J Intellect Disabil Res*, 42, 490–9.

Turner G, Robinson H, Wake S, Laing S and Partington M (1997). Case finding for the fragile X syndrome and its consequences. *Br Med J*, 315, 1223–6.

Usiskin SI, Nicolson R, Krasnewich DM et al. (1999). VCFS in childhood-onset schizophrenia. *J Am Acad Child Adolesc Psychiatry*, 38, 1536–43.

Vargha Khadem F, Watkins K, Alcock K, Fletcher P and Passingham R (1995). Praxic and non-verbal cognitive deficits in a large family with a genetically transmitted speech and language disorder. *Proc Natl Acad Sci USA*, 92, 930–3.

Vargha Khadem F, Watkins KE, Price CJ et al. (1998). Neural basis of an inherited speech and language disorder. *Proc Natl Acad Sci USA*, 95, 12695–700.

Verkerk AJ, Pieretti M, Sutcliffe JS et al. (1991). Identification of a gene (FMR-1) containing a CGG repeat coincident with a breakpoint cluster region exhibiting length variation in fragile X syndrome. *Cell*, 65, 905–14.

Weatherall D. (1999). From genotype to phenotype: genetics and medical practice in the new millennium. *Philos Trans R Soc Lond B Biol Sci*, 354, 1995–2010.

Wildenauer DB, Hallmayer J, Schwab SG et al. (1996). Searching for susceptibility genes in schizophrenia by genetic linkage analysis. *Cold Spring Harb Symp Quant Biol*, 61, 845–50.

Wildenauer D, Schwab S, Maier W and Detera-Wadleigh S (1999). Do schizophrenia and affective disorder share susceptibility genes? *Schizophr Res*, 39, 107–11.

Willard HF (1995). The sex chromosomes and X chromosome inactivation. In *The Metabolic and Molecular Bases of Inherited Disease*, Vol. 1, 7th edn, pp. 719–35. New York: McGraw Hill.

World Health Organization (1992). *The Tenth Revision of the International Classification of Diseases and Related Health Problems (ICD–10)*. Geneva: WHO.

Wright IC, McGuire PK, Poline JB et al. (1995). A voxel-based method for the statistical analysis of gray and white matter density applied to schizophrenia. *Neuroimage*, 2, 244–52.

Zinn AR and Ross JL (1998). Turner syndrome and haploinsufficiency. *Curr Opin Genet Dev*, 8, 322–7.

Part II

Brain development

3

Brain development: glial cells generate neurons — implications for neuropsychiatric disorders

Magdalena Götz

Max-Planck Institute of Neurobiology, Planegg-Martinsried, Germany

Introduction

A variety of neurological disorders may have their origin during development of the central nervous system (CNS) (see also Chapter 4 by Beasley et al.). In particular, disorders with displaced neurons are considered as a failure of neuronal migration and have therefore been named 'neuronal migration disorders' (NMD). NMDs occur rather frequently in the forebrain and comprise aberrations in the formation of gyri, heterotopia and dysplasia (Copp and Harding 1999; Walsh 1999; Lammens 2000; Clark 2001). In cases of heterotopia, neurons are located in the white matter (WM), the fibre tract of the CNS, where usually only somata of glial cells (astrocytes and oligodendrocytes) reside. Dysplasia is a focal malformation in the grey matter (GM) of the cerebral cortex (focal cortical dysplasia (FCD)), the dorsal part of the telencephalon. The grey matter contains the neurons that are arranged in horizontal layers in the cerebral cortex according to their functional properties and connectivity (Götz 1999). This layering is often distorted in dysplasia and large abnormal neurons can be detected (Cotter et al. 1999). Similarly, a variety of defects assigned to developmental stages have been detected in patients with schizophrenia, leading to the highly disputed 'neurodevelopmental hypothesis' of this complex disorder (Senitz 1984; Jakob and Beckmann 1994; Roberts et al. 1995; Hollister and Cannon 1998; Taylor 1998; see also Chapter 4 by Beasley et al.).

These malformations in the adult are assigned to developmental processes as smoke is considered an indication of a fire. We conclude from the displacement of neurons that migrational aberrations occur during development, since neurons are thought to acquire their final positions during development. Similarly, the large abnormal neurons in FCD that express traits of neurons and glial cells are interpreted as a result of erroneous neuronal differentiation during development.

These conclusions hinge on two dogmas that are currently being revised. In this chapter, I will discuss the evidence for these new views and consider their relevance for potential causes of neurological disorders.

A main dogma in neurobiology is that all neurons of the adult mammalian and in particular human CNS are generated during development and that no new neurons are added in adulthood (Gross 2000). Accordingly, misplaced neurons are thought to be at this position since the time of neuronal migration in embryogenesis, which ranges in the cerebral cortex of humans from gestational weeks 8–14 (Sidman and Rakic 1973; Copp and Harding 1999; Götz 1999). In contrast, neurogenesis continues into adulthood in the CNS of all other vertebrates. In lower vertebrates, such as fish and amphibia, parts of the brain continue to grow like other parts of the body and neurons are added continuously (Marcus et al. 1999). This massive neurogenesis is also reflected in an enormous capacity to regenerate entire parts of the CNS after lesions (Margotta and Morelli 1996; Zupanc and Ott 1999). Neurogenesis also continues into adulthood in reptiles and birds, even though it is much more limited to specific regions of the CNS (Alvarez-Buylla et al. 1990). Therefore the lack of adult neurogenesis has almost been considered as a trait of higher evolution in mammals with the justification that complex brains cannot easily incorporate new neurons. The increasing evidence for neurogenesis in the hippocampus and olfactory bulb of mammals (Kuhn et al. 1996; Doetsch et al. 1999) was thus for some time rejected for primates and humans, where neurogenesis was thought be absent or at least reduced to a very low level (Rakic 1985). By now, however, neurogenesis has been demonstrated not only in the olfactory bulb and hippocampus, but also in the neocortex of adult primates including humans (Eriksson et al. 1998; Gould et al. 1999; Kornack and Rakic 2001). Due to the increasing evidence for neurogenesis in the adult human brain (Gross 2000), we have to take into account that mistakes in neuronal migration and differentiation might be initiated not only during development but also during adulthood.

The second dogma about to fall is that neurons and glial cells are two rather separate cell classes in the CNS. Glial cells have been viewed as support cells for the neurons in the developing and adult CNS. Radial glial cells are the ubiquitous glial cell type in the developing CNS and are well known for their role in supporting migrating neurons (Rakic 1972). In this context they have already been considered as potentially relevant cell types involved in the aetiology of NMDs. It has now been shown, however, that these cells not only guide, but also generate, neurons in the developing mouse cortex (Malatesta et al. 2000; Noctor et al. 2001). I will review this evidence in this chapter with the focus on similarities and differences between rodent and human radial glial cells. Moreover, this novel role of glial cells – the generation of neurons – is not restricted to the developing nervous system. Astroglial cells have been identified as the source of the new neurons in the adult olfactory bulb, one of the regions known to produce new neurons into adulthood in both mice and men (Doetsch et al. 1999; Kornack and Rakic 2001). Astrocytes in this region of the adult CNS (the adult subventricular zone) are stem cells that maintain the capacity to generate all cell types of the CNS (Doetsch et al. 1999). These recent data therefore propose a new role of astroglial cells in the developing and adult CNS, namely the generation of neurons. Thus, changes in astroglial cells might impinge on the generation, location and differentiation of neurons in the adult brain and should therefore be considered as potential causes of NMDs.

What are radial glial cells?

Radial glial cells are a ubiquitous glial cell type throughout the developing vertebrate CNS, that are maintained into adulthood in all vertebrate classes, except mammals. They have been identified by their characteristic morphology since staining techniques have been available to reveal details of the cellular morphology. Camillo Golgi was the first to mention 'radial cells' in the developing chick embryo, and a few years later his colleague Magini coined the term 'radial cell' (Bentivoglio and Mazarello 1999). The characteristic radial processes of these cells span the entire thickness of the wall of the neural tube, the anlage of the CNS. The somata of precursor cells are located close to the ventricle of the neural tube where they undergo cytokinesis. All cells span the neural tube wall at early developmental stages, i.e. prior to the generation of neurons (Figure 3.1). When neurogenesis starts, however, most precursors are thought to lose the contact to the outer surface of the brain where the basal lamina is located underneath the meninges (Figure 3.1). Those cells that maintain their long radial processes start to express astroglial characteristics and are called radial glial cells (Figure 3.1). In 1980, Levitt and Rakic discovered the glial fibrillary acidic protein (GFAP) in radial cells of the developing primate cortex. Since GFAP is a hallmark for astrocytes in the CNS (for review see Eng et al. 2000), this was the first evidence for a glial nature of radial cells. Also at the ultrastructural level, similarities between radial glial cells and astrocytes, such as glycogen granules, were detected (Choi 1981). In addition, further astrocyte-specific molecules were found in radial glial cells, such as the astrocyte-specific glutamate transporter (GLAST; Shibata et al. 1997) or the brain lipid-binding protein (BLBP; Feng et al. 1994). Besides these molecular and ultrastructural similarities between radial glial cells and astrocytes, radial glial cells are directly linked to the formation of astrocytes since they transform into astrocytes at the end of development in the mammalian CNS (Schmechel and Rakic 1979a; Pixley and De Vellis 1984; Voigt 1989; Malatesta et al. 2000). As mentioned above, this transformation occurs only in mammals, since many radial glial cells persist without transformation into the adult CNS of other vertebrates.

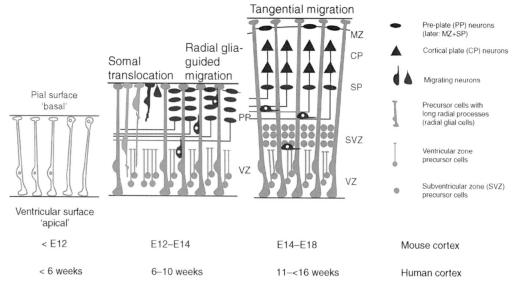

Figure 3.1   Schematic drawing of developmental stages in the cerebral cortex of mice and men. The sequence of precursor cells and radial glia is depicted and explained in the text, as well as the distinct modes of neuronal migration during development. For further details refer to the text. VZ, ventricular zone; MZ, marginal zone; SP, subplate.

Radial glial cells as guides for migrating neurons

The overall view of glial cells as support for neurons was once more confirmed by the finding that the radial processes of radial glia serve to support neuronal migration (Rakic 1972; Sidman and Rakic 1973). Pasko Rakic discovered by electron-microscope analysis of the developing primate cortex that neurons are closely attached to the radial processes of radial glial cells, and suggested that these processes might serve as guides to the cortical plate, the latter grey matter of the cerebral cortex (Rakic 1972; Figure 3.1). Long-distance migration is a hallmark of the developing CNS. Cells are generated in the layer lining the ventricle, the ventricular zone (VZ), and then migrate towards their final destination. The distance of neuronal migration increases during phylogeny due to the enlargement of the brain, in particular the cerebral cortex (Götz 1999; Kornack 2000). Neurons settle at the pial surface opposite to the ventricle and must therefore cross the entire thickness of the cortex. This distance increases during phylogeny. While neurons have to travel for days to bridge distances of several hundred micrometres in the developing rodent cortex, they migrate over distances of centimetres and take weeks to arrive at their final position in the human cortex (Sidman and Rakic 1973). Therefore neurons need a support or guiding structure most urgently in primate cortex. Nevertheless, the radial-glial guided mode of neuronal migration was then also detected in many other vertebrates and confirmed in live observations using time-lapse video microscopy (Hatten 1999).

However, neurons also use other modes of migration (Figure 3.1). In the 1970s, Ken Morest observed somata of cells attached by long radial processes to the pial surface seemingly translocating from the ventricular to the marginal zone while differentiating into neurons (Morest 1970). This mode of migration is referred to as 'perikaryal or somal translocation' and has also been observed directly in living tissue by time-lapse video microscopy (Book and Morest 1990; Nadarajah et al. 2001). Interestingly, cells undergoing somal translocation are immunoreactive for an antiserum directed against the phosphorylated form of GAP43 (Brittis et al. 1995), suggesting that phosphorylation of this growth-associated protein (GAP43) might turn out to be as important for somal translocation as it is for axonal outgrowth (Meiri et al. 1998). The somal translocation was actually the first hint that radial glial cells might transform into neurons while dislocating their somata towards the surface of the brain. This is in good agreement with the previously discovered neurogenic role of radial glial cells.

In addition to the radial dimension of neuronal migration, neurons (and oligodendrocytes, the myelinating glial cells of the CNS) migrate over large distances tangentially, i.e. parallel to the pial and ventricular surface, in the developing brain (Figure 3.1). These migrating cells have the capacity to cross between different brain regions that are otherwise strictly delineated during development (Lumsden and Krumlauf 1996). For example, a prominent border for most, but not all, migrating cells exists between dorsal and ventral regions in the developing telencephalon. The cerebral cortex with its layered cytoarchitecture originates from the dorsal while the modular basal ganglia arise from the ventral telencephalon anlage. These regions are specified at very early developmental stages, long before the first neurons are generated (Götz 1999). Transcription factors of the homeobox and paired box family are crucial for the dorsoventral patterning and instruct adhesive differences, as well as the formation of a boundary by a radial glial fascicle delineating the cerebral cortex and basal ganglia anlage (Stoykova et al. 1997). Some neurons, however, are able to cross this boundary. Increasing evidence suggests that mostly GABAergic interneurons migrate tangentially from ventral positions into the neocortex and further enter the hippocampus (Anderson et al. 1997; Pleasure et al. 2000). Thus, many if not most inhibitory interneurons of the cerebral cortex originate in the ventral telencephalon. A similar migration between brain regions has also been observed in primates from the telencephalon to the diencephalon (Rakic and Sidman 1969; Letinic and Rakic 2001). The substrate for tangentially migrating neurons is not known, even though some adhesion molecules influence specifically tangential, but not radial, cell migration (Heffron and Golden 2000).

Taken together, these data suggest an intricate link between the type of neuron and its mode of migration. Indeed, analyses using mouse chimera or cell lineage tracing showed clearly that GABAergic neurons disperse mostly in a tangential plane while glutamatergic projection neurons migrate in a more radial fashion in the developing cortex of rodents (Mione et al. 1997; Tan et al. 1998). Interestingly, radial migration becomes more dominant in primate cerebral cortex (see below). Subtle changes in the molecular specification of neuronal subtypes might thus be sufficient to cause changes between tangentially and radially migrating neurons and thereby affect the proportion of GABAergic neurons in different parts of the neocortex. Alterations in the number of GABAergic neurons in the lateral neocortex occur for example in temporal lobe epilepsy and schizophrenia (Roberts et al. 1995). Interestingly, mutations in patterning transcription factors often result in heterotopia of GABAergic neurons in lateral cortical regions (Schmahl et al. 1993; Chapouton et al. 1999; Fode et al. 2000). For example, the transcription factor Pax6 expressed in radial glial cells of the cerebral cortex, but absent in the basal ganglia, is essential for the formation of the boundary between these regions (Stoykova et al. 1997). In Pax6-mutant mice this boundary does not form and GABAergic neurons from ventral regions massively invade the cerebral cortex and accumulate in the lateral cortex of Pax6-mutant mice (Chapouton et al. 1999). At the same time, the loss of Pax6 function in these mutant mice also affects radial migration of neurons, even though to a lesser extent than tangential migration (Caric et al. 1997). The defects in radial migration are most likely due to the defects in radial glial cells in the Pax6-mutant mice (Götz et al. 1998). Thus, a point mutation of a single molecule expressed in radial glia, the transcription factor Pax6, affects the balance between tangential and radial migration and thereby causes an imbalance between excitatory and inhibitory neurons in lateral regions of the cerebral cortex in mice. Intriguingly, human patients with mutations in the Pax6 locus (called Aniridia; Pax6 is involved in the formation of eyes in all species analysed so far, from insects to mammals) exhibit cognitive defects suggesting that neurological aberrations might occur in the cerebral cortex (Heyman et al. 1999; Malandrini et al. 2001).

Heterotopia in lateral cortical regions occurs relatively frequently also in other mutant mice, and that might point to candidate genes for human patients. For example, the absence of the bHLH transcription factor Neurogenin2, which is expressed in the developing cerebral cortex, causes a leak of neurons from the cerebral cortex into the basal ganglia, a direction of migration that does not occur normally (Chapouton et al. 2001). This migrational defect results in prominent heterotopia in the lateral cortex of these mouse mutants (Fode et al. 2000). Interestingly, changes in the radial glial fascicle at the border between cortex and basal ganglia seem to be responsible for the migrational aberrations leading to heterotopia in both Ngn2- and Pax6-mutant mice (Stoykova et al. 1997; Chapouton et al. 1999; Chapouton et al. 2001). Thus, defects of radial glial cells contribute to all these different modes of migration, either as the radial guidance structure, as the cell transforming into a neuron and translocating its soma, or in their function as boundary structure delineating brain regions from each other.

Radial glial cells as precursor cells of neurons and glia

Besides the mechanical role of the radial processes as guides for migrating neurons, radial glial cells also have an active role as precursors. It has long been known that radial glia divides actively throughout development. Incorporation of DNA-base analogues such as ^{3}H-thymidine or bromo-desoxy-uridine can be used to visualize cells synthesizing DNA, i.e. cells in the S-phase of the cell cycle. Such analyses have shown that radial glial cells of primate and rodent cortex are dividing throughout development, including the phase of neurogenesis (Levitt et al. 1981; Misson et al. 1988; Hartfuss et al. 2001). Despite their proliferation during neurogenesis, radial glial cells have been viewed as glial progenitors based on their similarities to and later transformation into astrocytes. Radial glial cells dividing during neurogenesis were therefore considered to generate further radial glial cells and thereby provide a constant radial glial fibre density in the constantly increasing cortical volume during ontogeny (Misson et al. 1988). Accordingly, neurons were thought to derive from a morphologically and molecularly distinct set of precursor cells with short radial processes and lacking the astroglial characteristics (see Figure 3.1). However, the first direct analysis of the progeny of radial glial cells from rodent cerebral cortex showed that most radial glial cells generate exclusively neurons during the phase of neurogenesis (Malatesta et al. 2000). Radial glial cells become restricted to the generation of astrocytes only at later stages (from E18 in mouse cortex; Malatesta et al. 2000). This surprising neurogenic role has since been confirmed in time-lapse video microscopy of radial glial cells in slice preparations (Noctor et al. 2001) and transgenic fate-mapping analysis, demonstrating that even the majority of cortical neurons originates from radial glial cells (P. Malatesta and M. Götz, unpublished manuscript). Similar results have been obtained in the developing spinal cord (P. Malatesta and M. Götz, unpublished manuscript), implying that the neurogenic role of radial glial cells is not an exception of the cerebral cortex, but a rather general developmental feature. This implicates radial glial cells as a ubiquitous stem-cell-like progenitor in the developing CNS, responsible not only for the guidance of migrating neurons, but also for the generation and specification of most neurons in regions of high neurological relevance.

Radial glial cells form radial units in mammalian cerebral cortex

Radial glial cells not only generate neurons, but also seemingly guide their own 'daughter' cells during migration. This scenario was first proposed in 1988 by

P. Rakic and recently demonstrated in experiments in which the progeny of a single precursor cell can be followed by introduction of a genetic marker (Gray and Sanes 1992; Noctor et al. 2001). Neurons migrating along their own radial glial mother cell are supposed to form radial columns of clonally related cells in the developing cortex (Rakic 1988; Noctor et al. 2001). Thereby, clonal units might anticipate the functional organization of the adult cerebral cortex in radial columns (Rakic 1988). However, despite the migration of neurons along their clonally related radial glial mother, at least in rodent cortex there is also a considerable amount of tangential migration blurring the radial mapping (Grove et al. 1993; Reid et al. 1995; Tan et al. 1995). Indeed, this can be visualized in mouse chimera which inactivate a transgene at specific times during development (Tan et al. 1995, 1998). In these transgenics, for example, columns of blue cells that are all derived from a progenitor expressing the transgene showed a considerable degree of mixing with white cells, the progeny of precursors that inactivated the transgene. While radial units might be rather blurred in rodent cortex, however, the progeny of a single precursor cell is much more tightly radially aligned in primate cortex development (Kornack and Rakic 1995). Thus, radial units might be more frequent in primate cortex. This observation underlines again the importance of radial glial cells that generate and guide neurons. Moreover, it might be an interesting approach to consider molecular changes of radial glial cells between mammalian species in regard to the balance between radial and tangential migration. Obviously, one of the key questions is now to determine how similar or different radial glial cells are in mice and men.

Radial glial cells in mice and men — similarities and differences

The major features of radial glial cells seem to be very similar in mice and men. Radial glial cells exhibit astroglial traits such as electrolucent cytoplasm, glial filaments and glycogen granules. They appear at the onset of neurogenesis (7th–10th week fetal age; Choi and Lapham 1978; Choi 1981), they extend radial processes throughout the cortical wall until the end of neurogenesis and neuronal migration and then transform into astrocytes (17th/18th week; Choi and Lapham 1978). Moreover, a neurogenic role of human radial glial cells has been suggested by cells showing traits of radial glia and neurons observed in area 11 up to 6–9 months of age (Senitz 1994).

An obvious difference between radial glia in mice and anthropoid primates is, however, the length of the radial processes, spanning the entire cortical thickness of less than a millimetre in rodents but of several centimetres at late developmental stages in primates including humans (Sidman and Rakic 1973). This enormous length of the radial process is likely to influence cell division, since precursor cells might retract their processes preferentially in a certain mode of cell division

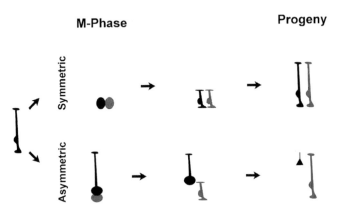

Figure 3.2   Schematic drawing of radial glial cells in two distinct modes of cell division. Note that radial glial cells seemingly do not retract their processes during an asymmetric mode of division (lower row) with a plane of division parallel to the ventricular surface (compare with Figure 3.1). For further details refer to the text.

(Figure 3.2). It is currently thought that neurons arise from an asymmetric mode of cell division, which is defined as a precursor generating two different daughter cells, namely a neuron that stops dividing and a precursor that continues to divide. Moreover, Chenn and McConnell (1995) suggested that the mode of division corresponds to the orientation of cell division with relation to the ventricular surface (Figure 3.2). Asymmetrically dividing precursors separate in a plane parallel to the ventricular surface, with the upper daughter cell losing contact with the ventricle and thereby differentiating into a neuron, while the lower daughter cell, which maintains contact with the ventricle, remains a precursor and continues to proliferate (Figure 3.2). In contrast, symmetrically dividing precursors would separate in a vertical angle to the ventricular surface and both persist as precursors. Since at least some radial glial cells transform into neurons that translocate their soma towards the brain surface, these cells obviously do not retract their radial processes. The lack of process retraction during M-phase is further consistent with immunostainings detecting the form of vimentin phosphorylated by Cdc2-kinase (Kamei et al. 1998) and recent time-lapse video microscopy of cell division in cortical slice preparations (Miyata et al. 2001; Noctor et al. 2001). The asymmetric mode of cell division might therefore be favoured in primate cortex where radial glia cells have very long processes, too long to retract during the G2-phase of the cell cycle. Since asymmetrically dividing cells generate neurons, these considerations would strengthen the suggestion that radial glial cells also generate neurons in humans.

A further consequence of the length of radial glial processes in primate cortex is the difference in their cytoskeleton composition compared with rodent radial glial cells. Radial glial cells in primate cortex contain GFAP, while rodent radial glial cells contain more flexible intermediate filament proteins such as vimentin and nestin, and start to express GFAP only at later stages when they transform into astrocytes (Levitt and Rakic 1980; Pixley and De Vellis 1984). However, as mentioned above, radial glial cells of rodent cortex express many other molecules characteristic of astroglial cells (e.g. GLAST). Only their intermediate filament composition corresponds more to immature muscle cells (Sultana et al. 2000). The reason why primate radial glia contains GFAP at earlier stages might be that it provides more stability and could be required to support the long radial extensions of primate radial glial cells. Indeed, its accumulation could even mediate a cessation of proliferation for some time (Schmechel and Rakic 1979b) by providing too much stability to the process for fast retraction during the cell cycle. Little is known so far, as to how intermediate filaments might influence proliferation during CNS development. Likewise, there is no evidence that intermediate filaments influence the progeny of precursor cells. However, from a phylogenetic point of view, a negative correlation between GFAP content and neurogenesis has been suggested (Margotta and Morelli 1997). Radial glia persist in all other vertebrates except mammals into adulthood. This persistence is correlated with the continuation of neurogenesis into adulthood in most vertebrate classes, except mammals. Thus, in most vertebrate species radial glial cells in the adult CNS are likely to contribute to neurogenesis as well as during development. Margotta and Morelli (1997) describe that the GFAP-content increases in radial glial cells of species with a lower regenerative potential, such as reptiles, while it is much lower in species with a higher regenerative potential, such as some amphibia. Other groups, however, find GFAP in radial glial cells of fish with a high neurogenetic potential (Onteniente et al. 1983). Thus, the simplest explanation of the species difference in GFAP content might be the different requirements for the stabilization of the cytoskeleton. A relation to the neurogenic potential of radial glial cells, however, can not be excluded and adverse effects of too high levels of GFAP in astrocytes are highlighted in the phenotype of patients with Alexander disease (Brenner et al. 2001).

Adult neurogenesis in mice and men — mediated by glial cells?

If radial glial cells also generate neurons in the primate cortex during development, do astrocytes also give rise to neurons in the adult? So far, the primate neocortex has been viewed as the region devoid of any neurogenesis in the adult (Rakic 1985), with neurogenesis only in the hippocampus and olfactory bulb (Eriksson et al. 1998; Kornack and Rakic 2001). However, recent evidence also demonstrates newly generated neurons in the adult primate neocortex (Gould et al. 1999). Since the precursors responsible for neurogenesis in the olfactory bulb have been identified as astrocytes in rodents (Doetsch et al. 1999) and astrocytes are in fact the only cell type capable of cell division in the adult CNS (both neurons and mature oligodendrocytes are postmitotic cell types), this is a good reason to believe that they also generate the new neurons in primates, including humans. Indeed, so far none of the differences postulated between primates and other mammals in regard to adult neurogenesis has survived direct experimental evidence (Gross 2000).

These new data suggest then that misplaced neurons discovered in schizophrenic, NMD and temporal lobe epilepsy might also arise during adulthood by defects in adult neurogenesis. Since astrocytes are involved in neurogenesis and are strongly affected in brain lesions, this cell type might be crucial in the aetiology of some of these neurological disorders. Many brain injuries, ranging from ischaemia and chemical toxins to various neurodegenerative paradigms, activate astrocytes to proliferate and to upregulate GFAP, a phenomenon classically known as gliosis. Interestingly, some of these paradigms also initiate dedifferentiation of astrocytes towards an earlier radial phenotype (Leavitt et al. 1999) and thereby might reiterate earlier neurogenic properties of these cells (Magavi et al. 2000; Malatesta et al. 2000). Moreover, brain injuries at early stages impair the transformation of radial glial cells into astrocytes (Miller and Robertson 1993; Rosen et al. 1994). These considerations would therefore suggest that astrocytes might be key to some neuronal defects in the adult CNS. These neuronal aberrations might have arisen during development when radial glial cells generate and guide neurons, or might have been caused at later stages by inappropriately activating or inhibiting neurogenesis from glial cells in the adult CNS. Indeed, cells with both neuronal and glial features found in several neurological disorders support the view that neurogenesis by astroglial cells might stop at an inappropriate point. For example, balloon neurons express neuronal and glial characteristics in cortical dysplasia and agyrophilic grain disease, a late-onset form of dementia (Tolnay and Probst 1998; Cotter et al. 1999). Moreover, glioblastoma cells also often exhibit features of neurons and glial cells (for review see Wechsler-Reya and Scott 2001), further in line with the suggestion that astrocytes in the adult brain retain not only the capacity to divide but also to differentiate at least somehow along a neuronal pathway. Interestingly, dysregulation of adult neurogenesis might also explain the features of dedifferentiation observed in brains of patients with Alzheimer's disease (Arendt 2000). Taken together, new insights into neurogenesis by radial glial cells during development and adulthood provide a new view on the potential origin of neurological aberrations in the adult human brain.

REFERENCES

Alvarez-Buylla A, Theelen M and Nottebohm F (1990). Proliferation "hot spots" in adult avian ventricular zone reveal radial cell division. *Neuron*, 5, 101–9.

Anderson SA, Eisenstat DD, Shi L and Rubenstein JLR (1997). Interneuron migration from basal forebrain to neocortex: dependence on *Dlx* genes. *Science*, 278, 474–6.

Arendt T (2000). Alzheimer's disease as a loss of differentiation control in a subset of neurons that retain immature features in the adult brain. *Neurobiol Aging*, 21, 783–96.

Bentivoglio M and Mazzarello P (1999). The history of radial glia. *Brain Res Bull*, 49, 305–15.

Book KJ and Morest DK (1990). Migration of neuroblasts by perikaryal translocation: role of cellular elongation and axonal outgrowth in the acoustic nuclei of the chick embryo medulla. *J Comp Neurol*, 297, 55–76.

Brenner M, Johnson AB, Boespflug-Tanguy O, Rodriguez D, Goldman JE and Messing A (2001). Mutations in *GFAP*, encoding glial fibrillary acidic protein, are associated with Alexander disease. *Nat Genet*, 27, 117–19.

Brittis PA, Meiri K, Dent E and Silver J (1995). The earliest patterns of neuronal differentiation and migration in the mammalian central nervous system. *Exp Neurol*, 134, 1–12.

Carić D, Gooday D, Hill RE et al. (1997). Determination of the migratory capacity of embryonic cortical cells lacking the transcription factor Pax-6. *Development*, 124, 5087–96.

Chapouton P, Gärtner A and Götz M (1999). The role of Pax6 in restricting cell migration between developing cortex and basal ganglia. *Development*, 126, 5569–79.

Chapouton P, Schuurmans C, Guillemot F and Götz M (2001). The transcription factor neurogenin2 restricts cell migration from the cortex to the striatum. *Development*, 128, 5149–59.

Chenn A and McConnell SK (1995). Cleavage orientation and the asymmetric inheritance of Notch1 immunoreactivity in mammalian neurogenesis. *Cell*, 82, 631–41.

Choi BH (1981). Radial glia of developing human fetal spinal cord: Golgi, immunohistochemical and electron microscopic study. *Brain Res*, 227, 249–67.

Choi BH and Lapham LW (1978). Radial glia in the human fetal cerebrum: a combined Golgi, immunofluorescent and electron microscopic study. *Brain Res*, 148, 295–311.

Clark GD (2001). Cerebral gyral dysplasias: molecular genetics and cell biology. *Curr Opin Neurol*, 14, 157–62.

Copp AJ and Harding BN (1999). Neuronal migration disorders in humans and in mouse models – an overview. *Epilepsy Res*, 36, 133–41.

Cotter DR, Honavar M and Everall I (1999). Focal cortical dysplasia: a neuropathological and developmental perspective. *Epilepsy Res*, 36, 155–64.

Doetsch F, Caille I, Lim DA et al. (1999). Subventricular zone astrocytes are neural stem cells in the adult mammalian brain. *Cell*, 97, 703–16.

Eng LF, Ghirnikar RS and Lee YL (2000). Glial fibrillary acidic protein: GFAP – thirty-one years (1969–2000). *Neurochem Res*, 25, 1439–51.

Eriksson PS, Perfilieva E, Björk-Eriksson T et al. (1998). Neurogenesis in the adult human hippocampus. *Nat Med*, 4, 1313–17.

Feng L, Hatten ME and Heintz N (1994). Brain lipid-binding protein (BLBP): a novel signaling system in the developing mammalian CNS. *Neuron*, 12, 895–908.

Fode C, Ma Q, Casarosa S et al. (2000). A role for neural determination genes in specifying the dorsoventral identity of telencephalic neurons. *Genes Dev*, 14, 67–80.

Götz M (1999). Cerebral cortex development. In *Encyclopedia of Life Sciences*. London: Nature Publishing Group.

Götz M, Stoykova A and Gruss P (1998). Pax6 controls radial glia differentiation in the cerebral cortex. *Neuron*, 21, 1031–44.

Gould E, Reeves AJ, Graziano MSA and Gross CG (1999). Neurogenesis in the neocortex of adult primates. *Science*, 286, 548–52.

Gray GE and Sanes JR (1992). Lineage of radial glia in the chicken optic tectum. *Development*, 114, 271–83.

Gross CG (2000). Neurogenesis in the adult brain: death of a dogma. *Nat Rev Neurosci*, 1, 67–73.

Grove EA, Williams BP, Li DQ, Hajihosseini M, Friedrich A and Price J (1993). Multiple restricted lineages in the embryonic rat cerebral cortex. *Development*, 17, 553–61.

Hartfuss E, Galli R, Heins N and Götz M (2001). Characterization of CNS precursor subtypes and radial glia. *Dev Biol*, 229, 15–30.

Hatten ME (1999). Central nervous system neuronal migration. *Ann Rev Neurosci*, 22, 511–39.

Heffron DS and Golden JA (2000). DM-GRASP is necessary for nonradial cell migration during chick diencephalic development. *J Neurosci*, 20, 2287–94.

Heyman I, Frampton I, Van Heyningen V et al. (1999). Psychiatric disorder and cognitive function in a family with an inherited novel mutation of the developmental control gene PAX6. *Psychiatr Genet*, 9, 85–90.

Hollister JM and Cannon TD (1998). Neurodevelopmental disturbances in the aetiology of schizophrenia. In *Disorders of Brain and Mind*, ed. MA Ron and AS David, pp. 280–302. Cambridge: Cambridge University Press.

Jakob H and Beckmann H (1994). Circumscribed malformation and nerve cell alterations in the entorhinal cortex of schiziphrenics. *J Neural Transm*, 98, 83–106.

Kamei Y, Inagaki N, Nishizawa M et al. (1998). Visualization of mitotic radial glial lineage cells in the developing rat brain by Cdc2 kinase-phosphorylated vimentin. *Glia*, 23, 191–9.

Kornack DR (2000). Neurogenesis and the evolution of cortical diversity: mode, tempo, and partitioning during development and persistence into adulthood. *Brain Behav Evol*, 55, 336–44.

Kornack DR and Rakic P (1995). Radial and horizontal deployment of clonally related cells in the primate neocortex: relationship to distinct mitotic lineages. *Neuron*, 15, 311–21.

Kornack DR and Rakic P (2001). The generation, migration, and differentiation of olfactory neurons in the adult primate brain. *Proc Natl Acad Sci USA*, 98, 4752–7.

Kuhn HG, Dickinson-Anson H and Gage FH (1996). Neurogenesis in the dentate gyrus of the adult rat: age-related decrease of neuronal progenitor proliferation. *J Neurosci*, 16, 2027–33.

Lammens M (2000). Neuronal migration disorders in man. *Eur J Morphol*, 38, 327–33.

Leavitt BR, Hernit-Grant CS and Macklis JD (1999). Mature astrocytes transform into transitional radial glia within adult mouse neocortex that supports directed migration of transplanted immature neurons. *Exp Neurol*, 157, 43–57.

Letinic K and Rakic P (2001). Telencephalic origin of human thalamic GABAergic neurons. *Nat Neurosci*, 4, 931–6.

Levitt P and Rakic P (1980). Immunoperoxidase localization of glial fibrillary acidic protein in radial glial cells and astrocytes of the developing rhesus monkey brain. *J Comp Neurol*, 193, 815–40.

Levitt P, Cooper ML and Rakic P (1981). Early divergence and changing proportions of neuronal and glial precursor cells in the primate cerebral ventricular zone. *Dev Biol*, 96, 472–84.

Lumsden A and Krumlauf R (1996). Patterning the vertebrate neuraxis. *Science*, 274, 1109–14.

Magavi SS, Leavitt BR and Macklis JD (2000). Induction of neurogenesis in the neocortex of adult mice. *Nature*, 405, 951–5.

Malandrini A, Mari F, Palmeri S et al. (2001). PAX6 mutation in a family with aniridia, congenital ptosis, and mental retardation. *Clin Genet*, 60, 151–4.

Malatesta P, Hartfuss E and Götz M (2000). Isolation of radial glial cells by fluorescent-activated cell sorting reveals a neuronal lineage. *Development*, 127, 5253–63.

Marcus RC, Delaney CL and Easter SSJ (1999). Neurogenesis in the visual system of embryonic and adult zebrafish (*Danio rerio*). *Vis Neurosci*, 16, 417–24.

Margotta V and Morelli A (1996). Encephalic matrix areas and post-natal neurogenesis under natural and experimental conditions. *Animal Biol*, 5, 117–31.

Margotta V and Morelli A (1997). Contribution of radial glial cells to neurogenesis and plasticity of central nervous system in adult vertebrates. *Animal Biol*, 6, 101–8.

Meiri KF, Saffell JL, Walsh FS and Doherty P (1998). Neurite outgrowth stimulated by neural cell adhesion molecules requires growth-associated protein-43 (GAP-43) function and is associated with GAP-43 phosphorylation in growth cones. *J Neurosci*, 18, 10429–37.

Miller MW and Robertson S (1993). Prenatal exposure to ethanol alters the postnatal development and transformation of radial glia to astrocytes in the cortex. *J Comp Neurol*, 337, 253–66.

Mione MC, Cavanagh JF, Harris B and Parnavelas JG (1997). Cell fate specification and symmetrical/asymmetrical divisions in the developing cerebral cortex. *J Neurosci*, 17, 2018–29.

Misson JP, Edwards MA, Yamamoto M and Caviness VSJ (1988). Mitotic cycling of radial glial cells of the fetal murine cerebral wall: a combined autoradiographic and immunohisto-chemical study. *Dev Brain Res*, 38, 183–190.

Miyata T, Kawaguchi A, Okano H and Ogawa M (2001). Asymmetric inheritance of radial glial fibers by cortical neurons. *Neuron*, 31, 727–41.

Morest DK (1970). A study of neurogenesis in the forebrain of the opposum pouch young. *Z Anat Entwicklungsgeschichte*, 130, 265–305.

Nadarajah B, Brunstrom JE, Grutzendler J et al. (2001). Two modes of radial migration in early development of the cerebral cortex. *Nat Neurosci*, 4, 143–50.

Noctor SC, Flint AC, Weissman TA et al. (2001). Neurons derived from radial glial cells establish radial units in neocortex. *Nature*, 409, 714–20.

Onteniente B, Kimura H and Maeda T (1983). Comparative study of the glial fibrillary acidic protein in vertebrates by PAP immunohistochemistry. *J Comp Neurol*, 215, 427–36.

Pixley SKR and De Vellis J (1984). Transition between immature radial glia and mature astrocytes studied with a monoclonal antibody to vimentin. *Dev Brain Res*, 15, 201–9.

Pleasure SJ, Anderson J, Hevner R et al. (2000). Cell migration from the ganglionic eminences is required for the development of hippocampal GABAergic interneurons. *Neuron*, 28, 727–40.

Rakic P (1972). Mode of cell migration to the superficial layers of fetal monkey neocortex. *J Comp Neurol*, 145, 61–83.

Rakic P (1985). Limits of neurogenesis in primates. *Science*, 227, 1054–6.

Rakic P (1988). Specification of cerebral cortical areas. *Science*, 241, 170–6.

Rakic P and Sidman RL (1969). Telencephalic origin of pulvinar neurons in the fetal human brain. *Z Anat Entwicklungsgeschichte*, 129, 53–82.

Reid CB, Liang I and Walsh C (1995). Systematic widespread clonal organization in cerebral cortex. *Neuron*, 15, 299–310.

Roberts GW, Royston MC and Götz M (1995). Pathology of cortical development and neuropsychiatric disorders. In *Development of the Cerebral Cortex*, Ciba Foundation Symposium 193, ed. GR Bock and G Cardew, pp. 296–316. Chichester: John Wiley and Sons.

Rosen GD, Sherman GF and Galaburda AM (1994). Radial glia in the neocortex of adult rats: effects of neonatal brain injury. *Dev Brain Res*, 82, 127–35.

Schmahl W, Knoedlseder M, Favor J and Davidson D (1993). Defects of neuronal migration and the pathogenesis of cortical malformations are associated with Small eye (Sey) in the mouse, a point mutation at the Pax-6-locus. *Acta Neuropathol*, 86, 126–35.

Schmechel DE and Rakic P (1979a). A Golgi study of radial glial cells in developing monkey telencephalon: morphogenesis and transformation into astrocytes. *Anat Embryol*, 156, 115–52.

Schmechel DE and Rakic P (1979b). Arrested proliferation of radial glial cells during midgestation in rhesus monkey. *Nature*, 277, 303–5.

Senitz D (1984). Neuronale strukturveränderungen im neocortex bei schizophrener psychose. In *Neurobiologische Aspekte in der Psychiatrie*, ed. GE Kühne, H Klepel and J Molcan, pp. 374–6. Bratislava: VEDA-Verlag der Slovakischen Akademie der Wissenschaften.

Senitz D (1994). Unusual morphological alterations of the radial glia cells in the human neocortex. *J Brain Res*, 35, 130–1.

Shibata T, Yamada K, Watanabe M et al. (1997). Glutamate transporter GLAST is expressed in the radial glia-astrocyte lineage of developing mouse spinal cord. *J Neurosci*, 17, 9212–19.

Sidman RL and Rakic P (1973). Neuronal migration, with special reference to developing human brain: A review. *Brain Res*, 62, 1–35.

Stoykova A, Götz M, Gruss P and Price J (1997). Pax6-dependent regulation of adhesive patterning, R-cadherin expression and boundary formation in developing forebrain. *Development*, 124, 3765–77.

Sultana S, Sernett SW, Bellin RM, Robson RM and Skalli O (2000). Intermediate filament protein synemin is transiently expressed in a subset of astrocytes during development. *Glia*, 30, 143–53.

Tan S-S, Faulkner-Jones BE, Breen SJ et al. (1995). Cell dispersion patterns in different cortical regions studied with an X-inactivated transgenic marker. *Development*, 121, 1029–39.

Tan S-S, Kalloniatis M, Sturm K et al. (1998). Separate progenitors for radial and tangential cell dispersion during development of the cerebral neocortex. *Neuron*, 21, 295–304.

Taylor E (1998). Early disorders and later schizophrenia: a developmental neuropsychiatric perspective. In *Disorders of Brain and Mind*, ed. MA Ron and AS David, pp. 255–79. Cambridge: Cambridge University Press.

Tolnay M and Probst A (1998). Ballooned neurons expressing αB-crystallin as a constant feature of the amygdala in agyrophilic brain disease. *Neurosci Lett*, 246, 165–8.

Voigt T (1989). Development of glial cells in the cerebral wall of ferrets: direct tracing of their transformation from radial glia into astrocytes. *J Comp Neurol*, 289, 74–88.

Walsh CA (1999). Genetic malformations of the human cerebral cortex. *Neuron*, 23, 19–29.

Wechsler-Reya R and Scott MP (2001). The developmental biology of brain tumors. *Annu Rev Neurosci*, 24, 385-428.

Zupanc GKH and Ott R (1999). Cell proliferation after lesions in the cerebellum of adult teleost fish: time course, origin, and type of new cells produced. *Exp Neurol*, 160, 78–87.

4

Brain development: the clinical perspective

Clare Beasley, Brenda Williams and Ian Everall

Institute of Psychiatry, De Crespigny Park, London, UK

Introduction

While the development of the brain may not at first glance appear to be relevant to psychosis, it is now widely acknowledged that schizophrenia may result from an abnormality of brain development. Although taken individually much of the evidence in support of this theory does not represent conclusive proof, an intriguing picture is emerging from a variety of approaches, including epidemiological and brain-imaging studies (reviewed by Murray and Woodruff 1995; Raedler et al. 1998). These, along with postmortem histological studies, have led to the 'neurodevelopmental hypothesis' of schizophrenia, which suggests that a brain abnormality is present early in life but does not fully manifest itself until late adolescence or early adulthood, perhaps following functional maturation (Weinberger 1987; Waddington 1993). However, the causes and timing of any such abnormality remain to be determined. The familial nature of schizophrenia implies that an interaction between genetic and environmental factors is likely, while the vulnerability period may extend from pregnancy to early adolescence.

There is less evidence to suggest that bipolar disorder may have a developmental aetiology. While studies of bipolar disorder are limited in number, in part due to diagnostic considerations, some shared epidemiological risk factors along with gross and microscopic pathologies have been identified (Torrey 1999). However, there are also important differences between the disorders. In this chapter evidence for a neurodevelopmental origin of both schizophrenia and bipolar disorder will be presented, along with possible implications for the timing and causes of these disorders.

Evidence for a neurodevelopmental origin of schizophrenia and bipolar disorder

Evidence from epidemiological studies

A number of observations have led to suggestions that events occurring either during gestation or early postnatally may contribute to the aetiology of schizophrenia and also possibly bipolar disorder. For example, it has been reported that patients with these disorders are more likely to have experienced obstetric complications in utero or during delivery. Increased reports of brain insult during pregnancy and delivery in psychiatric patients were first noted many decades ago. However, controversy continues regarding the association between obstetric complications and the risk of schizophrenia. While there have been reports confirming the presence of an excess of obstetric complications in the histories of patients with both schizophrenia and bipolar disorder (Lewis and Murray 1987; McNeil 1991), recent studies have failed to provide convincing evidence (Byrne et al. 2000; Crow and Waddington 2000; Kendell et al. 2000). In schizophrenia it has been suggested that a history of obstetric complications may be associated with an earlier onset and more chronic form of illness, poor treatment response and structural brain changes (Lewis 1989; Verdoux et al. 1997; McNeil et al. 2000*b*). However, it is difficult to distinguish if complications, such as perinatal hypoxia, are a cause of the problem, or if they are themselves sequelae of earlier events. One possibility is that perinatal difficulties could be secondary to an earlier event, for example viral infection during pregnancy. Mednick and colleagues (1988) have demonstrated an increased incidence of schizophrenia in the offspring of women who were in the second trimester of pregnancy during the 1957 influenza epidemic, suggesting that exposure to the influenza virus during this critical period may significantly increase the risk for schizophrenia in later life. However, this finding too is probably not specific to schizophrenia; recent reports suggest that prenatal exposure to viral infections may predispose to affective disorders (Machon et al. 1997).

Minor physical anomalies, such as high palates and low-set ears, are themselves considered to be indicators of in utero developmental abnormalities, and are reported to be more common in schizophrenia, although not in bipolar disorder, than in the general population (Green et al. 1994; McNeil et al. 2000*a*). These anomalies tend to be more common in males and are associated with a family history of the disorder. Furthermore, there is evidence that children who later develop schizophrenia have delayed motor milestones, poorer social development and poorer educational achievement (Jones et al. 1994) than the general population. This may or may not be true of children who go on to develop bipolar disorder (Crow et al. 1995; Gilvarry et al. 2000).

Evidence from structural imaging studies

In 1976 Johnstone et al. carried out the first computed tomography (CT) study in patients with chronic schizophrenia, reporting a significant increase in ventricular size. Over the following decade a substantial number of studies were undertaken which generally confirmed a small but significant increase in the volume of the lateral and third ventricles in this disorder (Raz and Raz 1990; Lewis 1991). Furthermore there are suggestions that brain size may be reduced in schizophrenia, in particular the volume of the frontal and temporal lobes (Andreasen et al. 1994; Bryant et al. 1999). Other studies have found significant reductions in cortical grey matter volume, again with the dorsolateral prefrontal cortex and superior temporal areas particularly affected (Sullivan et al. 1998; Zipursky et al. 1998).

While some of the structural brain abnormalities seen in schizophrenia have also been described in mood disorders (reviewed by Drevets 2001), it has been suggested that the magnitude and location of the pathology may be different. Ventricular enlargement has been described in some studies of bipolar disorder, although less than that observed in schizophrenia (Nasrallah et al. 1989; Raz and Raz 1990). Contrary to the reductions in brain size observed in schizophrenia, similar measurements in bipolar disorder have generally failed to find any reduction (Hoge et al. 1999), although deficits in cerebellar volume have been noted (Soares and Mann 1997). There are also indications that cortical grey matter volume is unchanged (Zipursky et al. 1997). The most consistent imaging finding in bipolar disorder is an increase in white matter hyperintensities (Altshuler et al. 1995). However, this finding is not specific to bipolar disorder and is observed in a number of other conditions including HIV, fuelling suggestions that hyperintensities may arise from environmental factors (McArthur et al. 1990).

Ventricular enlargement and reductions in brain volume are not specific to psychosis; indeed they are known to occur in neurodegenerative disorders such as Alzheimer's disease, so how do they provide evidence for a developmental origin? Basically, imaging studies of schizophrenics have shown that ventricular enlargement and reductions in brain volume are present at the onset of symptoms and do not progress throughout the course of the illness (DeLisi et al. 1991; Gur et al. 1998; Zipursky et al. 1998). Similarly, in bipolar disorder, one follow-up study has indicated an absence of progressive ventricular enlargement (Woods et al. 1990). This has led to suggestions that these structural brain changes are static, this being suggestive of a developmental, rather than a degenerative, origin (Lewis 1989). However, recent research has shown that some progressive worsening of structural brain changes may occur in specific patients, particularly those with childhood onset (Rapoport et al. 1997, 1999).

Evidence from postmortem findings

Despite over a century of research, the histopathology of schizophrenia has yet to be elucidated. While an early report described cytoarchitectural alterations in the cerebral cortex of patients with dementia praecox (Alzheimer 1897), by the 1970s it was widely considered that such pathological abnormalities were not present in schizophrenia. However, recent pathological investigations, particularly those using quantitative image-analysis techniques, are beginning to identify cytoarchitectural abnormalities, particularly in the frontal and temporal lobes (reviewed by Harrison 1999). Unfortunately, many of these findings have not been replicated consistently. Until recent years pathological studies of mood disorders have attracted less interest. In this volume Harrison and Gittins (see Chapter 14) present a review of postmortem studies of bipolar disorder and major depression undertaken over the last decade. Ultimately, the pathology of both schizophrenia and bipolar disorder is considered subtle and nonspecific. Furthermore, these findings are diverse and it is difficult to establish which (if any) constitute the primary pathology. However, continuing neuropathological studies will help to elucidate the pathology of these disorders and may give us clues about their aetiology.

Studies of glial cells in schizophrenia and bipolar disorder are relatively consistent. The epidemiological and imaging evidence described above has led to suggestions that schizophrenia and bipolar disorder result from abnormal brain development, occurring early in life, possibly prenatally and certainly before the onset of symptoms, and remaining stable throughout the course of the disease. If this were true it has been reasoned that postmortem studies would find no evidence of gliosis. Basically, any progressive process resulting in degenerative pathology, including inflammation, ischaemia, infection and classical neurodegeneration is widely considered to result in reactive gliosis. An absence of gliosis in the brain in schizophrenia and bipolar disorder would therefore be consistent with a developmental rather than an ongoing degenerative process. A number of studies have looked for evidence of reactive gliosis, or more specifically proliferation, activation and hypertrophy of astrocytes. This has typically been examined either using traditional histological stains, or by immunocytochemistry for the astrocytic marker GFAP. While one early report by Stevens (1982) described an increase in astrocytes in periventricular regions in schizophrenics compared with controls, virtually all other studies have found no evidence of reactive gliosis in schizophrenia (Falkai et al. 1999). The density of cortical glial cells has also been quantified using Nissl staining, and reductions in glial cell density reported in both schizophrenia and bipolar disorder (Ongur et al. 1998; Cotter et al. 2001; Rajkowska et al. 2001). Furthermore, there is also little evidence for the presence of neuritic plaques or neurofibrillary tangles, the hallmark pathology of Alzheimer's disease, in schizophrenia (Niizato et al. 1998).

Studies quantifying neuronal density are less conclusive. Reductions in neuronal density have been described in specific layers of the prefrontal cortex in both schizophrenia and bipolar disorder (Benes et al. 1986, 1991; Rajkowska et al. 2001); other groups have meanwhile reported that both neuronal density and the total number of neurons are unaltered (Pakkenberg 1993; Akbarian et al. 1995; Cotter et al. 2001). Further studies have described an elevation in neuronal density in this region. Selemon et al. (1995, 1998) found an increase in the density of neurons in layers III–VI in schizophrenia that was not specific to the prefrontal cortex, also being observed in the occipital cortex. Looking at specific populations of neurons the opposite may be true. A loss of presumptive interneurons in more superficial cortical layers has been noted in both schizophrenia and bipolar disorder (Benes et al. 1991, 2001) and a reduction in the density of interneurons expressing both specific calcium-binding proteins (Beasley and Reynolds 1997) and mRNA for glutamic acid decarboxylase (Akbarian et al. 1995; Volk et al. 2000) have been described in prefrontal regions in schizophrenia. There are also suggestions of neuronal loss in the thalamus in schizophrenia (Pakkenberg 1990; Young et al. 2000), which need further investigation. Cytoarchitectural studies in the cortex have described heterotopias, abnormalities in the position of neurons, in a variety of brain regions in schizophrenia. These include alterations in the position and orientation of neurons in the entorhinal cortex, hippocampus and subcortical white matter.

While most morphometric analyses of the cortex have failed to reveal any significant reductions in total neuronal number in schizophrenics compared with controls, there are indications that the cortex is thinner (Pakkenberg 1987; Gur et al. 1999). This evidence for reductions in cortical volume without cell loss has led to suggestions of a reduction in interneuronal neuropil (Selemon et al. 1995). The neuropil is comprised largely of axonal and dendritic processes; any reduction in this component would be expected to result in abnormal cortical circuitry. Studies have indeed found a loss of specific axons and a reduction in synaptic proteins in a number of brain regions in schizophrenia and bipolar disorder. Each of these findings provides further corroboration for the developmental hypothesis and will be discussed in more detail.

Brain development may provide clues for the cause and timing of the pathology of schizophrenia and bipolar disorder

While the development of the brain has been studied for many years, until recently relatively little was known about the molecular and biochemical signals that control processes such as pattern formation, proliferation and neuronal migration during normal cerebral cortical development. These signals are obviously influenced by a large number of developmental genes, and may conceivably be the site of interactions between genetic and environmental factors that predispose to schizophrenia and bipolar disorder. Knowledge of how the brain develops will help interpret information gained from postmortem and other studies with regard to timing and cause of any brain abnormalities. This chapter is not intended to be a comprehensive review of brain development, but aims to discuss specific aspects, in particular embryonic patterning, proliferation, neuronal migration, synaptogenesis and programmed cell death, with respect to how these processes might relate to postmortem findings in schizophrenia and bipolar disorder. Insights into current theories of neurogenesis and neuronal migration are presented in Chapter 3 by Götz.

Embryonic patterning

One of the earliest events in brain development is the specification of cells within the neural tube. Studies originally done on *Drosophila* have indicated that dorsal–ventral patterning depends on a series of genes that encode the homeobox (hox) family of transcription factors (Lumsden and Krumlauf 1996). While abnormalities of the homeobox system would lead to more severe changes than seen in schizophrenia, this does not rule out effects of other similar, but less well characterized, gene families. Such families are expressed later during development than hox genes and may be important in defining specific brain regions. While there are too many to mention here, the Otx and Emx genes, which play an important role in forebrain patterning (Ang et al. 1996), the Pax-6 and Dlx genes, which appear to define the boundary between the cortex and the corpus striatum (Porteus et al. 1994), and members of the POU family of transcription factors, such as Oct-6, may be of interest. Mutations in Pax-6 are known to cause aniridia in humans (Jordan et al. 1992), while mutations in Emx-2 lead to severe schizencephaly (Brunelli et al. 1996); thus these specific genes are unlikely to be involved in the aetiology of schizophrenia. However, there are indications that Oct-6 may be involved; preliminary studies have indicated that Oct-6 protein levels are increased in the cortex and hippocampus in schizophrenia (Ilia et al. 2002).

A further family of genes of interest in schizophrenia is the Wnt family. Wnt genes encode a family of secreted glycoproteins that play a vital role as intracellular signalling molecules both during early neural development and also in the mature nervous system. Wnt proteins have established roles in a number of diverse processes including embryonic patterning and the regulation of cell polarity and fate determination (reviewed by Brown and Moon 1998). There are indications that Wnt signalling may be affected in schizophrenia. Previous studies have noted that GSK-3β levels are reduced in the prefrontal cortex in schizophrenia (Kozlovsky et al. 2000), a finding that we have independently replicated (Beasley et al. 2001*b*). Other studies have shown that levels of GSK-3α are reduced in lymphocytes (Yang et al. 1994), while Wnt-1 is increased (Miyaoka et al. 1999) and β-catenin is reduced (Cotter et al. 1998) in the hippocampus in schizophrenia. Furthermore, we have previously demonstrated abnormalities of this pathway in focal cortical dysplasia, a neurodevelopmental brain disorder which presents with intractable epilepsy (Cotter et al. 1999). While the Wnt signalling pathway does not appear to be abnormal in bipolar disorder (Kozlovsky et al. 2000; Beasley et al. 2001*a*), defective signal transduction has been implicated in this disorder (Manji and Lenox 2000).

Changes in levels of Oct-6 and Wnt proteins may indicate faulty development, which could possibly be genetically determined. However, it has been suggested that these proteins may also have roles in the adult brain; for example, Wnt proteins may be involved in synaptic modulation and plasticity (Lucas and Salinas 1997);

these functions also need to be taken into account when interpreting such neuro-pathological findings.

Proliferation and differentiation

Another early event in development is a large increase in cell number inside the neural tube. The regulation of cell proliferation and differentiation is thought to depend on extracellular signals including growth factors and cytokines. A number of recent studies have suggested that abnormalities in the expression of specific neurotrophic factor are present in schizophrenia (reviewed by Nawa et al. 2000). These include increased levels of brain-derived neurotrophic factor (BDNF) and decreased levels of its receptor trkB in the hippocampus (Takahashi et al. 2000). Furthermore, levels of a number of the molecules regulated by BDNF, including reelin, synaptophysin and calbindin, have also been found to be abnormal in schizophrenia. Further studies have shown that levels of specific cytokines are also altered (Prolo and Licinio 1999). Abnormal levels of neurotrophic factors and cytokines may reflect aberrant proliferation and differentiation of neurons during development; relatively subtle changes in these processes may result in alterations in specific neuronal and glial cell populations. However, the action of cytokines and neurotrophic factors are also not limited to brain development and these factors are thought to be able to influence synaptic transmission and plasticity in the adult brain.

Migration

Following proliferation and fate determination the cell must migrate to its final position. Cortical lamination begins with the formation of the primordial plexiform layer (Marin-Padilla 1983). Following this stage neuronal precursors migrate from the periventricular origin towards the pial surface, guided by radial glial fibres, and accumulate to form the cortical plate. This structure divides the primordial plexiform layer into two parts, the most superficial being the presumptive cortical layer I, and the deepest part being the subplate layer.

The main types of cells in layer I are the Cajal–Retzius cells (CRCs), which are one of the earliest neuronal populations in the developing cortex. During cortico-genesis CRCs establish synaptic contacts with all migrating neuroblasts arriving at the cortical plate and play a vital role in the 'inside out' formation of the cortical layers. During later gestation CRC numbers reduce rapidly and in adulthood very few remain (Marin-Padilla 1998). Speculation exists as to what happens to CRCs but it is thought that they may change into other cell types or alternatively undergo programmed cell death. In a preliminary study Kalus et al. (1997) showed that schizophrenics display altered localization and type distribution of CRCs. Further studies have shown that protein and mRNA levels of reelin, a secreted glycoprotein which plays a vital role in normal cortical lamination and which is expressed preferentially by CRCs in layer I, are reduced in the prefrontal cortex, temporal cortex and hippocampus in both schizophrenia and bipolar disorder (Impagnatiello et al. 1998; Guidotti et al. 2000). Successful neuronal migration during development is also thought to depend on correct expression of a series of trophic factors and guidance molecules. One such family are the neural cell adhesion molecules (NCAMs), which are important during migration and also possibly in plasticity in the adult. It has been shown that the number of neurons expressing one specific form of NCAM are reduced in the hippocampus in schizophrenia (Barbeau et al. 1995).

The subplate forms below the cortical plate and consists of early-maturing neurons that also play a vital role in the orderly development of the overlying cortex as well as regulating the guidance of thalamocortical afferents (Kostovic and Rakic 1980; Allendoerfer and Shatz 1994). There is also evidence that the subplate may be involved in the gyrification of the cortex (Armstrong et al. 1995). In the late prenatal and early postnatal period the majority of subplate neurons die, leaving the interstitial neurons of the adult white matter (Chun and Shatz 1989; Ghosh and Shatz 1992). Further evidence for abnormal brain development in schizophrenia has been provided by Akbarian et al. (1993*a*, *b*, 1996), who described an altered distribution of interstitial cells in frontal and temporal subcortical white matter in schizophrenia. These studies reported a reduction in the density of white matter neurons in the superficial white matter, but an increased density in deeper white matter. These data were taken as an indication of aberrant neuronal migration or an abnormality of programmed cell death in schizophrenia. However, Anderson et al. (1996) essentially failed to replicate these results, finding an increased density of MAP-2 immunoreactive neurons only in the superficial white matter in schizophrenia, while recent studies of our own have indicated that the distribution of white matter neurons is not altered in the frontal lobe either in schizophrenia or in bipolar disorder (Beasley, Cotter and Everall, unpublished manuscript).

Abnormalities of the subplate and cortical layer I may result in the faulty migration of other, later-maturing neurons. Cytoarchitectural studies have described alterations in the position and orientation of neurons in a variety of brain regions in schizophrenia. In a widely cited study Kovelman and Scheibel (1984) reported a change in the orientation of pyramidal cells in the hippocampus in schizophrenia. This 'neuronal disarray' was present at the boundaries of CA1 with CA2 and with the subiculum. This study was crucial as it was the first to lead to the suggestion that abnormal early brain development occurs in schizophrenia. However, the findings of this original study have yet to be replicated. While a number of groups have also reported increased variability in the orientation of pyramidal neurons in other hippocampal regions (Conrad et al. 1991; Zaidel et al. 1997), further groups have found no evidence of hippocampal neuronal disarray (Christison et al. 1989; Cotter et al. 1997). An abnormal appearance of the pre-alpha cell clusters of the rostral entorhinal cortex has also been described in schizophrenia (Jakob and Beckmann 1986). While methodological flaws mean that this original study has been widely criticized, some further investigations of this region do support the finding. Falkai et al. (2000) have also described abnormalities in the position and size of pre-alpha cell clusters in the entorhinal cortex in schizophrenia, while Arnold and colleagues (1991, 1997) have twice reported alterations in cytoarchitecture in this region, the latter study using spatial pattern analysis. However, a number of other groups have failed to find any cytoarchitectural abnormalities in the entorhinal cortex in schizophrenia (Akil and Lewis 1997; Krimer et al. 1997; Bernstein et al. 1998). Comparable studies are extremely limited in bipolar disorder and are accordingly difficult to interpret. However, similar abnormalities in the position and size of entorhinal pre-alpha cell clusters have been noted in one small series of cases (Beckmann and Jakob 1991), which awaits replication.

While these early studies do indeed support a failure of migration, a process that occurs mainly during the second trimester, this may not be the whole story. It is documented that failures of neuronal migration do not typically lead to schizophrenia, but rather to severe heterotopias and dysplasias, which commonly result in mental retardation or epilepsy (Walsh 1999). However, this does not rule out more subtle abnormalities, possibly due to changes in pattern formation or differentiation or even abnormalities of programmed cell death, which could result in similar patterns of cytoarchitectural abnormalities to those noted in schizophrenia.

Formation of axonal connections and synaptogenesis

Once a neuron has reached its appropriate location it must establish axonal connections with other neurons. Recent biochemical, molecular and genetic studies have found a large number of specific axonal guidance molecules and receptors, such as the cell adhesion molecule limbic-associated membrane protein (LAMP) and growth-associated protein GAP-43, that are important in this process. Disruption of any of these may lead to the formation of abnormal cortical connections. Synaptogenesis begins during late gestation and continues to increase rapidly during the early postnatal period. At this stage of development the formation of connections is not specific. This is followed by a steady pruning of connections that is complete soon after birth in sensory areas such as the occipital cortex, but not until adolescence in association regions such as the prefrontal cortex (Huttenlocher 1979). This process is in part genetically modulated, although elimination of specific synapses may too have an environmental component.

The reduced-neuropil hypothesis (Selemon et al. 1995) suggests that cortical axonal and dendritic processes are reduced in schizophrenia, although which specific component is unknown. One candidate is local circuit connections; reductions in the density of chandelier cell axonal terminals, as identified using an antibody directed against the GABA membrane transporter GAT-1 have been observed in the prefrontal cortex in schizophrenia (Woo et al. 1998). There are also suggestions that thalamocortical inputs may be involved (Pierri et al. 1999). Cortico-cortical connections may also be diminished; a reduction in somal size, particularly of large cortical pyramidal cells, has been observed in schizophrenia and bipolar disorder (Rajkowska et al. 1998, 2001; Pierri et al. 2001). As somal size has been shown to correlate with the number, length and diameter of a cell's processes, as well as the number of synapses it receives (Jones and Cowan 1983), this could indicate faulty cortical connectivity.

Alongside reductions in axons, there is also evidence for a loss of synapses. Morphometric studies have indicated a reduction in the number of dendritic spines on pyramidal cells in the frontal and temporal cortex in schizophrenia (Garey et al. 1998), while levels of synaptic proteins such as synaptophysin, synapsin and SNAP-25 are reduced in the majority of studies, again mainly in the frontal and temporal lobes (Browning et al. 1993; Glantz and Lewis 1997; Young et al. 1998). As there is little evidence for increased neuronal density and decreased cortical width in bipolar disorder, a reduction in neuropil has not been hypothesized in this disorder. However, there is also evidence for reductions in synapse proteins in bipolar disorder, albeit restricted to a very small number of studies, including reductions in levels of complexins (Eastwood and Harrison 2000).

It was first suggested by Feinberg (1982) that aberrant pruning during adolescence could play a role in the aetiology of schizophrenia. More recently McGlashan and Hoffman (2000) have proposed the theory of 'developmentally reduced synaptic connectivity', suggesting that schizophrenia could arise from disturbances of synaptogenesis either during gestation or early postnatally or from abnormal synaptic pruning in adolescence. While abnormal synaptic pruning during adolescence could go some way to explaining why psychotic symptoms are typically not apparent until early adulthood, how this might be manifested is not understood.

Hemispheric laterality

The human brain develops asymmetrically. For example, the gyral pattern of the temporal lobe develops during the last trimester, with the left hemisphere developing 1–2 weeks later than the right. A number of hemispheric asymmetries have been described in the normal human brain. For example, the frontal lobe is wider on the right but the occipital is wider on the left, a phenomenon known as fronto-occipital torque (LeMay 1976). Asymmetry of the planum temporale and the Sylvian fissure are also pronounced (Geschwind and Levitsky 1968; LeMay 1976). The control of left–right asymmetry during organogenesis is not fully understood but may be under genetic control (Essner et al. 2000).

There are suggestions that this normal asymmetry is not present in schizophrenia. Following the hypothesis by Flor-Henry (1969) that schizophrenia may be associated with a dysfunction of the left rather than the right hemisphere, there has been a resurgence of interest in laterality in this disorder. Evidence from postmortem investigations suggests that both normal fronto-occipital torque and normal planum temporale asymmetry are reduced in schizophrenics (Falkai et al. 1995; DeLisi et al. 1997). There are also reports that ventricular enlargement is greater in the left temporal horn than the right (Crow et al. 1989). Cytoarchitectural and neurochemical studies have also revealed lateralized findings in schizophrenia; for example, synaptic protein is reduced in the left thalamus (Blennow et al. 1996), while changes in amygdala dopamine concentrations are confined to the left hemisphere (Reynolds 1983). There is currently no evidence to suggest that cerebral asymmetry is altered in bipolar disorder (Pearlson et al. 1997), although, interestingly, studies have shown altered asymmetry in dyslexia (Galaburda 1993). Anomalous asymmetry is compatible with an arrest of the normal development of the cerebrum before birth. However, how such a disturbance could arise is subject to debate. While it is likely that changes in asymmetry may have a genetic origin, environmental factors could also play a role.

Programmed cell death

Apoptosis is a physiological process of genetically programmed cell death. This process is vital for the regulation of brain morphology and connectivity. During development apoptosis is responsible for the elimination of up to 40% of cortical neurons, 60% of thalamic relay neurons and 80% of subplate neurons (Ferrer et al. 1992). Abnormalities of this process may therefore result in the reductions in cortical width, abnormal position of neurons, reductions in thalamic neurons and changes in thalamocortical connectivity described in schizophrenia (Catts and Catts 2000). The Bcl-2 gene family plays a vital role in the regulation of apoptosis. Recent studies have found reductions in Bcl-2 levels in the cortex in schizophrenia, supporting the notion that in schizophrenia neurons are more vulnerable to proapoptotic stimuli (Jarskog et al. 2000). However, deletions of Bcl-2 genes are known to cause more severe disturbances of cortical development than seen in schizophrenia (Motoyama et al. 1995).

Conclusion

Evidence from epidemiological, imaging and postmortem studies suggests that schizophrenia, and also possibly bipolar disorder, may result from abnormal brain development. However, the nature and timing of this problem are not known. A great deal of importance has been placed on suggestions that reactive gliosis is absent in schizophrenia and bipolar disorder, this finding being suggestive of a nonprogressive developmental aetiology. This lack of gliosis may also provide clues as to the timing of any abnormality, as any brain changes must have taken place before the onset of glial response. It is widely believed that this occurs in the second trimester in utero (Friede 1989), leading to the hypothesis that abnormalities of brain development would have to occur during midgestation or earlier (Roberts 1991). This may rule out birth injury or perinatal infection as major factors. While birth difficulties do give rise to infarcts that could lead to enlarged ventricles (Volpe 1989), such pathologies are accompanied by gliosis. However, it does not rule out changes in developmental processes such as embryonic patterning, differentiation, neuronal migration, synaptic pruning or even programmed cell death which does not lead to gliosis. While severe abnormalities of these processes may lead to more severe cytoarchitectural alterations than those seen in schizophrenia and bipolar disorder, more subtle abnormalities of any of these processes may result in aberrant patterns of connectivity, or 'miswiring' of the brain. How these changes may be manifested is not understood, although a genetic cause seems likely in the first instance. There is also evidence that the pathological process may occur later in life. In this volume Götz (Chapter 3) proposes that defects in adult neurogenesis may lead to the alterations in neuronal position that have been described in schizophrenia. Abnormal synaptic pruning during childhood or adolescence has also been proposed and could be due to environmental factors, such as stress. The resulting aberrant patterns of cortical connectivity ultimately may be responsible for the bizarre thought processes and cognitive dysfunction typical of schizophrenia and bipolar disorder.

REFERENCES

Akbarian S, Bunney WE Jr, Potkin SG et al. (1993a). Altered distribution of nicotinamide-adenine dinucleotide phosphate-diaphorase cells in frontal lobe of schizophrenics implies disturbances of cortical development. *Arch Gen Psychiatry*, 50, 169–77.

Akbarian S, Vinuela A, Kim JJ, Potkin SG, Bunney WE Jr and Jones EG (1993b). Distorted distribution of nicotinamide adenine dinucleotide phosphate-diaphorase neurons in temporal lobe of schizophrenics implies disturbances of cortical development. *Arch Gen Psychiatry*, 50, 178–87.

Akbarian S, Kim JJ, Potkin SG et al. (1995). Gene expression for glutamic acid decarboxylase is reduced without loss of neurons in prefrontal cortex of schizophrenics. *Arch Gen Psychiatry*, 52, 258–66.

Akbarian S, Kim JJ, Potkin SG, Hetrick WP, Bunney WE Jr and Jones EG (1996). Maldistribution of interstitial neurons in prefrontal white matter of the brains of schizophrenic patients. *Arch Gen Psychiatry*, 53, 425–36.

Akil M and Lewis DA (1997). Cytoarchitecture of the entorhinal cortex in schizophrenia. *Am J Psychiatry*, 154, 1010–12.

Allendoerfer KL and Shatz CJ (1994). The subplate, a transient neocortical structure: its role in the development of connections between thalamus and cortex. *Annu Rev Neurosci*, 17, 185–218.

Altshuler LL, Curran JG, Hauser P, Mintz J, Denicoff K and Post R (1995). T2 hyperintensities in bipolar disorder: magnetic resonance imaging comparison and literature meta-analysis. *Am J Psychiatry*, 152, 1139–44.

Alzheimer A (1897). Beitrage zur pathologischen anatomie der hirnrinde und zur anatomischen grundlage einiger psychosen. *Monatsschrift Psychiatrie Neurologie*, 2, 82–120.

Anderson SA, Volk DW and Lewis DA (1996). Increased density of microtubule associated protein 2-immunoreactive neurons in the white matter of schizophrenia subjects. *Schizophr Res*, 19, 111–19.

Andreasen NC, Flashman L, Flaum M et al. (1994). Regional brain abnormalities in schizophrenia measured with magnetic resonance imaging. *J Am Med Assoc*, 272, 1763–69.

Ang SL, Jin O, Rhinn M, Daigle N, Stevenson L and Rossant J (1996). A targeted mouse Otx2 mutation leads to severe defects in gastrulation and formation of axial mesoderm and to deletion of rostral brain. *Development*, 122, 243–52.

Armstrong E, Schleicher A, Omran H, Curtis M and Zilles K (1995). The ontogeny of human gyrification. *Cereb Cortex*, 5, 56–63.

Arnold SE, Hyman BT, Van Hoesen GW and Damasio AR (1991). Some cytoarchitectural abnormalities of the entorhinal cortex in schizophrenia. *Arch Gen Psychiatry*, 48, 625–32.

Arnold SE, Han L-Y and Ruscheinsky DD (1997). Further evidence of cytoarchitectural abnormalities of the entorhinal cortex in schizophrenia using spatial point pattern analysis. *Biol Psychiatry*, 42, 639–47.

Barbeau D, Liang JJ, Robitalille Y, Quirion R and Srivastava LK (1995). Decreased expression of the embryonic form of the neural cell adhesion molecule in schizophrenic brains. *Proc Natl Acad Sci USA*, 92, 2785–9.

Beasley CL and Reynolds GP (1997). Parvalbumin-immunoreactive neurons are reduced in the prefrontal cortex of schizophrenics. *Schizophr Res*, 24, 349–55.

Beasley C, Cotter D and Everall I (2001*a*). The Wnt signalling pathway and schizophrenia. *Schizophr Res*, 49, 50.

Beasley C, Cotter D, Khan N et al. (2001*b*). Glycogen synthase kinase-3β immunoreactivity is reduced in the frontal cortex in schizophrenia. *Neurosci Lett*, 302, 117–20.

Beckmann H and Jakob H (1991). Prenatal disturbances of nerve cell migration in the entorhinal region: a common vulnerability factor in functional psychoses? *J Neural Transm*, 84, 155–64.

Benes FM, Davidson J and Bird ED (1986). Quantitative cytoarchitectural analyses of the cerebral cortex of schizophrenics. *Arch Gen Psychiatry*, 43, 31–5.

Benes FM, McSparren J, Bird ED, SanGiovanni JP and Vincent SL (1991). Deficits in small interneurons in prefrontal and cingulate cortices of schizophrenic and schizoaffective patients. *Arch Gen Psychiatry*, 48, 996–1001.

Benes FM, Vincent SL and Todtenkopf M (2001). The density of pyramidal and nonpyramidal neurons in anterior cingulate cortex of schizophrenia and bipolar subjects. *Biol Psychiatry*, 50, 395–406.

Bernstein H-G, Krell D, Baumann B et al. (1998). Morphometric studies of the entorhinal cortex in neuropsychiatric patients and controls: clusters of heterotopically displaced lamina II neurons are not indicative of schizophrenia. *Schizophr Res*, 33, 125–301.

Blennow K, Davidsson P, Gottfries C-G, Ekman R and Heilig M (1996). Synaptic degeneration in thalamus in schizophrenia. *Lancet*, 348, 692–3.

Brown JD and Moon RT (1998). Wnt signaling: why is everything so negative? *Curr Opin Cell Biol*, 10, 182–7.

Browning MD, Dudek EM, Rapier JL, Leonard S and Freedman R (1993). Significant reductions in synapsin but not synaptophysin specific activity in the brains of some schizophrenics. *Biol Psychiatry*, 34, 529–35.

Brunelli S, Faiella A, Capra V et al. (1996). Germline mutations in the homeobox gene EMX2 in patients with severe schizencephaly. *Nat Genet*, 12, 94–6.

Bryant NL, Buchanan RW, Vladar K, Breier A and Rothman M (1999). Gender differences in temporal lobe structures of patients with schizophrenia: a volumetric MRI study. *Am J Psychiatry*, 156, 603–9.

Byrne M, Browne R, Mulryan N et al. (2000). Labour and delivery complications and schizophrenia. Case-control study using contemporaneous labour ward records. *Br J Psychiatry*, 176, 531–6.

Catts VS and Catts SV (2000). Apoptosis and schizophrenia: is the tumour supressor gene p53 a candidate susceptibility gene? *Schizophr Res*, 41, 405–15.

Christison GW, Casanova MF, Weinberger DR, Rawlings R and Kleinman JE (1989). A quantitative investigation of hippocampal pyramidal cell size, shape and variability of orientation in schizophrenia. *Arch Gen Psychiatry*, 1027–32.

Chun JJM and Shatz CJ (1989). Interstitial cells of the adult neocortical white matter are the remnant of the early generated subplate neuron population. *J Comp Neurol*, 282, 555–69.

Conrad AJ, Abebe T, Austen R, Forsythe S and Scheibel AB (1991). Hippocampal pyramidal cell disarray in schizophrenia as a bilateral phenomenon. *Arch Gen Psychiatry*, 48, 413–17.

Cotter D, Kerwin R, Doshi B, Martin CS and Everall IP (1997). Alterations in hippocampal non-phosphorylated MAP2 protein expression in schizophrenia. *Brain Res*, 765, 238–46.

Cotter D, Kerwin R, al-Sarraj S et al. (1998). Abnormalities of Wnt signalling in schizophrenia – evidence for neurodevelopmental abnormality. *Neuroreport*, 9, 1379–83.

Cotter D, Honavar M, Lovestone S et al. (1999). Disturbance of Notch-1 and Wnt signalling proteins in neuroglial balloon cells and abnormal large neurons in focal cortical dysplasia in human cortex. *Acta Neuropathol (Berl)*, 98, 465–72.

Cotter D, Mackay D, Landau S, Kerwin R and Everall I (2001). Reduced glial cell density and neuronal size in the anterior cingulate cortex in major depressive disorder. *Arch Gen Psychiatry*, 58, 545–53.

Crow TJ and Waddington JL (2000). Invited commentaries on: obstetric complications and schizophrenia/affective psychoses. *Br J Psychiatry*, 176, 527–30.

Crow TJ, Ball J, Bloom SR et al. (1989). Schizophrenia as an anomaly of development of cerebral asymmetry: a postmortem study and a proposal concerning the genetic basis of the disease. *Arch Gen Psychiatry*, 46, 1145–50.

Crow TJ, Done DJ and Sacker A (1995). Childhood precursors of psychosis as clues to its evolutionary origins. *Eur Arch Psychiatry Clin Neurosci*, 245, 61–9.

DeLisi LE, Stritzke PH, Holan V et al. (1991). Brain morphological changes in 1st episode cases of schizophrenia: are they progressive? *Schizophr Res*, 5, 206–8.

DeLisi LE, Sakuma M, Kushner M, Finer DL, Hoff AL and Crow TJ (1997). Anomalous cerebral asymmetry and language processing in schizophrenia. *Schizophr Bull*, 23, 255–71.

Drevets WC (2001). Neuroimaging and neuropathological studies of depression: implications for the cognitive-emotional features of mood disorders. *Curr Opin Neurobiol*, 11, 240–9.

Eastwood SL and Harrison PJ (2000). Hippocampal synaptic pathology in schizophrenia, bipolar disorder and major depression: a study of complexin mRNAs. *Mol Psychiatry*, 5, 425–32.

Essner JJ, Branford WW, Zhang J and Yost HJ (2000). Mesendoderm and left-right brain, heart and gut development are differentially regulated by pitx2 isoforms. *Development*, 127, 1081–93.

Falkai P, Bogerts B, Schneider T et al. (1995). Disturbed planum temporale asymmetry in schizophrenia: a quantitative post-mortem study. *Schizophr Res*, 14, 161–76.

Falkai P, Honer WG, David S, Bogerts B, Majtenyi C and Bayer TA (1999). No evidence for astrogliosis in brains of schizophrenic patients: a post-mortem study. *Neuropathol Appl Neurobiol*, 25, 48–53.

Falkai P, Schneider-Axmann T and Honer WG (2000). Entorhinal cortex pre-alpha cell clusters in schizophrenia: quantitative evidence of a developmental abnormality. *Biol Psychiatry*, 47, 937–43.

Feinberg I (1982). Schizophrenia: caused by a fault in programmed synaptic elimination during adolescence? *J Psychiatr Res*, 17, 319–34.

Ferrer I, Soriano E, Del Rio JA, Alcantara A and Auladell C (1992). Cell death and removal in the cerebral cortex during development. *Prog Neurobiol*, 39, 1–43.

Flor-Henry P (1969). Psychosis and temporal lobe epilepsy. A controlled investigation. *Epilepsia*, 10, 363–95.

Friede RL (1989). *Developmental Neuropathology*. Berlin: Springer Verlag.

Galaburda AM (1993). Neuroanatomic basis of developmental dyslexia. *Neurol Clin*, 11, 161–73.

Garey LJ, Ong WY, Patel TS et al. (1998). Reduced dendritic spine density on cerebral cortical pyramidal neurons in schizophrenia. *J Neurol Neurosurg Psychiatry*, 65, 446–53.

Geschwind N and Levitsky W (1968). Human brain: left-right asymmetries in temporal speech region. *Science*, 161, 186–7.

Gilvarry C, Takei N, Russell A, Rushe T, Hemsley D and Murray RM (2000). Premorbid IQ in patients with functional psychosis and their first-degree relatives. *Schizophr Res*, 41, 417–29.

Ghosh A and Shatz CJ (1992). Involvement of subplate neurons in the formation of ocular dominance columns. *Science*, 255, 1441–3.

Glantz LA and Lewis DA (1997). Reduction of synaptophysin immunoreactivity in the prefrontal cortex of subjects with schizophrenia. *Arch Gen Psychiatry*, 54, 660–9.

Green MF, Bracha HS, Satz P and Christenson CD (1994). Preliminary evidence for an association between minor physical anomalies and second trimester neurodevelopment in schizophrenia. *Psychiatry Res*, 53, 119–27.

Guidotti A, Auta J, Davis JM et al. (2000). Decrease in reelin and glutamic acid decarboxylase67 (GAD67) expression in schizophrenia and bipolar disorder: a postmortem brain study. *Arch Gen Psychiatry*, 57, 1061–9.

Gur RE, Cowell P, Turetsky BI et al. (1998). A follow-up magnetic resonance imaging study of schizophrenia. Relationship of neuroanatomical changes to clinical and neurobehavioral measures. *Arch Gen Psychiatry*, 55, 145–52.

Gur RE, Turetsky BI, Bilker WB and Gur RC (1999). Reduced gray matter volume in schizophrenia. *Arch Gen Psychiatry*, 56, 905–11.

Harrison PJ (1999). The neuropathology of schizophrenia. A critical review of the data and their interpretation. *Brain*, 122, 593–624.

Hoge EA, Friedman L and Schulz SC (1999). Meta-analysis of brain size in bipolar disorder. *Schizophr Res*, 37, 177–81.

Huttenlocher PR (1979). Synaptic density in human frontal cortex – developmental changes and effects of aging. *Brain Res*, 163, 195–205.

Ilia H, Beasley C, Meijer D et al. (2002). Expression of Oct-6, a PouIII domain transcription factor, in schizophrenia. *Am J Psychiatry* 159, 1174–82.

Impagnatiello F, Guidotti AR, Pesold C et al. (1998). A decrease of reelin expression as a putative vulnerability factor in schizophrenia. *Proc Natl Acad Sci USA*, 95, 15718–23.

Jakob H and Beckmann H (1986). Prenatal developmental disturbances in limbic allocortex of schizophrenics. *J Neural Transm*, 65, 303–26.

Jarskog LF, Gilmore JH, Selinger ES and Lieberman JA (2000). Cortical bcl-2 protein expression and apoptotic regulation in schizophrenia. *Biol Psychiatry*, 48, 641–50.

Johnstone EC, Crow TJ, Frith CD, Husband J and Kreel L (1976). Cerebral ventricular size and cognitive impairment in chronic schizophrenia. *Lancet*, 2, 924–6.

Jones EG and Cowan W (1983). Nervous tissue. In *The Structural Basis of Neurobiology*, ed. EG Jones. New York: Elsevier.

Jones P, Rodgers B, Murray R and Marmot M (1994). Child development risk factors for adult schizophrenia in the British 1946 birth cohort. *Lancet*, 344, 1398–402.

Jordan T, Hanson I, Zaletayev D et al. (1992). The human PAX6 gene is mutated in two patients with aniridia. *Nat Genet*, 1, 328–32.

Kalus P, Senitz D and Beckmann H (1997). Altered distribution of parvalbumin-immunoreactive local circuit neurons in the anterior cingulate cortex of schizophrenic patients. *Psychiatry Res*, 75, 49–59.

Kendell RE, McInneny K, Juszczak E and Bain M (2000). Obstetric complications and schizophrenia. Two case-control studies based on structured obstetric records. *Br J Psychiatry*, 176, 516–22.

Kostovic I and Rakic P (1980). Cytology and time of origin of interstitial neurons in the white matter in infant and adult human and monkey telencephalon. *J Neurocytol*, 9, 219–42.

Kovelman JA and Scheibel AB (1984). A neurohistological correlate of schizophrenia. *Biol Psychiatry*, 19, 1601–21.

Kozlovsky N, Belmaker RH and Agam G (2000). Low GSK-3β immunoreactivity in postmortem frontal cortex of schizophrenic patients. *Am J Psychiatry*, 157, 831–3.

Krimer LS, Herman MM, Saunders RC et al. (1997). A qualitative and quantitative analysis of the entorhinal cortex in schizophrenia. *Cereb Cortex*, 7, 732–9.

LeMay M (1976). Morphological cerebral asymmetries of modern man, fossil man, and non-human primate. *Ann N Y Acad Sci*, 280, 349–66.

Lewis SW (1989). Congenital risk factors for schizophrenia. *Psychol Med*, 19, 5–13.

Lewis S (1991). Computerised tomography in schizophrenia. *Br J Psychiatry*, 159, 158–9.

Lewis SW and Murray RM (1987). Obstetric complications, neurodevelopmental deviance, and risk of schizophrenia. *J Psychiatr Res*, 21, 413–21.

Lucas FR and Salinas PC (1997). WNT-7a induces axonal remodelling and increases synapsin I levels in cerebellar neurons. *Dev Biol*, 192, 31–44.

Lumsden A and Krumlauf R (1996). Patterning the vertebrate neuraxis. *Science*, 274, 1109–15.

Machon RA, Mednick SA and Huttunen MO (1997). Adult major affective disorder after prenatal exposure to an influenza epidemic. *Arch Gen Psychiatry*, 54, 322–8.

Manji HK and Lenox RH (2000). Signalling: cellular insights into the pathophysiology of bipolar disorder. *Biol Psychiatry*, 48, 518–30.

Marin-Padilla M (1983). Structural organization of the human cerebral cortex prior to the appearance of the cortical plate. *Anat Embryol*, 168, 21–40.

Marin-Padilla M (1998). Cajal–Retzius cells and the development of the neocortex. *Trends Neurosci*, 21, 64–71.

McArthur JC, Kumar AJ, Johnson DW et al. (1990). Incidental white matter hyperintensities on magnetic resonance imaging in HIV-1 infection. Multicenter AIDS Cohort Study. *J Acquir Immune Defic Syndr*, 3, 252–9.

McGlashan TH and Hoffman RE (2000). Schizophrenia as a disorder of developmentally reduced synaptic connectivity. *Arch Gen Psychiatry*, 57, 637–48.

McNeil TF (1991). Obstetric complications in schizophrenic parents. *Schizophr Res*, 5, 89–101.

McNeil TF, Cantor-Graae E and Ismail B (2000*a*). Obstetric complications and congenital malformation in schizophrenia. *Brain Res Brain Res Rev*, 31, 166–78.

McNeil TF, Cantor-Graae E and Weinberger DR (2000*b*). Relationship of obstetric complications and differences in size of brain structures in monozygotic twin pairs discordant for schizophrenia. *Am J Psychiatry*, 157, 203–12.

Mednick SA, Machon RA, Huttunen MO and Bonnet D (1988). Adult schizophrenia following prenatal exposure to an influenza epidemic. *Arch Gen Psychiatry*, 45, 189–92.

Miyaoka T, Seno H and Ishino H (1999). Increased expression of Wnt-1 in schizophrenic brains. *Schizophr Res*, 38, 1–6.

Motoyama N, Wang F, Roth KA et al. (1995). Massive cell death of immature hematopoietic cells and neurons in Bcl-x-deficient mice. *Science*, 267, 1506–9.

Murray RM and Woodruff PWR (1995). Developmental insanity or dementia praecox: a new perspective on an old debate? *Neurol Psych Brain Res*, 3, 167–76.

Nasrallah HA, Coffman JA and Olson SC (1989). Structural brain-imaging findings in affective disorders: an overview. *J Neuropsychiatry Clin Neurosci*, 1, 21–6.

Nawa H, Takahashi M and Patterson PH (2000). Cytokine and growth factor involvement in schizophrenia – support for the developmental model. *Mol Psychiatry*, 5, 594–603.

Niizato K, Arai T, Kuroki N, Kase K, Iritani S and Ikeda K (1998). Autopsy study of Alzheimer's disease brain pathology in schizophrenia. *Schizophr Res*, 31, 177–84.

Ongur D, Drevets WC and Price JL (1998). Glial reduction in the subgenual prefrontal cortex in mood disorders. *Proc Natl Acad Sci USA*, 95, 13290–5.

Pakkenberg B (1987). Post-mortem study of chronic schizophrenic brains. *Br J Psychiatry*, 151, 744–52.

Pakkenberg B (1990). Pronounced reduction of total neuron number in mediodorsal thalamic nucleus and nucleus accumbens in schizophrenics. *Arch Gen Psychiatry*, 47, 1023–8.

Pakkenberg B (1993). Total nerve cell number in neocortex in chronic schizophrenics and controls estimated using optical disectors. *Biol Psychiatry*, 34, 768–72.

Pearlson GD, Barta PE, Powers RE et al. (1997). Medial and superior temporal gyral volumes and cerebral asymmetry in schizophrenia versus bipolar disorder. *Biol Psychiatry*, 41, 1–14.

Pierri JN, Chaudry AS, Woo TU and Lewis DA (1999). Alterations in chandelier neuron axon terminals in the prefrontal cortex of schizophrenic subjects. *Am J Psychiatry*, 156, 1709–19.

Pierri JN, Volk CL, Auh S, Sampson A and Lewis DA (2001). Decreased somal size of deep layer 3 pyramidal neurons in the prefrontal cortex of subjects with schizophrenia. *Arch Gen Psychiatry*, 58, 466–73.

Porteus MH, Bulfone A, Liu JK, Puelles L, Lo LC and Rubenstein JL (1994). DLX-2, MASH-1, and MAP-2 expression and bromodeoxyuridine incorporation define molecularly distinct cell populations in the embryonic mouse forebrain. *J Neurosci*, 14, 6370–83.

Prolo P and Licinio J (1999). Cytokines in affective disorders and schizophrenia: new clinical and genetic findings. *Mol Psychiatry*, 4, 396.

Raedler TJ, Knable MB and Weinberger DR (1998). Schizophrenia as a developmental disorder of the cerebral cortex. *Curr Opin Neurobiol*, 8, 157–61.

Rajkowska G, Selemon LD and Goldman-Rakic PS (1998). Neuronal and glial somal size in the prefrontal cortex: a postmortem morphometric study of schizophrenia and Huntington disease. *Arch Gen Psychiatry*, 55, 215–24.

Rajkowska G, Halaris A and Selemon LD (2001). Reductions in neuronal and glial density characterize the dorsolateral prefrontal cortex in bipolar disorder. *Biol Psychiatry*, 49, 741–52.

Rapoport JL, Giedd J, Kumra S et al. (1997). Childhood-onset schizophrenia. Progressive ventricular change during adolescence. *Arch Gen Psychiatry*, 54, 897–903.

Rapoport JL, Giedd JN, Blumenthal J et al. (1999). Progressive cortical change during adolescence in childhood-onset schizophrenia. A longitudinal magnetic resonance imaging study. *Arch Gen Psychiatry*, 56, 649–54.

Raz S and Raz N (1990). Structural brain abnormalities in the major psychoses: a quantitative review of the evidence from computerized imaging. *Psychol Bull*, 108, 93–108.

Reynolds GP (1983). Increased concentration and lateral asymmetry of amygdala dopamine in schizophrenia. *Nature*, 305, 527–8.

Roberts GW (1991). Schizophrenia: a neuropathological perspective. *Br J Psychiatry*, 158, 8–17.

Selemon LD, Rajkowska G and Goldman-Rakic PS (1995). Abnormally high neuronal density in the schizophrenic cortex. *Arch Gen Psychiatry*, 52, 805–28.

Selemon LD, Rajkowska G and Goldman-Rakic PS (1998). Elevated neuronal density in prefrontal area 46 in brains from schizophrenic patients: application of a three-dimensional, stereologic counting method. *J Comp Neurol*, 392, 402–12.

Soares JC and Mann JJ (1997). The functional neuroanatomy of mood disorders. *J Psychiatr Res*, 31, 393–432.

Stevens JR (1982). Neuropathology of schizophrenia. *Arch Gen Psychiatry*, 39, 1131–9.

Sullivan EV, Lim KO, Mathalon D et al. (1998). A profile of cortical gray matter volume deficits characteristic of schizophrenia. *Cereb Cortex*, 8, 117–24.

Takahashi M, Shirakawa O, Toyooka K et al. (2000). Abnormal expression of brain-derived neurotrophic factor and its receptor in the corticolimbic system of schizophrenic patients. *Mol Psychiatry*, 5, 293–300.

Torrey EF (1999). Epidemiological comparison of schizophrenia and bipolar disorder. *Schizophr Res*, 39, 101–6.

Verdoux H, Geddes JR, Takei N et al. (1997). Obstetric complications and age at onset in schizophrenia: an international collaborative meta-analysis of individual patient data. *Am J Psychiatry*, 154, 1220–7.

Volk DW, Austin MC, Pierri JN, Sampson AR and Lewis DA (2000). Decreased glutamic acid decarboxylase$_{67}$ messenger RNA expression in a subset of prefrontal cortical gamma–aminobutyric acid neurons in subjects with schizophrenia. *Arch Gen Psychiatry*, 57, 237–45.

Volpe JJ (1989). Intraventricular hemorrhage and brain injury in the premature infant. Neuropathology and pathogenesis. *Clin Perinatol*, 16, 361–86.

Waddington JL (1993). Schizophrenia: developmental neuroscience and pathobiology. *Lancet*, 341, 531–6.

Walsh CA (1999). Genetic malformations of the human cerebral cortex. *Neuron*, 23, 19–29.

Weinberger DR (1987). Implications for normal brain development for the pathogenesis of schizophrenia. *Arch Gen Psychiatry*, 44, 660–9.

Woo TU, Whitehead RE, Melchitzky DS and Lewis DA (1998). A subclass of prefrontal gamma-aminobutyric acid axon terminals are selectively altered in schizophrenia. *Proc Natl Acad Sci USA*, 95, 5341–6.

Woods BT, Yurgelun-Todd D, Benes FM, Frankenburg FR, Pope HG Jr and McSparren J (1990). Progressive ventricular enlargement in schizophrenia: comparison to bipolar affective disorder and correlation with clinical course. *Biol Psychiatry*, 27, 341–52.

Yang SD, Yu JS, Lee TT, Yang CC, Ni MH and Yang YY (1994). Dysfunction of protein kinase FA/GSK-3 alpha in lymphocytes of patients with schizophrenic disorder. *J Cell Biochem*, 5, 108–16.

Young CE, Arima K, Xie J, Hu L, Beach TG, Falkai P and Honer WG (1998). SNAP-25 deficit and hippocampal connectivity in schizophrenia. *Cereb Cortex*, 8, 261–8.

Young KA, Manaye KF, Liang C, Hicks PB and German DC (2000). Reduced number of mediodorsal and anterior thalamic neurons in schizophrenia. *Biol Psychiatry*, 47, 944–53.

Zaidel DW, Esiri MM and Harrison PJ (1997). Size, shape, and orientation of neurons in the left and right hippocampus: investigation of normal asymmetries and alterations in schizophrenia. *Am J Psychiatry*, 154, 812–18.

Zipursky RB, Seeman MV, Bury A, Langevin R, Wortzman G and Katz R (1997). Deficits in gray matter volume are present in schizophrenia but not bipolar disorder. *Schizophr Res*, 26, 85–92.

Zipursky RB, Zhang-Wong J, Lambe EK, Bean G and Beiser M (1998). MRI correlates of treatment response in first episode psychosis. *Schizophr Res*, 30, 81–90.

Part III

New ways of imaging the brain

5

New directions in structural imaging

Xavier Chitnis[1] and Ian Ellison-Wright[1,2]

[1] Institute of Psychiatry, London, UK; [2] The Old Manor Hospital, Salisbury, UK

Introduction

Foucault commented that 'the medical gaze . . . contains within a single structure, different sensorial fields. The 'glance' has become a complex organisation with a view to the spatial assignment of the invisible' (Foucault 1963). During the last two decades, the structural brain image has been deconstructed using an increasing variety of analytic techniques in order to reveal previously invisible pathology.

Since the first major psychiatric computed tomography (CT) study published in 1976 (Johnstone et al. 1976), structural imaging has been utilized to investigate the major psychiatric disorders. It has become clear that many of these disorders are characterized by subtle structural brain changes. However, brain structure shows considerable variability between individuals, in terms of size, shape and composition (e.g. relative grey and white matter). Thus, the detection of a small neuropathological signal in the presence of loud noise (from neurodevelopment and other sources) has been a central problem for structural imaging studies and has provided the impetus for the development of a range of new analytic approaches. Several psychiatric and neurological disorders have been particularly important in terms of the development of structural imaging techniques, including schizophrenia, multiple sclerosis and epilepsy. In this chapter we illustrate new directions in structural imaging using research into brain changes in schizophrenia.

In addition to identifying the contributions of these new techniques, we highlight some of the problems that we believe have retarded progress in structural imaging. These need to be addressed by the neuro-imaging community, at both scientific and governance levels, if the full potential of these techniques is to be realized.

Meta-analyses

During the early 1980s there was a proliferation of CT studies of schizophrenia, followed in the later years of that decade by numerous magnetic resonance imaging

(MRI) studies. Typically, studies used a case–control design, comparing a sample of patients with schizophrenia and a sample of control subjects. Subjects underwent brain scanning and the area or volume of 'regions of interest' (ROIs), defined by anatomical criteria, were measured on the brain scans. The objective was to identify significant differences in the group means for the sizes of ROIs.

However, as the published literature on structural changes in schizophrenia expanded, it became apparent that there were problems in interpreting the literature. First, sample sizes in the case–control studies were generally small and, as the magnitudes of brain differences were also small, the results of individual studies were liable to be unduly influenced by sampling variation. Second, the results of the studies were generally reported with an emphasis on significance tests rather than confidence intervals, and this tended to give the misleading impression of a large number of inconsistent positive or negative findings. Third, many different brain regions were examined, but only a few of these were measured in each individual study. Finally, the results of some studies were reported in multiple publications.

A potential solution to this problem was provided by meta-analysis, a formal method for integrating quantitative data from multiple studies. It has the advantages that: (i) the results from individual studies are combined, improving the estimation of the overall effect size, (ii) statistical power is increased, (iii) confidence intervals for the overall effect size can be calculated, and (iv) factors causing heterogeneity in the results reported by individual studies can be investigated (Cooper and Hedges 1994). It is a method which contrasts with qualitative reviews (such as this book chapter), which do not use explicit criteria for selecting and analysing data and are therefore vulnerable to the subjectivity and biases of the authors.

The paper of Raz et al. (1988) was an important early meta-analysis in this field. They tested whether studies using a control group of normal subjects found different results from studies using a control group of medical/psychiatric patients. They ascertained 14 studies of schizophrenia using normal controls and 23 using medical/psychiatric patients. They calculated the 'effect size' for each study. This was simply the difference between patient and control group means in standard deviation units (Cohen's d). The overall effect size for studies using healthy controls (d = 0.85) was similar to studies using medical/psychiatric patients (d = 0.72). This showed that the lateral ventricles were larger in patients with schizophrenia whether the control group included healthy subjects or medical/psychiatric patients. Perhaps more importantly, it demonstrated that the meta-analytic method could be applied to brain structure in schizophrenia. A more recent meta-analysis has given a somewhat lower effect size (d = 0.49) for ventricular volume increase in schizophrenia, based on 30 MR studies using (mainly) healthy controls (Wright et al. 2000).

Van Horn and McManus (1992) analysed 39 studies of ventricular size in schizophrenia which measured the ventricle-to-brain ratio (VBR). This is the area of the ventricles (at the level on the scan at which the ventricles appear largest) expressed as a percentage of the total area of the brain scan. At that time VBR was the most widely used measure of ventricular size. For their meta-analysis, they used the difference in VBR between the patient and control groups as their measure of effect size. They found that in 92% of the studies, the mean VBR was greater in the schizophrenia group than the control group ($\chi^2 = 27.9$, 1 d.f., $P < 0.001$). This method of comparing results from studies has been called 'vote-counting', and is a technique that has been criticized in the meta-analytic literature as potentially misleading and inferior to the calculation of an overall effect size (Cooper and Hedges 1994). However, the main purpose of their study was the investigation of 'predictor variables' that might influence the VBR difference between patient and control groups. One of their statistically significant findings was that the year of publication had an effect on the VBR difference: the difference was less in later published studies. This result was important in leading researchers to question whether the early studies which found large VBR differences were a consequence of crude methodology, for example poor matching of subject and control groups.

The study of structural brain area and volume differences in schizophrenia was limited by the low spatial resolution of CT to large structures such as the ventricles, whole brain and brain lobes. However, a number of these studies suggested that while ventricular size was increased, whole brain size was reduced in schizophrenia. Ward et al. (1996) examined this literature in a meta-analysis. Their analysis included CT and MR and neuropathological studies and investigated extracranial and intracranial sizes as well as cerebral size. They included size measurements of volume, area, length, width or circumference. They calculated Cohen's d as their measure of effect size. For brain size, they identified 27 suitable studies (23 MRI, two CT and four neuropathological). The overall effect size was -0.26 (95% confidence intervals: -0.35 to -0.15, $P < 0.0001$), indicating that brain size was smaller in patients with schizophrenia. While intracranial size was also smaller in patients with schizophrenia ($d = -0.18$, $P = 0.0012$), there was no difference in extracranial size ($d = 0.14$, $P = 0.16$).

During the 1990s MR studies provided volume information about smaller brain structures including the limbic, subcortical and white matter structures which theorists believed were crucial in the pathology of schizophrenia. Particular regions of interest included the hippocampus, amygdala, superior temporal gyrus, thalamus, cerebellar vermis and corpus callosum. Major claims about the pathology of schizophrenia were supported by evidence from MR studies using small samples of patients and controls. This increased the need to integrate results from different neuro-imaging studies. Woodruff et al. (1995) conducted a meta-analysis of 11 published studies of corpus callosum morphology in schizophrenia, comprising 313 patients and 281 controls. They found that area of the corpus callosum was reduced in schizophrenia ($g = -0.18$, $P = 0.02$), although not the ratio of corpus callosum area to brain area (results not reported), leaving unanswered the question as to whether the corpus callosum reduction exceeded the whole brain volume reduction. Nelson et al. (1998) examined the volumes of the hippocampus and amygdala in schizophrenia. They included 18 studies with 522 patients and 426 controls. They found a bilateral reduction in hippocampal volume in schizophrenia (left: $d = -0.37$, $P < 0.001$; right $d = -0.39$, $P < 0.001$). The reduction was greater in studies which measured the combined amygdala–hippocampus (left $d = -0.67$, right $d = -0.72$). Konick and Friedman (2001) included 15 studies of thalamic volume or area (485 patients with schizophrenia and 500 control subjects). They found reduced thalamic size in schizophrenia ($d = -0.29$, $P < 0.0001$).

An emerging problem during the 1990s was that spatially distributed brain regions were found to show quantitative changes in schizophrenia. This was 'an embarrassment of riches', because the pathological consequences of schizophrenia appeared to spread throughout the brain, diminishing the hope that structural imaging would identify an atrophic (or underdeveloped) region which would prove to be the pathological focus of the disorder. If many brain regions were affected by schizophrenia were some nevertheless more affected than others? This was investigated by a multiregion quantitative review by Lawrie and Abukmeil (1998). Rather than calculate meta-analytic effect sizes for each region (such as Cohen's d), they used the percentage volume difference between the schizophrenia and control groups and then obtained the median value for the included studies. This technique had the advantages that it is easier to comprehend and compare percentage volume changes than standard deviation-based measures (e.g. Cohen's d), and the use of the median made it more robust against outlying results from individual studies. They concluded that while brain volume was reduced in schizophrenia (to 97% control volume), reductions in the amygdala (left 90%, right 90%) and hippocampus (left 93%, right 92.5%) exceeded the overall reduction.

Wright et al. (2000) extended the work of Lawrie and Abukmeil (1998) using more formal meta-analytic techniques, although retaining the percentage difference as the measure of effect size. They also used a technique to control for global volume changes (of whole brain for grey/white matter structures and total ventricular volume for ventricular structures). Their results confirmed the presence of global brain volume differences in schizophrenia: compared with comparison subjects, cerebral volume was lower in patients (97.8%) and total ventricular volume was higher (126%). Relative to the global differences, the cerebral regions with the lowest volumes in the patients with schizophrenia were: the amygdala (overall mean global-corrected effect size: left 94%, right 94%), hippocampus/amygdala (left 94%, right 95%), parahippocampus (left 93%, right 95%) and left anterior superior temporal gyrus (93%). Intriguingly, the distribution of ventricular volume changes (maximal increases in the body of the lateral ventricle bilaterally) appeared to differ from the pattern of cerebral changes (maximal reductions in frontal lobe and medial temporal regions bilaterally).

Laterality effects

Several theories of the pathogenesis of schizophrenia postulated that brain changes were predominantly left-sided (e.g. Lohr and Caligiuri 1997). These drew support from early neuropathological and CT studies, which found greater left than right temporal horn enlargement in schizophrenia and from neuropsychological evidence relating to the symptomatology of schizophrenia. It was also postulated that the genetic mechanism underlying normal left hemispheric dominance was abnormal in schizophrenia (Crow et al. 1989).

A particular focus of structural asymmetry studies was the planum temporale (PT). This is a small triangular region on the superior temporal lobe that is an important language area: on the left side of the brain it partly coincides with Wernicke's area. Shapleske et al. (1999) reviewed studies of planum temporale asymmetry in schizophrenia. Of 15 studies using MRI, there have been three broad claims: in schizophrenia (i) normal PT asymmetry (left >> right) is reduced (left > right) or reversed (left < right), (ii) PT asymmetry is unchanged (left >> right), or (iii) PT asymmetry is increased (left >>> right). Shapleske et al. (1999) identified 7 studies of PT area in schizophrenia (201 brains) and 21 studies of PT area in controls (607 brains). The overall effect size (Hedge's g) for PT area difference in controls was 0.67 (left >> right) but for patients with schizophrenia was −0.058 (left < right). There was a significant difference between these effect sizes ($F = 8.3$, $P < 0.008$) which reflected the larger surface area of the right PT in patients with schizophrenia.

Sommer et al. (2001) extended this investigation and performed meta-analysis on structural MR studies which investigated lateralized measurements of the planum temporale, Sylvian fissure, temporal horn of the lateral ventricle, superior temporal gyrus and posterior segment of the superior temporal gyrus. The planum temporale (11 samples) showed significant asymmetry favouring the left hemisphere in controls. However, as reported by Shapleske et al. (1999), asymmetry of the planum temporale was significantly reduced in patients. The Sylvian fissure (three samples) showed significant asymmetry favouring the left hemisphere in both controls and patients. Again, patients showed significantly decreased asymmetry compared with controls. The temporal horn of the lateral ventricle (12 samples) showed rightward asymmetry in patients and controls. Asymmetry was not significantly different between patients and controls. The superior temporal gyrus was larger in the right hemisphere in patients and controls (17 samples). Patients tended to have increased asymmetry of the superior temporal gyrus favouring the right hemisphere (although this was not significant). A separate analysis on five samples was performed to assess asymmetry of the posterior segment of the superior temporal gyrus. Rightward asymmetry was found for the patients and controls. Rightward asymmetry of the posterior segment of the superior temporal gyrus was significantly larger in patients. The authors argued that the decreased temporoparietal asymmetries in schizophrenia (i.e. involving the planum temporale and Sylvian fissure) probably reflected decreased language dominance in the patients, since planum temporale and Sylvian fissure asymmetries are believed to be strongly related to cerebral dominance (Gerschlager et al. 1998).

Further investigation of the asymmetry hypothesis will be assisted by the integration of structural and functional imaging results from individual patients (e.g. using functional MRI). This will permit a greater understanding of the relationship between language dominance and structural asymmetry.

The contribution of meta-analysis

Meta-analysis has permitted meaningful integration of the ROI data on schizophrenia. It has provided robust evidence for global structural differences in schizophrenia: reduced cerebral volume and increased total ventricular volume. In the ventricular system, the largest regional volume changes appear to be in the bodies of the lateral ventricles. In the cerebrum, regional volume reductions include the frontal lobes, lateral medial temporal lobe regions and the thalamus. Therefore, a general theory of the structural pathology of schizophrenia (if all these changes are due to pathology) must explain a complex pattern of cerebral changes, as well as ventricular changes with a different spatial distribution.

Meta-analyses have also highlighted the enormous research effort that was directed towards the investigation of structural brain changes in schizophrenia during the 1980s and 1990s. However, the majority of these neuro-imaging studies used small samples to detect small effects, with the risk of both Type 1 errors (false positive differences) and Type 2 errors (lack of power to detect true differences). In order to avoid 'brain data wastage' it has been argued that international researchers should pool both their results and brain images (Wright et al. 2000). Provision of the actual MR images to an electronic database would both facilitate the comparison of image analytic techniques and provide large samples for testing small effects. In contrast to the efforts of psychiatric geneticists, who have performed a number of important international collaborations involving data-sharing, psychiatric neuro-imagers have made little progress in this area.

However, there are also limitations of meta-analysis. First, the overall results of a meta-analysis are dependent on the quality of the primary studies. Second, some observations about the primary studies may be better made in a well-informed subjective review than in a statistical meta-analysis. For example, differences in the anatomical criteria for measuring ROIs may be identified as important in a subjective review, but there may be too few studies to have the power to test for this in a meta-analysis. Third, various types of publication bias may arise during publication of the primary studies (although there are some statistical techniques that can be used to detect the possibility of publication bias, e.g. funnel plots). Fourth, differences between groups detected by meta-analysis may be due to confounding factors rather than the pathology of schizophrenia (e.g. antipsychotic medication causing basal ganglia volume increases; Chakos et al. 1994).

Voxel-based morphometry

The results of the meta-analyses described above concluded that regional volume reductions were present in schizophrenia in: (i) medial temporal lobe regions, (ii) left superior temporal gyrus, (iii) bilateral frontal lobes and (iv) thalamus. These findings were consistent with a pathological process in schizophrenia involving distributed changes within the brain. However, studies employing ROI measurements usually only measure a small number of selected brain regions because the measurement process is very labour-intensive. For example, in the meta-analysis by Wright et al. (2000) most brain regions were only measured in a fraction of the total 1588 patients included in the analysis. Furthermore, because of the inherent difficulties in defining structurally complex and variable regions of cortex, ROI studies have tended to focus on structures that are easily definable, such as the hippocampus, at the expense of neocortical morphology, where intersubject variability in sulcal patterns may prove problematic. This has led to a distorted picture of the pattern of brain changes in schizophrenia, with an undue concentration of interest on a relatively few cerebral structures, at the expense of a more comprehensive assessment of brain structure.

The measurement problems associated with ROI analyses have led to the development of semi-automated 'whole-brain' techniques for analysing structural MR images. These methods have been called 'voxel-based morphometry' (VBM) because scans are analysed for structural change at the level of 'voxels' – the individual elements within a three-dimensional digital image.

These methods must overcome the problems posed by the complex three-dimensional anatomy of the brain and interindividual variability in brain size, shape and composition (such as the relative proportions of grey and white matter). The first published technique involved linear transformation of brain images into a 'bounding box' of constant size (Andreasen et al. 1994). Magnetic resonance images from patients and controls were transformed with a 'bounding box' to produce an 'average schizophrenic brain' and an 'average normal brain'. After image subtraction of the two averages, the areas of difference were displayed as an effect-size map. Specific regional abnormalities were observed in the thalamus and adjacent white matter. The authors argued that an abnormality in the thalamus and related circuitry explained the diverse symptoms of schizophrenia parsimoniously because they could all result from a defect in filtering or gating sensory input, which is one of the primary functions of the thalamus. Wolkin et al. (1998) used this 'image averaging' technique to compare MR scans from 25 patients with schizophrenia and 25 control subjects. Effect-size maps revealed widespread patchy signal intensity differences between the two groups in both cortical and periventricular areas, including major white matter tracts. Interestingly, unlike Andreasen's study, no differences were found within the thalamus. The authors suggested that their results were consistent with diffuse structural brain abnormalities occurring in both grey and white matter in schizophrenia.

An alternative VBM approach (Wright et al. 1995) used the solution to an analogous problem from positron emission tomography (PET). The analysis of PET functional images led to the development of a technique (Friston et al. 1995a) for the spatial transformation of images of regional cerebral blood flow into a standard stereotactic space (Talairach and Tournoux 1988). This was followed by three-dimensional analysis of radioactivity differences at each voxel of the image using a program called statistical parametric mapping (SPM; Friston et al. 1995b). When applied to MRI, images were segmented into maps of grey matter, white matter and cerebrospinal fluid (CSF). These images were spatially transformed into a standard space, permitting comparison of image voxel intensities at equivalent locations throughout the brain. The segmented images were spatially filtered ('smoothed') in order to improve the signal to noise ratio. Voxel intensity after spatial smoothing (weighting an individual voxel value by those of its neighbours) was assumed to represent a measure of the amount of grey (or white) matter at that point in the brain.

Wright et al. (1999a) applied this technique to MR scans of schizophrenics and controls. Using this method, it was possible to partition differences in grey matter distribution into global and regional changes, to construct a three-dimensional map of the regional changes on a voxel-by-voxel basis and to search for changes in a 'brain-wide' analysis rather than in a few preselected regions. In total, images from 42 subjects with schizophrenia and 52 controls were analysed from two previous schizophrenia–control studies. The statistical parametric map comparing regional grey matter between schizophrenia and control groups identified two regions of grey matter reduction in the schizophrenia group: (a) the right temporal pole, amygdala and insula and (b) the left temporal pole, insula and dorsolateral prefrontal cortex ($P < 0.01$) (Figure 5.1). There were no areas where the schizophrenia group had significantly more regional grey matter than the control group. A similar approach, adopted by Paillere-Martinot et al. (2001), examined white matter in addition to grey matter in 20 patients with schizophrenia and 20 control subjects.

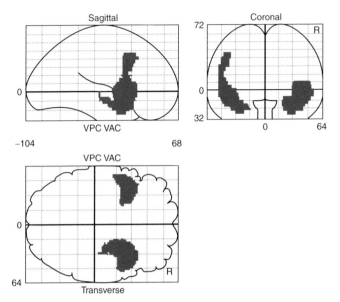

Figure 5.1   Regional grey matter reductions in schizophrenia. Statistical parametric map in three orthogonal projections showing voxels where the regional grey matter was reduced in schizophrenics relative to controls (SPM Z) thresholded at $Z > 2.33$ and $P < 0.01$ (corrected). The main regional differences were: (1) the right temporal pole, insula and amygdala, and (2) the left temporal pole, insula and perfrontal cortex. From Wright et al. 1999a.

Grey matter reductions in the patients included the left insula and left para-hippocampus; white matter reductions were present bilaterally in the frontal lobes (Figure 5.2). This VBM technique (Ashburner and Friston 2000) has now been applied to a variety of neurological and psychiatric disorders including depression (Shah et al. 1998), a genetic speech disorder (Vargha-Khadem et al. 1998), epilepsy (Richardson et al. 1997), and idiopathic headache syndrome (May et al. 1999).

Another approach, developed at the Institute of Psychiatry in London, UK, employed nonparametric techniques at the stage of statistical analysis (Bullmore et al. 1999), rather than the parametric statistics of SPM. The authors argued that this permitted the use of statistics incorporating three-dimensional spatial information which otherwise presented intractable analytic problems. Using this technique, Sigmundsson et al. (2001) investigated grey and white matter changes in 27 patients with schizophrenia and prominent negative symptoms, compared with 27 control subjects. The authors hoped that by examining a clinically homogeneous group of patients with primary and enduring negative symptoms they would detect a homogeneous pattern of brain changes. They found that whole brain volume

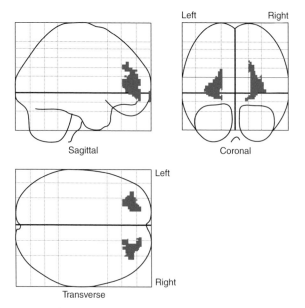

Figure 5.2   Statistical parametric maps for reductions in white matter in 20 patients with early-onset schizophrenia compared with 20 normal control subjects (height threshold $P = 0.01$; extent threshold = 800 voxels). From Paillere-Martinot et al. 2001.

was 4% smaller in the patients than in controls, grey and white matter were 5–6% smaller and CSF 7% greater. There were three regions of localized grey matter volume reduction: (i) left perisylvian (insula, and superior temporal and inferior frontal gyri), (ii) left medial temporal (gyrus) and (iii) anterior cingulate/medial frontal gyrus. There was also a white matter deficit in the patients in the left uncinate fasciculus. There was a region of grey matter excess in the patients in the left lentiform nuclei, which may have been attributable to antipsychotic drug treatment.

The contribution of voxel-based morphometry

Automated 'brain averaging' (Andreasen et al. 1994) or voxel-based methods (Ashburner and Friston 2000) have provided a technique for investigating the 'broader gestalt of morphologic deviation' (Wolkin et al. 1998). They may be useful in identifying changes in regions not easily measured by ROI studies. However, there is a danger that VBM studies will produce conflicting maps of brain changes in schizophrenia because of small sample sizes and (as with ROI studies) a reliance on significance testing in producing results. Furthermore, integrating the results of VBM research will be more difficult and complex than the meta-analyses required for ROI studies. Unless this integration can be achieved, their credibility is likely to diminish.

There are some important potential limitations of VBM techniques. Sigmundsson et al. (2001) point out that maps of voxel-based differences between two groups (i.e. the results of hypothesis testing) will reflect the size of test applied to the data. A stringent test reduces the possibility of Type 1 errors (false positives) but increases the risk of Type 2 errors (false negatives). Therefore maps of the results may show regions of significant difference but hide other regions of difference, which do not reach the statistical threshold. The power to detect differences may also vary within the image, depending on the methodology of image acquisition and analysis. For example, near the base of the brain there may be little power to detect differences because not all the images may contribute data to this region after spatial transformation. VBM maps generally do not reveal the regions where there is reduced power to detect differences – regions that might be considered 'black holes' for the test in question. In this respect their results can be misleading.

The image-processing steps employed in VBM are also controversial. In particular, the method is critically dependent on the type of registration used to map images into stereotactic space. Methods for image registration range from the simple rigid-body registration commonly used for the correction of head movement in functional MRI time-series analysis to high-dimensional techniques, such as fluid-deformation algorithms (Thompson and Toga 1997). Popular methods for VBM include affine registration, which corrects for differences in brain size and orientation, and low-frequency nonlinear registration, which additionally corrects for global differences in brain shape (Ashburner and Friston 2000).

The aim of image registration in VBM is to remove differences in brain structure due to 'uninteresting' variables, such as age and gender, while preserving as far as possible those differences that relate to the variable of interest, e.g. diagnosis. It is important that image registration does not exactly register images together. Most algorithms work by attempting to minimize the sum of squared differences of voxel values at each voxel between the template and input images. If two images are perfectly registered, then there will remain no differences in voxel values to be tested by VBM (Ashburner and Friston 2000). Some authors have questioned the validity of nonlinear image registration for VBM (Bookstein 2001). Indeed, it is possible that nonlinear deformations may either serve to reduce differences between groups by, for example, reducing the size of the ventricles in a group of schizophrenics, or alternatively, may introduce false differences through excessive warping in some regions.

In summary, the image-analytic steps employed in VBM can be approached in a variety of different ways. These steps include image acquisition, grey/white matter classification, spatial transformation (linear vs. nonlinear) and statistical analysis (parametric vs. nonparametric). Because of the possible number of alternative approaches, a difference map between two groups will generally represent one of many possible analytic solutions to the problem.

Shape, deformation and complexity studies

So far we have described techniques which test for size differences in the brains of patients with schizophrenia. An alternative approach focuses on shape changes. One of the limitations of traditional ROI studies is the specificity of the findings. Reduced hippocampal volume is one of the most consistent findings in the schizophrenia literature; however, reduced hippocampal volume has also been reported in Alzheimer's disease, depression and epilepsy (Barr et al. 1997; Shah et al. 1998; Krasuski et al. 1998). Clearly the neuropathology of these disorders (and the associated brain changes) must be different; however, ROI studies are severely limited in their ability to discriminate them. An alternative approach to simply studying volumetric changes is to look at differences in the shape and complexity of structures.

An important early example of this approach was a study by Bartley et al. (1993) of the shape of the Sylvian fissure in 10 normal monozygotic twin pairs and 10 twin pairs discordant for schizophrenia. Sylvian fissure shape was simply measured as its length and angle. They confirmed the expected asymmetries of length and angle of the Sylvian fissure in the normal monozygotic twin pairs. The length asymmetry was attributable to differences in the region of the PT. Within discordant pairs, affected and unaffected twins did not differ in asymmetry measures, suggesting no association between illness and diminished asymmetry. Moreover, the discordant twins did not differ from the normal twins, failing to confirm their hypothesis of a genetic association with abnormal asymmetry. These results are unexpected in view of the meta-analytic findings of Shapleske et al. (1999) and Sommer et al. (2001), of reduced PT asymmetry in schizophrenia.

Landmark-based morphometrics

An approach pioneered by Bookstein (1997) called geometric morphometrics (or landmark-based morphometrics – LBM) involves multivariate statistical analysis of landmark data from biomedical images. Structures are identified by a series of anatomical landmarks – e.g. at vertices – and these are used to generate a complete set of landmark-by-landmark deviations from an average shape. DeQuardo et al. (1999) used landmark-based morphometry to investigate midline brain shape in 20 patients with first-episode schizophrenia compared with 22 control subjects. They located 15 landmarks on the mid-sagittal brain slice for each subject. There was a significant difference between the two groups, which appeared to involve a shortening of the corpus callosum and displacement of the corpus callosum relative to the cerebellum. The authors argued that as well as midline abnormalities, these changes might reflect abnormalities in distal structures including the hippocampus,

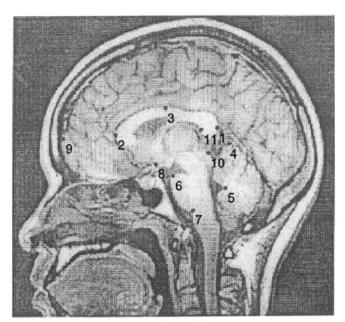

Figure 5.3　The locations of the landmarks used in the Garaibeh et al. (2000) study. 1, outside of splenium; 2, genu; 3, midpoint of corpus callosum; 4, top of cerebellum; 5, tip of fourth ventricle; 6, top of pons; 7, bottom of pons; 8, optic chiasm; 9, frontal pole (on the extension of a line from 1 to 2); 10, superior colliculus; 11, inside of splenium. (Modified from DeQuardo et al. 1996 and Bookstein 1995.)

amygdala and superior temporal gyrus. Gharaibeh et al. (2000) investigated whether deviations in the shape of midline brain structures were present at the time of onset of symptoms of schizophrenia and 3–5 years later. They located 11 landmarks on the mid-sagittal MR scan of 55 patients with schizophrenia and 22 control subjects (Figure 5.3). Geometric morphometric methods were used for the extraction of shape variables from landmark coordinates. Permutation tests were used to test effects including diagnosis and time elapsed since illness onset. They found that some anatomical abnormalities in patient brain morphology were present both at the time of diagnosis and at follow-up.

In an extension of this approach to the analysis of three-dimensional structures, Buckley et al. (1999) applied this method to 48 selected landmarks on the segmented ventricular system from MRI scans of 20 patients with schizophrenia and 20 control subjects. They found landmark changes in the proximal temporal horn of the lateral ventricles and in the region of the foramen of Munro. They predicted that these abnormalities would be associated with other neurodevelopmental changes, e.g. cranio-facial minor physical anomalies. Using LBM to explore the hypothesis that schizophrenia is a neurodevelopmental disorder, Deutsch et al. (2000) found cranio-facial dysmorphology in patients with schizophrenia. Embryologic-fate mapping studies related this cranio-facial region to the diencephalic–mesencephalic border in the brain, and hence they predicted brain midline maldevelopment at this border in schizophrenia. They analysed midline deviation in MR images from patients with schizophrenia and control subjects. Deviation scores were higher in the patients with schizophrenia and among the siblings of these schizophrenic patients. Brain and face dysmorphology scores cohered within subjects, providing further support to their embryologically derived model.

Deformation-based morphometry

Volz et al. (2000) used an interesting technique which they termed deformation-based morphometry (DBM). This can be viewed as a complementary method to VBM. They studied 75 patients with schizophrenia and 75 control subjects. Images were spatially transformed to standard space. However, rather than compare the image intensities at each voxel after transformation, they compared the low-frequency transformation vector maps for each subject. These vector maps described at each voxel the transformation or deformation field required to map a voxel of one brain onto its corresponding position in the template. To specify whether the change in each voxel was due to volume reduction or enlargement, they calculated the Jacobian determinant of the displacement vector. In the patients with schizophrenia, they found reduced volumes in the frontal lobe (superior frontal, middle and medial gyri), the left insula and superior temporal gyrus, the thalamus, the left cerebellar hemisphere and the right cerebellar vermis. There was an increase in volume in the right putamen. They argued that the deformation method allowed the detection of small subtle changes that may be invisible to manual segmentation procedures. However, they also acknowledged limitations of the technique. Regions where the variance of the deformation is high, e.g. in CSF, have the lowest sensitivity for detecting changes. This may be the reason why they were not able to detect ventricular enlargement in patients with schizophrenia compared with controls. Again, this highlights the point that global brain-image analytic techniques are vulnerable to Type 2 error problems. Their spatial vision is selective: they can identify some regions of change but risk missing others.

Gaser et al. (2001) compared DBM to semi-manual tracing of brain ventricles in 39 patients with schizophrenia. High-resolution T1-weighted MR scans were obtained and processed first with DBM and second with interactive tracing software. They evaluated the validity of the DBM by two different approaches. First, they divided subjects into two groups based on the mean ventricular/brain ratios and computed statistical maps of displacement vectors and their spatial derivatives. This analysis demonstrated consistency of the DBM and visual tracing results.

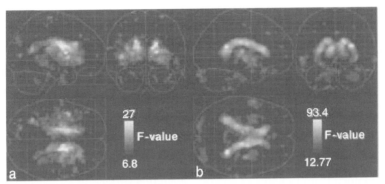

Figure 5.4   Maximum intensity projections (MIP) of categorical comparison of subgroups (24 vs. 15 patients) using deformation-based morphometry with the multivariate (image a; 3-variate F test with degrees of freedom of 3, 35) and the univariate Jacobian approach (image b; univariate F test with degrees of freedom of 1, 37). In both tests, only voxels with a threshold for significance of $P < 0.001$ are displayed. From Gaser et al. 2001.

They also showed that restricting the information about the deformation fields by computing the local Jacobian determinant (as a measure of volume change) provided evidence of the shape of ventricular deformation that was unavailable from ventricular volume measures alone (Figure 5.4). Second, they computed a mean measure of the Jacobian values over the entire ventricles and observed a correlation of $r = 0.96$ with visual tracing based ventricular/brain ratios. They concluded that their results supported the usefulness and validity of DBM for the local and global examination of brain morphology.

A number of ROI studies suggested that the size of the amygdala–hippocampal complex was reduced in schizophrenia. Csernansky et al. (1998) investigated whether one part of the hippocampus was more affected than the rest by examining shape changes. Their method (derived from principles of fluid mechanics) used transformations of a neuroanatomical template to the hippocampi within each brain. They compared MR scans from 15 patients with schizophrenia and 15 control subjects. There were shape differences between the two groups. In the patients with schizophrenia, the superior and lateral aspects of the hippocampal head were deformed on both the left and right sides. The authors suggested that since this subregion of the hippocampus was responsible for sending projections to the medial prefrontal cortex, their data provided support for the hypothesis that schizophrenia involves a disturbance of the connections between medial temporal and prefrontal cortical structures. More recently, this group investigated hippocampal asymmetry in schizophrenia (Wang et al. 2001). They were able to identify previously unknown patterns of local asymmetries, and to detect group differences in asymmetry localized to the subiculum.

The Laboratory of Neuroimaging (LONI) at UCLA, USA, has developed a number of algorithms for mapping local differences in cortical sulci, and structures such as the hippocampus, amygdala and corpus callosum (Thompson et al. 1996). Images are first scaled into standard stereotactic space. Structures or cortical sulci are manually traced. These outlines are then transformed into meshes of dense points, akin to a net being stretched over the object of interest. By matching corresponding points, it is possible both to quantify within-group variability and to test for between-group differences in shape parameters. As well as modelling shape parameters, a number of other potentially interesting geometric properties can be obtained from this sort of analysis, including surface area, curvature, asymmetry and cortical complexity.

Narr et al. (2000) applied this sort of analysis to study the corpus callosum in a group of patients with schizophrenia and normal controls. Their results showed shape differences between male patients and controls, with increased curvature of the corpus callosum in the patients, reflecting upward 'bowing'. They also noted gender differences in the degree of variability of corpus callosum shape. Narr et al. (2001*a*) extended this approach to the study of temporal lobe structures in schizophrenia. People with schizophrenia had local abnormalities in the posterior hippocampus, unexpected increases in amygdala volumes, but no differences in the superior temporal gyrus.

Lastly, Narr et al. (2001*b*) investigated overall cortical structure in 25 people with schizophrenia, compared with 25 controls. Curves following 12 major sulci (e.g. central sulcus, precentral sulcus) were outlined manually on magnified cortical surface models, in order to investigate their shape profile and asymmetry. They also applied a technique called 'surface based modelling', that extracts a very accurate map of the cortical surface of each subject. They parcellated each brain into four major lobar regions – superior frontal, inferior frontal, temporal and occipitoparietal – and used the cortical surface maps to study cortical complexity, which they measured by the frequency of sulcal/gyral convolutions. They found that the patients showed greater variability in frontal areas than the comparison subjects. Patients also had significant deviations in gyral complexity and asymmetry in the superior frontal regions. They argued that cortical variability and complexity identified regional abnormalities in the frontal cortex which were potentially specific to schizophrenia.

Complexity studies

The question of cortical complexity is potentially important to the study of schizophrenia. Formation of sulcal/gyral patterns occurs during prenatal development. Therefore, abnormal sulcal curvature or cortical complexity provides strong evidence for neurodevelopmental theories of structural brain changes in schizophrenia.

Bullmore et al. (1994) used fractal analysis to measure the complexity of the grey–white boundary in MR images. They measured the fractal dimension of the grey–white boundary in a study which included MR scans from 39 patients with schizophrenia and 31 control subjects. The mean fractal dimension was significantly reduced in patients with schizophrenia compared with control subjects. Bullmore et al. (1995) studied the 'radius of gyration' of the grey/white matter boundary within brain slices. The radius of gyration (Rg) is a statistic that has been widely used in engineering, physical and biological sciences to describe the extent to which points in a structure are dispersed about that structure's centre of gravity. Although there were no significant differences in Rg between 60 patients with schizophrenia and 36 control subjects, there were abnormal asymmetries of Rg in the male patients with schizophrenia.

Kulynych et al. (1997) postulated that schizophrenia caused an abnormality of cortical development resulting in a global reduction in cortical gyrification. They measured this using the gyrification index (GI – the ratio of the total to the superficially exposed cortical surface). They examined the GI in the left hemispheres of nine patients with schizophrenia and nine controls. They found significant reduction in the gyrification index in the schizophrenic patients, both in the frontal and posterior parts of the brain. Vogeley et al. (2001) measured the GI bilaterally in the prefrontal region. They studied 12 affected–unaffected sibling pairs from families multiply affected with schizophrenia or schizoaffective disorder. They found that the mean GI on the right side was significantly higher in siblings with schizophrenia or schizoaffective disorder than the unaffected siblings. They argued that this provided further support for a neurodevelopmental mechanism in the pathogenesis of schizophrenia.

The contribution of shape, deformation and complexity studies

Shape and deformation studies have some origins in dysmorphology, i.e. the characteristic deviations in physical features, for example, facial changes in certain genetic disorders. They have the potential to identify structural brain changes in schizophrenia which involve changes in spatial relationships rather than size changes. The paper by Deutsch et al. (2000) is particularly interesting by providing a strong theoretical model linking embryological development, via neurodevelopment, to structural pathology.

Landmark-based morphometry is dependent on the identification of homologous landmarks present in all brains. Identification of these landmarks is obviously susceptible to some degree of operator bias. The acceptance of the results of LBM will depend on either the acceptance of a standard atlas of landmarks to be used in replication studies, or the automation of the landmark-based approach.

The high-dimensional registration analyses typified by the studies of Csernansky et al. (1998) and Narr et al. (2000) offer the opportunity to identify structural abnormalities at the millimetre level. However, these methods are clearly exquisitely sensitive to the accuracy of manual tracings (where used), as they require expert knowledge of neuroanatomy to accurately delineate structures. Additionally, as with other methods described in this chapter, it will be difficult to bring together results from different studies.

Deformation-based morphometry may be viewed as a variation of automated LBM, with the advantage that it uses the global landmarks of the template image. DBM represents an analytic corollary to VBM, and it remains to be seen whether it will provide 'added value' in comparison with VBM analyses. The test will come when VBM and DBM analyses are performed on identical data. DBM, as thus far applied to schizophrenia, has only used low-frequency deformation fields. These low-frequency fields are capable of modelling only global shape differences. Therefore, it may only detect fairly large structural abnormalities, while missing more subtle changes. Whole-brain high-dimensional registration algorithms can model very local shape changes (Ashburner and Friston 2000), but they are computationally intensive, and have yet to be applied to the study of psychiatric disorders. One area in which DBM analyses may be important is in replacing ROI measurement with an automated technique. The results of Gaser et al. (2001) suggest that the tedious measurement of ROIs could be replaced by automatic parcellation of a template brain (for example, as described by Wright et al. 1999b) and computation of the mean Jacobian values over each parcellated ROI. This technique would have the potential to rejuvenate ROI studies within the field of structural analysis.

Multivariate analyses

Imaging studies, whether examining shape or size changes, have indicated that structural changes in schizophrenia are present in multiple brain regions. If this is the case, then can they be anatomically characterized as an abnormality at a supraregional level of brain organization?

A supraregional analysis is attractive for the investigation of brain changes in schizophrenia for two theoretical reasons. First, several theories of schizophrenia propose that the disorder results from pathological change in circuits of anatomically interconnected brain regions (Friston and Frith 1995). Second, there is considerable evidence in support of neurodevelopmental models for the pathogenesis of schizophrenia (Murray and Lewis 1987; Weinberger 1995). Since supraregional systems in biomorphological structures often share common developmental influences (Cheverud 1984), these systems may constitute the natural units for measuring subtle developmental abnormalities. Therefore a supraregional analysis of brain structure is relevant to both dysconnection and neurodevelopmental models of schizophrenia.

A supraregional analysis may reveal an underlying pattern of covariance in structural imaging data – a latent structure. Tien et al. (1996) noted that in the field of psychology the main tool for uncovering latent structures has been factor analysis. For example, analysis of population data from certain psychological tests by factor analysis has been interpreted in terms of latent structures relating to intelligence and personality traits such as extraversion. The same tool has been applied to imaging studies.

Cannon et al. (1989) postulated that patients with schizophrenia were subject to two possible aetiological factors: a genetic risk associated with distributed structural brain changes and birth complications associated with periventricular structural brain changes. To investigate this hypothesis, they performed CT scans on 34 subjects from a 'high-risk' sample (offspring of mothers with schizophrenia). Ten were diagnosed with schizophrenia, 10 with schizotypal personality disorder and 14 had no mental illness. They analysed six measurements on the CT scans including the Sylvian fissure, interhemispheric fissure, cortical sulci, third ventricle, ventricle–brain ratio and cerebellar vermis. They applied factor analysis to these measures and then related the factors to variables such as family history of schizophrenia and obstetric complication score. The first two factors accounted for over 60% of the variance. They interpreted the first factor as representing multisite neural deficits as reflected in abnormalities of the cerebellar vermis and widening of the Sylvian fissure, interhemispheric fissure and cortical sulci. The second factor was composed primarily of the ventricular measurements (third ventricle, and ventricle–brain ratio). The first factor correlated with genetic risk for schizophrenia while the second factor correlated with genetic risk, delivery complications and birth weight. These findings provided support for their hypotheses.

Tien et al. (1996) applied factor analysis to MR data from 44 patients with schizophrenia and 60 control subjects. The volumes of the superior temporal gyrus, medial temporal regions (amygdala, parahippocampal cortex, entorhinal cortex, hippocampus), basal ganglia regions (caudate, putamen, globus pallidus) and dorsolateral prefrontal cortex were measured by ROI methods. The authors considered two hypotheses regarding the factor structure of the schizophrenia and control data: (i) covariance structures were the same but sizes were different for some regions; (ii) the covariance structures were different because the brain areas that were larger (or smaller) in schizophrenia formed a factor that was not found in normal subjects. They found that the covariance structures of the schizophrenia and control groups were different. There seemed to be more overlap in the schizophrenia data between left–right pairs of items, for example left and right caudate loading onto the same factor as left and right superior temporal gyrus. The authors suggested that these abnormalities may reflect pathology in functional brain circuits involving these regions.

Wright et al. (1999b) argued that anatomical structures can generally be deconstructed into supraregional systems by principal components analysis (PCA) of the covariances or correlations in size between their regional elements (Olson and Miller 1958). Therefore they investigated whether PCA applied to regional brain measures would extract structural components which could be interpreted in terms of normal brain architecture and function and whether schizophrenia and control groups differed according to these 'normative' components. The authors used singular value decomposition of multiple regional measurements on MRI data from 64 subjects (37 patients with familial schizophrenia and 27 control subjects). They identified five principal components that collectively accounted for around 70% of total variance–covariance in the data. The patients with schizophrenia differed from controls in their scores on the two of these five components: a global change in grey matter/ventricular system and a frontotemporal system. The authors argued that since the variance components associated with these PCs were, by definition, orthogonal, this suggested that at least two processes of structural change were involved in schizophrenia.

The contribution of multivariate analyses

We have only reviewed three studies investigating brain structure in schizophrenia using multivariate analysis. This is an indication that it is an emergent field of research. It addresses the need to draw together the pattern of structural changes in schizophrenia into a meaningful whole. However, the studies so far utilize different approaches and should be viewed as exploratory, demonstrating methodologies rather than substantive results (unless they are subsequently replicated). The first major problem for these studies is that the most appropriate multivariate model for investigating the pathology of schizophrenia is unknown; therefore there is no guarantee that the model tested in a particular study is the most appropriate one. In the future, as more becomes known about the general relationships between brain pathology and brain structural change, it may become clearer which models are most useful to test. Wright et al. (1999b) suggested that it would be interesting to investigate other multivariate methods, such as path analysis (McIntosh et al. 1994) or the comparison of covariance matrices (Lofsvold 1986; Paulsen 1994), which might be able to account for the observed correlations between multiple brain regions measured from adult imaging data in terms of pre-existing theories of brain organization or development.

The second major problem is that it requires large samples and these have not generally been available. If larger samples become available, either through larger studies or pooling of data between studies, then testing sophisticated pathological models will become more realistic.

Genetic analyses

There is evidence from twin and family studies that the heritability of schizophrenia is high (around 65–85%), indicating the importance of genes in determining the variability of the disorder within the population. There is currently an intensive search for genes determining liability to schizophrenia. Researchers have also attempted to combine genetic information with structural-imaging data in order to establish the links between genes, pathology and symptoms in schizophrenia.

Twin studies

Twin studies provide a method to investigate genetic and environmental contributions to phenotypic variability. Whereas monozygotic twins have identical genotypes, dizygotic twins share only 50% of their genotype on average, permitting quantitative assessment of the genetic contribution to the phenotype (subject to a number of important assumptions). Twin studies have found that in normal subjects, cerebral volume, hemispheric volume (Bartley et al. 1997) and ventricular volume (Reveley et al. 1984) were highly heritable. This, and the evidence for structural brain changes in schizophrenia, suggests that brain structural measures may have a role as proxy measures for pathology in genetic studies of schizophrenia – such measures are known as 'endophenotypes'. Endophenotypic measures have some theoretical advantages in quantitative genetic studies over diagnostic status or symptomatology because they may represent more sensitive markers of underlying liability status. The potential value of structural endophenotypic markers has so far been limited by the difficulty of scanning the large numbers of subjects required for genetic studies.

Twin studies have been used to investigate the relative contributions of genetic and nongenetic factors to structural brain abnormalities in schizophrenia. These investigations have been based on the assumption that relatives of probands with schizophrenia share a genetic predisposition (varying according to their genetic relationship) but do not manifest the disorder because of a combination of genetic and nongenetic factors. For discordant monozygotic twins, who have (in theory) identical genotypes, discordance presumably results from environmental or epigenetic factors.

Noga et al. (1996) investigated 13 monozygotic twin pairs discordant for schizophrenia and nine normal monozygotic pairs. They measured brain hemisphere length, area and volume. They found that hemisphere volumes in the affected twin in the discordant pairs were significantly smaller bilaterally by about 3% compared with their unaffected co-twins, who did not differ from normal twins on this measure. This finding was consistent with previous reports of smaller brain size in schizophrenia and it suggested that the abnormality had, at least in part, an environmental origin. They also visually examined and rated the brains for developmental gyral abnormalities such as vertical temporal gyri or microgyria. These ratings did not differ between affected or unaffected discordant twins and normal twins. They concluded that if cortical maldevelopment is associated with schizophrenia it does not appear to disrupt gross gyral pattern formation.

Baare et al. (2001) carried out MR imaging on 15 monozygotic and 14 same-sex dizygotic twins discordant for schizophrenia and 29 healthy twins pair-wise matched for zygosity, sex, age and birth order. Irrespective of zygosity, discordant twins had smaller whole-brain (2%), parahippocampal (9%) and hippocampal (8%) volumes than healthy twins. Moreover, schizophrenics had smaller whole-brain volumes (2.2%) than their nonschizophrenic co-twins, who in turn had smaller brains (1%) than healthy twins. Lateral and third-ventricle volumes were increased in discordant dizygotic twins as compared with healthy dizygotic twins (60.6% and 56.6%, respectively). Finally, within discordant twins, lateral ventricles were larger (14.4%) in schizophrenics than in their nonschizophrenic co-twins. They concluded that smaller intracranial volumes in the monozygotic schizophrenics and their co-twins suggest that increased genetic risk to develop schizophrenia is related to reduced brain growth early in life. The additional reduction in whole-brain volume found in the schizophrenic twins suggests that the manifestation of the disorder is related to (neurodegenerative) processes that are most likely nongenetic in origin.

Family studies

The role of genetic factors has also been examined by several family studies. These have investigated probands with schizophrenia, their unaffected siblings and matched control subjects. For example, Cannon et al. (1998) found that both patients with schizophrenia and their full siblings showed significant reductions in frontal and temporal grey matter volumes compared with controls. Increased ventricular CSF volume and reduced white matter volume were found in the patients with schizophrenia but not their unaffected siblings. They concluded that this pattern of results suggests that frontal and temporal lobe grey matter reductions may reflect the influence of genetic (or shared environmental) factors whereas ventricular enlargement reflects environmental (nonshared) factors.

Association studies

The 'solution' to the problem of structural change in schizophrenia will probably define schizophrenia as a polygenic disorder, identify the relevant liability genes, characterize their influence on brain structure and determine the neurochemical mechanisms and neural systems by which they modify neurodevelopment or cause neurodegeneration. Unfortunately, this will not be achieved until the susceptibility genes for schizophrenia have been identified, and as yet they remain elusive. Until then, there are some studies of other disorders that provide models for future schizophrenia studies. For example, Eliez et al. (2000) have investigated structural brain changes in velo-cardio-facial syndrome. In most patients this results from a deletion of chromosome 22q11.2. Ten to twenty per cent of patients developed a psychiatric illness by the time they reached adulthood and in most cases the diagnosis was chronic paranoid schizophrenia (Shprintzen 2000). The clinical features of the disorder include cardiac malformations, cleft palate or velopharyngeal insufficiency, a characteristic facial appearance and learning difficulties. Eliez et al. (2000) investigated brain MR measurements in 15 children with velo-cardio-facial syndrome and 15 control subjects. Regional measurements were carried out by semi-automated methods. They found that in the patient group total brain volume was reduced by 11% but frontal lobe volumes were relatively spared. They suggested that velo-cardio-facial syndrome may have a characteristic pattern of regional brain changes related to the language and learning difficulties associated with the syndrome.

A study by Vargha-Khadem et al. (1998) of a family with an inherited verbal dyspraxia (associated with low IQ) provides a model for future schizophrenia studies. In this case the genetic abnormality had been localized to a 5.6-centiMorgan interval in the chromosomal band 7q31 (Fisher et al. 1998). The gene had autosomal dominant inheritance with full penetrance. They applied VBM to 34 MR scans from 17 family members (10 affected and 7 unaffected) and 17 control subjects. They also measured caudate nucleus volumes in these images using standard ROI techniques. In addition they used PET to investigate two affected family members and four normal control subjects during performance of verbal tasks. The PET study revealed functional abnormalities in both cortical and subcortical motor-related areas of the frontal lobe. The VBM analysis of MR scans revealed structural abnormalities in several of these same areas, particularly the caudate nucleus where grey matter was reduced in the affected relatives. ROI analysis confirmed that it was abnormally small bilaterally. Thus the authors integrated structural and functional imaging results with neuropsychology in a genetically well-characterized sample.

The contribution of genetic analyses

The structural analysis of twin studies has been an important influence on researchers' understanding of structural brain changes in schizophrenia, especially the study by Suddath et al. (1990). Nevertheless, twins are an atypical group of subjects and the interpretation of twin results according to genetic models depends on a number of assumptions, whose validity has been questioned (Phillips 1993).

As more twin and family studies are published there will be a need to integrate their results. Meta-analysis of ROI results will provide the first step in this integration. In the longer term, association studies are likely to become increasingly important, but this will depend on the clearer identification of schizophrenia-susceptibility loci.

The time dimension: longitudinal studies

Theories of the time course of structural brain abnormalities in schizophrenia fall into two main camps. Some authors have argued that brain changes are principally neurodevelopmental in origin, and reflect a 'static encephalopathy' (Raedler et al. 1998). These may reflect either genetic effects (Seidman et al. 1999) or environmental factors such as obstetric complications (Stefanis et al. 1999). Others have argued that brain changes are at least partially progressive in nature. The possibility of continuing brain changes after the onset of psychosis is not merely of scientific interest. If there is progressive neurodegenerative change – at least in a minority of schizophrenic patients – it may well have important clinical and cognitive correlates.

Most of the studies we have described this far have been cross-sectional, comparing brain structure in patients with schizophrenia with control subjects at one time point. Studies of patients early in their psychotic illness avoid potential confounds including medication effects, long-term institutionalization and possible neurodegenerative change. Although structural changes in patients with first-episode schizophrenia compared with chronic schizophrenia provide some indication as to whether the brain changes are static or progressive, several studies have attempted to investigate this question by rescanning patients and controls after a time interval.

Since ventricular enlargement is one of the best-established structural brain changes in schizophrenia and is of large magnitude, ventricular size has been the focus of several longitudinal studies. Vita et al. (1997) reviewed CT studies by their research group. In one study of 21 patients over 3 years, no change was seen in the ventricle–brain ratio at the time of the second scan. In a second sample, of nine patients who were scanned during their first episode of schizophrenia and rescanned 2–4 years later, again, there was no increase in ventricle–brain ratios. They concluded that ventricular enlargement remains stable, even in the initial phases of the disease. Conversely, Saijo et al. (2001) obtained MR scans in 15 schizophrenics and 12 controls at baseline and after 4- and 10-year follow-ups. After 10 years, a significant lateral ventricular enlargement was found in patients (mean percentage change: +22.9%) but not in controls (5.1%). They suggested that their results provided strong evidence that in schizophrenia progressive ventricular change occurs even in its chronic stage. Davis et al. (1998) obtained CT scans 4 years apart of a group of subjects with schizophrenia. One group termed 'Kraepelinian' on the basis of low social functioning and self-care, showed a marked increase in ventricular size over the 4 years. In contrast, the second group, termed 'Non-Kraepelinian' showed no significant change in ventricular size. Madsen et al. (1998) obtained serial CT scans of a group of initially drug-naïve patients with schizophrenia. After 5 years they noted significant frontal cortical atrophy. This was not related to illness progression, but surprisingly was associated with increasing dose of typical neuroleptic drugs.

More recently, Lieberman et al. (2001) obtained MRI scans for 107 patients in their first episode of schizophrenia or schizoaffective disorder and 20 healthy volunteers and clinical assessments for periods of up to 6 years. Their results confirmed the findings of ventricular enlargement and anterior hippocampal volume reductions in first-episode schizophrenia patients that have been previously reported. Consistent with the study of Davies et al. (1998), they found increases in ventricular volume that were associated with poor-outcome patients. Contrary to their hypothesis, there were no significant reductions in cortical and hippocampal volumes over time. Mathalon et al. (2001) studied brain structure in a group of patients with schizophrenia over a 4-year period. They observed progressive reductions in frontal and superior temporal lobe grey matter, and increasing volumes of frontal and temporal sulci. Rates of grey matter loss and sulcal expansion were associated with greater illness severity.

Although these studies offer strong evidence of some progressive change in brain structure in schizophrenia, they are limited in the information they provide. Longitudinal changes in regional volumes are subject to the same limitations as cross-sectional ROI studies, in terms of accurately mapping anatomical changes. One alternative is to look for local changes within individual subjects. For example, Puri et al. (2001) used subvoxel registration of serial MRI scans in first-episode schizophrenia to map changes in ventricular size. They coregistered subjects' serial scans together, and then used image subtraction to identify local changes. They examined baseline and follow-up (on average 8 months later) MRI scans from 24 patients with first-episode schizophrenia and 12 control subjects. They found no differences between patients and controls in mean change in ventricular volume. Although in a proportion of patients they found ventricular enlargement (supporting other studies indicating an ongoing neuropathological process in the early stages of schizophrenia), the reduction of ventricular size in the remaining patients was more difficult to explain. They suggested that this may reflect improvement in nutrition and hydration in those subjects following treatment.

In a recent advance, Thompson et al. (2001) conducted a sophisticated analysis of progressive cortical change in children with early-onset schizophrenia. They obtained three MR scans for 12 patients and 12 controls over a 5-year period. They accurately coregistered together maps of the cortex for each subject over three time points. The amount of grey matter at each voxel in the brain was calculated. By using a high-dimensional warping algorithm to exactly map subjects' individual cortical maps together, they calculated annual rates of grey matter change across the cortex. Individual subjects were mapped together into the same space, to facilitate group comparisons. The results showed a startling widespread progressive grey matter loss. They found that grey matter loss was first seen in parietal regions, but with increasing time, spread into frontal and temporal lobe regions, including the dorsolateral prefrontal cortex, and the superior temporal gyrus. Severity of positive symptoms was linked with the rate of temporal lobe grey matter loss, while negative symptoms were linked with the speed of frontal grey matter atrophy. These findings offer some tantalizing clues as to the origins and nature of structural brain changes in schizophrenia, and demonstrate the remarkable advances in computational neuroanatomy over the last two decades.

The contribution of longitudinal studies

Longitudinal studies have been used to investigate whether the structural pathology of schizophrenia is static or progressive after the onset of illness. As the results of these studies have been variable, there is a need to integrate their findings by meta-analytic techniques. One of the problems of these studies has been the presence of high variability in ROI measurements between baseline scan and rescan in individual subjects (in both patient and control groups). This suggests either that brain shape changes dynamically with time or that the measurement techniques used in these studies are not very reliable. The coregistration of individual subjects' serial scans (Puri et al. 2001; Thompson et al. 2001) should achieve more reliable measurement of structural changes over time and permit a better understanding of the factors influencing changes in brain shape. This technique may also be useful for identifying structural changes in individual subjects over time that may have prognostic or other clinical implications.

Conclusion

The progress of structural-imaging studies of schizophrenia during the last two decades has been characterized by two complementary developments. The first was the drive towards greater analytic sophistication in image analysis. The second was the attempt to integrate an ever-expanding and often confusing body of research findings. We would argue that these two developments have occurred in orthogonal rather than parallel directions, to the detriment of structural-imaging research.

Analytic sophistication has been pursued because of frustration with the limitations of the 'region-of-interest' approach which has been the main system of structural MR measurement since the 1980s. It is time consuming and of variable reliability because of the necessity for human intervention in interpreting the anatomical criteria. Usually only a few brain structures can be examined in each study because of the operator time required for measurement. Techniques to overcome these problems have tended to view the brain as a three-dimensional matrix amenable to spatial transformation and analysis. Increased automation of the analyses has improved reliability, reduced processing time and permitted a 'whole-brain' perspective on structural changes.

The integration of research findings has been attempted because of the difficulties of interpreting research using small samples to investigate effects of small magnitude. This has characterized the majority of structural-imaging studies of schizophrenia. The consequences were a confusing picture of inconsistent positive and negative findings and the unnecessary repetition of studies, wasting valuable resources, because of a failure to draw together the evidence from the previous literature. Meta-analyses have now been used to integrate the results of many ROI studies and may have some role in deterring researchers from unnecessary replication of established findings.

Unfortunately, whilst the more traditional ROI studies have been amenable to meta-analysis, the newer more sophisticated analytic techniques have been published in a form which is likely to resist integration with comparable studies. This is because the reports of newer techniques tend to summarize whole-brain results (comprising large data matrices) in a few tables or figures. Furthermore, there have been only limited efforts to compare results from different analytic techniques applied to the same data sets.

In the future, increasing utilization of the internet is likely to have important implications for structural-imaging research into schizophrenia. Already, a number of research groups make analytic programs available on web sites (Ashburner and Friston 2000; Mazziotta et al. 2001). Some published articles include extended data-sets on web sites (Wright et al. 2000). If more research groups publish raw data on web sites, this will permit much greater cross-validation of techniques as well as the integration of information from large samples. Automated analytic methods such as VBM and DBM will facilitate the rapid analysis of these large samples. Analysis of large samples may also allow meaningful genetic analyses, e.g. association studies determining the particular effect of single genes on brain morphometry. The identification of susceptibility genes for schizophrenia will lead to association studies to establish the effect of these genes on brain structure. Coregistration of structural and functional imaging data is likely to become increasingly a matter of routine. Finally, longitudinal studies of individual subjects using automated coregistration techniques may increase the importance of structural imaging in clinical practice, for example in determining subtle signs of regional neurodegeneration.

REFERENCES

Andreasen NC, Arndt S, Swayze V II et al. (1994). Thalamic abnormalities in schizophrenia visualized through magnetic resonance image averaging. *Science*, 14, 294–8.

Ashburner J and Friston KJ (2000). Voxel-based morphometry – the methods. *Neuroimage*, 6, 805–21.

Baare WF, van Oel CJ, Hulshoff Pol HE et al. (2001). Volumes of brain structures in twins discordant for schizophrenia. *Arch Gen Psychiatry*, 58, 33–40.

Barr WB, Ashtari M, Bilder RM, Degreef G and Lieberman JA (1997). Brain morphometric comparison of first-episode schizophrenia and temporal lobe epilepsy. *Br J Psychiatry*, 170, 515–19.

Bartley AJ, Jones DW, Torrey EF, Zigun JR and Weinberger DR (1993). Sylvian fissure asymmetries in monozygotic twins: a test of laterality in schizophrenia. *Biol Psychiatry*, 34, 853–63.

Bartley AJ, Jones DW and Weinberger DR (1997). Genetic variability of human brain size and cortical gyral patterns. *Brain*, 120, 257–69.

Bookstein FL (1995). How to produce a landmark point: the statistical geometry of incompletely registered images. In *Vision Geometry IV*. SPIE Proceedings, Vol. 2573, ed. R Matter, A Wu, F Bookstein and W Green, pp. 266–77. Bellingham, WA: SPIE Press.

Bookstein FL (1997). Landmark methods for forms without landmarks: morphometrics of group differences in outline shape. *Med Image Anal*, 1, 225–43.

Bookstein FL (2001). "Voxel-Based Morphometry" should not be used with imperfectly registered images. *Neuroimage*, 14, 1454–62.

Buckley PF, Dean D, Bookstein FL et al. (1999). Three-dimensional magnetic resonance-based morphometrics and ventricular dysmorphology in schizophrenia. *Biol Psychiatry*, 1, 62–7.

Bullmore E, Brammer M, Harvey I, Persaud R, Murray R and Ron M (1994). Fractal analysis of the boundary between white matter and cerebral cortex in magnetic resonance images: a controlled study of schizophrenic and manic-depressive patients. *Psychol Med*, 24, 771–81.

Bullmore E, Brammer M, Harvey I, Murray R and Ron M (1995). Cerebral hemispheric asymmetry revisited: effects of handedness, gender and schizophrenia measured by radius of gyration in magnetic resonance images. *Psychol Med*, 25, 349–63.

Bullmore ET, Suckling J, Overmeyer S, Rabe-Hesketh S, Taylor E and Brammer MJ (1999). Global, voxel, and cluster tests, by theory and permutation, for a difference between two groups of structural MR images of the brain. *IEEE Trans Med Imaging*, 18, 32–42.

Cannon TD, Mednick SA and Parnas J (1989). Genetic and perinatal determinants of structural brain deficits in schizophrenia. *Arch Gen Psychiatry*, 46, 883–9.

Cannon TD, van Erp TG, Huttunen M et al. (1998). Regional gray matter, white matter, and cerebrospinal fluid distributions in schizophrenic patients, their siblings, and controls. *Arch Gen Psychiatry*, 55, 1084–91.

Chakos MH, Lieberman JA, Bilder RM et al. (1994). Increase in caudate volumes of first-episode schizophrenic patients taking antipsychotic drugs. *Am J Psychiatry*, 151, 1430–6.

Cheverud JM (1984). Quantitative genetics and developmental constraints on evolution by selection. *J Theor Biol*, 110, 155–71.

Cooper H and Hedges LV (ed.) (1994). *The Handbook of Research Synthesis*. New York: Russell Sage Foundation.

Crow TJ, Ball J, Bloom SR et al. (1989). Schizophrenia as an anomaly of development of cerebral asymmetry. *Arch Gen Psychiatry*, 46, 1145–50.

Csernansky JG, Joshi S, Wang L et al. (1998). Hippocampal morphometry in schizophrenia by high dimensional brain mapping. *Proc Natl Acad Sci USA*, 95, 11406–11.

Davis KL, Buchsbaum MS, Shihabuddin L et al. (1998). Ventricular enlargement in poor-outcome schizophrenia. *Biol Psychiatry*, 43, 783–93.

DeQuardo JR, Bookstein FL, Green WDK, Brunberg JA and Tandon R (1996). Spatial relationships of the neuroanatomic landmarks in schizophrenia. *Psychiatry Res Neuroimaging*, 67, 81–95.

DeQuardo JR, Keshavan MS and Bookstein FL (1999). Landmark-based morphometric analysis of first-episode schizophrenia. *Biol Psychiatry*, 45, 1321–8.

Deutsch CK, Hobbs K, Price SF and Gordon-Vaugh K (2000). Skewing of the brain midline in schizophrenia. *Neuroreport*, 11, 3985–8.

Eliez S, Schmitt JE, White CD, Wellis VG and Reiss AL (2000). Children and adolescents with velocardiofacial syndrome: a volumetric MRI study. *Am J Psychiatry*, 157, 409–15.

Fisher SE, Vargha-Khadem F, Watkins KE, Monaco AP and Pembrey ME (1998). Localisation of a gene implicated in a severe speech and language disorder. *Nat Genet*, 18, 168–70.

Foucault M (1963). *The Birth of the Clinic*. (Translated from the French by AM Sheridan.) London: Tavistock Publications, 1986.

Friston K and Frith C (1995). Schizophrenia: a disconnection syndrome? *Clin Neurosci*, 3, 89–97.

Friston KJ, Ashburner J, Frith CD, Poline JB, Heather JD and Frackowiak RSJ (1995a). Spatial registration and normalization of images. *Hum Brain Mapp*, 2, 165–89.

Friston, KJ, Holmes AP, Worsley KJ, Poline JB, Frith CD and Frackowiak RSJ (1995b). Statistical parametric maps in functional imaging: a general approach. *Hum Brain Mapp*, 2, 189–210.

Gaser C, Nenadic I, Buchsbaum BR, Hazlett EA and Buchsbaum MS (2001). Deformation-based morphometry and its relation to conventional volumetry of brain lateral ventricles in MRI. *Neuroimage*, 6, 1140–5.

Gerschlager W, Lalouschek W, Lehrner J, Baumgartner C, Lindinger G and Lang W (1998). Language-related hemispheric asymmetry in healthy subjects and patients with temporal lobe epilepsy as studied by event-related brain potentials and intracarotid amobarbital test. *Electroencephalogr Clin Neurophysiol*, 108, 274–82.

Gharaibeh WS, Rohlf FJ, Slice DE and DeLisi LE (2000). A geometric morphometric assessment of change in midline brain structural shape following a first episode of schizophrenia. *Biol Psychiatry*, 48, 398–405.

Johnstone EC, Crow TJ, Frith CD, Husband J and Kreel L (1976). Cerebral ventricular size and cognitive impairment in chronic schizophrenia. *Lancet*, 2, 924–6.

Konick LC and Friedman L (2001). Meta-analysis of thalamic size in schizophrenia. *Biol Psychiatry*, 49, 28–38.

Krasuski JS, Alexander GE, Horwitz B et al. (1998). Volumes of medial temporal lobe structures in patients with Alzheimer's disease and mild cognitive impairment (and in healthy controls). *Biol Psychiatry*, 43, 60–8.

Kulynych JJ, Luevano LF, Jones DW and Weinberger DR (1997). Cortical abnormality in schizophrenia: an in vivo application of the gyrification index. *Biol Psychiatry*, 41, 995–9.

Lawrie SM and Abukmeil SS (1998). Brain abnormality in schizophrenia. A systematic and quantitative review of volumetric magnetic resonance imaging studies. *Br J Psychiatry*, 172, 110–20.

Lieberman J, Chakos M, Wu H et al. (2001). Longitudinal study of brain morphology in first episode schizophrenia. *Biol Psychiatry*, 49, 487–99.

Lofsvold D (1986). Quantitative genetics of morphological differentiation in Peromyscus. I. Tests of the homogeneity of genetic covariance structure among species and subspecies. *Evolution*, 40, 559–73.

Lohr JB and Caligiuri MP (1997). Lateralized hemispheric dysfunction in the major psychotic disorders: historical perspectives and findings from a study of motor asymmetry in older patients. *Schizophr Res*, 27, 191–8.

Madsen AL, Keidling N, Karle A, Esbjerg S and Hemmingsen R (1998). Neuroleptics in progressive structural brain abnormalities in psychiatric illness. *Lancet*, 352, 784–5.

Mathalon DH, Sullivan EV, Lim KO and Pfefferbaum A (2001). Progressive brain volume changes and the clinical course of schizophrenia in men: a longitudinal magnetic resonance imaging study. *Arch Gen Psychiatry*, 58, 148–57.

May A, Ashburner J, Buchel C et al. (1999). Correlation between structural and functional changes in brain in an idiopathic headache syndrome. *Nat Med*, 5, 836–8.

Mazziotta J, Toga A, Evans A et al. (2001). A probabilistic atlas and reference system for the human brain: International Consortium for Brain Mapping (ICBM). *Philos Trans R Soc Lond B Biol Sci*, 356, 1293–322.

McIntosh A, Grady C, Ungerleider L, Haxby JV, Rapoport SI and Horwitz B (1994). Network analysis of cortical visual pathways mapped with PET. *J Neurosci*, 14, 655–66.

Murray RM and Lewis SW (1987). Is schizophrenia a neurodevelopmental disorder? *Br Med J*, 295, 681–2.

Narr KL, Thompson PM, Sharma T, Moussai J, Cannestra AF and Toga AW (2000). Mapping morphology of the corpus callosum in schizophrenia. *Cereb Cortex*, 10, 40–9.

Narr KL, Thompson PM, Sharma T et al. (2001*a*). Three-dimensional mapping of temporo-limbic regions and the lateral ventricles in schizophrenia: gender effects. *Biol Psychiatry*, 50, 84–97.

Narr K, Thompson P, Sharma T et al. (2001*b*). Three-dimensional mapping of gyral shape and cortical surface asymmetries in schizophrenia: gender effects. *Am J Psychiatry*, 158, 244–55.

Nelson MD, Saykin AJ, Flashman LA and Riordan HJ (1998). Hippocampal volume reduction in schizophrenia as assessed by magnetic resonance imaging: a meta-analytic study. *Arch Gen Psychiatry*, 55, 433–40.

Noga JT, Bartley AJ, Jones DW, Torrey EF and Weinberger DR (1996). Cortical gyral anatomy and gross brain dimensions in monozygotic twins discordant for schizophrenia. *Schizophr Res*, 22, 27–40.

Olson E and Miller R (1958). *Morphological Integration.* Chicago: University of Chicago Press.

Paillere-Martinot M, Caclin A, Artiges E et al. (2001). Cerebral gray and white matter reductions and clinical correlates in patients with early onset schizophrenia. *Schizophr Res*, 50, 19–26.

Paulsen SM (1994). Quantitative genetics of butterfly wing color patterns. *Dev Genet*, 15, 79–81.

Phillips CIW (1993). Twin studies in medical research: can they tell us whether diseases are genetically determined? *Lancet*, 341, 1008–9.

Puri BK, Hutton SB, Saeed N et al. (2001). A serial longitudinal quantitative MRI study of cerebral changes in first-episode schizophrenia using image segmentation and subvoxel registration. *Psychiatry Res*, 106, 141–50.

Raedler TJ, Knable MB and Weinberger DR (1998). Schizophrenia as a developmental disorder of the cerebral cortex. *Curr Opin Neurobiol*, 8, 157–61.

Raz S, Raz N and Bigler ED (1988). Ventriculomegaly in schizophrenia: is the choice of controls important? *Psychiatry Res*, 24, 71–7.

Reveley AM, Reveley MA, Chitkara B and Clifford C (1984). The genetic basis of cerebral ventricular volume. *Psychiatry Res*, 13, 261–6.

Richardson MP, Friston KJ, Sisodiya SM et al. (1997). Cortical grey matter and benzodiazepine receptors in malformations of cortical development: a voxel-based comparison of structural and functional imaging data. *Brain*, 120, 1961–73.

Saijo T, Abe T, Someya Y et al. (2001). Ten year progressive ventricular enlargement in schizophrenia: an MRI morphometrical study. *Psychiatry Clin Neurosci*, 55, 41–7.

Seidman LJ, Faraone SV, Goldstein JM et al. (1999). Thalamic and amygdala-hippocampal volume reductions in first-degree relatives of patients with schizophrenia: an MRI-based morphometric analysis. *Biol Psychiatry*, 46, 941–54.

Shah PJ, Ebmeier KP, Glabus MF and Goodwin GM (1998). Cortical grey matter reductions associated with treatment-resistant chronic unipolar depression. Controlled magnetic resonance imaging study. *Br J Psychiatry*, 172, 527–32.

Shapleske J, Rossell SL, Woodruff PW and David AS (1999). The planum temporale: a systematic, quantitative review of its structural, functional and clinical significance. *Brain Res Brain Res Rev*, 29, 26–49.

Shprintzen RJ (2000). Velo-cardio-facial syndrome: a distinctive behavioral phenotype. *Ment Retard Dev Disabil Res Rev*, 6, 142–7.

Sigmundsson T, Suckling J, Maier M et al. (2001). Structural abnormalities in frontal, temporal, and limbic regions and interconnecting white matter tracts in schizophrenic patients with prominent negative symptoms. *Am J Psychiatry*, 158, 234–43.

Sommer I, Ramsey N, Kahn R, Aleman A and Bouma A (2001). Handedness, language lateralisation and anatomical asymmetry in schizophrenia: meta-analysis. *Br J Psychiatry*, 178, 344–51.

Stefanis N, Frangou S, Yakeley J et al. (1999). Hippocampal volume reduction in schizophrenia: effects of genetic risk and pregnancy and birth complications. *Biol Psychiatry*, 46, 697–702.

Suddath RL, Christison GW, Torrey EF, Casanova MF and Weinberger DR (1990). Anatomical abnormalities in the brains of monozygotic twins discordant for schizophrenia. *N Engl J Med*, 322, 789–94.

Talairach J and Tournoux P (1988). *Co-planar Stereotaxic Atlas of the Human Brain.* Stuttgart: Thieme Verlag.

Thompson PM and Toga AW (1997). Detection, visualization and animation of abnormal anatomic structure with a deformable probabilistic brain atlas based on random vector field transformations. *Med Image Anal*, 1, 271–94.

Thompson PM, Schwartz C, Lin RT, Khan AA and Toga AW (1996). Three-dimensional statistical analysis of sulcal variability in the human brain. *J Neurosci*, 16, 4261–74.

Thompson PM, Vidal C, Giedd JN et al. (2001). Mapping adolescent brain change reveals dynamic wave of accelerated gray matter loss in very early-onset schizophrenia. *Proc Natl Acad Sci USA*, 98, 11650–5.

Tien AY, Eaton WW, Schlaepfer TE et al. (1996). Exploratory factor analysis of MRI brain structure measures in schizophrenia. *Schizophr Res*, 19, 93–101.

Van Horn JD and McManus IC (1992). Ventricular enlargement in schizophrenia. A meta-analysis of studies of the ventricle:brain ratio (VBR). *Br J Psychiatry*, 160, 687–97.

Vargha-Khadem F, Watkins KE, Price CJ et al. (1998). Neural basis of an inherited speech and language disorder. *Proc Natl Acad Sci USA*, 95, 12695–700.

Vita A, Dieci M, Giobbio GM, Tenconi F and Invernizzi G (1997). Time course of cerebral ventricular enlargement in schizophrenia supports the hypothesis of its neurodevelopmental nature. *Schizophr Res*, 23, 25–30.

Vogeley K, Tepest R, Pfeiffer U et al. (2001). Right frontal hypergyria differentiation in affected and unaffected siblings from families multiply affected with schizophrenia: a morphometric MRI study. *Am J Psychiatry*, 158, 494–6.

Volz H, Gaser C and Sauer H (2000). Supporting evidence for the model of cognitive dysmetria in schizophrenia – a structural magnetic resonance imaging study using deformation-based morphometry. *Schizophr Res*, 46, 45–56.

Wang L, Joshi SC, Miller MI and Csernansky JG (2001). Statistical analysis of hippocampal asymmetry in schizophrenia. *Neuroimage*, 14, 531–45.

Ward KE, Friedman L, Wise A and Schulz SC (1996). Meta-analysis of brain and cranial size in schizophrenia. *Schizophr Res*, 22, 197–213.

Weinberger DR (1995). From neuropathology to neurodevelopment. *Lancet*, 346, 552–7.

Wolkin A, Rusinek H, Vaid G et al. (1998). Structural magnetic resonance image averaging in schizophrenia. *Am J Psychiatry*, 155, 1064–73.

Woodruff PW, McManus IC and David AS (1995). Meta-analysis of corpus callosum size in schizophrenia. *J Neurol Neurosurg Psychiatry*, 58, 457–61.

Wright IC, McGuire PK, Poline J-B et al. (1995). A voxel-based method for the statistical analysis of grey and white matter applied to schizophrenia. *Neuroimage*, 2, 244–52.

Wright IC, Ellison ZR, Sharma T, Friston KJ, Murray RM and McGuire PK (1999*a*). Mapping of grey matter changes in schizophrenia. *Schizophr Res*, 35, 1–14.

Wright IC, Sharma T, Ellison ZR et al. (1999*b*). Supra-regional brain systems and the neuro-pathology of schizophrenia. *Cereb Cortex*, 9, 366–78.

Wright IC, Rabe-Hesketh S, Woodruff PW, David AS, Murray RM and Bullmore ET (2000). Meta-analysis of regional brain volumes in schizophrenia. *Am J Psychiatry*, 157, 16–25.

6

The application of neuropathologically sensitive MRI techniques to the study of psychosis

Maria A Ron and Jacqueline Foong

Institute of Neurology, University College London, London, UK

Introduction

Magnetic resonance imaging (MRI) has become the technique of choice to study subtle structural brain abnormalities and its value is well established in psychiatric research. Early studies aimed at detecting diffuse volumetric changes in patient populations have recently been superseded by advances in image analysis (e.g. voxel-based morphometry) that make it possible to detect minor, but functionally significant, focal volumetric changes (see Chapter 5 by Chitnis and Ellison-Wright). The yield of conventional MRI for psychiatry is not yet exhausted, but even with the help of sophisticated methods of image analysis some drawbacks will always limit its value. The first of these drawbacks is the lack of pathological specificity that makes it impossible to separate such diverse pathological processes as oedema, inflammation or gliosis. The second, especially relevant to psychiatry, is the fact that neuropathological abnormalities, whether developmental or degenerative, can be detected only when they are severe enough to cause loss of volume. These limitations make the use of these MRI techniques compelling, because of their potential to provide more specific neuropathological information and their ability to detect abnormalities invisible on conventional MRI. The two main techniques are magnetization transfer imaging (MTI) and diffusion tensor imaging (DTI). Here we describe these techniques, the neuropathological insights they can provide and their application to the study of psychiatric disease, schizophrenia in particular.

The principles of magnetization transfer imaging and diffusion tensor imaging

Protons in brain tissue can be 'bound' to macromolecules in myelin or cell membranes or 'free' in tissue water, and there is an exchange of water molecules between

Bound and Free Water

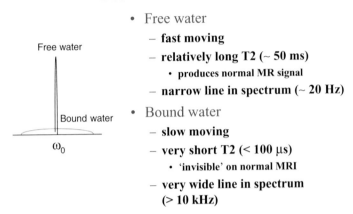

- Free water
  - **fast moving**
  - **relatively long T2 (~ 50 ms)**
    - **produces normal MR signal**
  - **narrow line in spectrum (~ 20 Hz)**
- Bound water
  - **slow moving**
  - **very short T2 (< 100 μs)**
    - **'invisible' on normal MRI**
  - **very wide line in spectrum (> 10 kHz)**

Figure 6.1   Characteristics of free and bound protons.

these two compartments. The rate of the exchange reflects the relative sizes of the two compartments and the tissue types. The magnetic resonance (MR) signal on conventional MRI is produced by the fast-moving, free water protons with long T2 relaxation times (~50 milliseconds). By contrast, slow-moving, bound water protons have very short T2 relaxation times (less than 100 microseconds) and are essentially 'invisible' on conventional MRI. Magnetization in the pool of bound water protons is characterized by a broad spectral line centred on the water resonance frequency, while magnetization of free water protons has a narrow, sharp spectral peak (Figure 6.1).

Magnetization transfer imaging

MTI is based on the interactions between protons in a relatively free environment and those with restricted motion. In the brain, free protons in tissue water and protons bound to the macromolecules of myelin and cell membranes comprise these two compartments. MTI uses an off-resonance radio frequency (RF) pulse, that is, one whose central frequency is well away from that of water, to saturate bound protons selectively without directly altering the mobile proton pool. This results in the transfer of magnetization from the saturated, bound protons to the mobile proton pool, with reduction in the nuclear magnetic resonance (NMR) signal arising from mobile protons. The degree of signal loss, measured as a percentage, is the magnetization transfer ratio or MTR. The MTR is, therefore, determined by the size of the bound pool and it depends on the density of the macromolecules in a given tissue. It follows that pathological processes that damage these macromolecules, axonal membranes and myelin in particular, will result in reductions of the MTR.

Different MTR values are observed in different normal brain tissues, with the highest values in the white matter (30–50%), medium in grey matter (20–40%) and very low in cerebrospinal fluid (close to 0%). Regional variations in white matter MTR reflect the density of myelinated fibres, with the highest values in the corpus callosum and frontal regions, and higher values in the left hemisphere than in the right (Silver et al. 1997). The MTR does not appear to vary greatly with age and gender, although there is some evidence from cross-sectional studies that increasing age is associated with MTR reductions in frontal white matter, corpus callosum (Silver et al. 1997) and cortical grey matter (Traboulsee et al. 2001). MTR measurements are highly reproducible in normal subjects rescanned after various intervals (Barker et al. 1996).

MTIs are obtained by subtraction of images obtained with and without saturation of the bound proton pool. The overall effect of magnetization transfer (MT) – reducing the observed intensity of brain and other tissues, while leaving blood 'unsuppressed' – is the basis of MT angiography, which allows the visualization of vasculature that is invisible with conventional MRI. The combination of MTI and contrast agents (gadolinium–DTPA) increases the detection of enhancing lesions (e.g. MS lesions and brain tumours) (Mehta et al. 1996; Silver et al. 1997).

The neuropathological counterparts of MTR changes

Only a couple of postmortem studies, both in patients with multiple sclerosis (MS), have tried to examine these neuropathological changes directly. Van Waesberghe et al. (1999), using brain slices, found a close correlation between MTR reduction and axonal loss in normal-appearing white matter, and a less close correlation with severity of myelin loss. Mottershead et al. (1998) found a similar correlation with reduced axonal density in the spinal cord. Correlations between MTR reduction and loss of myelin and axonal loss also show up in studies of animals with experimental allergic encephalitis (Dousset et al. 1992); toxic demyelination (Deloire-Grassin et al. 2000), Wallerian degeneration after ablation of the visual cortex (Lexa et al. 1994) and traumatic brain injury (Kimura et al. 1996).

Apart from these few studies, neuropathological counterparts have been inferred from the application of MT to patients with diseases of known pathology. In MS, where axonal loss is known to occur in the so-called normal-appearing white matter, several studies have found a reduced MTR (Gass et al. 1994; Davie et al. 1999; Filippi et al. 2000). MTR reduction also appeared to be related to loss of NAA (N-acetyl-aspartate), a marker of neuronal and axonal integrity, giving further credence to the idea that axonal loss may determine MTR values in MS (Davie et al. 1999). A close correlation between MTR reduction and cognitive and physical impairment in MS patients further suggests that MTR is a good index of axonal loss, the key determinant of disability. MTR reductions have also been reported in other conditions that lead to axonal damage and myelin loss, such as cerebral ischaemia (Pendleburyab et al. 2000; Kado et al. 2001), white matter hyperintensities of presumed vascular origin (Fazekas et al. 2000), systemic lupus erythematosus (Bosma et al. 2000), HIV infection (Dousset et al. 1997), immune-mediated diseases (Rovaris et al. 2000) and after cerebral trauma (Liu et al. 1999). Much less is known about the grey matter abnormalities underlying MTR reductions. Wallerian neuronal degeneration triggered by distant axonal damage, and microscopic grey matter plaques, were thought to be responsible for cortical MTR reduction in a recent study of MS patients (Cercignani et al. 2001).

Diffusion tensor imaging

All molecules in liquids and gases undergo random motion as a result of interactions with other molecules. The distance travelled during diffusional motion in a given time is the self-diffusion coefficient. In biological systems, molecules are confined to finite spaces by partially permeable barriers (e.g. cellular membranes and subcellular organelles) that hinder diffusion (Figure 6.2). This leads to a situation where the diffusion coefficient (the so-called 'apparent diffusion coefficient', or ADC) is always lower than that of water (Le Bihan et al. 2001). In a typical diffusion experiment, with a diffusion time around 40–60 ms, protons may travel a distance of 5–20 microns, which is in the range of cell and fibre diameters. ADC increases when there is damage to these diffusion barriers and decreases when there is a shift of protons between tissue compartments (e.g. cytotoxic oedema). Isotropic diffusion occurs when tissues have identical diffusion properties in all directions. In other words, during the diffusion experiment, molecules from the same location would be spatially distributed over a three-dimensional sphere. For other

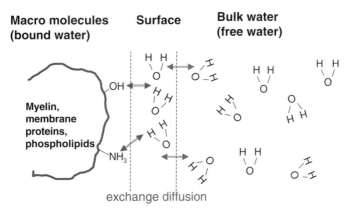

Figure 6.2   Schematic representation of the principles of diffusion.

cellular structures, such as axons, diffusion is much less restricted when motion occurs along, rather than across, the axis, and the resulting distribution of water molecules becomes ellipsoidal rather than circular during the diffusion experiment. Diffusion that has a strong directional component is said to be anisotropic and can be characterized by different ADCs in different directions (Hajnal et al. 1991). DTI, by measuring the interaction between tissue water and cellular structures, provides information about the orientation, size and geometry of brain structures. The diffusion 'tensor', first described by Basser et al. in 1994, contains information about the three-dimensional geometry, orientation and shape of the diffusion ellipsoid, and thus fully characterizes the diffusion system. The tensor provides information about mean diffusivity and fractional anisotropy, the most robust measure of anisotropy. In grey matter, diffusion is isotropic when averaged on a voxel scale, while in white matter it is extremely anisotropic because of the directionality of fibre tracts. The range of anisotropy within white matter is variable, with the highest values in organized fibre tracts such as the corpus callosum and lowest where fibres cross or have different orientations. Studies in infants at various stages of myelination have established that both myelin and axons contribute to anisotropy (Miranda et al. 1998). The differences in fractional anisotropy between white and grey matter make it possible to use this parameter to detect the boundary between the two. Tissues with a high ADC (e.g. CSF) appear dark on DTI, while those with restricted diffusion and, therefore, a low ADC have a high signal intensity. The directionality of diffusion for each voxel can be displayed on colour-coded maps, which reveal the trajectories of fibre tracts. This technique is known as tractography (Basser et al. 2000).

The neuropathological counterparts of DTI

Decreases in ADC occur when water protons from the extracellular compartment enter the cell (as in cytotoxic oedema) and their diffusion is restricted by cell membranes. Cytotoxic oedema is a feature of cerebral ischaemia, in which blood flow is reduced and the membrane ion pump fails, allowing excessive sodium and water to enter the cells. After a stroke, changes in ADC can be detected in the first 30 minutes; values are halved in the first few hours and remain low for several days. At the same time, DTI shows high signal intensity in the ischaemic area (Schwamm et al. 1998), long before changes become detectable with conventional MRI. A similar mechanism may explain the low ADCs seen in encephalitis (Golomb et al. 2001), acute traumatic brain injury (Liu et al. 1999; Marmarou et al. 2000) and anoxic/ischaemic encephalopathy (Chalela et al. 2001). Cerebral abscesses are also characterized by a low ADC and a hyperintense DTI signal, as a result of the increased cellularity and the viscosity of pus. In the early stages of Creutzfeldt–Jakob disease, vacuolation and prion deposition, impeding diffusion, probably account for the hyperintense

DTI lesions that later disappear when neuronal loss and fibrillary gliosis become prominent (Matoba et al. 2001). Transient reductions in diffusivity immediately after epileptic attacks have also been described (Wieshmann 1998).

Chronic brain disease, on the other hand, often results in breakdown of the barriers that normally restrict diffusion and this breakdown often leads to increased diffusivity and reduced fractional anisotropy. DTI can also detect abnormalities before they become apparent on conventional MRI. Thus, in MRI-negative epileptic patients with focal EEG abnormalities, DTI identified EEG-congruent focal abnormalities (Rugg-Gunn et al. 2001). Abnormalities in mean diffusivity and fractional anisotropy in patients with focal epilepsy have also been reported in normal-appearing white matter, beyond the cortical malformations detected with conventional MRI (Eriksson et al. 2001). In these patients, increased extracellular space due to failure of neurogenesis or neuronal loss could explain the increased diffusivity, while reduced anisotropy could result from abnormal myelination or ectopic grey matter.

Increased diffusivity and low fractional anisotropy also occur in MS lesions, with oedema, demyelination and axonal loss accounting for the former (Werring et al. 1999) and axonal degeneration for the latter (Ciccarelli et al. 2001). DTI abnormalities are also present in the normal-appearing white and grey matter – in the latter, perhaps, following Wallerian degeneration and/or undetected cortical lesions (Filippi et al. 2000). The close correlation between indices of disability and DTI abnormalities adds support to the idea that DTI is a sensitive measure of myelin and axonal damage, the key neuropathological abnormalities responsible for loss of function.

The application of neuropathologically sensitive techniques to the study of schizophrenia

Aberrant neurodevelopment is now considered to be central to the causation of schizophrenia (Murray and Lewis 1987; Weinberger 1987). The best support for this hypothesis accrues from the key neuropathological findings that include cytoarchitectural abnormalities and absence of gliosis (Harrison 1999). This hypothesis, however, does not specify a time or mechanism for these abnormalities and it remains uncertain whether aberrant neurodevelopment is necessary or sufficient in all patients. Evidence from functional and structural imaging studies has led to the view that abnormal functional connectivity between different brain regions may provide an explanation for the cluster of symptoms that typify schizophrenia (Friston and Frith 1995). Although aberrant functional connectivity may occur in the absence of an anatomical substrate, the integration of abnormalities in structure and function is still central to our understanding of the cause and pathophysiological mechanisms of schizophrenia. Harrison (1999) has suggested that the neuronal, synaptic and dendritic abnormalities reported in schizophrenia are consistent with aberrant functional connectivity. White-matter abnormalities have been less well documented, but they are also likely to play a role in the disordered connectivity.

The application of neuropathologically sensitive MRI techniques to the study of schizophrenia is just starting. The few available studies have taken forward the information that conventional techniques can provide and have yielded results that are in keeping with current neuropathological knowledge. In the future, these techniques will be more widely used and will provide much-needed information about the phenotypic diversity and evolution of brain abnormalities in psychosis.

Grey matter abnormalities
Evidence from conventional MRI

Cortical abnormalities have long been recognized in schizophrenia. Conventional MRI studies have described widespread loss of cortical volume (Harvey et al. 1993), particularly marked in the amygdala, hippocampus, parahippocampus and superior temporal gyrus (Lawrie and Abukmeil 1998; Wright et al. 2000). The possibility that cortical abnormalities occur in interconnected areas with common developmental influences has recently received considerable attention (see Chapter 5 by Chitnis and Ellison-Wright). Wright et al. (1999) have addressed this question in patients with chronic schizophrenia by doing cerebral parcellation of MRI segmented grey matter maps, registered to a standard space. This procedure, which allowed the detection of volumetric changes in the major Brodmann areas, made it possible to identify loss of volume in interconnected inferior frontal, temporal (hippocampus, parahippocampus, inferior and superior temporal gyri and auditory cortex) and insular cortices. Palliere-Martinot et al. (2001) have replicated these findings in a group of 20 male schizophrenics using the same methodology. Sigmundsson et al. (2001) reported similar findings in a group of chronic schizophrenics with predominantly negative symptoms using nonparametric voxel-based morphometry. In this study, volumetric losses were more evident in the left hemisphere and were detected in the superior temporal gyrus and insular cortex, medial temporal lobe (including the hippocampus and parahippocampus), anterior cingulate and medial frontal gyri. The coexistence of volumetric loss in the large white matter tracts connecting these areas adds further support to the evidence of abnormalities in large-scale neural networks.

The abnormalities detected by these studies are, by definition, severe enough to have caused measurable volume loss and would otherwise have gone undetected.

Evidence from novel MRI techniques

The application of neuropathologically sensitive techniques that can detect more subtle changes is still in its infancy, and only a handful of psychiatric studies are so far available. The most interesting findings so far have accrued from studies using MTI. In our first study (Foong et al. 2001), we examined a group of patients with chronic schizophrenia and a control group of healthy volunteers matched for age, gender and parental social class. A voxel-based group analysis (statistical parametric maps; SPM) detected widespread areas of cortical MTR reduction in the schizophrenic group (Figure 6.3). These abnormalities were predominantly cortical and were more prominent in the inferior and middle frontal, inferior and middle temporal and superior occipital gyri, although they also extended to parieto-occipital regions. In the temporal lobes, MTR abnormalities extended into the adjacent white matter of the fasciculus uncinatus. These findings add support to the hypothesis that abnormalities in frontotemporal circuits are central to schizophrenia (Weinberger et al. 1992; Wright et al. 1999; Sigmundsson et al. 2001). The interest of this work also rests on the fact that these abnormalities were present in patients with minimal volumetric losses limited to the left inferior frontal cortex. The MTR abnormalities were more widespread than those reported in recent conventional MRI studies.

Recent neuropathological studies in schizophrenia (Harrison 1999) provide a tentative explanation for these imaging abnormalities. Studies using objective stereological techniques have reported a cortical increase in neuronal density in the presence of volume reduction. This has led to the hypothesis that reduction in the neuropil (mainly consisting of dendrites, axons and synapses) may account for the reduction of volume detected by conventional imaging and may be a key neuropathological feature of schizophrenia (Selemon et al. 1998; Selemon and Goldman-Rakic 1999; Glantz and Lewis 2000). In keeping with this hypothesis are the loss of dendritic spines in layer-III pyramidal cells in the prefrontal cortex (Glantz and Lewis 1997) and subicular apical dendrites in the hippocampus (Rosoklija et al. 2000), and the reduction of dendritic (MAP2) (Arnold et al. 1991) and synaptic markers in the hippocampus (Harrison and Eastwood 1998) and dorsolateral prefrontal cortex (Glantz and Lewis 1997). Neuropil reduction, even if subtle enough not to cause detectable volume loss, would lead to MTR reduction by reducing the size of the bound proton pool. Neuropil abnormalities may also explain the aberrant interneuronal connectivity postulated to be the key functional abnormality in schizophrenia (Selemon et al. 1998).

Other subcortical grey matter structures can also be studied using a region-of-interest methodology. Bagary et al. (in press) used this procedure to explore the integrity of the prefrontal-thalamic-cerebellar circuit subserving attention, sensory gating and information processing. Thalamic pathology disrupting this circuit has been put forward as an explanation for the complex cognitive changes and symptoms of schizophrenia (Andreasen et al. 1998), although previous neuropathological and MRI studies have failed to provide unequivocal support for this theory. We sampled areas in the dorsomedial and pulvinar nuclei in the same group of chronic schizophrenics known to have extensive cortical abnormalities (Foong et al. 2001)

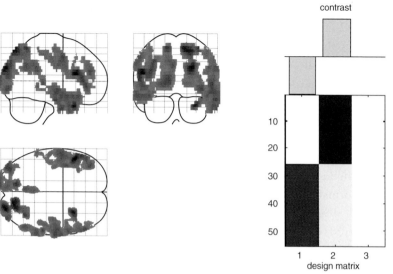

P values and statistics:

Set-level {c}	Cluster-level {k,Z}	Voxel-level {Z}	Uncorrected k and Z		x,y,z {mm}		
0.000 (10)	0.002 (1780, 5.46)	**0.001 (5.46)**	0.000	0.000	−52	21	20
		0.046 (4.48)		0.000	−57	31	15
		0.113 (4.25)		0.000	−52	38	0
	0.000 (3734, 5.29)	**0.001 (5.29)**	0.000	0.000	26	−93	30
		0.004 (5.08)		0.000	14	−76	60
		0.006 (4.96)		0.000	23	−77	55
	0.000 (5486, 5.10)	**0.003 (5.10)**	0.000	0.000	31	17	−30
		0.077 (4.35)		0.000	65	−11	−20
		0.108 (4.26)		0.000	66	−2	−35
	0.000 (3534, 4.68)	**0.021 (4.68)**	0.000	0.000	−13	−75	60
		0.061 (4.42)		0.000	−38	−89	25
		0.065 (4.40)		0.000	−36	−85	35
	0.007 (1462, 4.35)	**0.078 (4.35)**	0.001	0.000	60	38	0
		0.239 (4.02)		0.000	61	32	10
		0.455 (3.79)		0.000	62	18	15
	0.025 (981, 4.26)	**0.110 (4.26)**	0.004	0.000	−40	44	25
		0.638 (3.62)		0.000	−44	39	35
		0.939 (3.27)		0.001	−41	33	45
	0.000 (3326, 4.17)	**0.147 (4.17)**	0.000	0.000	−61	−3	−15
		0.153 (4.16)		0.000	−41	7	−15
		0.195 (4.09)		0.000	−49	25	−15

Height threshold {u} = 3.09, P = 0.001   Volume {S} = 434010 voxels or 471.2 Resels
Extent threshold {k} = 6.926663e + 02 voxels, P = 0.012   Degrees of freedom due to error = 53.0
Expected voxels per cluster, E{n} = 97.7   Smoothness {FWHM mm} = 14.9, 15.3, 17.7
Expected number of clusters, E{m} = 0.1   {voxels} = 6.3, 6.5, 7.5

Figure 6.3   Relative MTR reduction in patients with chronic schizophrenia compared with healthy controls. Widespread cortical abnormalities are present in the patient group. MTR abnormalities also extend into the temporal white matter.

and in a group of normal controls matched for age, gender and parental social class. These nuclei are potentially relevant because of their connections to the amygdala and prefrontal cortex (for the dorsomedial nucleus) and to the auditory association cortex (for the pulvinar). In contrast with the report of Andreasen et al. (1998), we failed to find abnormalities in the dorsomedial and pulvinar thalamic nuclei in this group of schizophrenic patients, although the possibility remains that prefrontal-thalamic-cerebellar circuits might be abnormal in other schizophrenic subgroups.

There is increasing evidence that the structural brain abnormalities detected in schizophrenia may be progressive, at least in subgroups of patients (DeLisi et al. 1995; Puri et al. 2001). A few recent longitudinal studies using sophisticated image-analysis techniques provide the strongest evidence (see Chapter 5 by Chitnis and Ellison-Wright). Progressive ventricular enlargement is the most consistent finding, although widespread cortical volume loss has also been reported even in young patients (Thompson et al. 2001). Neuropathological studies have established that Alzheimer's disease pathology is not increased in schizophrenia (Harrison 1999) and progressive structural abnormalities require a different explanation. Longitudinal studies of large numbers of patients with schizophrenia observed from the onset of their illness are needed to determine whether progression of brain abnormalities is a hallmark of schizophrenia or occurs only in subgroups of patients with specific clinical and cognitive phenotypes. Longitudinal data using neuropathologically sensitive MRI are not yet available, but comparison between cross-sectional studies in first-episode and chronic patients suggests that progressive neuropathological changes are likely.

Thus, in first-episode patients, we found MTR reductions in the insula, antero-medial frontal cortex extending into the anterior cingulate and the right superior and middle temporal gyri (MS Bagary, MR Symms, G Barker et al. unpublished manuscript) (Figure 6.4). Cortical abnormalities were far less widespread early in the disease than those detected in chronic schizophrenics using the same technique (Foong et al. 2001). As in chronic patients, white matter abnormalities were detected in first-episode schizophrenic patients in the fasciculus uncinatus connecting frontotemporal cortices. The relevance of these findings is two-fold. First, they provide further evidence that abnormalities in a fronto-temporal supraregional system are already present early in the disease. Second, by comparison with the more widespread abnormalities detected in our study of chronic patients, they suggest that brain abnormalities may be progressive, at least in some patients. Cortical abnormalities are known to be present in first-episode patients (Zipursky et al. 1998) and a recent study using conventional MRI (Thompson et al. 2001) gives strong support to the possibility that they may be progressive, at least in some patients. In their study, Thompson and colleagues detected progressive loss of grey matter in

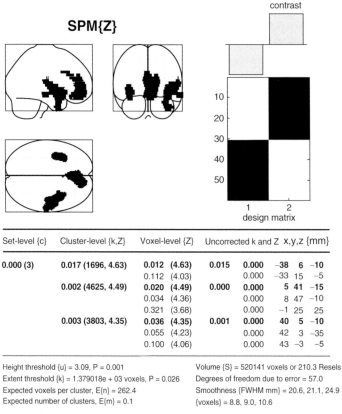

Figure 6.4   Relative MTR reductions in first-episode schizophrenic patients compared with healthy controls. MTR reductions occurred in the insula, anteromedial frontal cortex (including the anterior cingulate) and the right, superior and middle temporal gyri.

12 patients with severe, early-onset schizophrenia scanned three times over a 5-year period. The grey matter loss, estimated to be 5% per year, first occurred in parietal and sensorimotor regions and later extended to include temporal and dorsolateral prefrontal cortices. Cortical loss was far more severe in schizophrenic patients than in other patients with psychoses.

White matter abnormalities in schizophrenia

Few neuropathological studies have been devoted to the study of white matter abnormalities in schizophrenia, although there is empirical evidence to suggest that myelin abnormalities may be relevant. Benes et al. (1994) considered delayed hippocampal myelination as a likely aetiological factor in schizophrenia. Clinical observation of patients with metachromatic leukodystrophy (Hyde et al. 1992) also suggests that schizophrenia-like symptoms are a frequent accompaniment of this white matter disease of early life. More recently, Hakak et al. (2001) have reported altered expression levels of five genes functionally clustered and implicated in the formation and maintenance of myelin sheaths, in the dorsolateral prefrontal cortex of chronic schizophrenics. Dysregulation of these genes, which are critical for efficient axonal conduction and for the development and long-term survival of axons, suggests abnormal oligodendrocyte function.

Evidence from conventional MRI

Few conventional imaging studies have studied white matter abnormalities in schizophrenia. MRI hyperintensities are known to occur and to occupy larger brain areas than in matched controls (Persaud et al. 1997). Recent methods of voxel-based morphometry that permit the fractionation of white and grey matter have also suggested that regional white matter abnormalities may be present in schizophrenia. Sigmundsson et al. (2001), using voxel-based morphometry in chronic patients with prominent negative symptoms, found a 13% loss of volume in white matter localized to the left hemisphere, involving the uncinate fasciculus and extending posteriorly into the inferior longitudinal fasciculus and inferior parietal lobe. Palliere-Martinot et al. (2001) have also detected bilateral loss of frontal white matter volume using similar methods.

Evidence from novel MRI techniques

A few studies using diffusion imaging have tried to explore abnormalities in anatomical connectivity by measuring fractional anisotropy, or related measures, that could indicate changes in directionality or structure of white matter fibre tracts. The different methodologies and the small samples used in these studies require considerable caution when interpreting their findings.

Buchsbaum et al. (1998) examined relative anisotropy in five patients with chronic schizophrenia and six age- and gender-matched controls. Relative anisotropy, a robust but insensitive measure of anisotropy, was measured using a voxel-based analysis in two axial slices. Significantly lower white matter anisotropy in the inferior prefrontal region and in the area adjacent to the putamen was found in schizophrenic patients than in the controls. These abnormalities did not appear to be related to age, duration of pharmacological treatment or cognitive impairment. Using positron emission tomography (PET) in the same medication-naïve subjects, schizophrenic patients did not show the significant correlations between metabolic rates in the prefrontal regions and putamen exhibited by healthy controls. These results were interpreted as indicating abnormalities in the interconnecting regional white matter between the frontal lobe and striatum.

Lim et al. (1999) examined fractional anisotropy in eight contiguous slices covering cortex and a large area of white matter that included the corpus callosum and the centrum semiovale. The median fractional anisotropy was measured in 10 male patients with chronic schizophrenia maintained on atypical neuroleptics and in 10 age-matched controls. Structural MRI demonstrated a volume reduction in grey but not white matter in the patient group. By contrast, fractional anisotropy was reduced in white but not grey matter in the schizophrenic group. The lower white matter fractional anisotropy persisted when white and grey matter volumes and age were controlled for. Within the patient group, fractional anisotropy changes extended from the frontal to the occipital regions and were similar in the two hemispheres. The dissociation between fractional anisotropy and volumetric abnormalities in white and grey matter was interpreted as suggesting compromised white matter connectivity caused by cortical abnormalities (e.g. abnormally small neurons or loss of neuropil) that could explain the reduction of cortical volume in the absence of diffusion changes. These findings confirmed those of Buchsbaum et al. (1998) and earlier ones from their own group (Hedehus et al. 1998). More recently, Agartz et al. (2001), using methods that allowed whole-brain analysis, also found widespread diffusion abnormalities in the white matter of a group of 20 chronic schizophrenics compared with normal controls. Changes in diffusivity were not related to age or gender. Conventional MRI did not detect differences between the two groups.

Other studies, however, have failed to find white matter abnormalities. Thus, Steel et al. (2001) examined the prefrontal white matter of 10 patients with established DSM–IV schizophrenia and 10 controls, using a more powerful, 2-tesla magnet. In order to increase the chances of finding detectable abnormalities in connectivity, the two groups had been selected to show minor differences in brain and ventricular volume. Despite this study design, no significant differences were found between patients and controls in any DTI parameters. Moreover, DTI and volumetric measurements were not closely correlated. Our own study (Foong et al. 2000) explored differences in DTI parameters in the corpus callosum of chronic schizophrenics and normal controls using a region-of-interest methodology. Mean diffusivity was increased and fractional anisotropy decreased in the splenium but not in the genu of the corpus callosum in the patient group. These findings were interpreted as indicating disruption in the packing and organization of the inter-hemispheric fibres connecting the inferotemporal and occipital regions that traverse the splenium. Using a more stringent, voxel-based analysis in the same group of patients, we failed to detect widespread white matter abnormalities. Our findings are similar to those of Agartz et al. (2001), who also reported abnormalities in the splenium of the corpus callosum. The callosal abnormalities were not related to age, gender or duration of illness, and their focal nature made it unlikely that they could have been due to medication effects. Changes in axonal density in the corpus callosum have been described in postmortem studies (Nasrallah et al. 1983; Highley et al. 1999), and they have also been described in a meta-analysis of structural MRI studies (Woodruff et al. 1995).

Relationship between brain abnormalities and symptomatology

A handful of investigators using novel image analysis methods have tried to correlate clinical symptomatology and specific structural abnormalities. The severity of negative symptoms, a stable deficit intimately related to cognitive abnormalities, correlates best with structural abnormalities across a number of recent studies using conventional MRI. Thus, Sigmundsson et al. (2001) described a relationship between the presence of severe negative symptoms and volumetric losses in left temporal gyrus, insular cortex, medial temporal lobe, anterior cingulate and medial frontal gyri and related white matter tracts. Similar results have also been reported by Palliere-Martinot et al. (2001), who found negative symptoms to correlate with loss of white matter volume in the cingulate and right internal capsule. Thompson et al. (2001), in a longitudinal study of patients with young-onset, severe schizophrenia, found an association between frontal cortical loss and negative symptoms, but, in contrast with the findings of Sigmundsson et al. (2001), the severity of positive symptoms was associated with loss of temporal grey matter.

The exploration of these correlations using neuropathologically sensitive imaging techniques is just beginning, but their ability to detect abnormalities earlier than conventional MRI is likely to prove advantageous. In a group of chronic schizophrenics, without evidence of volumetric reductions, compared with a control group, Foong et al. (2001) found a correlation between the severity of negative symptoms and MTR reductions in the parieto-occipital cortex and the genu of the corpus callosum. Future studies using similar methodology in larger populations are likely to clarify clinical–cognitive–neuropathological correlations.

The application of novel MRI techniques to the study of bipolar disorder

Current diagnostic classifications separate schizophrenia from bipolar disorder, but it is increasingly evident that they share clinical and epidemiological features and that some genetic and environmental determinants may also be common to both conditions. Neuropathological similarities between the two are also becoming clearer. The neuropathology of bipolar disorder is reviewed elsewhere in this book (see Chapter 14 by Harrison and Gittins). Abnormalities in the prefrontal cortex (anterior cingulate and ventromedial and dorsolateral prefrontal cortex) have been consistently reported. A decrease in glial density, particularly in the anterior cingulate, and reduced density and size in other neuronal populations have been the most important and consistent findings. There is now enough evidence to suggest that abnormalities in neural circuitry, particularly those involving the prefrontal

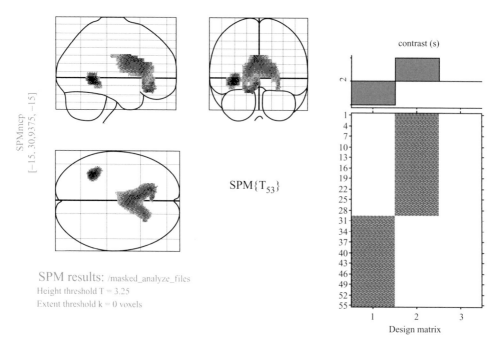

SPM{T$_{53}$}

SPM results: /masked_analyze_files
Height threshold T = 3.25
Extent threshold k = 0 voxels

contrast (s)

Design matrix

Statistics: volume summary (p–values corrected for entire volume)

Set-level		Cluster-level			Voxel-level				x, y, z {mm}		
p	c	p$_{corrected}$	k$_I$	p$_{uncorrected}$	p$_{corrected}$	T	(Z$_\blacksquare$)	p$_{uncorrected}$			
0.184	4	0.160	927	0.079	0.298	4.03	(3.75)	0.000	−33	−48	0
					0.409	3.88	(3.62)	0.000	−39	−44	−5
		0.000	7677	0.000	0.407	3.88	(3.62)	0.000	−15	31	−15
					0.437	3.84	(3.59)	0.000	−4	16	25
					0.467	3.81	(3.56)	0.000	−5	6	30
		0.838	20	0.821	0.810	3.39	(3.21)	0.001	58	−20	30
		0.854	12	0.869	0.835	3.35	(3.17)	0.001	−34	−39	45

Figure 6.5   Relative MTR reductions in bipolar patients compared with healthy controls in the anterior cingulate.

cortex, are likely to be relevant in bipolar disorder. The cause and evolution of these abnormalities remain to be determined.

Imaging studies of patients with bipolar disorder have also reported ventricular and sulcal enlargement (Elkis et al. 1995; Strakowski et al. 1999; Kumra et al. 2000) and hippocampal volume loss in chronic and first-episode bipolar patients (Velakoulis et al. 1999). These abnormalities tend to be less severe than those described in schizophrenia, but there is also indirect evidence that some of them, in particular loss of hippocampal volume, may be progressive (Sapolsky 2000). Other imaging abnormalities appear to be different from or more severe than those reported in schizophrenia. Thus, amygdalar enlargement (Altshuler et al. 2000), reduction in anterior cingulate volume (Drevets et al. 1997) and white matter hyperintensities (Altshuler et al. 1995) may be more specific to bipolar disorder, may appear early in the disease (Stoll et al. 2000) and may be genetically determined (Botteron et al. 1992).

Preliminary data from the first MTI study of patients with bipolar disorder, carried out by our group (Bruno et al. 2001), suggest that this technique is also sensitive to the presence of neuropathological abnormalities in these patients. Using a voxel-based analysis (SPM), a significant reduction of the MTR was found in the supracallosal region of the anterior cingulate and surrounding areas in 29 chronic patients fulfilling DSM–IV criteria for bipolar disorder and 28 healthy, matched controls (Figure 6.5). Conventional MRI had failed to detect volumetric changes between the two groups of subjects. In contrast with our findings in patients with chronic schizophrenia, patients with bipolar disorder did not exhibit widespread cortical MTR changes. These preliminary findings are an illustration of the similarities (pathological changes in the anterior cingulate) and differences (absence of cortical abnormalities) between bipolar disorder and schizophrenia.

Conclusions

In the past 30 years, imaging has, without doubt, provided the main impetus for research into the psychoses. This has also led to the resurgence of neuropathological research. The yield of conventional MRI is not yet exhausted, but its inherent limitations make the application of neuropathologically sensitive techniques all that more interesting. So far, these techniques have been applied to small groups of patients, and findings await replication in larger samples by other research groups.

The studies available so far suggest that MTI and DTI can detect abnormalities not visible with conventional MRI. Widespread cortical abnormalities in the absence of significant volume loss are a feature of chronic schizophrenia but not of bipolar disorder. The lack of widespread cortical abnormalities in patients with first-episode schizophrenia also suggests that these abnormalities may be progressive, at least in some patients. These abnormalities are in keeping with the theory of neuropil reduction in schizophrenia. Finally, there is emerging evidence that localized white matter abnormalities may also be present.

REFERENCES

Agartz I, Andersson JLR and Skare S (2001). Abnormal brain white matter in schizophrenia: a diffusion tensor imaging study. *Neuroreport*, 12, 2251–4.

Altshuler LL, Curran JG, Hauser P, Mintz J, Denicoff K and Post R (1995). T2 hyperintensities in bipolar disorder: magnetic resonance imaging comparison and literature meta-analyis. *Am J Psychiatry*, 152, 1139–44.

Altshuler LL, Bartzokis G, Grieder T et al. (2000). An MRI study of temporal lobe structures in men with bipolar disorder or schizophrenia. *Biol Psychiatry*, 48, 147–62.

Andreasen NC, Paradiso S and O'Leary DS (1998). 'Cognitive dysmetria' as an integrative theory of schizophrenia: a dysfunction in cortical-subcortical-cerebellar circuitry? *Schizophr Bull*, 24, 203–18.

Arnold SE, Lee VM-Y, Gur RE and Trojanoski JQ (1991). Abnormal expression of two microtubule-associated proteins (MAP2 and MAP5) in specific subfields of the hippocampal formation in schizophrenia. *Proc Natl Acad Sci USA*, 88, 10850–4.

Bagary MS, Foong J, Maier M et al. (in press). A magnetization transfer analysis of the thalamus in schizophrenia. *J Neuropsychiatry Clin Neurosci.*

Barker GJ, Tofts PS and Gass A (1996). An interleaved sequence for accurate and reproducible clinical measurement of magnetization transfer ratio. *Magn Reson Imaging*, 14, 403–11.

Basser P, Mattiello J and LeBihan D (1994). Estimation of the effective self-diffusion tensor from the NMR spin-echo. *J Magn Reson*, 103, 247–54.

Basser PJ, Pajevic S, Pierpaoli C, Duda J and Aldroubi A (2000). In vivo fiber tractography using DT-MRI data. *Magn Reson Med*, 44, 625–32.

Benes FM, Turtle M, Khan Y and Farol P (1994). Myelination of a key relay zone in the hippocampal formation occurs in the human brain during childhood, adolescence and adulthood. *Arch Gen Psychiatry*, 51, 477–84.

Bosma GP, Rood MJ, Zwinderman AH, Huizinga TW and van Buchem MA (2000). Evidence of central nervous system damage in patients with neuropsychiatric systemic lupus erythematosus, demonstrated by magnetization transfer imaging. *Arthritis Rheum*, 43, 48–54.

Botteron KN, Figiel GS, Wetzel MW, Hudziak J and Van Eerdewegh M (1992). MRI abnormalities in adolescent bipolar affective disorder. *J Am Acad Child Adolesc Psychiatry*, 31, 258–61.

Bruno SD, Bagary MS, Symms M and Ron MA (2001). An in-vivo MRI study of neuropathology of bipolar disorder using diffusion weighted imaging and magnetisation transfer imaging. *Schizophr Res*, 49 (Suppl. 1), 151.

Buchsbaum MS, Tang CY, Peled S et al. (1998). MRI white matter diffusion anisotropy and PET metabolic rate in schizophrenia. *Neuroreport*, 9, 425–30.

Cercignani M, Bozzali M, Iannucci G, Comi G and Fillippi M (2001). Magnetization transfer ratio and mean diffusivity of normal appearing white and grey matter from patients with multiple sclerosis. *J Neurol Neurosurg Psychiatry*, 70, 311–17.

Chalela JA, Wolf RL, Maldjian JA and Kasner SE (2001). MRI identification of early white matter injury in anoxic-ischemic encephalopathy. *Neurology*, 56, 481–5.

Ciccarelli O, Werring DJ, Wheeler-Kingshott CA et al. (2001). Investigations of MS normal-appearing brain using diffusion tensor MRI with clinical correlations. *Neurology*, 56, 926–33.

Davie CA, Silver NC, Barker GJ et al. (1999). Does the extent of axonal loss and demyelination from chronic lesions in multiple sclerosis correlate with the clinical subgroup? *J Neurol Neurosurg Psychiatry*, 67, 710–15.

DeLisi LE, Tew W, Xie S et al. (1995). A prospective follow-up study of brain morphology and cognition in first episode schizophrenic patients: preliminary findings. *Biol Psychiatry*, 38, 349–60.

Deloire-Grassin MS, Brochet B et al. (2000). In vivo evaluation of remyelination in rat brain by magnetization transfer imaging. *J Neurol Sci*, 178, 10–16.

Dousset V, Grossman RI, Ramer KN et al. (1992). Experimental allergic encephalomyelitis and multiple sclerosis: lesion characterization with magnetization transfer imaging. *Radiology*, 182, 483–91.

Dousset V, Armand JP, Lacoste D et al. (1997). Magnetization transfer study of HIV encephalitis and progressive multifocal leukoencephalopathy. *Am J Neuroradiol*, 18, 895–901.

Drevets WC, Price JL, Simpson JR Jr et al. (1997). Subgenual prefrontal cortex abnormalities in mood disorders. *Nature*, 386, 824–7.

Elkis H, Friedman L, Wise A and Meltzer H (1995). Meta-analysis of studies of ventricular enlargement and cortical sulcal prominence in mood disorders. *Arch Gen Psychiatry*, 52, 735–46.

Eriksson SH, Rugg-Gunn FJ, Symms MR, Barker GJ and Duncan JS (2001). Diffusion tensor imaging in patients with epilepsy and malformations of cortical development. *Brain*, 124, 617–26.

Fazekas F, Ropele S, Bammer R, Kapeller P, Stollberger R and Schmidt R (2000). Novel imaging technologies in the assessment of cerebral ageing and vascular dementia. *J Neural Transm*, 59, 45–52.

Filippi M, Inglese M, Rovaris M et al. (2000). Magnetization transfer imaging to monitor the evolution of MS: a 1-year follow-up study. *Neurology*, 55, 940–6.

Foong J, Maier M, Barker GJ, Miller DH and Ron MA (2000). In vivo investigation of white matter pathology in schizophrenia with magnetization transfer imaging. *J Neurol Neurosurg Psychiatry*, 68, 70–4.

Foong J, Symms MR, Barker GJ et al. (2001). Neuropathological abnormalities in schizophrenia: evidence from magnetization transfer imaging. *Brain*, 124, 882–92.

Friston KJ and Frith CD (1995). Schizophrenia: a disconnection syndrome? *Clin Neurosci*, 3, 89–97.

Gass A, Barker GJ, Kidd D et al. (1994). Correlation of magnetization transfer ratio and clinical disability in multiple sclerosis. *Ann Neurol*, 36, 62–7.

Glantz LA and Lewis DA (1997). Reduction of synaptophysin immunoreactivity in the prefrontal cortex of subjects with schizophrenia: regional and diagnostic specificity. *Arch Gen Psychiatry*, 54, 943–52.

Glantz LA and Lewis DA (2000). Decreased dendritic spine density on prefrontal cortical pyramidal neurons in schizophrenia. *Arch Gen Psychiatry*, 57, 65–73.

Golomb MR, Durand ML, Schaefer PW, McDonald CT, Maia M and Schwamm LH (2001). A case of immunotherapy-responsive eastern equine encephalitis with diffusion-weighted imaging. *Neurology*, 56, 420–1.

Hajnal JV, Doran M and Hall AS (1991). MR imaging of anisotropically restricted diffusion of water in the nervous system: technical, anatomic and pathological considerations. *J Comput Assist Tomogr*, 5, 1–18.

Hakak Y, Walker JR, Li C et al. (2001). Genome-wide expression analysis reveals dysregulation of myelination-related genes in chronic schizophrenia. *Proc Natl Acad Sci USA*, 98, 4746–51.

Harrison PJ (1999). The neuropathology of schizophrenia: a critical review of the data and their interpretation. *Brain*, 122, 593–624.

Harrison PJ and Eastwood SL (1998). Preferential involvement of excitatory neurons in medial temporal lobe in schizophrenia. *Lancet*, 352, 1669–73.

Harvey I, Ron MA, Du Boulay G, Wicks D, Lewis SW and Murray RM (1993). Reduction of cortical volume in schizophrenia on magnetic resonance imaging. *Psychol Med*, 23, 591–604.

Hedehus M, de Crespigny A, Menon V, Moseley M and Lim KO (1998). Mapping of white matter tracts in schizophrenics using diffusion tensor imaging. *Proc Int Soc Magn Reson Med*, 1342.

Highley JR, Esiri MM, McDonald B, Cortina-Borja M, Herron BM and Crow TJ (1999). The size and fibre composition of the corpus callosum with respect to gender and schizophrenia: a post mortem study. *Brain*, 122, 99–110.

Hyde TM, Ziegler JC and Weinberger DR (1992). Psychiatric disturbances in metachromatic leukodystrophy: insights into the neurobiology of psychosis. *Arch Neurol*, 49, 401–6.

Kado H, Kimura H, Tsuchida T, Yonekura Y, Tokime T and Tokuriki Y (2001). Abnormal magnetization transfer ratios in normal-appearing white matter in conventional MR images of patients with occlusive cerebrovascular disease. *Am J Neuroradiol*, 22, 922–7.

Kimura H, Meaney DF, McGowan JC et al. (1996). Magnetization transfer imaging of diffuse axonal injury following experimental brain injury in the pig: characterisation by magnetization transfer and histopathological correlation. *J Comput Assist Tomogr*, 20, 540–6.

Kumra S, Giedd JN, Vaituzis AC et al. (2000). Childhood-onset psychotic disorders: magnetic resonance imaging of volumetric differences in brain structure. *Am J Psychiatry*, 157, 1467–74.

Lawrie SM and Abukmeil SS (1998). Brain abnormality in schizophrenia – a systematic and quantitative review of volumetric magnetic resonance imaging studies. *Br J Psychiatry*, 172, 110–20.

Le Bihan D, Mangin JF, Poupon C et al. (2001). Diffusion tensor imaging: concepts and applications. *J Magn Reson Imaging*, 13, 534–46.

Lexa FJ, Grossman RJ and Rosenquist AC (1994). MR of wallerian degeneration in the feline visual system: characterisation by magnetization transfer rate with histopathological correlation. *Am J Neuroradiol*, 15, 201–12.

Lim KO, Hedehus M, Moseley M, de Crespigny A, Sullivan E and Pfeferbaum A (1999). Compromised white matter tract integrity in schizophrenia inferred from diffusion tensor imaging. *Arch Gen Psychiatry*, 56, 367–74.

Liu AY, Maldjian JA, Bagley LJ, Sinson GP and Grossman RI (1999). Traumatic brain injury: diffusion-weighted MR imaging findings. *Am J Neuroradiol*, 20, 1636–41.

Marmarou A, Portella G, Barzo P et al. (2000). Distinguishing between cellular and vasogenic edema in head injured patients with focal lesions using magnetic resonance imaging. *Acta Neurochir*, 76 (Suppl.), 349–51.

Matoba M, Tonami H, Miyaji H, Yokota H and Yamamoto I (2001). Creutzfeld–Jakob disease: serial changes on diffusion weighted MRI. *J Comput Assist Tomogr*, 25, 274–7.

Mehta RC, Pike GB and Enzmann DR (1996). Measure of magnetization transfer in multiple sclerosis demyelinating plaques, white matter ischemic lesions, and edema. *Am J Neuroradiol*, 17, 1051–5.

Miranda MJ, Born P and Wiegell MR (1998). White matter tract visualisation in infants by diffusion tensor MRI. *Proc Int Soc Magn Reson Med*, 528.

Mottershead JP, Thornton JS, Clemence M et al. (1998). Correlation of spinal cord axonal density with post mortem NMR measurements in multiple sclerosis and controls. *Proc Int Soc Magn Reson Med*, 2163.

Murray RM and Lewis SW (1987). Is schizophrenia a neurodevelopmental disorder? *Br Med J*, 295, 681–2.

Nasrallah HA, McCalley-Whitters M, Bigelow LB and Rauscher FP (1983). A histological study of the corpus callosum in chronic schizophrenia. *Psychiatry Res*, 8, 251–60.

Pailliere-Martinot M, Caclin A, Artiges E et al. (2001). Cerebral gray and white matter reductions and clinical correlates in patients with early onset schizophrenia. *Schizophr Res*, 50, 19–26.

Pendleburyab ST, Lee MA, Blamire AM, Styles P and Matthews PM (2000). Correlating magnetic resonance imaging markers of axonal injury and demyelination in motor impairment secondary to stroke and multiple sclerosis. *Magn Reson Imaging*, 18, 369–78.

Persaud R, Russow H, Harvey I et al. (1997). Focal signal hyperintensities in schizophrenia. *Schizophr Res*, 27, 55–64.

Puri BK, Hutton SB, Saeed N et al. (2001). A serial longitudinal quantitative MRI study of cerebral changes in first episode schizophrenia using image segmentation and subvoxel registration. *Psychiatry Res*, 106, 141–50.

Rosoklija G, Toomayan G, Ellis SP et al. (2000). Structural abnormalities of subicular dendrites in subjects with schizophrenia and mood disorders. *Arch Gen Psychiatry*, 57, 349–56.

Rovaris M, Viti B, Ciboddo G et al. (2000). Brain involvement in systemic immune mediated diseases: magnetic resonance and magnetization transfer imaging study. *J Neurol Neurosurg Psychiatry*, 68, 170–7.

Rugg-Gunn FJ, Eriksson SH, Symms MR, Barker GJ and Duncan JS (2001). Diffusion tensor imaging of cryptogenic and acquired partial epilepsy. *Brain*, 124, 627–36.

Sapolsky R (2000). Glucocorticoids and hippocampal atrophy in neuropsychiatric disorders. *Arch Gen Psychiatry*, 57, 925–35.

Schwamm LH, Koroshetz WJ, Sorensen AG et al. (1998). Time course of lesion development in patients with acute stroke: serial diffusion and hemodynamic-weighted magnetic resonance imaging. *Stroke*, 29, 2268–76.

Selemon LD and Goldman-Rakic PS (1999). The reduced neuropil hypothesis: a circuit based model of schizophrenia. *Biol Psychiatry*, 45, 17–25.

Selemon LD, Rajkowska G and Goldman-Rakic PS (1998). Elevated neuronal density in prefrontal area 46 in brains from schizophrenic patients: application of a three dimensional, stereologic counting method. *J Comp Neurol*, 392, 402–12.

Sigmundsson T, Suckling J, Maier M et al. (2001). Structural abnormalities in frontal, temporal and limbic regions and interconnecting white matter tracts in schizophrenic patients with prominent negative symptoms. *Am J Psychiatry*, 158, 234–43.

Silver NC, Barker GJ, MacManus DG, Tofts PS and Miller DH (1997). Magnetization transfer ratio of normal brain white matter: a normative database spanning four decades of life. *J Neurol Neurosurg Psychiatry*, 62, 223–38.

Steel RM, Bastin ME, McConnell S et al. (2001). Diffusion tensor imaging (DTI) and proton magnetic resonance spectroscopy (1H MRS) in schizophrenic subjects and normal controls. *Psychiatry Res*, 106, 161–70.

Stoll L, Renshaw P, Yurgelum-Todd D and Cohen B (2000). Neuroimaging in bipolar disorder: what have we learned? *Biol Psychiatry*, 48, 505–17.

Strakowski SM, DelBello MP, Sax KW et al. (1999). Brain magnetic resonance imaging of structural abnormalities in bipolar disorder. *Arch Gen Psychiatry*, 56, 254–60.

Thompson PM, Vidal C, Giedd JN et al. (2001). Mapping adolescent brain change reveals dynamic wave of accelerated gray matter loss in very early-onset schizophrenia. *Proc Natl Acad Sci USA*, 98, 11650–5.

Traboulsee A, Chard DT, Dehmeshki J, Foong J, Barker GJ, Miller DH (2001). Age and gender effects on segmented brain fractions and MTR histograms in a normal control population. *Multiple Sclerosis*, 7 (Suppl.1), S87.

Van Waesberghe JH, Kamphorst W, De Groot CJ et al. (1999). Axonal loss in multiple sclerosis lesions: magnetic resonance imaging insights into substrates of disability. *Ann Neurol*, 46, 747–54.

Velakoulis D, Pantelis C, McGorry PD et al. (1999). Hippocampal volume in first-episode psychosis and chronic schizophrenia: a high-resolution magnetic resonance imaging study. *Arch Gen Psychiatry*, 56, 133–41.

Weinberger DR (1987). Implications of normal brain development for the pathogenesis of schizophrenia. *Arch Gen Psychiatry*, 44, 660–9.

Weinberger DR, Berman KF, Suddath RL and Torrey EF (1992). Evidence of dysfunction of a prefrontal-limbic network in schizophrenia: a magnetic resonance imaging and regional cerebral blood flow study of discordant monozygotic twins. *Am J Psychiatry*, 149, 890–7.

Werring DJ, Clark CA, Barker GJ, Thompson AJ and Miller DH (1999). Diffusion tensor imaging of lesions and normal-appearing white matter in multiple sclerosis. *Neurology*, 52, 1626–32.

Wieshmann UC, Symms MR, Franconi F, Clark CA, Barker GJ and Shorvon SD (1998). Reduced diffusion anisotropy in malformations of cortical development. *Proc Int Soc Magn Reson Med*, 1245.

Woodruff PWR, McManus IC and David AS (1995). Meta-analysis of corpus callosum size in schizophrenia. *J Neurol Neurosurg Psychiatry*, 58, 457–61.

Wright IC, Sharma T, Ellison ZR et al. (1999). Supra-regional brain systems and the neuropathology of schizophrenia. *Cereb Cortex*, 9, 366–78.

Wright IC, Rabe-Hesketh S, Woodruff PW, David AS, Murray RM and Bullmore ET (2000). Meta-analysis of regional brain volumes in schizophrenia. *Am J Psychiatry*, 157, 16–25.

Zipursky RB, Lambe EK, Kapur SK and Mikulis DJ (1998). Cerebral gray matter volume deficits in first episode psychosis. *Arch Gen Psychiatry*, 55, 540–6.

Part IV

Imaging the normal and abnormal mind

7

Functional neuro-imaging and models of normal brain function

R J Dolan

Institute of Neurology, London, UK

Introduction

Functional neuro-imaging techniques provide an unparalleled window on the living human brain. Using neuro-imaging techniques it has, for the first time, become possible to address fundamental questions regarding the neurobiological underpinnings of core human psychological functions, such as memory, attention and emotion. The present chapter will illustrate basic principles of normal brain function by considering how the brain processes a particular class of object, namely the human face. This example will be used to illustrate two distinct, though complementary, modes of brain function involving functional specialization and functional integration respectively. Evidence for functional specialization, a fundamental principle of brain organization, will be illustrated by consideration of neuro-imaging studies which show that a circumscribed region of inferior temporal cortex, the fusiform cortex, is selectively responsive to presentation of faces relative to other classes of objects. By contrast, functional integration, the idea that during complex psychological functions there is coordination of activity among functionally specialized brain regions, will be illustrated by considering the influence of selective attention and emotional content on patterns of activation in functionally specialized regions that mediate face processing.

Functional specialization

Humans are remarkably adept at recognizing individuals by their faces, an ability that may rely on specialized neural circuits (Bruce and Young 1986). Findings from 'prosopagnosic' brain-damaged patients with deficient face processing (Damasio et al. 1982), as well as physiological data from nonhuman primates (Rolls 1992), have now been supplemented by functional imaging results. These data indicate

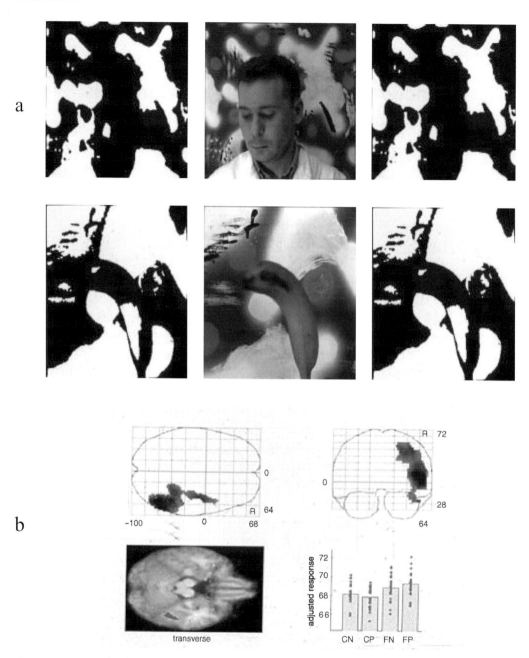

Figure 7.1   Example of a perceptual learning paradigm (a). The side panels represent degraded
figures of a face and object respectively. On initial viewing of these stimuli distinguishing
the face and the banana is difficult. However, following exposure to the full grey-scale
versions of the stimuli there is a rapidly acquired, and lasting, enhancement of perception.
In the lower panel (b) (upper section) is displayed a glass brain which shows regions of

that ventral occipito-temporal areas of the human brain, around the fusiform gyrus, respond more strongly to faces than to other classes of visual stimuli (De Renzi et al. 1994).

It is noteworthy that many neuro-imaging studies of face processing have adopted a general approach of comparing activations elicited by faces with activations elicited by other classes of objects, such as houses (see for example Kanwisher et al. 1997). It needs to be acknowledged that such an approach, while providing evidence for functional specialization in relation to face processing, leaves open the question of whether activation differences represent category-specific differences (faces versus houses) or simply differences due to distinct low-level visual features that characterize faces and other classes of objects.

One powerful approach to the issue of functional specialization that avoids a confound of differences in low-level visual features between stimuli is the use of perceptual learning paradigms. The benefits of this approach include the fact that there is absolute control over the visual input coupled with either phenomenological or behavioural evidence of enhanced stimulus processing. One assumption, underlying this type of experimental approach, is that enhanced processing evidenced either phenomenologically or behaviourally, is mediated by regions that are functionally specialized for the object under investigation. An example of such an experimental approach is the use of a perceptual learning paradigm to address a perceptual facilitation for objects or faces from degraded versions presented in binarized images. This is illustrated in Figure 7.1a.

Note that the experimental design involved four conditions comprising either two-tone (i.e. black and white) images of objects or faces before and after exposure to their associated grey scale. Thus, the experiment comprised four conditions: (a) two-tone images of objects, before learning (the learning phase consisted of the presentation of the grey-scale images); (b) two-tone images of objects, post-learning; (c) two-tone images of faces, prelearning; (d) two-tone images of faces, postlearning. A control experiment, conducted in a separate group of subjects, involved presenting exactly the same sequence of stimuli as above, to account for order effects, but without exposure to the relevant grey-scale image, resulting in an absence of learning. It can be seen that prior to exposure to the grey-scale

Figure 7.1 (*cont.*) the brain where there is greater activity in response to faces compared to houses. An extensive region within the right temporal lobe extending down to the inferior temporal cortex is highlighted. The left lower section shows the region within the above volume where there is a specific perceptual learning-related activation for faces while the right lower panel shows the condition-specific adjusted blood flow responses for this same region.

images there is a low probability of a visual percept. However, after exposure to the associated grey-scale images, which act as visual primes, there is a high probability of a rich percept. This change in phenomenological experience indicates that rapid perceptual learning has taken place. The key question is where in the brain is this form of perceptual learning expressed.

Using positron emission tomography (PET) to index brain activity, the principal finding was that perceptual learning for objects and faces was associated with regionally specific enhanced neuronal responses (Dolan et al. 1997). Thus, learning-dependent effects due to enhanced object perception were seen in the left fusiform region while learning-dependent effects due to faces demonstrated a similar effect in the right fusiform gyrus (see Figure 7.1b). Thus, the important observation was that for both classes of objects there was an enhanced response in fusiform gyri (left for objects and right for faces) to an identical visual input when it elicited a rich visual percept. The observation that the right fusiform region alone alters its response profile as a result of perceptual learning for faces is strong evidence for a high degree of face-specific processing in this region. Note that as the same visual inputs were used across all conditions (pre- and postlearning) the findings specifically address what brain areas are activated when faces or objects are *perceived*.

A similar approach to the study of category-specific brain responses is the use of a related form of learning paradigm referred to as repetition priming. Repetition priming is one of the most basic forms of memory in higher nervous systems and has been studied extensively by cognitive psychologists. Repetition priming is usually indexed behaviourally as faster reaction times or improved identification accuracy following repetition (Schacter and Buckner 1998). A well-established neurophysiological index of repetition priming is a relative decrease in neuronal firing with repeated stimulus presentations – referred to as repetition suppression (Miller et al. 1991) – as found, for example, in inferotemporal regions of monkey cortex (Brown et al. 1987). In an extension of the study described above we determined neuronal responses associated with learning expressed behaviourally as repetition priming.

The methodology used in this study involved event-related functional magnetic resonance imaging (fMRI). This approach allows the measurement of neuronal responses to single events of interest. The experimental design involved studying normal volunteer subjects while they viewed a baseline image that was replaced by either a face or a symbol (see Figure 7.2a). Each stimulus was either familiar (a famous face or meaningful symbol) or unfamiliar (a nonfamous face or meaningless symbol). In separate experiments stimuli were presented twice (Experiments 1 and 2) or five times (Experiments 3 and 4) in a randomly intermixed design. Participants were required to press a key only if the stimulus was a prespecified target (an inverted face or symbol), so that the events of interest, the nontarget stimuli (faces and symbols), were uncontaminated by motor-response requirements. This use of an indirect task

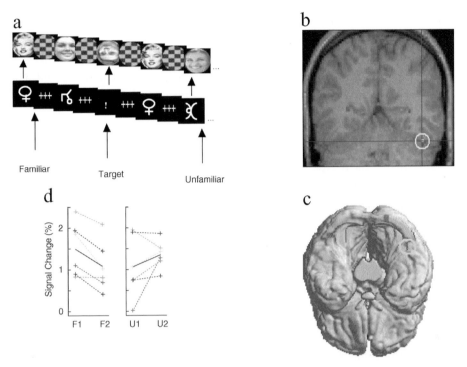

Figure 7.2   On the top left (a) is displayed the experimental layout consisting of consecutive runs of either faces or symbols. The focus here is upon the response to faces. Note that the faces are either familiar or unfamiliar. The occasional inverted face constitutes a target to which the subject was required to respond. The images on the right show two views of the fusiform cortex. The top right image (b) shows the region of brain where there was an enhanced response to familiar compared with unfamiliar faces; the right lower (c) where there was a repetition-related change in neural response involving a decreased response to familiar and an increased response to unfamiliar faces. The left lower figure (d) provides plots of signal change to first and second presentation of faces for familiar and unfamiliar faces respectively.

removes any explicit requirement for differential attention to stimulus familiarity or repetition. Both experiments employed a two-by-two factorial design in which the events of interest were the first or repeated presentation of familiar (F1 and F2) and unfamiliar (U1 and U2) stimuli.

The only regions exhibiting a greater response to familiar than unfamiliar faces were bilateral fusiform cortices (Figure 7.2b), close to what has been referred to as the face area (Kanwisher et al. 1997). This suggests that the neuronal response in the fusiform is sensitive to whether or not a face is recognized, perhaps reflecting activation of face recognition units (FRUs) (Bruce and Young 1986). A right fusiform region (Figure 7.2c) also showed an interaction between familiarity and repetition.

This interaction reflected a decreased response to repetition of familiar stimuli, as observed in most previous imaging studies of repetition priming. In contrast, an increased response was seen to repetition of unfamiliar stimuli, a repetition enhancement effect. These dissociable responses are illustrated in Figure 7.2d. The interpretation of these data is that repetition suppression reflects more efficient processing of repeated familiar stimuli, whereas repetition enhancement reflects neuronal responses associated with a qualitative change in the perception of repeated unfamiliar stimuli.

In terms of the issue of functional specialization, the key finding in the study is the demonstration that a highly circumscribed region of inferior temporal cortex is sensitive to an index of learning, repetition priming, with respect to a distinct class of object, namely faces. More generally, the observed neuronal responses, both enhancements and decrements, to repetition of stimuli can be conceptualized as an expression of a rapidly acquired form of plasticity. The findings reinforce a view of functional specialization within this region for faces but also illustrate that neuronal responses to identical classes of stimuli can be modulated by subtle psychological influences. In the current instance the pattern of neuronal response was influenced as a function of whether there is a prior representation for that stimulus as exemplified by the dimension of familiarity. Thus, patterns of neuronal response are not a simple function of the visual input but are susceptible to higher-order influences.

The functional role of face-specific activations

An important issue raised by a finding of regional specialization is its functional significance. Functional specialization begs the question as to what set of operations are performed by a particular brain region that account for its responsiveness to a particular environmental attribute. In the case of faces it is known that familiar individual faces cannot be recognized solely on the basis of low-level two-dimensional information about spatial frequencies or edges. Instead, such recognition usually requires perception of the three-dimensional surface structure for each face, based on shape-from-shading cues (Kemp et al. 1996; Biederman and Kalocsai 1997). Faces can be readily recognized in a two-tone format that omits all colour and grey-scale information, where there is preservation solely of critical surface shading. The crucial role of shading cues is further illustrated by the well-known difficulty of recognizing faces when contrast polarity is reversed, as in photographic negatives (Bruce and Humphreys 1994) (see Figure 7.3a). Since shadows appear as brighter regions in negatives, the three-dimensional percept of shape-from-shading is lost, even though the edges and spatial frequencies remain unchanged. Consequently, while negatives can still be classified as a face, the depicted individual can no longer be recognized, unless the positive of the same image is shown shortly before, in effect acting as a 'prime'.

We exploited these psychological phenomena to test whether the computational role of face-responsive brain areas in the fusiform gyrus is to extract three-dimensional surface properties for the recognition of individuals (George et al. 1999). If so, three predictions can be made. First, there should be a stronger neural response to positive than negative two-tone images, in brain areas coding the surface structure of faces via shape-from-shading, as only positives yield appropriate three-dimensional shading cues. Second, this advantage for positives over negatives should be more pronounced for known than unknown faces, since only known positives yield recognition of a familiar individual. Finally, the negatives of known faces should become more recognizable, and thus induce a stronger neuronal response, when the corresponding positive is shown before in a manner that 'primes' subsequent recognition. An important psychological observation in this regard is that recognition of a particular individual in a negative is facilitated by previously successful recognition of that same face, but not by a previous exposure in which the face was unidentified (Bruce 1986; Bruce and Humphreys 1994). Since unknown faces cannot yield identification even in positive form, the predicted increase in neural responses for primed (relative to unprimed) negatives should only be observed for known faces and not for unknown faces.

To address these questions we used two-tone pictures of faces that were either of known (famous) individuals, or unknown (nonfamous) people (Figure 7.3a). Positive and negative two-tones were made for each face where shadows appeared as dark-red in the positives, and as light-green in the negatives. Crucially, the total area of dark and light was equal in every picture, thus holding overall luminance constant. These stimuli were presented in a blocked factorial fMRI design, with epochs of famous positives, unknown positives, famous negatives, and unknown negatives, each separated by a baseline period of fixation, in counterbalanced order. For half the epochs ('unprimed'), the particular face-pictures shown had not been seen in previous epochs. For the other epochs ('primed'), the particular face-pictures had appeared before, but with the reverse contrast polarity. Comparing these conditions allowed determination of priming effects.

The first prediction, of a stronger response for positive than negative two-tones, was confirmed by enhanced activation in bilateral posterior fusiform gyri. This profile of activation was more extensive in the left hemisphere, peaking in the posterior border of the fusiform gyrus and extending anteriorly. In the right hemisphere, the activation peaked in the lateral border of the fusiform gyrus (see Figures 7.3b and 7.3c). It needs to be emphasized that the stronger response for positives than negatives cannot be due to edge or spatial frequency differences between the stimuli,

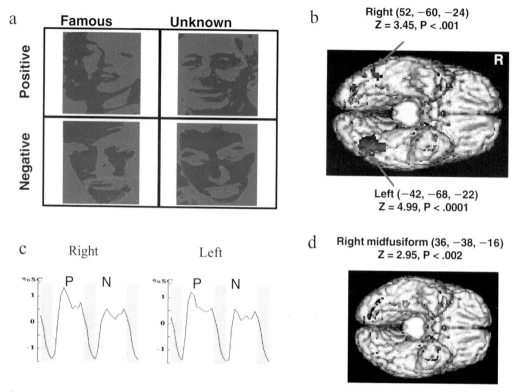

Figure 7.3   On the upper left (a) shows the experimental stimuli and design, which crossed polarity (positive versus negative) of face stimuli with fame (famous or nonfamous). On the upper right (b) shows regions where activations were greater to positive than negative stimuli. The activations are rendered on to a structural MRI projection of the inferior surface of the brain and show regions of focal activation involving the right and left fusiform gyrus. On the lower left (c) shows the time series of the evoked response in the right and left fusiform gyrus to either positive (P) or negative stimuli (N). On the lower right (d) highlights the region where there was an interaction between fame and polarity, involving a larger positive versus negative difference for famous than nonfamous faces (numbers in parentheses refer to coordinates in standard space).

since these two-dimensional cues were identical for positive and negative versions of each face. The critical psychological difference here was the richer percept of three-dimensional face-structure for positives than negatives, due to shading cues. The finding clearly illustrates that the activated brain areas are sensitive to those shape-from-shading cues, which are known to be critical for face recognition.

Our second prediction was that for brain areas involved in the recognition of particular individuals from their faces, the advantage of positives over negatives should be stronger for the known (famous) faces, as only familiar faces can yield true recognition. This was tested by the interaction between positive versus negative, and famous versus unknown. As predicted, stronger activation was found for famous positive faces, with a focus in the right mid-fusiform gyrus (Figure 7.3d). Thus, this region of the fusiform is sensitive to whether a positive face is recognizable as a known individual. The positive and negative of each stimulus always shared these low-level features exactly, yet the right mid-fusiform response was no greater for famous faces among the negatives, only for famous faces among the positives. This confirms that the increased activation for famous positive faces in right mid-fusiform was specifically due to recognition of familiar individuals from three-dimensional surface structure, not to any difference in two-dimensional features. This activation was more anterior than that found for the comparison of positive versus negative faces overall. Note that the latter main effect includes activation due to unknown positive faces, and thus emphasizes just the richer three-dimensional face-percept for positives, rather than the recognition processes isolated by the interaction. The results support proposals that posterior regions of fusiform gyrus are primarily concerned with encoding the structure of faces, whereas more anterior regions use this to contact long-term representations of known faces (Damasio et al. 1990; Ungerleider 1995; Courtney et al. 1997).

The final analysis addressed priming effects arising when a particular face that had appeared in one epoch subsequently reappeared in a later epoch, but now with the reverse contrast polarity. Recall that previous experience with a positive should facilitate subsequent recognition of its negative, but only for the famous faces. We therefore examined famous-face epochs for a simple effect showing greater activation for primed negatives (previously seen as positive) than unprimed negatives (not previously seen). This analysis revealed bilateral fusiform activations for primed famous negatives. The right hemisphere activation peaked at the lateral border of the fusiform gyrus, and extended into the mid-fusiform gyrus. The left hemisphere activation peaked more posteriorly in the fusiform. Thus, the very same negatives of famous faces produced more fusiform activation when they had previously been seen as positives, which make them more identifiable.

These results suggest that face-responsive areas, along the fusiform gyrus, process the three-dimensional shape-from-shading information required for recognition of individuals from their faces. Moreover, activation in specific fusiform regions is stronger for a given face when it is recognized as a known individual, as shown by the interaction with familiarity, and by the effect of priming on famous negatives. The use of contrast-polarity reversal controls means that these findings cannot be attributed to low-level influences from edge or spatial-frequency differences between stimuli. The observed neuronal responses depend on a shading-derived three-dimensional face-percept, and on whether the particular face was identifiable as a known individual from this, regardless of the low-level features. Consequently, these results thus allow face-selective responses in the fusiform gyrus to be directly linked to a putative computational function involving the extraction of three-dimensional surface properties for the recognition of individual faces.

Higher order influences on sensory processing

Adaptive behaviour requires the brain to deal with opposing demands: the selection of goal-relevant stimuli for privileged processing by mechanisms of attention, but also the detection of potentially significant events that may occur unpredictably outside the focus of attention. Competing demands on the brain require specialized processing but also coordination of function between specialized regions in the service of coherent behaviour. In the case of the human face it is evident that any of a number of attributes, for example identity or emotion, may be selected for further processing. Attention is a term used for the generic set of psychological processes that enable this type of selection.

The influence of selective attention on visual processing has been studied from a number of perspectives. While neuro-imaging studies have established that faces can activate relatively specific areas in the fusiform gyrus (Puce et al. 1995; Kanwisher et al. 1997; George et al. 1999) the degree of activation in these regions appears to depend on the degree of attention towards faces, whether they are recognized (Dolan et al. 1997) or task-relevant (Henson et al. 2001). Evidence from functional neuro-imaging in humans (Corbetta et al. 1990; Buchel et al. 1998; Kastner et al. 1998; Rees and Frith 1998) and single-cell recording in monkeys (Moran and Desimone 1985; Chelazzi et al. 1998) also indicate that neuronal responses to unattended stimuli are greatly reduced or even suppressed as compared with attended stimuli. Similarly, at the psychological level, stimuli that are unattended are often perceived less accurately, and may even escape awareness (Newby and Rock 1998). From the perspective of neuro-imaging this suggests a threshold effect, in terms of degree of activation, below which a stimulus is not amenable to conscious awareness.

By contrast to the above consideration there is compelling psychological evidence to suggest that information about stimuli with emotional significance may be processed outside the focus of attention, or even in the absence of awareness for stimulus occurrence. Psychophysical studies have shown that normal observers exhibit fast involuntary responses to emotional stimuli, in particular when these are related to potential threats, such as faces with fearful expressions, or aversive pictures (Ohman 1995; Globisch et al. 1999). Thus, masked fear-conditioned faces can elicit skin conductance changes even when subjects fail to report these stimuli (Ohman 1995). Such automatic, apparently 'preattentive' processing of emotional stimuli might serve to prioritize responses towards particularly significant stimuli. In keeping with this, behavioural studies in normal (Pratto and John 1991; Bradley et al. 1997) and brain-damaged patients with deficits in attention such as spatial neglect (Vuilleumier and Schwartz 2001*a*) have found that emotional stimuli may capture attention more readily than neutral stimuli.

Given the importance of emotionality and attention a crucial question is how each influences face processing. What needs to be emphasized is that attention and emotion are processes that involve regions quite distinct from the fusiform cortex. Thus, it is known that emotional expressions in faces activate brain regions such as the amygdala, anterior cingulate gyrus, orbitofrontal cortex and other prefrontal areas (Breiter et al. 1996; Morris et al. 1996; Blair et al. 1999). The amygdala in particular is consistently activated by fearful faces (Breiter et al. 1996; Morris et al. 1996; Morris et al. 1998*b*; Whalen et al. 1998). By contrast regions involved in selective attention include dorsolateral prefrontal cortex and posterior parietal cortices.

The effect of selective attention on the brain response to faces

To address how attention and emotionality influence face processing we used event-related functional magnetic resonance imaging (fMRI) that examined neural responses to emotional face stimuli during a manipulation of spatial attention. Our specific goals were to determine whether processing a fearful expression in faces occurs automatically, even when attention is directed elsewhere. Evidence that such processing may be relatively 'automatic' includes the fact that amygdala activation to fearful faces is seen even without any requirement for explicit judgement of facial expression (e.g. as when subjects make gender judgements; Morris et al. 1996) or without actual awareness of the faces (i.e. when faces are masked; Morris et al. 1998*b*). In the latter studies, however, subjects were still required to direct spatial attention to the location of the effective stimuli, without any concurrent competing distracters in the scene. On this basis it can be argued that subliminal responses to fear-related stimuli therefore do not necessarily imply that emotional processing will be immune to modulation by spatial attention (Lavie 1995; Maruff et al. 1999). The crucial question consequently is the degree to which any automatic processing for emotional faces is modulated by an attentional manipulation.

The design of our study manipulated attention (i.e. whether stimuli appeared at task-relevant or task-irrelevant locations) and facial expression as independent factors, allowing us to examine the effects on neural processing produced by each factor separately, and to test for a possible interaction. The basic layout of the experiment is illustrated in Figure 7.4a. Twelve healthy volunteers were studied while they viewed brief visual displays that, across all experimental conditions, always contained four stimuli, two faces and two houses, arranged in vertical and horizontal pairs. The two faces in each display had either a neutral or a fearful expression. Stimulus position (vertical pairs of faces and horizontal pairs of houses, or vice versa) and emotional expression (fearful or neutral faces) varied in a counterbalanced and

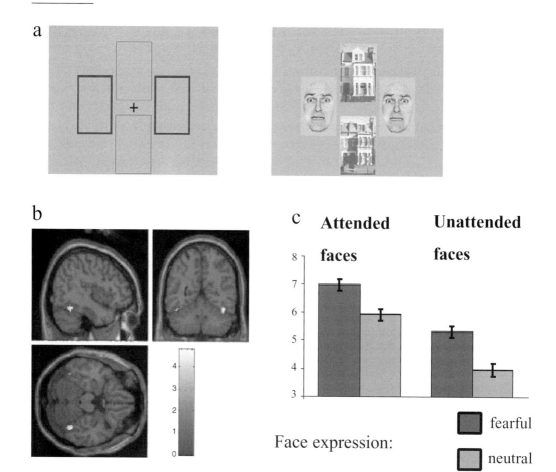

Figure 7.4   The experimental design is illustrated in the top panel (a). Before each experimental run subjects saw a stimulus layout as shown on the left that indicated they had to perform a speeded matching task (same or different) on stimuli appearing at this location. The right-hand panel shows a typical stimulus array that always involved faces and houses. Either of these categories could appear at task-relevant locations (in the example this is the horizontal but on other runs it could be at the vertical positions). In the example provided fearful faces appear at task-relevant locations. Note that faces could also show neutral expressions. On the lower left (b) the brain region, involving bilateral fusiform gyri, which shows a greater response to faces appearing at attended compared with unattended locations, is superimposed on a structural MRI scan. The MRI scan provides transverse, sagittal (right-sided) and coronal views through the fusiform cortex. On the lower right, (c) shows the parameter estimates for face-evoked responses in right fusiform cortex for faces at attended and unattended locations. Note that for both attended and unattended locations the activation to fearful faces is greater than that for neutral.

randomized order. During four successive series of trials subjects had to attend selectively either to the vertical pair of stimuli, or to the horizontal pair of stimuli, and perform a demanding same-different matching judgement for these two stimuli. The two experimental factors of interest (i.e. effects of *attention*, with either faces or houses appearing at the relevant locations, and effects of *emotion*, with fearful versus neutral expressions in faces) were varied independently, and thus were entirely unpredictable on a trial-by-trial basis. This 2×2 factorial design allowed for a direct comparison of the effects of emotional expression for faces presented at task-relevant versus irrelevant locations.

We first determined which brain regions showed an effect of attention in relation to face processing. In other words, we compared all events where the face stimuli appeared at the task-relevant location versus houses occurring at task-relevant sites, regardless of any emotional effect due to fearful expression in the faces. Attending to faces at relevant locations produced a marked increase of activity in the fusiform gyrus in the right hemisphere, as well as in the fusiform and inferior temporo-occipital gyri of the left hemisphere (see Figure 7.4b). These fusiform areas were remarkably symmetrical and correspond to regions previously found to respond more to faces than other classes of stimuli (Puce et al. 1995; Kanwisher et al. 1997). Note that here activation was purely driven by attentional modulation of stimulus processing, in this case faces, with the visual displays themselves being equivalent across conditions. Thus, these findings indicate an effect of higher-order brain processes, in this case selective attention, on patterns of brain activity in regions showing functional specialization for processing distinct attributes of the perceptual world.

Right fusiform activity also increased when faces were fearful, an effect that was additive to that of attention. Such an additive pattern suggests independent sources for these two influences of attention and emotionality. This pattern seen in humans is highly consistent with enhanced responses of face-selective neurons to emotional versus neutral expressions seen in the monkey (Sugase et al. 1999). Fusiform cortex receives prominent feedback projections from the amygdala (Amaral and Price 1984) and such connections could act to enhance processing of emotional stimuli detected by the amygdala (Morris et al. 1998b; Armony and LeDoux 2000). Indeed, an enhancing influence from the amygdala upon the fusiform response to faces with emotional expressions could underlie the particular saliency of such stimuli, as observed in previous behavioural studies (Bradley et al. 1997; Vuilleumier and Schwartz 2001b). The independent effects of emotion and attention on right fusiform activity suggest separate modulatory processes that can mediate competitive influences on visual processing in extrastriate areas. Indeed, evidence from patients with amygdala lesions suggests that a possible behavioural correlate of this modulation is an enhanced perceptual sensitivity for sensory items with emotional value (Anderson and Phelps 2001).

Measuring contextual influences on brain responses to faces

The independent effect of emotionality and attention on fusiform responses to faces is evidence for a substantial influence of psychological context on evoked neuronal responses to sensory inputs. The effect of attention is likely to be mediated via influences from regions such as prefrontal and parietal cortices. For example, in the experiment described above on perceptual priming, activity in the right fusiform showed face-specific responses when, and only when, parietal activity was high. This influence of parietal cortex on fusiform cortex is illustrated in Figure 7.5a. These context-specific effects can be interpreted as an attentional-related difference in face-specific responses in the fusiform cortex mediated through a direct influence from the parietal cortex (Dolan et al. 1997).

By the same token the emotional content-related enhancement of fusiform cortex activity is likely to be mediated via modulatory back-projections from the amygdala (Amaral et al. 1992). Evidence in support of this suggestion comes from a study of emotional face processing where activation of fusiform cortex was predicted by activity in the amygdala when the visual input involved fearful as opposed to happy faces (Morris et al. 1998a) (see Figure 7.5b).

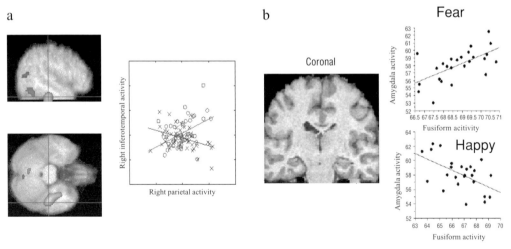

Figure 7.5   Examples of higher-level modulatory influences on lower-level brain processing from two separate experiments. On the left (a) is illustrated the fusiform gyrus region where activity in relation to face presentation is enhanced when, and only when, parietal activity is also high. On the plot, circles represent faces and crosses represent objects. On the right (b) is a similar region of fusiform where enhanced activity is predicted by activity in the amygdala only when subjects are processing fearful as opposed to neutral faces. Both findings can be conceptualized in terms of contextual influences from higher brain regions on processing in lower-level regions.

Both the above findings suggest that an important aspect of dynamic brain organization is mediated via contextual effects. This idea can be taken further to suggest that a major contribution to the specialization of a region derives from influences from backward as opposed to forward anatomical connections (Friston and Price 2001). It is noteworthy that computational models of brain function, particularly as embodied in what is termed generative models, also emphasize the role of backward connections in mediating responses at lower input levels based on the activity of units in higher levels (Hinton et al. 1995).

The effect of emotionality on face processing

Given evidence for attentional modulation of face processing in fusiform cortex a remaining question is whether distinct attributes of face stimuli, such as emotionality, are processed by brain regions distinct from those processing faces themselves. A related question is the degree to which such processing is influenced by attention. In the experiment described the question of where emotion (in this case fear) is processed can be determined by identifying brain regions activated irrespective of the condition of spatial attention. Thus, comparing displays with fearful and neutral faces revealed peaks of activation in the left amygdala. This finding of increased amygdala activation is consistent with a crucial role for this structure in emotional processing, indicated by evidence from animal studies (LeDoux 2000), from patients with focal brain damage (Adolphs et al. 1995; Young et al. 1995), and from functional neuro-imaging in normal humans (Breiter et al. 1996; Morris et al. 1996; LaBar et al. 1998). Previous studies using PET (Morris et al. 1996) or blocked fMRI (Breiter et al. 1996; Whalen et al. 1998) found preferential activation of the left amygdala by fearful as opposed to neutral faces. This accords with the present event-related results, showing left amygdala activity as a main effect of fearful faces in the visual field, regardless of the attentional condition, and thus of the allocation of spatial attention. The broader relevance of these findings is that it demonstrates that distinct attributes of face stimuli are processed in separate brain regions.

The key question here is whether processing of emotional face stimuli in the amygdala is susceptible to attentional modulation, as demonstrated for the fusiform gyrus. Recall that attentional effects with respect to faces leads to enhancement of fusiform activation. The critical issue is whether the response to fearful versus neutral faces, expressed in the amygdala, is also modulated by an attentional manipulation. The most direct test for an effect of attention on the response to fearful expressions is to identify brain regions showing a significant interaction between the two factors (attention and valence) across all trial conditions. In this analysis three distinct areas responded more to fearful faces when these appeared at

feed-forward and backward anatomical connectivity. The wider relevance of the findings presented in this chapter relates to the likely level of dysfunction that underlies serious psychiatric disorder. It is tempting to speculate that a fundamental deficit in these conditions may be expressed at the level of integration.

REFERENCES

Adolphs R, Tranel D, Damasio H and Damasio AR (1995). Fear and the human amygdala. *J Neurosci*, 15, 5879–91.

Amaral DG and Price JL (1984). Amygdalo-cortical projections in the monkey (*Macaca fascicularis*). *J Comp Neurol*, 230, 465–96.

Amaral DG, Price JL, Pitkanen A and Carmichael ST (1992). Anatomical organization of the primate amygdaloid complex. In *The Amygdala: Neurobiological Aspects of Emotion, Memory and Mental Dysfunction*, ed. J Aggleton, pp. 1–66. New York: Wiley-Liss.

Anderson AK and Phelps EA (2001). Lesions of the human amygdala impair enhanced perception of emotionally salient events. *Nature*, 411(6835), 305–9.

Armony J and LeDoux J (2000). How danger is encoded: towards a systems, cellular, and computational understanding of cognitive-emotional interactions in fear. In *The New Cognitive Neurosciences*, ed. M Gazzaniga. Cambridge, MA: MIT Press.

Biederman I and Kalocsai P (1997). Neurocomputational bases of object and face recognition. *Philos Trans R Soc London B Biol Sci*, 352(1358), 1203–19.

Blair RJ, Morris JS, Frith CD, Perrett DI and Dolan RJ (1999). Dissociable neural responses to facial expressions of sadness and anger. *Brain*, 122, 883–93.

Bradley BP, Mogg K and Lee SC (1997). Attentional biases for negative information in induced and naturally occurring dysphoria. *Behav Res Ther*, 35, 911–27.

Breiter HC, Etcoff NL, Whalen PJ et al. (1996). Response and habituation of the human amygdala during visual processing of facial expression. *Neuron*, 17, 875–87.

Brown MW, Wilson FA and Riches IP (1987). Neuronal evidence that inferomedial temporal cortex is more important than hippocampus in certain processes underlying recognition memory. *Brain Res*, 409, 158–62.

Bruce V (1986). Influences of familiarity on the processing of faces. *Perception*, 15, 387–97.

Bruce V and Humphreys GW (1994). Recognizing objects and faces. *Vis Cogn*, 1, 141–80.

Bruce V and Young AW (1986). Understanding face recognition. *Br J Psychology*, 77, 305–27.

Buchel C, Josephs O, Rees G, Turner R, Frith CD and Friston KJ (1998). The functional anatomy of attention to visual motion. A functional MRI study. *Brain*, 121, 1281–94.

Chelazzi L (1995). Neural mechanisms for stimulus selection in cortical areas of the macaque subserving object vision. *Behav Brain Res*, 71, 125–34.

Chelazzi L, Duncan J, Miller EK and Desimone R (1998). Responses of neurons in inferior temporal cortex during memory-guided visual search. *J Neurophysiol*, 80, 2918–40.

Corbetta M, Miezin FM, Dobmeyer S, Shulman GL and Petersen SE (1990). Attentional modulation of neural processing of shape, color, and velocity in humans. *Science*, 248, 1556–9.

Courtney SM, Ungerleider LG, Kell K and Haxby JV (1997). Transient and sustained activity in a distributed neural system for human working memory. *Nature*, 386, 608–11.

Damasio AR, Damasio H and Van Hoesen GW (1982). Prosopagnosia: anatomical basis and behavioural mechanisms. *Neurology*, 32, 331–41.

Damasio AR, Tranel D and Damasio H (1990). Face agnosia and the neural substrates of memory. *Annu Rev Neurosci*, 13, 89–109.

De Renzi E, Perani D, Carlesimo GA, Silveri MC and Fazio F (1994). Prosopagnosia can be associated with damage confined to the right hemisphere – an MRI and PET study and a review of the literature. *Neuropsychologia*, 32, 893–902.

Dolan RJ, Fink GR, Rolls E, Booth M, Frackowiak RSJ and Friston KJ (1997). How the brain learns to see objects and faces in an impoverished context. *Nature*, 389, 596–9.

Friston, KJ and Price CJ (2001). Dynamic representation and generative models of brain function. *Brain Res Bull*, 54, 273–85.

George N, Dolan RJ, Fink GR, Baylis GC, Russell C and Driver J (1999). Contrast polarity and face recognition in the human fusiform gyrus. *Nat Neurosci*, 2, 574–80.

Globisch J, Hamm O, Esteves F and Ohman A (1999). Fear appears fast: temporal course of startle reflex potentiation in animal subjects. *Psychophysiology*, 30, 66–7.

Henson R, Gorno-Tempini M, Shallice T and Dolan RJ (2001). Face repetition effects in implicit and explicit memory tasks. *Cereb Cortex* (in press).

Hinton GE, Dayan P, Frey BJ and Neal RM (1995). The wake-sleep algorithm for unsupervised neural networks. *Science*, 268, 1158–61.

Kanwisher N, McDermott J and Chun MM (1997). The fusiform face area: a module in human extrastriate cortex specialized for face perception. *J Neurosci*, 17, 4302–11.

Kastner S, De Weerd P, Desimone R and Ungerleider LG (1998). Mechanisms of directed attention in the human extrastriate cortex as revealed by functional MRI. *Science*, 282, 108–11.

Kemp R, Pike G, White P and Musselman A (1996). Perception and recognition of normal and negative faces: the role of shape from shading and pigmentation cues. *Perception*, 25, 37–52.

LaBar KS, Gatenby JC, Gore JC, LeDoux JE and Phelp EA (1998). Human amygdala activation during conditioned fear acquisition and extinction: a mixed-trial fMRI study. *Neuron*, 20, 937–45.

Lavie N (1995). Perceptual load as a necessary condition for selective attention. *J Exp Psychol: Hum Percept Perform*, 21, 451–68.

LeDoux JE (2000). Emotion circuits in the brain. *Annu Rev Neurosci*, 23, 155–84.

LeDoux JE, Cicchetti P, Xagoraris A and Romanski LM (1990). The lateral amygdaloid nucleus: sensory interface of the amygdala in fear conditioning. *J Neurosci*, 10, 1062–9.

Maruff P, Danckert J, Camplin G and Currie J (1999). Behavioral goals constrain the selection of visual information. *Psychol Sci*, 10, 522–5.

Miller EK, Li L and Desimone R (1991). A neural mechanism for working and recognition memory in inferior temporal cortex. *Science*, 254, 1377–9.

Moran J and Desimone R (1985). Selective attention gates visual processing in the extrastriate cortex. *Science*, 229, 782–4.

Morris JS, Frith D, Perrett DI, et al. (1996). A differential neural response in the human amygdala to fearful and happy facial expressions. *Nature*, 383, 812–15.

Morris JS, Friston KJ, Buchel C et al. (1998*a*). A neuromodulatory role for the human amygdala in processing emotional facial expressions. *Brain*, 121, 47–57.

Morris JS, Ohman A and Dolan RJ (1998*b*). Conscious and unconscious emotional learning in the human amygdala. *Nature*, 393, 467–70.

Morris JS, Ohman A and Dolan RJ (1999). A subcortical pathway to the right amygdala mediating unseen fear. *Proc Nat Acad Sci USA*, 96, 1680–5.

Morris JS, DeGelder B, Weiskrantz L and Dolan RJ (2001). Differential extrageniculostriate and amygdala responses to presentation of emotional faces in a cortically blind field. *Brain*, 124, 1241–52.

Newby E A and Rock I (1998). Inattentional blindness as a function of proximity to the focus of attention. *Perception*, 27, 1025–40.

Ohman A (1995). Preparedness and preattentive associative learning: electrodermal conditioning of masked stimuli. *J Psychophysiol*, 9, 99–108.

Pratto F and John OP (1991). Automatic vigilance: the attention-grabbing power of negative social information. *J Pers Soc Psychol*, 61, 380–91.

Puce A, Allison T, Gore JC and McCarthy G (1995). Face-sensitive regions in human extrastriate cortex studied by functional MRI. *J Neurophysiol*, 74, 1192–9.

Rees G and Frith CD (1998). How do we select perceptions and actions? Human brain imaging studies. *Philos Trans R Soc Lond B Biol Sci*, 353, 1283–93.

Rolls ET (1992). Neurophysiological mechanisms underlying face processing within and beyond the temporal cortical visual areas. *Philos Trans R Soc Lond*, 335, 11–21.

Schacter DL and Buckner RL (1998). Priming and the brain. *Neuron*, 20, 185–95.

Sugase Y, Yamane S, Ueno S and Kawano K (1999). Global and fine information coded by single neurons in the temporal visual cortex. *Nature*, 400, 869–73.

Ungerleider LG (1995). Functional brain imaging studies of cortical mechanisms for memory. *Science*, 270, 769–75.

Vuilleumier P and Schwartz S (2001*a*). Beware and be aware: capture of spatial attention by fear-related stimuli in neglect. *Neuroreport*, 12, 1119–22.

Vuilleumier P and Schwartz S (2001*b*). Emotional facial expressions capture attention. *Neurology*, 56, 153–8.

Whalen PJ, Rauch SL, Etcoff NL, McInerney SC, Lee MB and Jenike MA (1998). Masked presentations of emotional facial expressions modulate amygdala activity without explicit knowledge. *J Neurosci*, 18, 411–18.

Young AW, Aggleton JP, Hellawell DJ, Johnson M, Broks P and Hanley JR (1995). Face processing impairments after amygdalotomy. *Brain*, 118, 15–24.

8

Functional magnetic resonance imaging in psychiatry: where are we now and where are we going?

Ed Bullmore

University of Cambridge, Addenbrooke's Hospital, Cambridge, UK

Introduction

As a technique for measuring changes in oxygenated cerebral blood flow related to local neuronal activity, functional magnetic resonance imaging (fMRI) is approximately 10 years old. As an instrument of psychiatric research, it is even younger – perhaps 7 years old by the time this book is published.

Already it is clear that fMRI has some outstanding technical advantages compared with previously available methods for functional neuro-imaging, such as positron- and single photon-emission tomography (PET and SPET). (For a general introduction to fMRI physics, experimental design and data analysis, see review articles by Bullmore and Suckling (2000, 2001).) First and foremost, it is remarkably safe. There is no requirement for exposure to ionizing radiation or radioisotopes and, at static magnetic field strengths of 3 tesla or less, the only significant health and safety risks are posed by the loud acoustic noise of most scanners (subjects must wear ear-protectors) and by deposition of radiofrequency energy (which limits scanning time in a single session to 45 minutes in some centres). This degree of safety considerably relieves any ethical concerns about scanning patients and usefully favours study designs entailing multiple repeated measures on each subject. The second major advantage of fMRI is that it has superior spatial resolution (in the order of mm) and temporal resolution (in the order of s) compared with any single alternative modality for investigation of living human brain function. This has allowed the recent development of event-related methods using fMRI, by which the physiological response to a few dozen brief, discrete stimuli or cognitive trials can be precisely mapped (Friston et al. 1999). A third major advantage is that fMRI is closely related to other magnetic resonance-based techniques for imaging brain structure and cerebrovascular function which potentially facilitates, for example, the integration of fMRI data with complementary data more sensitive to white matter tract organization (Werring et al. 1998).

Of course no neuro-imaging technique is perfect and functional MRI is not without its limitations. The scanning environment is restrictive, indeed some people find it intolerably claustrophobic, and there are often pragmatic limits on how stimuli may be presented and/or how subjects may register their responses during scanning. Some areas of the brain are poorly visualized due to susceptibility artefacts, which affect particularly regions such as inferior temporal cortex and orbitofrontal cortex which lie in close proximity to tissue (bone or air-filled sinus) with very different magnetization properties. The signal is exquisitely sensitive to movement of the head during scanning. Head movements of less than 1 mm may create disproportionately large, cognitively spurious signal changes; and patient groups may be more prone to head movement than normal comparison subjects (Bullmore et al. 1999*a*). Perhaps most fundamentally, fMRI measures the haemodynamic response to neuronal activation rather than neuronal activity per se and this 'vascular confound' might be thought to complicate interpretation of signal changes such as those observed before and after treatment with psychoactive drugs like methylphenidate that also have effects on systemic and cerebral vasculature (Rao et al. 2000). However, recent work combining fMRI and single-unit recording in anaesthetized monkeys has emphasized the strong linear association between magnitude of the fMRI signal and local field potentials generated in visual cortex by photic stimulation (Logothetis et al. 2001), suggesting that a straightforward interpretation of fMRI signal change in terms of local synaptic activity may often be plausible.

On balance, it seems that the technical advantages of fMRI clearly outweigh its disadvantages. So how has this potentially important technique been applied so far to investigation of psychiatric disorder? And how can we imagine the application of fMRI to psychiatry will develop in future?

fMRI and psychiatry: where are we now?

The majority of published studies have inherited an apparently simple case–control design from the prior PET literature. A group of patients, usually defined by an operationalized diagnosis of disorder, is scanned during performance of a cognitive task or during sensory stimulation. The presentation of the stimulating or demanding *activation* condition is contrasted with a relatively undemanding *baseline* condition; more than one activation condition may be presented in the course of a single experiment. (For a recent account of the logic of cognitive subtraction, originally developed by FC Donders in the nineteenth century and widely used in functional neuro-imaging since *c.* 1985, see Sternberg (2001).) A statistical model for signal change determined by the contrast between baseline and activation condition(s) is fitted to the fMRI time series observed at each voxel of the image, yielding a parametric map of some test statistic(s) for functional activation. Exactly the same procedures are used to measure task-specific brain activation in a group of comparison subjects. Analysis of variance or covariance is used to identify voxels or regions of the image where there is a significant difference between groups in functional activation. Multiple-hypothesis tests may be conducted using frequentist parametric or nonparametric methods (Bullmore et al. 2001; Nicholls and Holmes 2001); Bayesian approaches to inference in fMRI are also under active development (Genovese 2000).

Functional MRI studies conducted along these lines have already demonstrated abnormalities, usually deficiencies, of functional activation under diverse cognitive conditions in patients with schizophrenia, bipolar disorder, obsessive–compulsive disorder, autism, attention-deficit hyperactivity disorder, etc. (Curtis et al. 1997; Ring et al. 1999; Rubia et al. 1999; Yurgelun-Todd et al. 2000). The high prevalence of such positive results indicates the sensitivity of fMRI, especially in light of the modest-sized samples studied (typically $n < 20$ per group), but it may also raise questions about the specificity of findings. For example, if a group of patients performs a given task more slowly or less accurately than the subjects with whom they are compared, can any difference in physiological activation be attributed specifically to the presence of disorder rather than to the more general effects of impaired performance (Weinberger and Berman 1996)? A comparable problem is posed by the fact that the majority of patients with severe mental illness will have been treated with antipsychotics or other drugs which may have significant effects on functional activation in their own right. In short, fMRI is sensitive to many nonpathological variables which can easily mimic or obscure any disease-specific effects on brain physiology (Bullmore et al. 1999b).

Besides these methodological and pioneering case–control studies, the existing fMRI literature has also begun to explore some conceptual issues that are likely to prove important in formulating functional anatomical models of psychiatric disorder. Some basic concepts of particular relevance are connectivity, activation capacity and cognitive load-response. Connectivity refers to the fact that the human brain is densely, often reciprocally, interconnected and that most 'higher order' functions that might be abnormal in psychiatric disorders are subserved not by one or a few specialized brain modules but by large-scale neurocognitive networks (Mesulam 2000). The integrated function of large-scale neurocognitive networks can be explored and modelled by applications of various multivariate statistical methods to analysis of functional MRI data (Bullmore et al. 1996, 2000). These methods range from simple estimation of the correlation between two time series sampled from different brain regions, to techniques such as principal components analysis which are useful in exploring a large number of inter-regional relationships simultaneously, to more model-based or confirmatory techniques such as path analysis. Abnormal states of integrated network function, in short states of functional dysconnectivity, have been theoretically predicted as neural correlates of psychiatric disorder since the work of Carl Wernicke and other nineteenth century 'diagram-makers' (Bullmore et al. 1997). The conjunction of fMRI and multivariate data analysis potentially allows this very early idea in psychiatry to develop into a more rigorous, empirically based and quantitative formulation of disorders in terms of dysconnectivity.

One other key concept is that the brain normally has a finite capacity for functional activation (Handy 2001) and increasing cognitive demands will tend to use a greater proportion of this capacity to support appropriately specialized processing, i.e. the brain has load-response properties (Braver et al. 1997). These basic principles can inform psychiatric fMRI in various ways. For example, we might want to say that endogenous, psychopathological states, such as auditory–verbal hallucinations, can *compete* with exogenous, experimentally controlled demands for activation of the same processing systems. Given the finite capacity available to meet total demand, such a competition predicts attenuated activation by exogenous demands in the presence of competitive symptoms. We might also want to conceive of reduced functional activation by patients in terms of flattening or shifting of the cognitive load-response curves that define the local relationships between experimental demand and neurocognitive supply (Fletcher et al. 1998; Callicott et al. 1999).

fMRI and psychiatry: where next?

One likely development in the immediate future is the further refinement of case–control methodology for fMRI. There will be more studies using patients with other disorders as control groups, or untreated or never-treated patient groups (Barch et al. 2001), to isolate the effects of medication. There will be more widespread use of various techniques intended to match task performance between groups. For example, there will probably be greater use of graded or parametric experiments, which ideally allow a cognitive task to be presented over a continuously variable range of difficulty, so that activation between groups can be compared at possibly different levels of task difficulty associated with equivalent performance (Fletcher et al. 1998; Callicott et al. 1999, 2000). Event-related experiments promise a similar benefit in that incorrectly performed trials can simply be omitted from analysis and two groups can then be compared on the basis of their response to an equal number of correctly performed trials.

Another development which may help to focus our understanding of physiological effects specific to diagnosis will be the greater use of meta-analysis and data-sharing to compare and combine results across many small case–control studies. Currently, meta-analytic techniques have been applied to structural MRI case–control studies of schizophrenia (Wright et al. 2000) but not yet extended to the more complex problems of integrating results over several fMRI studies which may differ in numerous, possibly significant details of design. An illustration of the feasibility and interest of combining results across fMRI studies is provided by a recent report highlighting the commonality of prefrontal and anterior cingulate cortical activations by a variety of experimental designs (Duncan and Owen 2000). However, it may be that more formal meta-analysis of psychiatric fMRI data will not be possible based on results published in traditional format but will need to await the establishment of digital data repositories where 'raw' imaging data can be stored and accessed via the internet (Koslow 2000; OHBM 2001).

More radically, it is likely that there will be a thorough reappraisal of case–control designs for fMRI in relation to at least two questions. First, if we wish to make a between-group comparison, is 'caseness' or diagnosis always the best grouping variable for the patients? Second, do we need to make cross-sectional comparisons between groups to use fMRI incisively in psychiatry? The short answer to both questions is probably no.

Many diagnostic categories in psychiatry subsume a tremendous heterogeneity of clinical states and outcomes. None of the major diagnoses is yet articulated in terms of cognitive neuroscience. It would perhaps be surprising if fMRI studies designed on the basis of traditional diagnostic categories provided proof of their specific neural correlates. One emerging reaction to this problem is to investigate patients in terms of symptoms, or dimensions of correlated symptoms, rather than classical diagnostic entities (Kircher et al. 2001; Menon et al. 2001*b*; Perlstein et al. 2001). Another important future trend, involving fMRI but extending beyond it, will likely be a neurocognitive reformulation of the phenomena of psychiatry (Halligan and David 2001). One example of this process that has already proved fruitful in fMRI is the concept of auditory hallucinations as a manifestation of disordered monitoring of inner speech (Frith 1996). This model cuts across the diagnostic boundaries between varieties of psychosis and is based on an established body of work concerning normal frontoparietal and frontotemporal systems for articulatory rehearsal, auditory–verbal imagery and self-monitoring (Shergill et al. 2000). Comparable recent initiatives include investigation of dysexecutive and abulic psychotic symptoms in relation to disordered function of fronto-striato-thalamic circuits (Manoach et al. 2000; Menon et al. 2001*a*) and a characterization of obsessive and compulsive symptoms in relation to the functional neuroanatomy of disgust and other cardinal emotions (Phillips et al. 2000). Hopefully, these are just the beginnings of a major effort using fMRI to test models of psychiatric phenomena that are rooted in contemporary cognitive neuroscience rather than the (admittedly acute) nosological acumen of psychiatry's founding fathers.

In any case, there is no immediate need to restrict fMRI designs to a cross-sectional comparison between groups, however defined. Unlike PET, fMRI is sufficiently sensitive to map functional neuroanatomy quite reliably in a single individual. This potentially allows a case study approach, whereby individual patterns of functional activation can be understood in relation to individual profiles of symptoms and cognitive impairment (David et al. 1996). More ambitiously, it opens the door to possible clinical applications. Abnormal activation patterns might be normalized by drug or psychological treatments before there is an overt clinical response, providing a role for fMRI in treatment planning or monitoring. Probabilistic diagnosis by fMRI is also conceivable. A single patient could be scanned under standard conditions and these imaging data referred to a large normative database to assign a probability of normal brain function at each voxel. Serial measurements of brain function on the same patient at intervals of one or more years could be compared to age-matched norms to provide an index of neurocognitive maturation or developmental trajectory (Rubia et al. 2000). These major clinical benefits of fMRI may currently seem somewhat fanciful but are not inconceivable in the medium term. However, any application of functional (or structural) MRI to diagnostic or prognostic questions in clinical psychiatry must properly be underpinned by an epidemiologically scaled, comprehensive and quantitative engagement with general population variability of brain structure and function over the course of the life cycle. Whatever the sophistication of our neuro-imaging devices, we will need to know more about the appearances of *normality* before abnormalities associated with psychiatric disorder, however defined, become clinically salient.

All of these incipient or imagined developments entail using fMRI to achieve a clearer understanding of dysfunctional neurocognitive systems correlated with abnormal psychological states. In other words, they are all aspects of fMRI as part of a new phenomenology; yet one of the most exciting future prospects is that fMRI may also contribute to a new aetiology. A particularly promising strategy is the combination of fMRI with recent developments in molecular genetics and developmental neurobiology to understand the consequences for human brain function of polymorphism in genes for neurotransmitters, neurodevelopmental control factors, cell adhesion molecules and other products that are critical to normal brain development or integrated function in animal models. There are so far only a few examples of this approach in the literature (Egan et al. 2001) but there will be more. A complementary approach that may also become more widely adopted is investigation of rare and relatively neglected disorders, such as Fragile X syndrome (Kwon et al. 2001), velo-cardio-facial syndrome (van Amelsvoort et al. 2001) or tuberous sclerosis (Ridler et al. 2001), which share clearly defined genetic lesions and a risk for psychopathology. In both studies of normal genetic polymorphisms and neurogenetic syndromes, fMRI is in a strong position to provide a crucial explanatory link between genetic and behavioural levels of understanding.

Finally, there is also the potential contribution of fMRI to therapeutics. The effects of several psychoactive compounds on functional activation have already been measured by fMRI (Vaidya et al. 1998; Furey et al. 2000; Mattay et al. 2000). For example, patients with schizophrenia receiving risperidone were found to have enhanced frontal cortical activation by a working-memory task compared with patients taking typical antipsychotic drugs (Honey et al. 1999). Functional MRI cannot currently compete with PET as a tool for receptor-binding studies (see Chapter 9 by Grasby), although MR-contrast-inducing agents can be attached to receptor-specific ligands, so receptor mapping without radioactivity may be possible in future. At present, however, the main value of pharmacological fMRI (or phMRI as it is sometimes called) is to investigate the neurocognitive effects of psychoactive compounds, perhaps exploiting the safe repeatability of fMRI to study several active compounds or the same compound at several doses in the same subject. More futuristically, phMRI may be coupled with developments in pharmacogenomics to explain genetically determined variability of behavioural response to drugs or to assist post-genomic processes of drug development that start with a gene product (putative target) of unknown function rather than a possible drug of unknown toxicity and efficacy (Leslie and James 2000).

Conclusions

These are admittedly enthusiastic thoughts but I want to emphasize in closing that I am not primarily enthusiastic about the technology of fMRI. I do not believe that scanners are inherently smart, or that bigger magnets are necessarily better, or that further technological advances in neuro-imaging will automatically resolve the problems of psychiatry. However, used decisively in conjunction with contemporary neurosciences and sound experimental design, there is surely much that fMRI can show us about the brain that will have a progressive influence on psychiatry.

REFERENCES

Barch DM, Carter CS, Braver TS et al. (2001). Selective deficits in prefrontal cortex function in medication-naïve patients with schizophrenia. *Arch Gen Psychiatry*, 58, 280–8.

Braver TS, Cohen JD, Nystrom LE, Jonides J, Smith EE and Noll DC (1997). A parametric study of prefrontal cortex involvement in human working memory. *Neuroimage*, 5, 49–62.

Bullmore ET and Suckling J (2000). Functional MRI. In *The New Oxford Textbook of Psychiatry*, ed. M Gelder, NC Andreasen and J Lopez-Ibor, Vol. 1, pp. 218–23. New York: Oxford University Press.

Bullmore ET and Suckling J (2001). Functional magnetic resonance imaging. *Int Rev Psychiatry*, 13, 24–33.

Bullmore ET, Rabe-Hesketh S, Morris RG et al. (1996). Functional magnetic resonance image analysis of a large-scale neurocognitive network. *Neuroimage*, 4, 16–33.

Bullmore ET, Frangou S and Murray RM (1997). The dysplastic net hypothesis: an integration of developmental and dysconnectionist theories of schizophrenia. *Schizophr Res*, 28, 143–56.

Bullmore ET, Brammer MJ, Rabe-Hesketh S et al. (1999*a*). Methods for diagnosis and treatment of stimulus correlated motion in generic brain activation studies using fMRI. *Hum Brain Mapp*, 7, 38–48.

Bullmore ET, Brammer MJ, Williams SCR et al. (1999*b*). Functional MR imaging of confounded hypofrontality. *Hum Brain Mapp*, 8, 86–91.

Bullmore ET, Horwitz B, Honey GD, Brammer MJ, Williams SCR and Sharma T (2000). How good is good enough in path analysis of fMRI data? *Neuroimage*, 11, 289–301.

Bullmore ET, Long C, Suckling J et al. (2001). Colored noise and computational inference in neurophysiological (fMRI) time series analysis: resampling methods in the time and wavelet domains. *Hum Brain Mapp*, 12, 61–78.

Callicott JH, Mattay VS, Bertolino A et al. (1999). Physiological characteristics of capacity constraints in working memory as revealed by functional MRI. *Cereb Cortex*, 9, 20–6.

Callicott JH, Bertolino A, Mattay VS et al. (2000). Physiological dysfunction of the dorsolateral prefrontal cortex in schizophrenia revisited. *Cereb Cortex*, 10, 1078–92.

Curtis VA, Bullmore ET, Wright IC et al. (1997). Attenuated frontal activation during verbal fluency in schizophrenia. *Am J Psychiatry*, 155, 1056–63.

David AS, Woodruff PWR, Howard R et al. (1996). Auditory hallucinations inhibit exogenous activation of auditory cortex. *Neuroreport*, 7, 932–6.

Duncan J and Owen AM (2000). Common regions of the human frontal lobe recruited by diverse cognitive demands. *Trends Neurosci*, 23, 475–83.

Egan MF, Goldberg TE, Kolachana BS et al. (2001). Effect of COMT Val (108/158) Met genotype on frontal lobe function and risk for schizophrenia. *Proc Natl Acad Sci USA*, 98, 6917–22.

Fletcher PC, McKenna PJ, Frith CD, Grasby PM, Friston KJ and Dolan RJ (1998). Brain activations in schizophrenia during a graded-memory task studied with functional neuroimaging. *Arch Gen Psychiatry*, 55, 1001–8.

Friston KJ, Zarahn E, Josephs O, Henson RNA and Dale AM (1999). Stochastic designs in event-related fMRI. *Neuroimage*, 10, 607–19.

Frith CD (1996). The role of the prefrontal cortex in self-consciousness: the case of auditory hallucinations. *Philos Trans R Soc B*, 351, 1505–12.

Furey M, Pietrini P and Haxby JV (2000). Cholinergic enhancement and increased selectivity of perceptual processing during working memory. *Science*, 290, 2315–19.

Genovese CR (2000). A Bayesian time-course model for functional magnetic resonance imaging data. *J Am Stat Assoc*, 95, 691–703.

Halligan PW and David AS (2001). Cognitive neuropsychiatry: towards a scientific psychopathology. *Nat Rev Neurosci*, 2, 209–15.

Handy TC (2001). Capacity theory as a model of cortical behavior. *J Cogn Neurosci*, 12, 1066–9.

Honey GD, Bullmore ET, Soni W, Varatheesan M, Williams SCR and Sharma T (1999). Differences in frontal cortical activation by a working memory task following substitution of risperidone for typical antipsychotic drugs in schizophrenic patients. *Proc Natl Acad Sci USA*, 96, 13432–7.

Kircher TTJ, Liddle PF, Brammer MJ, Williams SCR, Murray RM and McGuire PK (2001). Neural correlates of formal thought disorder in schizophrenia – preliminary findings from a functional magnetic resonance imaging study. *Arch Gen Psychiatry*, 58, 769–74.

Koslow S (2000). Should the neuroscience community make a paradigm shift to sharing primary data? *Nat Neurosci*, 3, 863–5.

Kwon H, Menon V, Eliez S et al. (2001). Functional neuroanatomy of visuospatial working memory in fragile X syndrome: relation to behavioral and molecular measures. *Am J Psychiatry*, 158, 1040–51.

Leslie RA and James MF (2000). Pharmacological magnetic resonance imaging: a new application for functional MRI. *Trends Pharmacol Sci*, 21, 314–18.

Logothetis NK, Pauls J, Augath M, Trinath T and Oeltermann A (2001). Neurophysiological investigation of the basis of the fMRI signal. *Nature*, 412, 150–7.

Manoach DS, Gollub RL, Benson ES et al. (2000). Schizophrenic subjects show aberrant fMRI activation of dorsolateral prefrontal cortex and basal ganglia during working memory performance. *Biol Psychiatry*, 48, 99–109.

Mattay VS, Callicott JH, Bertolino A et al. (2000). Effects of dextroamphetamine on cognitive performance and cortical activation. *Neuroimage*, 12, 268–75.

Menon V, Anagnoson RT, Glover GH and Pfefferbaum A (2001*a*). Functional magnetic resonance imaging evidence for disrupted basal ganglia function in schizophrenia. *Am J Psychiatry*, 158, 646–9.

Menon V, Anagnoson RT, Mathalon DH, Glover GH and Pfefferbaum A (2001*b*). Functional neuroanatomy of auditory working memory in schizophrenia: relation to positive and negative symptoms. *Neuroimage*, 13, 433–46.

Mesulam M-M (2000). *Principles of Behavioural and Cognitive Neurology*. New York: Oxford University Press.

Nicholls TE and Holmes AP (2001). Nonparametric permutation tests for functional neuroimaging: a primer with examples. *Hum Brain Mapp*, 15, 1–25.

OHBM [Council for Organisation of Human Brain Mapping] (2001). Neuroimaging databases. *Science*, 292, 1673–6; see also *http://www.humanbrainmapping.org*.

Perlstein WM, Carter CS, Noll DC and Cohen JD. (2001). Relation of prefrontal cortex dysfunction to working memory and symptoms in schizophrenia. *Am J Psychiatry*, 158, 1105–13.

Phillips ML, Marks IM, Senior C et al. (2000). A differential neural response in obsessive-compulsive disorder patients with washing compared with checking symptoms to disgust. *Psychol Med*, 30, 1037–50.

Rao SM, Salmeron BJ, Durgerian S et al. (2000). Effects of methylphenidate on functional MRI blood oxygen level dependent contrast. *Am J Psychiatry*, 157, 1697–9.

Ridler K, Bullmore ET, de Vries PJ et al. (2001). Widespread anatomical abnormalities of grey and white matter in tuberous sclerosis. *Psychol Med*, 31, 1437–46.

Ring HA, Baron-Cohen S, Wheelwright S et al. (1999). Cerebral correlates of preserved cognitive skills in autism: a functional magnetic resonance imaging study of embedded figures task performance. *Brain*, 122, 1305–15.

Rubia K, Overmeyer S, Taylor E et al. (1999). Hypofrontality in attention deficit hyperactivity disorder during higher order motor control: a study with functional MRI. *Am J Psychiatry*, 156, 891–6.

Rubia K, Overmeyer S, Taylor E et al. (2000). Functional frontalisation with age: mapping neurodevelopmental trajectories with fMRI. *Neurosci Biobehav Rev*, 24, 13–19.

Shergill SS, Bullmore ET, Simmons A, Murray RM and McGuire PK (2000). The functional anatomy of auditory-verbal imagery in patients with auditory hallucinations. *Am J Psychiatry*, 157, 1691–3.

Sternberg S (2001). Separate modifiability, mental modules, and the use of pure and composite measures to reveal them. *Acta Psychologica*, 106, 147–246.

Vaidya CJ, Austin G, Kirkorian G et al. (1998). Selective effects of methylphenidate in attention deficit hyperactivity disorder: a functional magnetic resonance imaging study. *Proc Natl Acad Sci USA*, 95, 14494–9.

Van Amelsvoort T, Daly E, Robertson D et al. (2001). Structural brain abnormalities associated with deletion at chromosome 22q11 – quantitative neuroimaging study of adults with velo-cardio-facial syndrome. *Br J Psychiatry*, 178, 412–19.

Weinberger DR and Berman KF (1996). Prefrontal function in schizophrenia: confounds and controversies. *Phil Trans R Soc B*, 351, 1495–503.

Werring DJ, Clark CA, Barker GJ et al. (1998). The structural and functional mechanisms of motor recovery: complementary use of diffusion tensor and functional magnetic resonance imaging in a traumatic injury of the internal capsule. *J Neurol Neurosurg Psychiatry*, 65, 863–9.

Wright IC, Rabe-Hesketh S, Woodruff PWR, David AS, Murray RM and Bullmore ET (2000). Regional brain structure in schizophrenia: a meta-analysis of volumetric MRI studies. *Am J Psychiatry*, 157, 16–25.

Yurgelun-Todd DA, Gruber SA, Kanayam G, Killgore WDS, Baird AA and Young AD. (2000). fMRI during affect discrimination in bipolar affective disorder. *Bipolar Disord*, 2, 237–48.

9

Positron emission tomography (PET) neurochemistry: where are we now and where are we going?

P M Grasby

Hammersmith Hospital, London, UK

Introduction

A basic neuroscientist reading about 'brain functional mapping' might be forgiven for thinking all PET-based (positron emission tomography) investigations of brain function have been superseded by functional magnetic resonance imaging (fMRI). Nothing could be further from the truth. Certainly, in many circumstances fMRI is replacing PET for imaging regional cerebral blood-flow changes induced by cognitive tasks – the basis of brain functional mapping paradigms where blood flow is used to index neuronal activation (Raichle 1987). However, brain PET is first and foremost a technique for imaging neurochemistry in the living brain (Pike 1993; Grasby et al. 1996; Grasby 2000). As such it is unrivalled in the potential diversity of imageable neurochemical targets and the sensitivity of detection. Neurochemical targets can be measured at very low concentrations with PET; thus many central nervous system (CNS) receptor systems, typically at concentrations of nmoles/g or pmoles/g tissue, can be investigated.

PET methodology and application to psychiatry

PET is a technologically and financially demanding tool, which has restricted its widespread application in the UK, although there are estimated to be over 250 PET centres worldwide. Briefly, a successful PET programme requires a flexible medical cyclotron to produce short-lived radioisotopes, particularly ^{11}C, ^{18}F and ^{15}O. In addition, an adequate automated radiochemistry resource is necessary to incorporate these short-lived radioisotopes into molecules of biological interest that can be injected into humans at subpharmacological 'tracer' doses (typically microgram amounts). These positron-emitting radiotracers are typically high-affinity, selective antagonists for receptors or substrates for specific enzymes. A PET camera, consisting of multiple rings of crystal-based gamma ray detectors connected to photomultiplier tubes and linked in coincidence circuits, localizes the decaying positrons which emit (on annihilation) two high-energy gamma rays 180 degrees to each other. Finally, information about the radiotracer's fate in the brain, obtained from the PET camera images of positron decay, acquired over a timescale of typically 1–2 hours, is incorporated into biologically plausible mathematical models of the radiotracer's interaction with the neurochemical target, be it receptor or enzyme. Thus, a modern PET imaging programme requires much technology and diverse scientific skills from engineers, physicists, chemists, mathematicians, pharmacologists and clinicians. However, the scientific rewards are potentially high given the unique in vivo neurochemical information accessible with this technique.

For psychiatry, the merit of being able to sample neurochemical aspects of the living brain is immediately obvious. Neurochemical transmission is a fundamental element of brain functional organization and psychopharmacological interventions form the basis of specific treatments for schizophrenia, bipolar disorder and many mood and anxiety disorders. At present it appears difficult to conceive of pathophysiological explanations for the major psychiatric illnesses that do not posit a central role for neurochemical factors – even suggestions that schizophrenia is a high-level disorder of functional or effective connectivity, between brain areas at a systems level (Friston 1996), must have an underlying neurochemical substrate.

Given these considerations, what contribution is PET making to our understanding of psychiatric illness and treatment, and what prospects are there for providing a robust description of psychiatric diagnoses, syndromes or symptoms at a PET neurochemical level?

Mapping psychotropic drug action

The most successful contribution of PET neurochemistry, to date, has been to index pharmacokinetic and pharmacodynamic properties of psychotropic agents in vivo. In particular, the determination of the central dopamine D_2 receptor occupancy achieved by specific neuroleptic treatments for schizophrenia has been notable (Farde et al. 1988, 1992; Sedvall and Farde 1995). PET studies have consistently demonstrated appreciable neuroleptic occupancy of striatal dopamine D_2 receptors in vivo as a defining characteristic of all successful treatments for schizophrenia – there is no known marketed neuroleptic that fails to occupy striatal dopamine D_2 receptors in vivo. Furthermore, very high levels of striatal occupancy (80% or more) are quite conclusively associated with extrapyramidal side effects (EPS) (Farde et al. 1992; Kapur et al. 2000). These PET imaging findings are sufficiently robust such that all novel neuroleptics in clinical development are routinely examined for their in vivo occupancy at dopamine D_2 receptors. There are some caveats to these findings, however, as occupancy at the striatal dopamine D_2 receptor per se is certainly not a sufficient explanation for the mechanism of action of neuroleptics. Theoretically, dopamine D_2 receptors in cortical or limbic, rather than simply striatal, areas might be the critical targets for neuroleptic action (Lidow et al. 1998). Experimentally, striatal D_2 occupancy occurs within hours of a single neuroleptic dose but time to achieve clinical efficacy is obviously much longer. Moreover occupancy does not distinguish responders from nonresponders and some atypical neuroleptics have relatively low striatal D_2 occupancy (40% for clozapine) but are as efficacious as neuroleptics with high striatal occupancy (65% or more for many typicals). Finally, occupancy declines in days when a neuroleptic is stopped but relapse may take many months to manifest. Thus, striatal dopamine D_2 occupancy may well be necessary, but not sufficient, for fully predicting successful drug responses.

With this realization other dopamine receptor sites are being studied for occupancy effects with much attention currently being focused on cortical D_2 sites. Estimations of occupancy at cortical dopamine D_2 sites are now feasible with the development of very-high-affinity (pmolar) radiotracers such as ^{11}C-FLB 457, and the single photon emission tomography (SPET) tracer, ^{123}I-epipride, which provide reasonable signal-to-noise characteristics in cortical regions (Farde et al. 1997) where D_2 receptors are only about 1–10% of the concentration in the basal ganglia. These novel tracers have overcome many of the inherent difficulties of quantifying small cortical signals. Intriguingly, some studies comparing striatal D_2 versus cortical D_2 receptor occupancies have reported that atypical neuroleptics show a preferential occupancy at cortical sites, implying that saturation will occur at cortical sites before striatal sites (Pilowsky et al. 1997; Xiberas et al. 2001). These studies suggest that atypical neuroleptics may achieve a beneficial side-effect profile, especially of low EPS, by this selectivity and that the therapeutic site of neuroleptic action may be more clearly related to cortical rather than striatal occupancy. However, other PET studies have failed to demonstrate 'limbic selectivity' using the same neuroleptic (e.g. clozapine) but with different radiotracers (Talvik et al. 2001). The disparity between studies might relate to the different radiotracers being employed, and uncertainties in the determination of equilibrium conditions of the specific radiotracer in areas of high signal intensity. If radiotracer equilibrium is not attained in high-signal areas (striatum) compared with low-signal regions (cortex), occupancy values may be underestimated in striatal areas. To clarify this controversial question of so-called 'limbic selectivity', consensus as to the most appropriate radiotracers to be used is needed.

Other receptor sites of some interest in understanding neuroleptic drug action include the 5-HT$_{2A}$, 5-HT$_{1A}$, 5-HT$_{2C}$, alpha$_2$ adrenoceptor, dopamine D_3 and D_1 sites (Sedvall and Farde 1995; Kapur et al. 1999; Bantick et al. 2001). For certain sites, there are no specific radiotracers yet available (e.g. alpha$_2$) but others, such as the 5-HT_{2A} or 5-HT_{1A} sites, can be investigated in vivo. For example, two atypicals with high affinity for the 5-HT_{1A} site, clozapine and ziprasidone, are currently being examined for occupancy at this site using the novel radiotracer ^{11}C WAY 100635 (Pike et al. 1996). In nonhuman primates, clozapine occupies the 5-HT_{1A} site at clinical doses (Chou et al. in press); if confirmed in humans such occupancy might be relevant to the theoretical role of 5-HT_{1A} agonism to reduce EPS and negative symptoms and increase prefrontal dopamine release (Bantick et al. 2001).

Occupancy at the 5-HT_{2A} site, a common target of many 'atypicals', is probably not associated with clinical response as receptor saturation occurs at subtherapeutic doses of neuroleptic (Kapur et al. 1999) and MDL 100907, a selective 5-HT_{2A} receptor antagonist, is ineffective in the treatment of schizophrenia (see Kapur et al. 1999). However, saturation at this site may specifically confer a degree of protection against EPS. The relatively low incidence of EPS in clinical trials with atypicals is present even when low doses (rather than the more usual high dose) of the comparator (often haloperidol) are given (Geddes et al. 2000). Protection against EPS is not absolute, however, as some atypicals at higher doses will induce EPS in the presence of complete 5-HT_{2A} site occupancy. Clinically, it is of interest that low doses of haloperidol (2–3 mg/day) can be used to achieve reasonable degrees of striatal D_2 occupancy (65% but less than 80%), without a high incidence of EPS and in the absence of any 5-HT_{2A} blockade (Kapur et al. 2000).

Another notable example of where in vivo occupancy studies have helped to confirm, or at least clarify, mechanisms of drug action include the recent demonstration that therapeutic doses of the selective serotonin reuptake inhibitors (SSRIs) paroxetine and citalopram practically saturate the cortical 5-HT reuptake site in depressed patients (Meyer et al. in press) – although here again this may be a necessary but not sufficient explanation for efficacy, as high occupancy occurs after a single dose but therapeutic effects are delayed. Occupancy studies of the 5-HT_{1A} site have recently demonstrated that the putative antidepressant effect of augmenting SSRI action with pindolol, a beta-blocker with nanomolar affinity for the 5-HT_{1A} site, is unlikely to be mediated via an antagonist action of pindolol at the raphe 5-HT_{1A} site as proposed theoretically, because the dose of pindolol used in clinical trials is too low to achieve consistent occupancy at this site (Martinez et al. 2000; Rabiner et al. 2000, in press). Other receptor mechanisms might need to be evoked to explain pindolol's claimed efficacy.

These examples illustrate how PET can meaningfully test mechanisms of drug action and in some cases provide a clear rationale for further drug developments. They also highlight, however, the commonly held view that understanding neurochemical change downstream of the receptor site will be critical for explaining how many psychotropic drug treatments work. More pragmatically, however, it is not too fanciful to conceive of a time in the near future when most new psychotropic treatments will be titrated against PET in vivo measures, obtained at a putative target site, as a means to decide on drug dosage, timing, possible mechanism of action, and likely side-effect profile.

Mapping psychiatric illness

PET has been disappointing in identifying clearly distinct changes of receptor populations in psychiatric illness, despite many postmortem studies. There are some notable negative results, however. For example, early well-conducted base-line dopamine D_2 receptor measurements strongly suggested there were no substantial increases in striatal dopamine D_2 receptors in drug-naïve schizophrenia (Farde et al. 1990; Nordstrom et al. 1995). Two recent meta-analyses have concluded that increases of dopamine D_2 receptors, if indeed present, are generally of modest effect size (0.54 and 1.6) and overlap considerably with normal values (Laruelle 1998; Zakzanis and Hansen 1998). These PET findings suggest the frequently reported substantial postmortem increases of D_2 receptors most likely reflect previous neuroleptic exposure, which in many cases upregulate dopamine D_2 receptors in animals treated subchronically with such drugs.

Similarly, for major depression, neuroreceptor changes in the clinical syndrome remain unclear. Of the monoamine systems, the 5HT system is a prime candidate for an association with depressive illness. Thus, neuroendocrine challenge experiments suggest a deficit of 5HT neurotransmission in depressive illness, tryptophan depletion induces depressive symptoms in recovered depressives and many antidepressant treatments enhance 5HT neurotransmission in animal studies (Smith and Cowen 1997). The 5HT receptor system had generally lacked highly specific PET radiotracers until the recent introduction of ^{11}C WAY 100635 (Pike et al. 1996) and ^{11}C MDL 100907 (Hiroshi et al. 1998) for the delineation of $5HT_{1A}$ and $5HT_{2A}$ receptor populations, respectively. Major depressive disorder may well be associated with reduced $5HT_{1A}$ receptor number (Drevets et al. 1999; Sargent et al. 2000a) but similar findings are seen in panic disorder (Sargent et al. 2000b), suggesting this neurochemical signal cannot be specific for a DSM–IV diagnosis of major depression. Furthermore, the depressed state per se is probably not the common factor driving these receptor changes, as state measures of depression (BDI and HAM-D) did not correlate with receptor number in two separate studies (Drevets et al. 1999; Sargent et al. 2000a). In addition, changes of $5HT_{2A}$ receptors may also occur in depressive disorders, although this finding is somewhat inconsistent depending on the exact population studied and radiotracer used (see Fujita et al. 2000). Thus, for example, a reduction of $5HT_{2A}$ receptor binding was found in drug-free depressed patients using ^{18}F altanserin and ^{18}F fluoro-ethyl-spiperone in two studies, whilst a SPET study using ^{123}I ketanserin found an *increase* in 5HT$_{2A}$ receptor binding sites. When suicidal patients were excluded in one study, no alteration of 5HT$_{2A}$ receptor binding was found in drug-free depressed patients using ^{18}F setoperone. A mitigating factor has been that the radiotracers used in these PET 5HT$_{2A}$ studies have not been optimal, thus studies with the highly selective radioligand ^{11}C MDL 100907 are eagerly awaited.

These brief examples clearly show that a PET-based endophenotype of any psychiatric illness is far from being established. Of course, this failure is predicated on assumptions that psychiatric 'illness' can be directly expressed at the level of receptors or enzymes and that there is sufficient pathophysiological homogeneity within a diagnostic category to allow a consistent neurochemical signal to manifest. Whilst the former assumption may be reasonable, the latter is contentious given the ambiguities and uncertainties of diagnostic criteria and conventions. Certainly, functional mapping studies (using blood-flow-based signals) have not yet conclusively defined a consistent pattern of altered neural activation (e.g. hypofrontality) that is pathognomonic of a single diagnostic category (e.g. schizophrenia) (Dolan et al. 1993; Chua and McKenna 1995; Weinberger and Berman 1996; Spence et al. 1998) although more sophisticated mathematical treatments of functional mapping data (e.g. functional connectivity estimates) may offer some promise in this regard (Meyer-Lindenberg et al. 2000; Spence et al. 2000). Many authors have suggested that the patterns of altered neural activation seen in many brain-mapping studies of patients more likely represents the neural correlates of individual symptoms or syndromes than the diagnosis per se. Intriguingly, results mapping syndromes or symptoms to altered neural activation have been frequently reported in the last 10 years (Liddle et al. 1992; Bench et al. 1993; Dolan et al. 1993; McGuire et al. 1993; Silbersweig et al. 1995; Spence et al. 1997; Woodruff et al. 1997) but these require replication (including sensitivity and specificity measures) before an unequivocal neural marker of a specific symptom or syndrome is usefully defined.

In contrast, attempts to map PET neurochemistry on to individual syndromes or symptoms are still uncommon but certainly represent one obvious solution to the problem of finding neurochemical correlates of specific diagnoses. Representative of this trend are a few reports linking dopamine signals and behaviour; thus, dopamine D$_2$ receptor number correlated with the behavioural traits of personal detachment in normal volunteers (Farde et al. 1997; Breier et al. 1998; but also see Kestler et al. 2000) and with the degree of 'pleasant effects' experienced with psychostimulants (Volkow et al. 1999). Similarly, 5HT$_{1A}$ receptor number has recently been correlated with a trait marker of anxiety (Tauscher et al. 2001). Whether such seemingly striking links can be seen between other neurochemical signals and symptoms or syndromes remains to be established.

Linking PET neurochemistry directly with behaviour

More direct links between behaviour and neurochemistry may be possible, making use of a particular property of two chemically related dopamine radiotracers, ^{123}I IBZM and ^{11}C-raclopride, whose binding is sensitive to endogenous levels of dopamine. Thus, pretreatment with the dopamine releaser amphetamine will reduce the binding of ^{123}I IBZM and ^{11}C-raclopride in human brain (Volkow et al. 1994; Laruelle et al. 1995). The simplest explanation for this effect is that there are fewer binding sites available to bind to the radiotracer in the presence of increased levels of synaptic dopamine. Using this method, patients with schizophrenia have been shown to have increased baseline striatal dopamine levels (Abi-Dargham et al. 2000) and an exaggerated amphetamine-induced release of dopamine compared with normal controls (Laruelle et al. 1996; Breier et al. 1997). In one of the two studies reporting an exaggerated release, it was not the presence of symptoms per se that was associated with increased release but rather the appearance or change in symptom intensity that was predictive of increased dopamine release. These observations must provide some of the most direct evidence to date that schizophrenia (as diagnosed by DSM–IV) can be associated with dysfunction of the dopamine system, although the extent to which this abnormality represents the core pathophysiological deficit is uncertain given that it is may only be relapsing patients that show this abnormality. Certainly, it appears unlikely to represent some nonspecific effect of psychiatric illness per se, as depressed patients do not show such exaggerated responses (Parsey et al. 2001).

Using a similar PET methodology there are a few reports that behavioural manipulations also cause dopamine release. Thus a video-game paradigm with novelty, reward and motor learning releases dopamine in normal volunteers (Koepp et al. 1998) as does placebo administration (Fuente-Fernandez et al. 2001) and possibly psychological 'stress' (Pruessner et al. 2000). Whether this subtle PET methodology will allow a more precise dissection of behavioural factors controlling dopamine release is yet to be fully established, not least because of controversies over the influence of potential confounding factors such as changes of blood flow and head movement on detection of radioligand displacement effects. These specific problems may be overcome using modified PET designs such as bolus/infusion protocols (to remove flow effects) or re-binning of emission data according to head movement (to remove head-movement artefacts). Certainly, this methodology would be of generic use if a range of radiotracers could be found that demonstrate sensitivity to endogenous neurotransmitter release. Surprisingly, simple pharmacological factors such as the receptor affinity of the radiotracer per se may be less important than levels of baseline occupancy, amounts of neurotransmitter released, receptor localization and receptor internalization (Laruelle 2000). If multiple neurotransmitter 'sensitive' radiotracers could be found, this would open up the field of in vivo 'cognitive neurochemistry', where direct links between cognition and neurotransmitter release might be established. Of course, a major challenge for all PET neurochemical studies, including those of release, is to understand the appropriate level at which neurochemistry will correlate with behaviour or cognition. For example, dopamine is known to have seemingly diverse effects on distinct cognitive functions such as working memory, reward and motor control (Robbins and Everitt 1992; Luciana and Collins 1997; Schultz et al. 1997). To what extent these seemingly diverse roles can be understood at the resolution of PET neurochemistry is unknown.

Attempts to measure neurotransmitter synthesis continue, but as yet there is no radiotracer that can directly and quantitatively measure neurotransmitter synthesis rate. Thus, the accumulation of the radiotracer ^{18}F-DOPA predominantly samples the aromatic amino-acid decarboxylase enzyme activity that converts DOPA to dopamine, rather than measuring the rate-limited step of dopamine synthesis, which is the hydroxylation of tyrosine. Similarly, ^{11}C-alphamethyltryptophan accumulation in man probably samples the brain uptake of tryptophan rather than the synthesis of serotonin. The formation of ^{11}C-alphamethylserotonin might have been used to infer serotonin synthesis rates if sufficient amounts of ^{11}C-alphamethyltryptophan were converted to ^{11}C-alphamethylserotonin during the time course of a human PET experiment. Unfortunately, however, this does not seem to be the case on the basis of nonhuman primate work (Shoaf et al. 2001).

Imaging beyond the receptor

Other major neurochemical targets of interest are the neuro-imaging and quantitation of second messenger systems and gene expression. Limited success has been achieved in imaging second messenger systems, probably because of the difficulties of developing a radiotracer that will selectively allow a specific component of second messenger biochemistry to be indexed. In brief, to be useful the radiotracer has to penetrate the cell, interact with a specific second messenger neurochemical process and accumulate rapidly as a product of that process without further metabolism to allow quantitation of the signal and separation of nonspecific components within a few half-lives of the radiotracer. In contrast, significant progress has been achieved in imaging aspects of gene activity. One promising approach is of a PET 'reporter gene' strategy (see Herschman et al. 2000 for a review). Here a reporter gene is complexed with another 'therapeutic' gene such that when the therapeutic gene is active the reporter gene itself becomes active. Imaging is used to detect the product of the expression of the reporter gene. Typically, the product may be a receptor such as the dopamine D_2 receptor or an enzyme such as thymidine kinase. Hence, if a PET radiotracer is employed which binds to the

D_2 receptor it becomes possible to image the body tissues or brain areas where the therapeutic gene is active by following the specific binding of the D_2 radiotracer, taking account, of course, of the normal background regional levels of expression of the receptor. One early example of this pioneering work involved inserting a D_2 receptor coding sequence after a cytomegalovirus early promoter sequence and inserting this complex into a replication-deficient adenovirus. Following injection of this modified adenovirus into mice, a PET D_2 receptor probe ([18]FESP) was used to image the subsequent expression of D_2 receptors in the mouse liver, reflecting the site of activity of the injected adenovirus. Similarly ^{18}F-fluroganciclovir has been used as a probe for herpes simplex thymidine kinase gene expression. Although PET reporter genes are yet to be used in humans it is not impossible to imagine that such reports might appear in the mid-future.

The future of PET neurochemistry?

One critical issue for the long-term future of neurochemical imaging will be to develop improved and diverse radiotracers. Currently, only a small fraction of the numerous neuroreceptors and neurochemicals in the human brain can be imaged (Sedvall and Farde 1995). Any one imaging centre can only have limited success in developing new radioligands; optimistically, only a few totally new radiotracers will prove to be useful in any one year in any one centre. A solution proposed for many years, but not yet fully realized, is to establish closer links with large pharmaceutical companies such that the powers of combinatorial chemistry can be fully utilized for radiotracer development. In addition, more detailed knowledge is required of the exact physiochemical or pharmacological parameters that predict a useful radiotracer. Some factors are known, such as moderate lipophilicity, ability to cross the blood–brain barrier, high affinity and low nonspecific binding, but many other factors are unknown. In particular, databases and algorithms are needed that allow prediction of usefulness (Abrunhosa et al. 2001). Such a predictive database may be a major challenge, as relatively subtle quantitative changes in radiotracer properties can convert a useful to useless radiotracer (Pike 1993). As many investigators have stated, finding a novel useful radiotracer is almost as hard as finding novel therapeutic drugs.

Another issue that remains to be tackled systematically is to bring the information obtained from functional brain mapping (which defines the regional neuroanatomy of higher cognitive processes) together with that provided by neurochemical mapping (which quantifies regional receptor or enzyme populations). Although multidimensional databases may be part of the answer, where patterns of functional brain activations can be potentially correlated with regional receptor distributions, the real challenge will be directly and experimentally to relate in vivo neuronal circuitry underlying specific cognitive operations with in vivo neurochemical information obtained with PET in the same individual. Many different imaging approaches may be useful here. These include conjoint psychopharmacological activation where regional cognitive activations are examined for the modulatory effects of drugs (Friston et al. 1992; Grasby et al. 1992; Mehta et al. 2000) and ligand displacement studies where cognitive tasks are used to provoke neurotransmitter release (Koepp et al. 1998), imaged with neurotransmitter-sensitive PET radiotracers. Combined transcranial magnetic stimulation (TMS) and PET may also be useful, where TMS is used to stimulate specific brain areas to provoke neurotransmitter release, thereby testing the functional neurochemical integrity of particular pathways (Strafella et al. 2001). Finally and more speculatively, combined pharmacokinetic/pharmacodynamic (PK/PD) studies may be indicated where PET occupancy of a drug is directly related to a functional measure (Malizia et al. 1996) such as the activation effect of the drug, perhaps measured with fMRI in the same individual.

Conclusions

All the PET neurochemical imaging methods discussed above can be seen as being part of a continuum along which all aspects of receptor activation from receptors, second messengers, gene expression, neuronal activation and brain circuitry is potentially imageable. Progress towards this goal of 'cognitive neurochemistry' is being made, albeit at a rate that is too much determined, at present, by the slow availability of novel radiotracers. Despite this limitation, the versatility and chemical sensitivity of the technique will ensure PET remains a significant methodology for exploring the pathophysiology of psychiatric illness for the foreseeable future.

REFERENCES

Abi-Dargham A, Rodenhiser J, Printz D et al. (2000). Increased baseline occupancy of D2 receptors by dopamine in schizophrenia. *Proc Natl Acad Sci USA*, 97, 8104–9.

Abrunhosa AJ, Brady F, Luthra S, De Lima JJ and Jones T (2001). Preliminary studies of computer aided ligand design for PET. In *Physiological Imaging of the Brain with PET*, ed. A Gjedde, SB Hansen, GM Knudesen and OB Paulson, pp. 51–6. New York: Academic Press.

Bantick RA, Deakin JFW and Grasby PM (2001). The 5-HT1A receptor in schizophrenia: a promising target for novel atypical neuroleptics? *J Psychopharmacol*, 15, 37–46.

Bench CJ, Friston KJ, Brown RG, Frackowiak RS and Dolan RJ (1993). Regional cerebral blood flow in depression measured by positron emission tomography: the relationship with clinical dimensions. *Psychol Med*, 23, 579–90.

Breier A, Su TP, Saunders R et al. (1997). Schizophrenia is associated with elevated amphetamine-induced synaptic dopamine concentrations: evidence from a novel positron emission tomography method. *Proc Natl Acad Sci USA*, 94, 2569–74.

Breier A, Kestler L, Adler C et al. (1998). Dopamine D2 receptor density and personal detachment in healthy subjects. *Am J Psychiatry*, 155, 1440–2.

Chou-YH, Farde L and Halldin C (in press). Occupany of 5-HT1A receptors by clozapine in the monkey brain: a PET study. *Neuropsychopharmcology*, in press.

Chua SE and McKenna PJ (1995). Schizophrenia, a brain disease? A critical review of structural and functional cerebral abnormality in the disorder. *Br J Psychiatry*, 166, 563–82.

Dolan RJ, Bench CJ, Liddle PF et al. (1993). Dorsolateral prefrontal cortex dysfunction in the major psychoses: symptom or disease specificity? *J Neurol Neurosurg Psychiatry*, 56, 1290–4.

Drevets WC, Frank E, Price JC et al. (1999). PET imaging of serotonin 1A receptor binding in depression. *Biol Psychiatry*, 46, 1375–87.

Farde L, Wiesel FA, Halldin C and Sedvall G (1988). Central D2-dopamine receptor occupancy in schizophrenic patients treated with antipsychotic drugs. *Arch Gen Psychiatry*, 45, 71–6.

Farde L, Wiesel F-A, Stone-Elander S et al. (1990). D2 dopamine receptors in neuroleptic naive schizophrenic patients. *Arch Gen Psychiatry*, 47, 213–19.

Farde L, Nordstrom A-L, Wiesel FA, Pauli S, Halldin C and Sedvall G (1992). Positron emission tomographic analysis of central D1 and D2 dopamine receptor occupancy in patients treated with classical neuroleptics and clozapine. Relation to extrapyramidal side effects. *Arch Gen Psychiatry*, 49, 538–54.

Farde L, Suhara T, Nyberg S et al. (1997). A PET-study of [11C] FLB 457 binding to extra-striatal D2-dopamine receptors in healthy subjects and antipsychotic drug-treated patients. *Psychopharmacology*, 133, 396–404.

Friston KJ (1996). Theoretical neurobiology and schizophrenia. *Br Med Bull*, 52, 644–55.

Friston KJ, Grasby PM, Frith CD et al. (1992). Measuring the neuromodulatory effects of drugs in man with positron emission tomography. *Neurosci Lett*, 141, 106–10.

Fuente-Fernandez R de al, Ruth TJ, Sossi V, Schulzer M, Calne DB and Stoessl AJ (2001). Expectation and dopamine release: mechanism of the placebo effect in Parkinson's disease. *Science*, 293, 1164–6.

Fujita M, Charney DS and Innis RB (2000). Imaging serotonergic neurotransmission in depression: hippocampal pathophysiology may mirror global brain alterations. *Biol Psychiatry*, 48, 801–12.

Geddes J, Freemantle N, Harrison P and Bebbington P (2000). Atypical antipsychotics in the treatment of schizophrenia: systematic overview and meta-regression analysis. *Br Med J* 321, 1371–6.

Grasby PM (2000). Functional PET. In *New Oxford Textbook of Psychiatry*, ed. M Gelder, J Lopez-Ibor Jr and NC Andreasen, Vol. 1, pp. 206–12. Oxford: Oxford University Press.

Grasby PM, Friston KJ, Bench C et al. (1992). The effect of apomorphine and buspirone on regional cerebral blood flow during the performance of a cognitive task – measuring neuromodulatory effects of psychotropic drugs in man. *Eur J Neurosci*, 4, 1203–12.

Grasby PM, Malizia A and Bench C (1996). Psychopharmacology – in vivo neurochemistry and pharmacology. *Br Med Bull*, 52, 513–26.

Herschman HR, MacLaren DC, Iyer M et al. (2000). Seeing is believing: non-invasive quantitative and repetitive imaging of reporter gene expression in living animals, using positron emission tomography. *J Neurosci Res*, 59, 699–705.

Hiroshi I, Nyberg S, Halldin C, Lundkvist C and Farde L (1998). PET imaging of central 5-HT2A receptors with carbon-11-MDL 100,907. *J Nucl Med*, 39, 208–14.

Kapur S, Zipursky RB and Remington G (1999). Clinical and theoretical implications of 5-HT2 and D2 receptor occupancy of clozapine, risperidone and olanzapine in schizophrenia. *Am J Psychiatry*, 156, 286–93.

Kapur S, Zipursky R, Jones C, Remington G and Houle S (2000). Relationship between dopamine D2 occupancy, clinical response and side effects: a double-blind PET study of first-episode schizophrenia. *Am J Psychiatry*, 157, 514–20.

Kestler LP, Malhotra AK, Finch C, Adler C and Breier A (2000). The relation between dopamine D2 receptor density and personality: preliminary evidence from the NEO personality inventory–revised. *Neuropsychiatry Neuropsychol Behav Neurol*, 13, 48–52.

Koepp MJ, Gunn RN, Lawrence AD et al. (1998). Evidence for striatal dopamine release during a video game. *Nature*, 393, 266–8.

Laruelle M (1998). Imaging dopamine transmission in schizophrenia: a review analysis. *Q J Nucl Med*, 42, 211–21.

Laruelle M (2000). Imaging synaptic neurotransmission with in vivo binding competition techniques: a critical review. *J Cereb Blood Flow Metab*, 20, 423–51.

Laruelle M, Abi-Dargham A, van Dyck CH et al. (1995). SPECT imaging of striatal dopamine release after amphetamine challenge. *J Nucl Med*, 36, 1182–90.

Laruelle M, Abi-Dargham A, van Dyck CH et al. (1996). Single photon emission computerised tomography imaging of amphetamine-induced dopamine release in drug free schizophrenia subjects. *Proc Natl Acad Sci USA*, 93, 9235–40.

Liddle PF, Friston KJ, Frith CD, Hirsch SR, Jones T and Frackowiak RSJ (1992). Patterns of cerebral blood flow in schizophrenia. *Br J Psychiatry*, 160, 179–86.

Lidow MS, Williams GV and Goldman-Rakic PS (1998). The cerebral cortex: a case for a common site of action of antipsychotics. *Trends Pharmacol Sci*, 19, 136–40.

Luciana M and Collins PF (1997). Dopaminergic modulation of working memory for spatial but not object cues in normal volunteers. *J Cogn Neurosci*, 9, 330–47.

Malizia A, Gunn RN, Wilson SJ et al. (1996). Benzodiazepine site pharmacokinetic/pharmacodynamic quantification in man: direct measurement of drug occupancy and effects on the human brain in vivo. *Neuropharmacology*, 35, 1483–91.

Martinez D, Broft A and Laruelle M (2000). Pindolol augmentation of antidepressant treatment: recent contributions from brain imaging studies. *Biol Psychiatry*, 48, 844–53.

McGuire PK, Shah GMS and Murray RM (1993). Increased blood flow in Broca's area during auditory hallucinations in schizophrenia. *Lancet*, 342, 703–6.

Mehta MA, Owen AM, Sahakian BJ, Mavaddat N, Pickard JD and Robbins TW (2000). Methylphenidate enhances working memory by modulating discrete frontal and parietal lobe regions in the human brain. *J Neurosci*, 20, RC65 (1–6).

Meyer JH, Wilson AA, Ginovart N et al. (in press). Occupancy of serotonin transporters by paroxetine and citalopram during treatment of depression: a [11C] DASB PET imaging study. *Am J Psychiatry*, in press.

Meyer-Lindenberg A, Kohn P, Holt J, Egan M, Weinberger D and Berman KF (2000). Disturbed connectivity in schizophrenia: PET studies. *Neuroimage*, 11, S186.

Nordstrom A-L, Farde L, Eriksson L and Halldin C (1995). No elevated D2 dopamine receptors in neuroleptic naive schizophrenic patients revealed by PET and 11C-NSMP. *Psych Res*, 61, 67–83.

Parsey RV, Oquendo MA, Zea-Ponce Y et al. (2001). Dopamine D2 receptor availability and amphetamine-induced dopamine release in unipolar depression. *Biol Psychiatry*, 50, 313–22.

Pike V (1993). Positron emitting radioligands for studies in vivo – probes for human psychopharmacology. *J Psychopharmacol*, 7, 139–58.

Pike V, McCarron JA, Lammerstma AA et al. (1996). Exquisite delineation of 5-HT1A receptors in human brain with carbonyl 11C-WAY-100635. *Eur J Pharmacol*, 301, R5–7.

Pilowsky LS, Mulligan RS, Acton PD, Ell PJ, Costa DC and Kerwin RW (1997). Limbic selectivity of clozapine. *Lancet*, 350, 490–1.

Pruessner JC, Champagne F, Meaney MJ and Dagher A (2000). Evidence for striatal dopamine release during an anxiety inducing stress task measured with [11C]raclopride and high resolution positron emission tomography. *Neuroimage*, 11, S22.

Rabiner E, Gunn RN, Sargent PA et al. (2000). Beta-blocker binding to human 5-HT1A receptors in vivo and in vitro: implications for antidepressant therapy. *Neuropsychopharmacology*, 23, 285–93.

Rabiner EA, Bhagwagar Z, Gunn RN et al. (in press). Pindolol augmentation of antidepressant SSRI efficacy: PET evidence suggests the dose used in clinical trials is too low. *Am J Psychiatry*.

Raichle ME (1987). Circulatory and metabolic correlations of brain function in normal humans. In *Handbook of Physiology. Section 1: The Nervous System. Vol 5: Higher Functions of the Brain*, ed. F Plum, pp. 643–74. New York: Oxford University Press.

Robbins TW and Everitt BJ (1992). Functions of dopamine in the dorsal and ventral striatum. In *Seminars in the Neurosciences*, ed. TW Robbins, pp. 119–28. London: Saunders Scientific Publishers.

Sargent PA, Husted Kjaer K, Bench CJ et al. (2001*a*). Brain serotonin1A receptor binding measured by positron emission tomography with [11C]WAY-100635: effects of depression and antidepressant treatment. *Arch Gen Psychiatry*, 57, 174–80.

Sargent P, Nash J, Hood S et al. (2000*b*). 5-HT1A receptor binding in panic disorder; comparison with depressive disorder and healthy volunteers using PET and [11C]WAY-100635. *Neuroimage*, 11, S189.

Schultz W, Dayan P and Montague PR (1997). A neural substrate of prediction and reward. *Science*, 275, 1593–9.

Sedvall G and Farde L (1995). Chemical brain anatomy in schizophrenia. *Lancet*, 346, 743–9.

Shoaf SE, Carson RE, Hommer D et al. (2001). [α-11C]methyl-L-tryptophan in anesthetized rhesus monkeys: a tracer for serotonin synthesis of tryptophan uptake. In *Physiological Imaging of the Brain with PET*, ed. A Gjedde, SB Hensen, GM Knudsen and OB Paulson, pp. 229–35. New York: Academic Press.

Silbersweig DA, Stern E, Frith CD et al. (1995). A functional neuroanatomy of hallucinations in schizophrenia. *Nature*, 378, 176–9.

Smith KA and Cowen PJ (1997). Serotonin and depression. In *Depression: Neurobiological, Psychopathological and Therapeutic Advances*, ed. A Hening and HM van Praag, pp. 129–46. Chichester: John Wiley and Sons.

Spence SA, Brooks DJ, Hirsch SR, Liddle PF, Meehan J and Grasby PM (1997). A PET study of voluntary movement in schizophrenic patients experiencing passivity phenomena (delusions of alien control). *Brain*, 120, 1997–2011.

Spence SA, Hirsch SR, Brooks DJ and Grasby PM (1998). Prefrontal cortex activity in people with schizophrenia and control subjects. Evidence from positron emission tomography for remission of 'hypofrontality' with recovery from acute schizophrenia. *Br J Psychiatry*, 172, 316–23.

Spence SA, Liddle PF, Stephan MD et al. (2000). Functional anatomy of verbal fluency in people with schizophrenia and those at genetic risk. *Br J Psychiatry*, 176, 52–60.

Strafella AP, Paus T, Barrett J and Dagher A (2001). Repetitive transcranial magnetic stimulation of the human prefrontal cortex induces dopamine release in the caudate nucleus. *J Neurosci*, 21, RC157.

Talvik M, Nordstrom AL, Nyberg S, Olsson H, Halldin C and Farde L (2001). No support for regional selectivity in clozapine-treated patients: a PET study with [11C]Raclopride and [11C]FLB 457. *Am J Psychiatry*, 158, 926–30.

Tauscher J, Bagley RM, Javanmard M, Christensen BK, Kasper S and Kapur S (2001). Inverse relationship between serotonin 5-HT1A receptor binding and anxiety: a [11C]WAY-100635 PET investigation in healthy volunteers. *Am J Psychiatry*, 158, 1326–28.

Volkow ND, Wang G-J, Fowler JS et al. (1994). Imaging endogenous dopamine competition with 11C-raclopride in the human brain. *Synapse*, 16, 255–62.

Volkow ND, Wang GJ, Fowler JS et al. (1999). Prediction of reinforcing responses to psycho-stimulants in humans by brain dopamine D2 receptor levels. *Am J Psychiatry*, 156, 1440–43.

Weinberger DR and Berman KF (1996). Prefrontal function in schizophrenia: confounds and controversies. *Philos Trans R Soc Lond B Biol Sci*, 351, 1495–503.

Woodruff PWR, Wright IC, Bullmore ET et al. (1997). Auditory hallucinations and the temporal cortical response to speech in schizophrenia: a functional magnetic resonance imaging study. *Am J Psychiatry*, 154, 1676–82.

Xiberas X, Martinot J-L, Mallet L et al. (2001). In vivo extrastriatal and striatal D2 dopamine receptor blockade by amisulpride in schizophrenia. *J Clin Psychopharmacol*, 21, 207–14.

Zakzanis KK and Hansen KT (1998). Dopamine D2 densities and the schizophrenic brain. *Schizophr Res*, 32, 201–6.

Part V

Consciousness and will

10

The scientific study of consciousness

Chris Frith

Institute of Neurology, University College London, London, UK

Introduction

Scientists rediscover consciousness

In one of the most striking developments to occur at the end of the twentieth century scientists became increasingly eager to study the physiological basis of consciousness. This was a dramatic change in attitude since for much of the early part of that century consciousness was not considered an appropriate topic for scientific study. This attitude held even for psychologists (or at least for experimental psychologists) who switched from the study of the mind to the study of behaviour on the grounds that only behaviour could be studied objectively. As is often the case, the change in attitude which led to the study of consciousness was driven by advances in technology. The development of information theory (Shannon and Weaver 1949) enabled the construction of digital computers and had a strong influence on psychology (Attneave 1959). Computers were 'electronic brains'. Computer engineers were not restricted to studying the behaviour of these thinking machines. They could study directly mechanisms of memory and perception both in terms of the computations that achieved these functions and in terms of the electronic hardware that made the computations. Psychologists applied the same ideas to the study of thinking people. They began to speculate about the invisible processes that enabled behaviour to occur. This new study of 'information processing' led on to the development of cognitive psychology, now the dominant approach.

Consciousness and unconsciousness

From attempts to develop artificial intelligence it rapidly became clear that many apparently simple processes were actually very complex in terms of the computations needed to make them possible. The prime example was visual perception. In the 1960s almost no one realized that machine vision was difficult (Marr 1982). We now know that it is very difficult. There are many problems. A fundamental question is how to work out which edges go with which object in a typical cluttered scene containing many overlapping objects. The reason that no one thought visual perception was difficult was because it is so easy for us. I look out of the window and I see all the trees, flowers and people in the square. I am not aware of making inferences or other difficult thought processes. I am instantly and directly aware of all these objects. Thus the computational approach to vision revealed the existence of a cognitive unconscious (Kihlstrom 1987) upon which our effortless perception of the world depends. Such unconscious processes are not restricted to vision, but underlie all perceptual modalities and especially the perception of speech. Later in this chapter I shall discuss in more detail the unconscious processes that underlie movement and action. In terms of information processing consciousness is just the tip of an iceberg. Indeed it has been proposed that we are not conscious of any cognitive process, but only of the products of that process (Nisbett and Wilson 1977).

There is now ample evidence that these processes can influence our behaviour even when we are unaware of them or their products (Milner and Rugg 1992). The most robust example is unconscious priming. The decision as to whether the letter string BUTTER is a word or not will occur faster if the string was preceded by the word BREAD. This facilitation will occur even if the subject is not aware that the word BREAD has been presented because it appeared very briefly and was immediately followed by a visual mask (Marcel 1983). The effects of unconscious processes on behaviour are seen in their most striking form in certain neurological patients such as those with 'blindsight' (Weiskrantz 1986). These patients have lesions in primary visual cortex and claim to see nothing in that part of the visual field served by the damaged area. Nevertheless, if asked to guess, they are able to detect simple visual properties such as movement far better than would be expected by chance. They have no conscious visual experience of the objects in their blind field, and yet information about these objects is available to guide their behaviour.

These studies show that there are two classes of behaviour. There is the behaviour, and it is probably most of our behaviour, that occurs in the absence of any conscious experience and there is the behaviour that is associated with conscious experience. The behaviour that occurs in the absence of conscious experience is straightforward. This is the kind of behaviour shown by any information processing device whether it is a computer or a thermostat. We know in principle how such devices work. The mystery is why some behaviour is associated with conscious experience. There are a number of questions to be answered. (1) Are there some types of behaviour that can only occur when associated with conscious experience? (2) Can these types of behaviour be distinguished from other types without reference to the co-occurrence of conscious experience? (3) Is conscious experience a necessary property of certain kinds of information-processing systems? (4) How can conscious experience emerge from a physical system, like a brain? Such questions are at the heart of the scientific study of consciousness.

In my opinion these developments have very little to do with the ideas about the unconscious popularized by Freud. Freud was not talking about the cognitive unconscious. He was concerned to demonstrate that much of our behaviour is controlled by motivations, attitudes and primitive thought processes of which we are unaware. Furthermore, he believed that there were powerful unconscious mechanisms designed to prevent those motivations and attitudes that civilized people would wish to disown from becoming conscious. For Freud the mystery to be explained was the functioning of this unconscious system. Today's neuroscientists have demonstrated that much of our behaviour is controlled by *stimuli* of which we are unaware. For us the mystery to be explained is the purpose and functioning of *consciousness*. Why do we need to be conscious of anything when we can achieve so much without awareness?

The neural correlates of consciousness

The second technological advance that changed attitudes to the study of consciousness was the development of noninvasive brain imaging. The earliest method for imaging brain function was the electroencephalogram (EEG) which was reported by Berger in 1929. Probably the greatest triumph of this technique in relation to the neural correlates of consciousness was the discovery of sleep stages. On the basis of measures of EEG and electromyogram (EMG), sleep can be divided into several clear stages. In one of these stages the EEG shows the low-voltage, fast activity characteristic of waking, but the muscle tone is actively inhibited and the person remains asleep. Stereotypic bursts of saccadic eye movements called rapid eye movements (REM) occur, giving this state the name REM sleep (Aserinsky and Kleitman 1953); 90–95% of the time, when a person is aroused from REM sleep and asked to report immediately he or she will describe dreams. Dreams are characterized by vivid hallucinatory imagery, usually in the visual modality along with illusions of self-motion (Hobson 1988). Even though they occur when we are asleep dreams are a form of conscious experience. They are also perhaps the only form of conscious experience for which we have such a reliable physiological marker. After the discovery of REM sleep it was possible to answer questions about dreams that would have previously seemed unanswerable because dreams are entirely subjective and private. For example, how many of our dreams do we remember? Less than 5%. How quickly does the memory of a dream fade? Within 5 minutes of the termination of a period of REM sleep, awakening yields no report of dreaming. So the memory of a dream has faded to nothing in less than 5 minutes unless we can rehearse our recollection (Hobson 1988).

As a consequence of this reliable physiological marker we are happy to accept that most mammals dream, because they also show the characteristic pattern of fast-activity EEG, rapid eye movements and inhibited muscle tone. Furthermore it is possible to make lesions which remove the paralysis normally associated with REM sleep (Jouvet 1979). Cats with such lesions get up during REM sleep and appear to an observer to be acting out dreams. Because we are able to study REM sleep in animals, we have learned a great deal about the underlying physiology of this state and are beginning to develop clear hypotheses as to its function in the consolidation of memories (Stickgold 1998). Paradoxically, although we can accept that mammals dream just like us, we are much more uncertain as to whether the conscious experiences that they have while awake are anything like ours. This caution arises simply because we do not yet have a reliable physiological marker of conscious experiences associated with the waking state. Unlike the dream state we do not have any clear idea of the function of conscious experience. Many believe that it has no function and is simply an irrelevant side-show and byproduct of certain kinds of information processing. I shall return to the problem of the function of consciousness at the end of this chapter.

However, EEG measures have made their major contribution to studies of information processing through the event-related potential (ERP). The ERP is a characteristic signal in the EEG associated with an event, whether it be a stimulus or a response, that is revealed by averaging across many trials (see for example Kutas and Dale 1997). Measurement of ERPs to stimuli revealed the effects of top-down processes on attention in the brain. There is larger response to a stimulus when it is attended to even though the physical properties of the stimulus do not change (Hillyard et al. 1973). In other words, by a deliberate act of will (attending to one stimulus rather than another) we can alter the way our brain processes sensory signals. Since that observation the brain mechanisms underlying selective attention have been studied intensively. Recent functional-imaging studies suggest strongly that there is a very close relation between selective attention and the conscious experience of stimuli (Rees and Lavie 2001).

Of direct relevance to the discovery of the neural correlates of consciousness are ERP studies of memory. In these experiments volunteers study lists of words which they try to remember. Subsequently they are shown sequences of words, some of which are old (i.e. were in the study lists), while some are new. Inevitably the volunteer will misidentify some of the words from the study lists and erroneously classify them as new. However, there is evidence that these words have been processed since they may show priming effects. Indeed, patients with amnesia may completely fail to distinguish between the old and the new words, but will still show priming effects from the unrecognized old words (Schacter 1992). The ERPs elicited by the words clearly distinguish between old words that are not detected and new words. This is a marker of unconscious memory. The ERPs also distinguish between old words correctly identified and those which are not (Rugg et al. 1998). In this comparison the stimuli are identical (previously studied words). The difference arises because one stimulus elicits a conscious recollection while the other does not, providing a marker of conscious recollection. However, the pattern of differences was different for the two kinds of memory. Conscious memories showed the greatest effects at frontal electrode sites while unconscious memories showed the greatest effect at parietal electrode sites.

Although EEG measurement techniques have been available for decades it took a long time for them to be applied to the neural basis of cognitive processes. Many of the key studies were published after the meteoric rise of functional brain imaging, perhaps because of the competition and because of the new paradigms that were developed to exploit these new techniques.

While EEG measurements had been ahead of their time, the techniques of functional brain imaging arrived on the scene at exactly the right moment to take full advantage of the developments of cognitive neuropsychology. On the basis of their studies of patients with discrete cognitive problems, cognitive neuropsychologists had developed the well-known box and arrow diagrams (Morton 1980) which purported to illustrate the discrete cognitive processes underlying tasks such as reading and spelling (Figure 10.1). Neurological cases could be found in which some of these discrete processes were impaired while the others remained intact. The assumption was that each of the cognitive boxes corresponded to a particular module in the brain, but where were these modules? The series of papers published by Posner and his colleagues in 1988 showed us how positron emission tomography (PET) could be used to write the brain region into the boxes (Petersen et al. 1988; Posner et al. 1988). Within a very short time the even more powerful technique of functional magnetic resonance imaging (fMRI) had been developed (Turner and Jezzard 1994). The growth of studies using these techniques was exponential and had a major impact on the search for the neural correlates of consciousness.

One reason for the increasing interest in consciousness is derived from the constraints imposed by the new techniques. The imaging environment is so restricting for the volunteer that experiments in which he or she just lies in the machine and thinks have a particular attraction. In one of the earliest experiments volunteers were asked to imagine leaving their house and walking through the streets taking a left turn at each choice point (Roland and Friberg 1985). This purely mental activity was associated with changes in blood flow in many regions. Subsequently a series of more exact experiments have been conducted to identify the neural activity associated with making imaginary movements. These show that when a volunteer imagines moving his hand, activity is seen in a subset of the motor system activated by real movements of the hand (Jeannerod 1994). More recently, fMRI has been used to study visual imagery in much the same way. In response to a cue volunteers were asked to imagine a face or a house they had recently seen (O'Craven and Kanwisher 2000). Imagining these objects activated the same regions as are activated

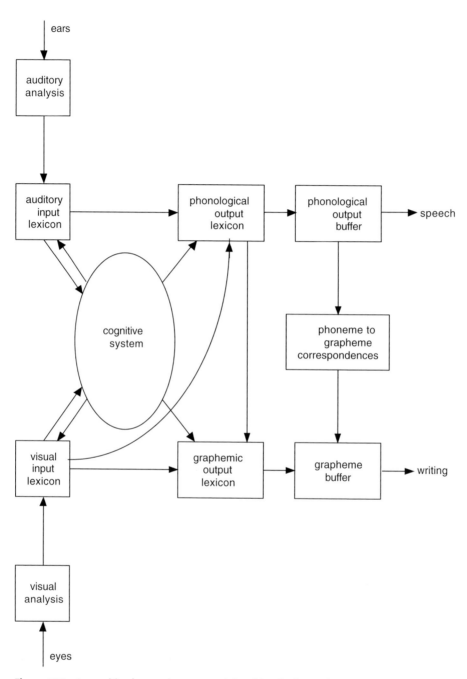

Figure 10.1   A cognitive box and arrow model waiting for instantiation in the brain (redrawn from Morton 1980).

by the actual presentation of these items (the fusiform gyrus and the parahippocampal gyrus respectively). In all these experiments no behaviour can be observed. To an outside observer the volunteer is lying in the scanner doing nothing. We hope he or she is obeying our instructions to imagine things, but how can we tell? With the new imaging techniques we have, for the first time, an objective marker of this mental activity.

The motor control system

So far, by far the most attention in terms of imaging and behavioural studies has been paid to consciousness in the visual system (Rees 2001). However, I believe that an understanding of the role of consciousness in the motor system will be particularly important if we are to understand various neurological and psychiatric disorders (Frith et al. 2000*b*).

How do we know about the state of our motor system? There are two sources of information. First there is sensory information. Signals about where our arm is arise from the visual system, from touch receptors in the skin and from kinaesthetic receptors in joints and muscles. However, this information is not enough. Information about our arm position can also be inferred from the motor commands that have recently been generated to control that arm. Using these two sources of information an estimate of the current state of the motor system can be derived, but this is only an estimate. The CNS has no direct information about the exact state of the system.

On its own, having a good estimate of the current state of our motor system is not sufficient for us to actually do anything. In order to reach for the wineglass I must issue a series of motor commands. Which commands are appropriate depends upon where my arm is now (the current state of the system), but also on where my arm should be after the movement has been made (the desired state of the system). From the current and desired state of the system a suitable controller can compute the appropriate sequence of motor commands (this is sometimes know as inverse modelling). Through experience the controller can learn to make more and more accurate computations of the appropriate motor-command sequence. However, on its own such a system would still not be very efficient. One problem is that there are large delays in the system. Sensory feedback giving some indication of the success of a movement will not arrive until ∼100 ms after the movement has been completed. Another problem is that it is difficult to compute the appropriate sequence of motor commands since there are many different ways of achieving the same end. To overcome these and other problems we also represent the predicted state of the motor system. The sequence of motor commands computed by a controller are used to predict, first, where our arm would be if the commands were carried out

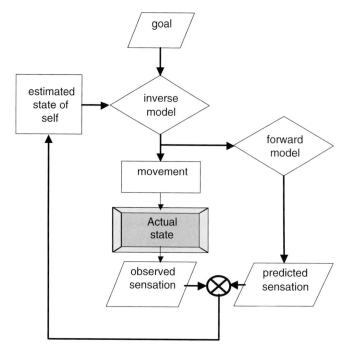

Figure 10.2 An engineering model of motor control. What is the role for consciousness? (Redrawn from Frith et al. 2000*b.*)

and, second, what sensory feedback will occur in consequence. This computation is not so difficult. For a given sequence of motor commands, there is only one possible outcome. These predictions are sometimes referred to as the forward model.

In our simplified model of motor control (see Figure 10.2) three states are represented: the current state of the system, the desired state of the system and the predicted state of the system. There are two types of computational device: controllers which compute the appropriate motor commands to achieve the desired state and predictors which use these commands to compute the predicted state. Both the controllers and the predictors can learn to improve their performance on the basis of errors; that is, the discrepancies between the various states. For example, a discrepancy between the desired state and the predicted state indicates an error in the motor command sequence even before the command has been issued to the muscles. On the basis of this discrepancy errors can be corrected very rapidly without the need to wait for sensory feedback.

The model I have just outlined provides a very useful framework for discussing motor control. However, I have not yet said anything about the place of consciousness in this system. Just because various states of the system are represented in the CNS, it does not follow that we are conscious of these states.

Actions without awareness

We know, for example, that quite complex movements can be made without any awareness at all. A well-studied example of action without awareness is the double-step task (Prablanc and Jeannerod 1975). The volunteer fixates a light spot A bearing in mind the instruction that an eye movement must be made as soon as this spot is extinguished and a new one (B) appears. On some trials, as soon as the volunteer's eye moves towards spot B, this disappears and spot C appears. Volunteers initially move their eyes towards spot B, but rapidly correct their movement in order to finish by fixating on spot C. However, they are not aware of making a corrective eye movement towards spot C, or that an intermediate target (B) appeared. Even when an arm movement is made at the same time as the eye movement, volunteers are unaware of the double-step movement (Péllison et al. 1986). Castiello et al. (1991) used a version of this task in which volunteers had to reach and grasp one of three rods. As soon as one of the rods was illuminated the volunteer had to reach and grasp it. On some trials (20%) the middle rod was illuminated, but as soon as the subject reached for it, one of the outer rods was illuminated in its place. Volunteers made smooth adjustments of their hand movements with reaction times of ~110 ms, but this detection of the target change and adjustment of the movement both happened well before the subject could report that the target rod had changed (~420 ms). Clearly no consciousness of any aspect of the motor system was needed for computing the appropriate movement correction in these circumstances.

The timing of awareness

Castiello et al. (1991) were not the first to show that awareness of action often occurs *after* the action has been selected. Libet et al. (1983) measured EEG during a task in which volunteers had to lift a finger from time to time, 'whenever the urge came upon them'. As had already been demonstrated by Deecke (1987), each time a finger was lifted there was an associated readiness potential (RP) occurring in the second or so prior to the moment that the finger was lifted. Libet et al. also asked their volunteers to indicate, using a clock-like device, precisely when they had the urge to lift their finger. The striking result, recently replicated by Haggard and Eimer (1999), was that the onset of the readiness potential could be detected several hundred milliseconds before the report of the urge to lift the finger. Although the observation that the readiness potential precedes the experience of the urge is interesting it does not of itself tell us about the relationship between the RP and the experience of the urge. Haggard and Eimer (1999) have argued that, if there is a close relationship between them, then there should be a correlation in time between the physical and the mental event. In other words, it should be possible to predict the time of the urge from the time of the RP onset (and vice versa). Haggard and Eimer (1999) examined this relationship for both early and the late component of the RP. This distinction can be made by measuring the lateralized readiness potential (LRP). While the early stages of the RP show their strongest effects centrally, the later stages become lateralized, showing greater activity on the side contralateral to the finger to be lifted. Haggard and Eimer (1999) found that it was the onset of this later, lateralized component of the RP that predicted the time of the 'urge' to lift the finger. In terms of our model of motor control, this result suggests that a movement has to be fully specified by a controller before we can be aware of it.

Libet et al. (1983) also asked volunteers to indicate the time at which they were aware of actually initiating the movement (i.e. lifting their finger). In contrast to the 'urge', awareness of initiation preceded the actual moment of initiation by ~80 ms. Haggard et al. (1999) have also replicated this result. This observation demonstrates that our awareness of initiation cannot be based on the tactile and kinaesthetic sensations associated with lifting the finger. These sensations could not reach the cortex until ~100 ms after initiation and yet we perceive initiation occurring before the movement begins. In terms of our model, this result implies that, around the moment of initiation of a movement, what we are aware of is the predicted state of the system, not the actual state of the system. Experiments (Haggard and Magno 1999) with transcranial magnetic stimulation (TMS) suggest that the awareness of the initiation of an action is not associated with activity in primary motor cortex, but in more anterior regions, possible the supplementary motor area (SMA).

There is much more direct evidence to show that we can have very limited awareness of the actual state of our motor system. Fourneret and Jeannerod (1998) asked volunteers to draw a straight line away from the body. The volunteers could see the line they were drawing on a computer monitor, but could not see their hand or arm. Distortions were introduced into the drawing system so that, in order to produce the correct line on the screen, the hand and arm had to deviate to the left or the right. Volunteers could easily compensate for these distortions, but were not aware of the deviations in their arm movements. If they were asked to repeat the movement without visual feedback while hand and arm remained unseen, then they generated a straight forward movement, rather than the deviant movement that they had made a few seconds before. This observation suggests that if our action is successful, as indicated by visual feedback in this study, then we presume that the predicted state of the motor matches the actual state of the system. In this case there is no need to modify our estimate of the actual state of the system on the basis of kinaesthetic and tactile signals concerning the exact position of our arm.

In contrast, dramatic updating of our estimates of the actual state of the system occurs when our predictions are wrong. We have all experienced the trick milk bottle which is empty, but has been painted white inside. On picking this up we suddenly find that our arm has shot up because we used too much force. We predicted the bottle was much heavier than it actually was. Meanwhile the trickster is amused to see how long it takes us to respond to the discrepancy.

As long as nothing goes wrong the motor system runs autonomously and automatically with minimal awareness. Only when our predictions are not met and things go wrong is our attention directed to the motor system. At this point certain aspects of the system enter awareness.

Awareness of agency

When we perform a deliberate, voluntary act (as in the experiment by Libet) we have a strong sense of agency. It is my 'urge' to lift my finger at this moment, which causes the finger lifting to occur. However, as Wegner has pointed out, all we are actually experiencing is a contingency (Wegner and Wheatley 1999). The urge to lift the finger always precedes the finger lifting. However, this correlation need not imply causation. As a result our sense of having generated an act can sometimes be false. In one study a volunteer and a stooge both placed their fingers on a modified mouse that controlled the position of a pointer on the screen. As with the old Ouija board, the movement of the pointer could be controlled by the volunteer or the stooge or both. Various objects were displayed on the screen and the volunteer heard a series of words through earphones which included names of the objects on the screen. Meanwhile, unbeknown to the volunteer, the stooge heard a series of instructions to move the pointer to particular objects on the screen. The soundtracks were arranged so that the volunteer might hear the word 'red square' and shortly afterwards the stooge would move the pointer to the red square. If the interval was sufficiently short (∼500 ms) then the volunteer would report that he or she had deliberately moved the pointer to the red square, even though the movement had actually been made by the stooge. Such false experiences of agency did not occur if the interval was long, or if the movement of the pointer started at the same time or earlier than the moment at which the volunteer's attention was drawn to the target. In another experiment, volunteers falsely denied their role in a movement. The task used was based on the technique of 'facilitated communication'. In this task the stooge has her fingers resting on a keyboard while the volunteer rests her fingers lightly on top of the stooge's fingers. By this procedure the volunteer is supposed to be able to 'help' the stooge make appropriate responses. Questions appear on a screen, which the stooge is supposed to answer. However, unbeknown to the volunteer the questions the stooge sees are different from the questions the volunteer sees. The volunteer believes that it is the stooge who is making the movements, but, since the answers given correspond to the volunteer's questions, it was in fact the volunteer who was generating the movements. Both these studies show that, given the appropriate context, we can be misled about our role in the production of action. If we think about making an action and the action occurs, then we think we have made it. If we think about someone else making an action, and the action occurs, then we think that the other person made it.

In summary, these various studies show that there are many aspects of action of which we are unaware. When we are aware of actions then this awareness is often determined more by our expectations and predictions than by sensory feedback about the state of our motor system.

Abnormalities in the awareness of action

Given these observations about awareness of action in the normal case, many apparently bizarre abnormalities seem much less surprising.

Phantom limbs

How, we might ask, is it possible to experience a phantom limb (Ramachandran and Hirstein 1998) when there is no actual limb from which sensory signals can arise? As we have seen, estimations of the current position of a limb are also based on the motor commands issued to move the limb to that position. Even when the limb is missing such motor commands can still be issued. On the basis of these we can be aware of the position of the limb, and we can also experience the limb as moving. We predict where the limb should be as a result of the motor commands and it is this predicted position of the limb that is the basis of the experience of a phantom. Of course the predictor will eventually learn that issuing the motor commands does not result in any actual movement. In consequence the patient will no longer be able to move his phantom limb. Sometimes the phantom becomes 'stuck' in a position that feels very painful, so that the patient has a great desire to move the limb into a less painful position. Ramachandran and Rogers-Ramachandran (1996) have shown that the ability to move the phantom can sometimes be reinstated. To achieve this, the patient views his intact limb in a mirror arranged in such a way that he sees the reflection of the intact limb in the position where the missing limb should be. When he tries to move both limbs in concert then he will get visual feedback that appears to indicate that the missing limb and the intact limb are both moving. This false feedback recalibrates the system. The predictor now indicates that the motor commands will lead to movement and the phantom is experienced as moving even when the mirror arrangement is no longer present.

Anosognosia

Even more bizarre is the observation that some patients, usually after right-hemisphere lesions, will deny that they are paralysed and may claim that they have moved their paralysed limb when this is not actually the case (Ramachandran 1996). As with the phantom limb the motor system is still able to compute the motor commands needed to achieve the desired movement and can predict what the consequences of these commands will be. Thus the patient can experience a movement based on prediction. The damage on the right parietal lobe may well include regions where sensory feedback is processed. As a result signals indicating that the movement has not occurred may no longer be available. It is also possible that the regions that monitor and respond to discrepancies between expected and actual outcome are no longer properly functioning. Sirigu et al. (1996) have shown that patients with parietal lesions, but without anosognosia, will accept as veridical false visual feedback suggesting that they are making normal movements even though their actual movements are grossly impaired.

Prediction in the motor system

Many studies (Fourneret and Jeannerod 1998) suggest that when the actual outcome of a movement matches the predicted outcome we have minimal awareness of the sensory consequences of our own movements. Presumably this effect reflects an attenuation of the sensory feedback associated with the movement. If the actual feedback matches the predicted feedback it is cancelled out. This mechanism enables us to distinguish between sensations caused by external events and those caused by our own movements. We are strongly aware of the sensation if our arm comes in contact with an unexpected object in the course of a movement. The phenomenon of tickling provides a useful paradigm for studying this mechanism. Tactile stimulation applied to the palm of our hand by someone else feels intense and 'ticklish'. When we tickle ourselves the tactile signals are felt as far less intense (Weiskrantz et al. 1971). This is because we can predict the sensory consequences of our own movements. These subjective feelings have their counterpart at the physiological level. The reduced sensation is associated with reduced activity in primary (SI) and secondary somatosensory (SII) cortices (Blakemore et al. 1998). Volunteers lay in a MRI scanner and were tickled by the experimenter or tickled themselves by using their right hand to move a stimulator across their left palm. Tickling by the experimenter caused increases in activity in SI and SII. Self-tickling produced significantly less activity. Indeed, self-tickling did not produce any more activity than movements of the right hand that did not cause any stimulation of the left palm. Of course we do not have to tickle ourselves in order to produce sensations when we move. Any movement will generate sensory signals in the limb that is moved. However, passive movements of limb are associated with greater sensation than active movements. Passive movements are associated with greater activity in parietal cortex than the same movements made actively (Weiller et al. 1996).

How precise is the prediction that is needed to attenuate our experience of the sensory consequences of our own movements? It could simply be that our sensations are attenuated whenever we are moving. Blakemore et al. (1999) demonstrated that this is not the case. Volunteers tickled themselves with a system of robots. Their right hand moved a robot arm through which the movements they made could be accurately recorded. This record of the movements was transmitted to a second robot arm. This second robot arm tickled the subject's left palm, using precisely the movements made by the volunteer's right hand. In the baseline condition this was like tickling oneself with a rigid rod. This experience was significantly less intense than being tickled by the robot arm. (In this experiment the movements could be very precisely matched. The movements made by the robot arm were identical to those produced by the volunteer on a previous trial.) With this system it was possible to produce small and precise distortions in the transmission of the signal from one hand to the other. For example, the tactile stimulation could be delayed. The movements of the rod on the left palm would occur after the movements generated by the right hand. As this delay was increased the tactile sensation that was experienced also increased. With a 200 ms delay the sensation was as great as when the tickling was not self-generated by the right hand, but independently generated by the robot. The same result was obtained when the movement was distorted in space rather than time. If the volunteer's right hand moved vertically up and down, but the robot arm moved at 45 degrees, then the tickling sensation increased. These results suggest that the attenuation of sensations associated with self-generated movements depends upon a very precise prediction about these sensations.

We still do not know how the brain makes the predictions that allow the attenuation of self-generated sensations. It is clearly necessary for there to be some sort of interaction between the brain regions in the frontal lobe that generate the movements and the more posterior regions including the parietal cortex where sensations associated with movements are processed. However, this interaction is undoubtedly mediated through many brain regions. It has long been held that the cerebellum has a special role in predicting the consequences of movement on both theoretical (Ito 1970; Wolpert et al. 1998) and empirical (Gellman et al. 1985; Simpson et al. 1996) grounds. Using the system of robots described above, Blakemore et al. (2001) observed that activity in the cerebellum increased as the delay between movement and sensation increased. I am optimistic that over the next few years it will possible to specify fairly precisely the brain system that underlies our ability to predict the sensory consequences of our own movements. As we shall see in the next section, such a specification may well have important implications for our understanding of schizophrenia.

Problems identifying self and other in schizophrenia

It is important to distinguish between sensations caused by our own actions and those caused by independent events in the outside world. Independent events may indicate that we need to change our plans and therefore they require our attention. The mechanism by which the sensory signals associated with our own actions are attenuated ensures that independent events will engage our attention more than self-generated events. If this mechanism went wrong then our attention might be inappropriately attracted by our own actions and we might have difficulty in distinguishing between signals about the self and signals about other agents. Many accounts of schizophrenia have proposed precisely these kinds of problem. In particular it has been proposed that passivity experiences, such as delusions of control, reflect a confusion between the self and the other such that self-generated actions are attributed to another (Frith et al. 2000a: see Spence 2002 for a review of such theories). There is now preliminary evidence that these symptoms are associated with a failure to attenuate responses to sensations caused by self-generated actions. Patients with these kinds of symptoms experience self-generated tactile stimulation as being as intense as the same stimulation applied by someone else (Blakemore et al. 2000). At the physiological level these patients show abnormal overactivity in areas including parietal cortex when making active movements (Spence et al. 1997; see also Chapter 11 by Spence). These regions can plausibly be associated with the processing of sensory signals relating to movement. In normal volunteers these are the regions which show more activity in passive rather than active movements (Weiller et al. 1996). Thus, at both the psychological and the physiological level the patients behave as if active movements are indistinguishable from passive movements. Such an abnormal experience could explain why the patient experiences his own active movements as if they were being made for him by someone else. Given this account there are a number of experiments that could be extremely informative. Are there particular kinds of movement that are more likely to induce the delusion? I would predict that the delusion should be more likely to occur when a movement is highly practised rather than when it is novel. Does the problem associated with schizophrenia arise at a particular point in the circuitry by which self-generated sensations are attenuated? Or, is the problem associated with a more general mechanism that modulates the long-range interactions between the components of the system?

Awareness of high level executive control

So far my discussion of awareness of the motor control system has been largely restricted to a consideration of simple actions often involving a single limb movement. However, one might expect that there would be a much greater role for awareness when performing complex tasks, which require flexible coordination between multiple response components. These are the kinds of task which can only be performed with the help of the kind of executive control system widely believed to be instantiated in the frontal cortex (Shallice 1988). In studies of executive control an important distinction is made between novel tasks and routine or automatic tasks. Almost any task that has never been performed before is likely to engage executive processes and thus cause difficulty to patients with 'frontal' problems. But, with practice, almost any task can become routine and automatic and will no longer engage these processes. As part of this change we become far less conscious of what we are doing. An operational definition of an automatic task is that we can do something else at the same time without impairing performance of the task. In other words, we no longer have to think about the performance of an automatic task and can devote our thoughts to something else. This ability to perform a task without awareness provides an elegant way to identify some of the neural correlates of awareness in motor control.

Jueptner et al. (1997) taught volunteers to perform a sequence of button presses using four buttons and the fingers of the right hand. The task was paced by a tone and initially the volunteers had to learn by trial and error which button to press next. After about 90 min of practice volunteers could perform this task automatically in the sense that they could do something else at the same time without impairing their performance. At the beginning of practice there was much activation in the frontal lobe including dorsolateral prefrontal cortex (DLPFC) and anterior cingulate cortex (ACC). However, after practice there was no more activity in these frontal areas than in a rest condition. The most interesting condition was one in which the volunteers performed the automatic task, but were asked to think about what they were doing. Specifically they were told that each time they pressed a button they should think about the next button in the sequence. In this condition reaction times became slightly slower. In addition there was an increase in activity in left DLPFC and in ACC. Activity in these regions is clearly associated with awareness of task performance, but note that in this example the awareness certainly did not improve task performance.

The same brain areas have been implicated by other studies in which awareness of task performance was manipulated in different ways. For example, button sequences like those used by Jueptner et al. (1997) can be learned without the volunteer realizing that there is anything to learn (Nissen and Bullemer 1987). The volunteer believes he is performing a choice reaction-time task in which he has to press one of four buttons in response to a signal light. He is not aware that the lights are coming on in a fixed sequence, but nevertheless his reaction time gets shorter because implicit learning enables him to predict which button to press next. Such implicit learning does not engage frontal regions any more than performance of sequences that are entirely random (Grafton et al. 1995; Hazeltine et al. 1997). Comparison of explicit with implicit learning of the same sequence shows increased activity in right DLPFC and ACC when volunteers are aware that they are learning. In this example, while the sequence was being learned, performance was better and learning was faster when volunteers were aware that they were learning a sequence.

It has long been thought that DLPFC and ACC have major roles in executive control, but the precise nature of these roles remains controversial. Cameron Carter and his colleagues (MacDonald et al. 2000) suggest that DLPFC maintains top-down control of task-appropriate behaviour while ACC is involved in evaluative processes (such as conflict monitoring) and can thus indicate when control needs to be more strongly engaged. My major concern here is not to argue about the role of these regions in the executive system, but to consider how their functions relate to awareness of action. Towards this end it will be particularly useful to consider tasks which never become automatic, however much we practice them. There must be a special feature of such tasks that necessitates the use of executive control.

One such task is random-number generation (Baddeley 1966). The volunteer is asked to generate a sequence of random numbers between 1 and 9. To give some idea of the nature of such a sequence, he is told to imagine he is picking slips of paper with the numbers written on them out of a hat and replacing each number after he has called it out. The randomness of the sequence produced can be measured and typically deviates from true randomness because volunteers avoid repetitions (1–1, 3–3, etc.) and runs (1–2, 5–6, 9–8) more than they should. However, performance in the sense of the randomness of the sequence does not improve with practice and, however much you practice, the task does not become automatic. Jahanshahi et al. (2000) studied the neural correlates of random generation (compared with counting) and found the expected activations in DLPFC and in ACC. In this study the random-number generation was paced and volunteers were required to produce the numbers at six different rates. In confirmation of previous studies (Baddeley 1966; Robertson et al. 1996) performance deteriorated at high rates since increasing numbers of runs (1–2, 5–6, etc.) were produced at these rates. For me, the problem at high rates is that I do not have time to find a suitable number before the pacing tone forces me to give a response. Because counting is so well learned, the first number that comes into my head is the next one in the sequence. This is just what I am trying to avoid, but often this is the only number available for me to give. This is precisely the situation in which there are demands upon some high-level executive control system.

How do we cope with this dual-task situation in which the requirement to make a response now competes with the process of choosing an appropriate response? Which brain areas are brought into play in these difficult circumstances? The results of Jahanshahi's study were very clear. The DLPFC is not this high-level executive area. Activity in this area *decreased* at high rates of generation when the randomness of the sequence decreased. Decreases in DLPFC activity have been observed in other studies where the need to do two tasks at once has led to an impairment of performance (Fletcher et al. 1995; Goldberg et al. 1998). ACC, in contrast, did not show a decrease and, in the study of Fletcher et al. (1995), showed a significant increase when two tasks had to be done at once. If there is a higher-level executive area it is more likely to be ACC than DLPFC.

On the basis of this result and others, I have argued that the role of DLPFC is to specify a class of responses that are suitable for the tasks at hand (Frith 2000). The probability of making responses within this class is increased while the probability of making responses outside the category is reduced (sculpting the response space). If this class of responses is fixed for a particular task, then this biasing effect will eventually be elicited directly by the task context, and the intervention of DLPFC is no longer required. The task has then become automatic. For the random-number generating task the class of appropriate responses has to be updated each time a response is made. As a result it can never become automatic.

This formulation of the role of DLPFC resembles a number of other accounts (Shallice 1988). However, my concern is not so much with the exact role of DLPFC, but with the extent to which we are aware of its operations. I have already mentioned the general principle that we are not aware of cognitive processes, but only of the outcome of these processes (Nisbett and Wilson 1977). If this principle is correct then we would not be aware of the processing of selecting appropriate responses, but only of which response had been selected. On the other hand a number of authors (Marcel 1980) have proposed that conscious awareness is necessary for the strategic control of intentional action. A major component of such strategic control is the selection of appropriate responses in novel situations. I am arguing that we are not aware of this selection process, only the results of the selection. Some kind of active process associated with awareness, often referred to as working memory, does seem to be required to maintain the selection. The main function of this process seems to be to prevent task-irrelevant stimuli or thoughts from interfering with the current selection (de Fockert et al. 2001). However, there is now evidence that, at least at the moment the selection is implemented, initiation of responses can be achieved without awareness.

Varraine et al. (2002) had volunteers walking on a treadmill which was driven by this walking activity. The resistance of the treadmill could be varied continuously and volunteers were asked to detect changes in this resistance. In addition the volunteers were told how to respond to the change in resistance. In one condition they were instructed to maintain their initial walking speed. This requires an increase in the force of the step to compensate for the increase in resistance of the treadmill. In another condition they were instructed to keep the force of their step constant. This requires a reduction in walking speed. The volunteers had no difficulty carrying out these instructions. These changes in movement were intentional and were not automatic. Yet the changes occurred well before the volunteers were aware of the change in the resistance of the treadmill. When the resistance was gradually increased, changes in walking occurred with 2 seconds of the change beginning, while reports of the change in resistance were not given for another 4 seconds. This is an example of strategic control in which there is no awareness either of the stimulus eliciting the action or of the action itself. In this task, at least, once the arbitrary contingencies between stimulus and response have been put in place, strategic control can occur without awareness.

Hypnosis provides a more extreme and, possibly, more controversial example of strategic control without awareness (Smith et al., reported in Kopelman and Morton 2001). Volunteers were hypnotized and then performed a word-association task, giving the first word that came into their head in response to a list of words read out by the experimenter. While still under hypnosis they were instructed that they could not remember the task they had just performed. The task was then repeated with the same list of words. A 'truly' amnesic patient in these circumstances would not be able to recall the list of words just presented to him, but would still show normal priming effects. He would show a strong tendency to produce the same words that he had generated the first time and would probably generate them slightly faster. This was not the behaviour of the normal volunteers under hypnosis. To the second presentation of the word list they tended to produce different words somewhat more slowly. For this behaviour to occur at least two requirements must be met. First the volunteer has to apply his knowledge, in this case faulty, about what would happen if he couldn't remember the first presentation of the list. He believes that different words are likely to be given. (This is reminiscent of people generating random numbers who believe, falsely, that repetitions should not occur in random sequences.) Second, during performance of the task the volunteer has to reject the first word that comes into his head when this is the word he gave last time and give another one instead. Thus, under hypnosis, all this strategic control happens, to some degree, in the absence of awareness. In this study the volunteers were not only unaware of applying the contingencies, as in the treadmill experiment, but also were unaware of setting up the contingencies in the first place.

We have only just started to explore the extent to which the executive control of action can take place without awareness. The preliminary evidence is that much of such control can occur without awareness. This has, I believe, relevance for the understanding of hysteria or, more specifically, hysterical conversion. A hysterical paralysis can be seen as an example of strategic control without awareness. The patient has determined that a certain category of responses shall not be emitted although he or she is not aware of having deliberately set up this category. As in the hypnosis experiment described above, the responses produced by the hysteric patient reflect his or her beliefs (beliefs that may be false) about what behaviour should occur as a result of some physical damage. One implication of this idea is that hysterical behaviour looks like a wilful act and can only be distinguished from such behaviour at the physiological level (Spence 1999; Spence et al. 2000). If this unconscious wilful behaviour is also possible in 'normal' volunteers, then there are great opportunities for studying experimentally the cognitive and physiological mechanisms that underlie the phenomena of strategic control without awareness.

What is the function of awareness in the motor control system?

I have argued that we are aware of very little of the workings of our motor control system. At the bottom level, by which I mean the level at which movements are being generated, we have little or no awareness of the precise details of the movements we are making or of the associated muscle activity. What we do seem to be aware of is a rather abstract representation of the movement we are about to make and an awareness of making the movement. What is perhaps surprising is that this awareness is based on prediction rather than sensory feedback. In the case of well-practised actions, attention to the action and particularly to the details of the action will usually impair performance. So there does seem to be an advantage of a lack of awareness of these low levels of the motor system. However, I have also argued that we have very little awareness of the highest levels of the system. We are not aware of how our responses are selected, but only of the responses themselves. If asked we may produce a story about how we are able to control some complex system, but this may not correspond to what we are actually doing (Berry and Broadbent 1984).

This raises a question about the function of consciousness. If we do not need to be conscious of the process or the stimuli to achieve high-level strategic control, then what function, if any, does consciousness serve? Our awareness of motor control seems to be focused at a middle level, the level of discrete intentions and the actions that follow them. It is at this level of the motor control system that a strong sense of agency is possible. There is a close contingency in time (a few hundred milliseconds) between the intention and the action. Furthermore, this contingency is enhanced in awareness. The delay in awareness of the response selected and the premature awareness of the initiation of that response brings even closer together the two components that underlie our sense of agency (see Figure 10.3). Perhaps the purpose of awareness of our own motor control system is to create and enhance this sense of our own agency: the experience that our actions are determined by our wishes and intentions and that we can choose what we will do next. I have suggested (Frith 1995; see also Humphrey 1978) that this awareness of our own sense of agency is critical for adopting an 'intentional stance' (Dennett 1987), that is, to understand that other people also act on the basis of their wishes and intentions.

This is all very speculative, but support for these ideas comes from at least two sources. First, there is the evidence from neuropsychological studies that there is a single brain system which is involved both with our own actions and with the

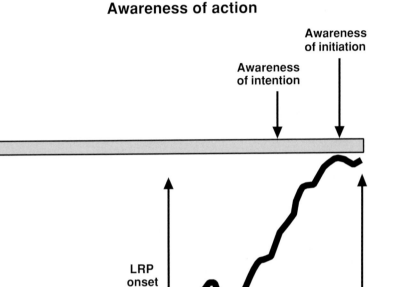

Figure 10.3 Awareness emphasizes the link between intention and action (drawn from data in Haggard and Eimer 1999).

actions of others. In monkeys there are 'mirror neurons' which respond when the monkey makes a response and when the monkey sees someone else making the same response (Rizzolatti et al. 1996). In humans there is a system including medial prefrontal cortex that is active when we attend to our own mental states or to the mental states of others (Frith and Frith 1999). Second, there is the evidence from studies of psychopathology that, in the case of schizophrenia, abnormalities in the awareness of the patient's own actions are intimately associated with abnormalities in the awareness of agency in others. Patients with delusions of control do not simply say that they feel that they are not in control of their actions. They also believe that these actions are being controlled by another agent. Such beliefs about the influence of other agents are a common thread running though many of the symptoms of schizophrenia (see Chapter 11 by Spence).

I believe that these observations in normal and abnormal cases give us vital clues about the nature and purpose of awareness of action. Following up these clues with carefully controlled empirical studies of consciousness and its physiological basis now has the potential to greatly increase our understanding of psychotic states in particular and of the human condition in general.

Conclusions

In this chapter I have made the case that it is possible to study the physiological basis of consciousness as rigorously as that of any other psychological process. I hope I have also shown that a full understanding of many neurological and psychiatric disorders must depend upon elucidating the physiological basis of consciousness. Phantom limbs, delusions of control and hysterical paralysis all reflect abnormalities of consciousness at different levels in a system for the control of action. The awareness we have of our motor system is intimately associated with the sense of agency which, in turn, is the basis for the concept of free will. Many seem to believe that the study of the physiological basis of agency somehow eliminates free will and, with it, any belief that we have a moral responsibility for our own actions. On the contrary I believe that these investigations will not only help us to understand some very distressing neurological and psychiatric disorders, but also will give us a better understanding of the nature of free will and responsibility.

REFERENCES

Aserinsky E and Kleitman N (1953). Regularly occurring periods of eye motility and concomitant phenomena during sleep. *Science*, 118, 273–4.

Attneave F (1959). *Applications of Information Theory to Psychology*. New York: Henry Holt.

Baddeley AD (1966). The capacity for generating information by randomisation. *Q J Exp Psychol*, 18, 119–29.

Berger H (1929). Uber das Elektrekephalogramm des Menschen. *Arch Psychiatrie Nervenkrankheiten*, 87, 527–70.

Berry DC and Broadbent DE (1984). On the relationship between task performance and associated verbalisable knowledge. *Q J Exp Psychology*, 36, 209–31.

Blakemore S-J, Wolpert DM and Frith CD (1998). Central cancellation of self-produced tickle sensation. *Nat Neurosci*, 1, 635–40.

Blakemore S-J, Frith CD and Wolpert DW (1999). Spatiotemporal prediction modulates the perception of self-produced stimuli. *J Cogn Neurosci*, 11, 551–9.

Blakemore S-J, Smith J, Steel R, Johnstone EC and Frith CD (2000). The perception of self-produced sensory stimuli in patients with auditory hallucinations and passivity experiences: evidence for a breakdown in self-monitoring. *Psychol Med*, 30, 1131–9.

Blakemore S-J, Frith CD and Wolpert DM (2001). The cerebellum is involved in predicting the sensory consequences of action. *Neuroreport*, 12, 1879–84.

Castiello U, Paulignan Y and Jeannerod M (1991). Temporal dissociation of motor responses and subjective awareness. A study in normal subjects. *Brain*, 114, 2639–55.

Deecke L (1987). Bereitschaftspotential as an indicator of movement preparation in supplementary motor area and motor cortex. In *Motor Areas of the Cerebral Cortex: CIBA Symposium 132*, ed. G Bock, pp. 231–50. London: John Wiley and Sons.

Dennet DC (1987). *The Intentional Stance*. Cambridge, MA: MIT Press.

Fletcher P, Frith CD, Grasby P, Shallice T, Frackowiak RSJ and Dolan RJ (1995). Brain systems for encoding and retrieval of auditory-verbal memory. *Brain*, 118, 401–16.

de Fockert JW, Rees G, Frith CD and Lavie N (2001). The role of working memory in visual selective attention. *Science*, 291, 1803–6.

Fourneret P and Jeannerod M (1998). Limited conscious monitoring of motor performance in normal subjects. *Neuropsychologia*, 36, 1133–40.

Frith CD (1995). Consciousness is for other people. *Behav Brain Sci*, 18, 682–3.

Frith CD (2000). The role of dorsolateral prefrontal cortex in the selection of action as revealed by functional imaging. In *Control of Cognitive Processes. Attention and Performance XVlll*, ed. S Monsell and J Driver, pp. 549–65. Cambridge, MA: MIT Press.

Frith CD and Frith U (1999). Interacting minds – a biological basis. *Science*, 286, 1692–5.

Frith CD, Blakemore S-J and Wolpert DM (2000*a*). Explaining the symptoms of schizophrenia: abnormalities in the awareness of action. *Brain Res Rev*, 31, 357–63.

Frith CD, Blakemore S-J and Wolpert DM (2000*b*). Abnormalities in the awareness and control of action. *Philos Trans R Soc Lond B*, 355, 1771–88.

Gellman R, Gibson AR and Houk JC (1985). Inferior olivary neurons in the awake cat – detection of contact and passive body displacement. *J Neurophysiol*, 54, 40–60.

Goldberg TE, Berman KF, Fleming K et al. (1998). Uncoupling cognitive workload and prefrontal cortical physiology, *Neuroimage*, 7, 296–303.

Grafton ST, Hazeltine E and Ivry R (1995). Functional mapping of sequence learning in normal humans. *Hum Brain Mapp*, 1, 221–34.

Haggard P and Eimer M (1999). On the relation between brain potentials and awareness of voluntary movements. *Exp Brain Res*, 126, 128–33.

Haggard P and Magno E (1999). Localising awareness of action with transcranial magnetic stimulation. *Exp Brain Res*, 127, 102–7.

Haggard P, Newman C and Magno E (1999). On the perceived time of voluntary actions. *Br J Psychol*, 90, 291–303.

Hazeltine E, Grafton ST and Ivry R (1997). Attention and stimulus characteristics determine the locus of motor-sequence encoding. *Brain*, 120, 123–40.

Hillyard SA, Hink RF, Schwent VL and Picton TW (1973). Electrical signs of selective attention in the human brain. *Science*, 182, 177–80.

Hobson JA (1988). *The Dreaming Brain*. New York: Basic Books.

Humphrey N (1978). Nature's psychologists. *New Scientist*, 78, 900–3.

Ito M (1970). Neurophysiological aspects of the cerebellar motor control system. *Int J Neurol*, 7, 126–76.

Jahanshahi M, Dirnberger G, Fuller R and Frith CD (2000). The role of the dorsolateral prefrontal cortex in random number generation. *Neuroimage*, 12, 713–25.

Jeannerod M (1994). The representing brain – neural correlates of motor intention and imagery. *Behav Brain Sci*, 17, 187–202.

Jouvet M (1979). What does a cat dream about? *Trends Neurosci*, 2, 15–16.

Jueptner M, Stephan KM, Frith CD, Brooks DJ, Frackowiak RS and Passingham RE (1997). Anatomy of motor learning. I. Frontal cortex and attention to action. *J Neurophysiol*, 77, 1313–24.

Kihlstrom JF (1987). The cognitive unconscious. *Science*, 237, 1445–52.

Kopelman M and Morton J (2001). Psychogenic amnesias – functional memory loss. In *Recovered Memories: The Middle Ground*, ed. G Davies and T Dalgleish, pp. 219–43. Chichester: John Wiley and Sons.

Kutas M and Dale A (1997). Electrical and magnetic readings of mental functions. In *Cognitive Neuroscience*, ed. MD Rugg, pp. 197–242. Hove: Psychology Press.

Libet B, Gleason CA, Wright EW and Pearl DK (1983). Time of conscious intention to act in relation to onset of cerebral activity (readiness potential): the unconscious initiation of a freely voluntary act. *Brain* 106, 623–42.

MacDonald AW, Cohen JD, Stenger VA and Carter CS (2000). Dissociating the role of the dorso-lateral prefrontal and anterior cingulate cortex in cognitive control. *Science*, 288, 1835–8.

Marcel AJ (1980). Conscious and preconscious recognition of polysemous words: locating the selective effects of prior verbal context. In *Attention and Performance VIII*, ed. RS Nickerson, pp. 435–57. Hillsdale, NJ: Lawrence Erlbaum Associates.

Marcel AJ (1983). Conscious and unconscious perception: experiments on visual masking and word recognition. *Cogn Psychol*, 15, 197–237.

Marr D (1982). *Vision*. San Francisco: Freeman.

Milner AD and Rugg MD (1992). *The Neuropsychology of Consciousness*. London: Academic Press.

Morton J (1980). The logogen model and orthographic structure. In *Cognitive Approaches in Spelling*, ed. U Frith, pp. 117–33. London: Academic Press.

Nisbett RE and Wilson TD (1977). Telling more than we can know: verbal reports on mental processes. *Psychol Rev*, 84, 231–59.

Nissen MJ and Bullemer P (1987). Attentional requirements of learning: evidence from perfor-mance measures. *Cogn Psychol*, 19, 1–32.

O'Craven KM and Kanwisher N (2000). Mental imagery of faces and places activates correspond-ing stimulus-specific brain regions. *J Cogn Neurosci*, 12, 1013–23.

Péllison D, Preblanc C, Goodale MA and Jeannerod M (1986). Visual control of reaching move-ments without vision of the limb. II. Evidence of fast unconscious processes correcting the trajectory of the hand to the final position of a double step stimulus. *Exp Brain Res*, 62, 303–11.

Petersen SE, Fox PT, Posner MI, Mintun M and Raichle ME (1988). Positron emission tomo-graphic studies of the cortical anatomy of single word processing. *Nature*, 331, 585–9.

Posner MI, Petersen SE, Fox PT and Raichle ME (1988). Localisation of cognitive operations in the human brain. *Science*, 240, 1627–31.

Prablanc C and Jeannerod M (1975). Corrective saccades: dependence on retinal reafferent signals. *Vision Res*, 15, 465–9.

Ramachandran VS (1996). What neurological syndromes can tell us about human nature: some lessons from phantom limbs, Capgras syndrome, and anosognosia. In *Cold Spring Harbor Symposium on Quantitative Biology, Vol. 61*, pp. 115–34. New York: Cold Spring Harbor Laboratory Press.

Ramachandran VS and Hirstein W (1998). The perception of phantom limbs. *Brain* 121, 1603–30.

Ramachandran VS and Rogers-Ramachandran D (1996). Synaesthesia in phantom limbs induced with mirrors. *Proc R Soc Lond Biol B Sci*, 263, 377–86.

Rees G (2001). Neuroimaging of visual awareness in patients and normal subjects. *Curr Opin Neurobiol*, 11, 150–6.

Rees G and Lavie N (2001). What can functional imaging reveal about the role of attention in visual awareness? *Neuropsychologia*, 39, 1343–53.

Rizzolatti G, Fadiga L, Gallese V and Fogassi L (1996). Premotor cortex and the recognition of motor actions. *Cogn Brain Res*, 3, 131–41.

Robertson C, Hazelwood R and Rawson MD (1996). The effects of Parkinson's disease on the capacity to generate information randomly. *Neuropsychologia*, 14, 1069–78.

Roland PE and Friberg L (1985). Localization of cortical areas activated by thinking. *J Neurophysiol*, 53, 1219–43.

Rugg MD, Mark RE, Walla P, Schloerscheidt AM, Birch CS and Allen K (1998). Dissociation of the neural correlates of implicit and explicit memory. *Nature*, 392, 595–8.

Schacter DL (1992). Consciousness and awareness in memory and amnesia. In *The Neuropsychology of Consciousness*, ed. AD Milner and MD Rugg, pp. 179–200. London: Academic Press.

Shallice T (1988). *From Neuropsychology to Mental Structure*. Cambridge: Cambridge University Press.

Shannon CE and Weaver W (1949). *The Mathematical Theory of Information*. Urbana, IL: University of Illinois Press.

Simpson JI, Wylie DR and De Zeeuw CI (1996). On climbing fiber signals and their consequence(s). *Behav Brain Sci*, 19, 384.

Sirigu A, Duhamel JR, Cohen L, Pillon B, Dubois B and Agid Y (1996). The mental representation of hand movements after parietal cortex damage. *Science*, 273, 1564–8.

Spence SA (1999). Hysterical paralyses as disorders of action. *Cogn Neuropsychiatry*, 4, 203–26.

Spence SA (2002). Alien control: from phenomenology to cognitive neurobiology. *Philos Psychiatry Psychol*, in press.

Spence SA, Brooks DJ, Hirsch SR, Liddle PF, Meehan J and Grasby PM (1997). A PET study of voluntary movement in schizophrenic patients experiencing passivity phenomena (delusions of alien control). *Brain*, 120, 1997–2011.

Spence SA, Crimlisk HL, Cope H, Ron MA and Grasby PM (2000). Discrete neurophysiological correlates in prefornal cortex during hysterical and feigned disorder of movement. *Lancet*, 355, 1243–4.

Stickgold R (1998). Sleep: off-line memory reprocessing. *Trends Cogn Sci*, 2, 484–92.

Turner R and Jezzard P (1994). How to see the mind. *Physics World*, 29–34.

Varraine E, Bonnard M and Pailhous J (2002). The top down and bottom up mechanisms involved in the sudden awareness of low level sensori-motor behaviour. *Cogn Brain Res*, 13, 357–61.

Wegner DM and Wheatley T (1999). Apparent mental causation – sources of the experience of will. *Am Psychol*, 54, 480–92.

Weiller C, Juptner M, Fellows S et al. (1996). Brain representation of active and passive movement. *Neuroimage*, 4, 105–10.

Weiskrantz L (1986). *Blindsight*. Oxford: Oxford University Press.

Weiskrantz L, Elliot J and Darlington C (1971). Preliminary observations of tickling oneself. *Nature*, 230, 598–9.

Wolpert DM, Miall RC and Kawato M (1998). Internal models on the cerebellum. *Trends Cogn Sci*, 2, 338–47.

11

Cognitive neurobiology of volition and agency in schizophrenia

Sean A Spence

University of Sheffield, Sheffield, UK

Introduction

Since its initial description, schizophrenia has been known to affect *volition*: voluntary movement (Kraepelin 1919; Zec 1995; McKenna et al. 1998). But such abnormality is not restricted to the *way* that a movement is performed, it also affects its *purpose*. Patients may do things abnormally – they may also choose to do abnormal things. In this chapter we address the neural substrates of disordered action performance and the disturbed sense of agency that may occur in some patients with this disabling condition.

Volition and will

Volition encompasses a spectrum of voluntary behaviours and some of these ('willed', 'intended' or 'freely chosen') seem to us to be quintessentially human. The 'will' refers to our capacity to choose. We may 'choose' to 'control' some of our involuntary impulses. We may choose to attend to one stream of competing information over another. We may initiate conversations, many of which may be structurally unique and unpredictable. We may create a sequence for performing even the most mundane tasks. What we choose to do is an 'action'; the one who chooses it is an 'agent' (Macmurray 1991). One influential theory characterized schizophrenia as a 'disorder of action' (Frith 1987). By making action central to schizophrenia, Frith's early theory made the latter a disorder of *higher* volition – of that which is willed (or chosen) over that which is automatic (Frith 1987; Liddle 1993; see Chapter 10 by Frith). Frith's theories have undergone changes and he currently uses 'action' to refer to *all* movements. However, in this essay I shall retain the original use of the word, to denote 'chosen' responses to the world. As I will demonstrate, such actions implicate higher (executive) motor control processes. Clinically, this distinction is meaningful: the patient who cannot generate willed actions exhibits 'negative' symptomatology ('avolition'), yet they may still perform automatic behaviours (e.g. stereotypies).

Whether the will is 'free' is a problem pertaining as much to 'normal' volition as to the behaviours performed by people with schizophrenia (Spence 1996a; Dilman 1999). Such freedom may refer to the intra- or extrapersonal. In the former we are interested in whether the 'feeling' or *experience* of freedom (agency) is justified: is agency 'just' an illusion? It is this *sense* of agency that may be so radically altered in the phenomenology of schizophrenia, e.g. in those experiencing 'alien control' (see below). In 'extrapersonal' freedom, we are referring to the constraints placed upon the agent by outside forces; this is also of special relevance to people affected by schizophrenia, who may be detained in hospitals 'against their will'.

Free will and consciousness

An elegant and accessible overview of the philosophy of 'free will' has been provided by Dilman (1999); and the brain mechanisms supporting volition have been subjected to interdisciplinary critique (Libet et al. 1999). The timing of neural activity relative to conscious 'intention' and its implications for intrapersonal freedom have been debated previously (Libet et al. 1983; Frith 1996; Spence 1996a, b; Libet 1996; see Chapter 10 by Frith). Essentially, the onset of predictive trains of neural activity (as detected by electroencephalogram (EEG)), preceding the subjective experience of a conscious intention to move, suggests that the latter intention is not causally related to the ensuing act (Spence 1996a). Intention may be a corollary to, but it is not synonymous with, the initiation of an action. This poses a difficult 'problem'. Why do we experience a sense of agency, consciously, if our responses are generated prior to our awareness of them? Frith attempts to answer this question (Chapter 10).

In this essay my purpose is to summarize those findings from cognitive neuroscience and functional neuro-imaging that impact specifically upon volition in schizophrenia. I shall not address *involuntary* movements, which have been reviewed elsewhere (Barnes and Spence 2000). Catatonia, comprising a mix of voluntary and involuntary behaviours, is also excluded; the subject has been revivified by Rogers (1985, 1991) and is thoughtfully reviewed by McKenna et al. (1998). The forensic aspects of psychotic action have likewise been addressed elsewhere by Taylor (1998).

A cognitive neurobiology of volition

Neural control of volition may be cognitively specified in terms of motor planning, preparation, programming and execution (Passingham 1993; Jeannerod 1997). In this scheme it is the prefrontal cortex that supports planning and 'choice' of action, while preparing and programming movement are 'delegated' to premotor and basal ganglia regions, utilizing sensory data analysed in posterior association cortices.

The execution of motor tasks (especially those requiring manual precision) involves the motor cortices. Hence, when a 'routine' motor task is being performed it may be conceptualized as a 'programme' being run by the premotor cortices and basal ganglia (Passingham 1993); automatic tasks becoming 'default' settings (Goldman-Rakic and Selemon 1997). Higher centres may intervene when a task is difficult, requires a novel response or involves something new being learned (explicitly). In one contemporary model, this intervening 'supervisory attentional system' has been equated with the 'will'; it has been hypothesized to be a (multicomponent) function of prefrontal cortex (Shallice and Burgess 1996).

Integration of brain function is exemplified by cortico-cortical connections between cortical regions and the thalamo-cortico-basal ganglia loops, linking cortical sites to specific subcortical regions (Alexander et al. 1986). A 'cognitive' loop projects to the dorsolateral prefrontal cortex and a 'motor' loop to the supplementary motor area (Masterman and Cummings 1997). Though not addressed in detail here, any fully specified model of volition must incorporate the functioning of these distributed systems (Spence and Frith 1999).

If schizophrenia were 'just' a disorder of higher volition (action), then we might expect motor abnormalities to be confined to the performance of novel or 'chosen' movements, reflecting an underlying dysfunction of the prefrontal cortex. But if the volitional disorder of schizophrenia were *not* restricted to action then we should expect abnormalities of other, 'lower' motor regions to impede less complex movements.

Motor cortex in schizophrenia

Schizophrenic volitional disturbance clearly extends to such 'lower' movements and motor regions. It has long been recognized that the illness is associated with *involuntary* movements (seen before the neuroleptic era) and abnormalities of *voluntary* movement such as: clumsiness, muscle force instability and impaired finger grip and dexterity (Puri et al. 1996). Some neurological 'soft' signs of the disorder are also of this type (Flashman et al. 1996). Such abnormalities are found in children at high genetic risk for schizophrenia (Manschreck 1986; Fish et al. 1992), in those who later develop the disorder (Walker et al. 1994) and in adult schizotypals (Neumann and Walker 1999). Functional neuro-imaging studies of patients have consistently revealed relative failure of motor cortical activation during voluntary movement, irrespective of neuroleptic treatment (Guenther et al. 1994; Kotrla et al. 1995; Schroder et al. 1995; Spence et al. 1997). Studies using EEG have also found signal abnormalities over sensorimotor regions (Chiarenza et al. 1985). In addition, transcranial magnetic stimulation (TMS) has revealed abnormalities in evoked potentials over motor cortex (Puri et al. 1996). Taken together, these findings suggest that motor cortex is functionally abnormal in schizophrenia. Hence, we should expect even simple movements to be potentially affected.

Premotor cortex in schizophrenia

In premotor cortex, the predominant finding is one of hypofunction during limb movement, especially in the supplementary motor area (SMA; Guenther et al. 1994; Schroder et al. 1995). This medial structure is implicated in the preparation and programming of movements, particularly when there is an element of choice, complexity or the requirement for bimanual coordination. It is also activated during verbal fluency. The medial frontal lobe, in the region of SMA, is thought to give rise to one of the characteristic EEG signals preceding movement: the readiness potential (see Chapter 10 by Frith). This signal is abnormal in schizophrenia, again suggesting an abnormality of motor programming (Karaman et al. 1997; Dreher et al. 1999).

However, there is probably less uniformity among patients with respect to pre-motor dysfunction than there is for that of motor cortex. While the latter appears underactive in each patient group reported, this is not the case with SMA, especially in studies involving verbal material (Frith et al. 1995; Fletcher et al. 1996; Dye et al. 1999; Spence et al. 2000). Thus, while those who experience auditory verbal halluci-nations (when ill) exhibit trait hypofunction of SMA during covert verbal imagery (when stable), other ('schizophrenic') patients do not do so (McGuire et al. 1995). Also, chronically institutionalized patients with reality distortion syndrome (delu-sions and hallucinations) exhibit hyperactivation of SMA during overt verbal flu-ency, while other patients from the same institution (Frith et al. 1995; Spence et al. 1995) and stable community samples do not (Dye et al. 1999; Spence et al. 2000). Acutely ill patients with passivity phenomena, performing limb movements, exhibit hyperactivation of SMA during stereotypic movements, compared with 'normals', other acutely ill patients, and themselves when recovering (Spence et al. 1997).

Similarly, the readiness potential may vary with symptomatology: positive symp-toms being associated with reduction of its early component; negative symptoms with reduction of its late component (Karaman et al. 1997).

Hence, premotor cortical dysfunction is found in some, but not all, patients affected by schizophrenia. It is uncertain whether this is trait- or state-related. Further, detailed studies are required.

Prefrontal cortex in health and disease

Prefrontal cortex in action

Many strands of evidence point to prefrontal cortex being implicated in normal and abnormal 'action'. Those regions particularly relevant are dorsolateral prefrontal cortex (DLPFC) and anterior cingulate cortex (ACC) (Passingham 1997; Spence and Frith 1999; see Chapter 10 by Frith).

Neuropsychological and functional neuro-imaging studies in 'normals' and neuropsychiatric patients support the contention that DLPFC has a role in the

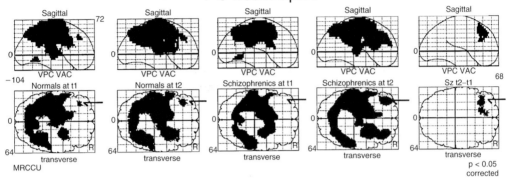

Figure 11.1   Brain areas activated in control subjects and schizophrenic patients during a motor task involving the paced movement of a joystick in freely chosen directions at two points in time (t1 and t2), 4–6 weeks apart. The patients were recovering from a schizophrenic relapse ('Schizophrenics' at t1 and t2). Brain regions showing a significantly greater neuronal response to the free selection of joystick movement with the right hand compared with the resting state are shown in black. In normal controls there is a similar pattern of activation on both occasions (there is no statistically significant difference between the maps at t1 and t2). Controls activate left prefrontal cortex on both occasions. The right-hand figure shows areas exhibiting greater neuronal response at t2 in patients with schizophrenia (compared to t1). Patients exhibit a recovery of prefrontal function coinciding with symptomatic recovery. These figures show statistical parametric maps (SPMs) thresholded for display purposes at $P < 0.05$ (corrected for multiple comparisons). Although prefrontal activation is not seen in subjects with schizophrenia at t1, it is present at t2 (the comparison of these SPMs revealing statistically greater activation in left prefrontal cortex at t2). Sagittal sections are views from the right side of the brain; transverse sections are views from above. In each image the arrow points to the left dorsolateral prefrontal cortex (adapted from Spence et al. 1998).

selection (or choice) of novel motor output (including words and numbers), while focal pathology impairs such performance (Luria 1966; Perret 1974; Fuster 1980; Frith et al. 1991*a*, *b*, 1995; Ingvar 1994; Shallice and Burgess 1996; Goldman-Rakic and Selemon 1997; Jahanshahi et al. 1997; Jeannerod 1997; Passingham 1997; de Zubicaray et al. 1997, 1998; Desmond et al. 1998; Spence et al. 1998, 2000; Knight et al. 1999). In brief, DLPFC is activated when subjects generate novel or self-chosen responses (actions; see Figure 11.1). Transient 'experimental lesions' induced by TMS (over DLPFC) impair the generation of such actions, leading to the emergence of stereotypic response patterns (Jahanshahi et al. 1998). The role of DLPFC in action is reviewed at length elsewhere (Spence and Frith 1999).

ACC comprises two divisions, cognitive (dorsal) and emotional (ventral) (Bush et al. 2000). The cognitive division is particularly involved in attention to action, response selection and tasks in which there are competing streams of incoming stimulus information. The affective division is activated by emotional stimuli and may play a role in motivation and analysis of stimulus salience. Cells in the ACC are also engaged in monitoring errors in performance (Gehring and Knight 2000). This region has been linked to an EEG signal specifically related to error detection ('error-related negativity'; Gehring and Knight 2000).

Respective contributions to the relationship between DLPFC and ACC in the context of action generation are difficult to fully differentiate. They are frequently coactivated by tasks requiring attention to action, generation of novelty or dual task performance (Passingham 1997; Duncan and Owen 2000). Hence, they are frequently coactivated by 'action' (Macmurray 1991). But in normal subjects performing very difficult tasks, activations in these regions may become 'decoupled', with concomitant deterioration in task performance (Goldberg et al. 1998). Thus, DLPFC may exhibit a 'lawful' pattern of response whereby local activity increases with task demand (Rypma et al. 1999) but diminishes if that demand becomes too great (Goldberg et al. 1998). As we shall see, this may be pertinent to deficits in prefrontal function exhibited in schizophrenia.

Prefrontal cortical dysfunction in schizophrenic avolition

Prefrontal cortex exhibits structural and functional abnormalities in schizophrenia (Goldman-Rakic and Selemon 1997). Negative symptoms, such as alogia (lack of spontaneous speech), suggest impaired prefrontal activation, as does the corresponding executive dysfunction on formal cognitive testing (i.e. reduced verbal fluency; Liddle 1993; Joyce et al. 1996).

Functional neuro-imaging has revealed 'hypofrontality' in schizophrenia: reduced activity at rest, and a failure to activate on cognitive challenge (Chua and McKenna 1995; Weinberger and Berman 1996). Despite methodological and theoretical constraints a consensus has emerged that failure to activate is not simply a consequence of exposure to neuroleptic medication (Weinberger and Berman 1996). One important factor is patient symptomatology during scanning.

'Psychomotor poverty', incorporating alogia and avolition, has been found to be associated with reduced prefrontal blood flow at rest (relative to other patients) (Liddle et al. 1992). This relationship may be independent of the schizophrenia syndrome since combined analysis of these data with those from a resting-state study of depressed patients revealed alogia to be associated with reduced blood flow in left DLPFC, irrespective of diagnosis (Dolan et al. 1993). Hence, those who fail to generate spontaneous speech outside the scanner (irrespective of diagnosis) exhibit reduced blood flow to left DLPFC while at rest inside the scanner.

The finding that psychomotor poverty is associated with prefrontal dysfunction has been replicated in people with schizophrenia (Ebmeier et al. 1993) and has also been extended to an apparent reduction of prefrontal grey matter volume (associated with psychomotor poverty on a voxel-based analysis of structural MRI data; Chua et al. 1997). Hence, the failure of patients to initiate speech spontaneously (alogia) may reflect both structural and functional deficits of prefrontal cortex.

Negative symptoms share features with those of Parkinson's disease and are compatible with reduced prefrontal dopaminergic neurotransmission. Of interest is the finding that nonpsychotic relatives of people with schizophrenia may also exhibit 'negative symptoms', and that these are associated with reduced plasma levels of homovanillic acid (HVA), the major dopamine metabolite and indicator of brain dopaminergic activity (Amin et al. 1999). Plasma HVA is inversely correlated with severity of negative symptoms in these relatives. Hence, the propensity to negative symptoms may involve a genetic diathesis, implicating dopamine transmission.

As in Parkinson's disease, dopaminergic agonists have had some therapeutic effect on negative symptoms in schizophrenia (albeit at the risk of exacerbating positive symptomatology; Liddle 1993; Mortimer and Spence 2001). In organic brain disorders, dopamine agonists have been used to treat 'abulia' ('absence of the will'; Barrett 1999). The role of dopamine in restoring volition is also supported by the finding that the atypical antipsychotic clozapine increases dopamine levels in DLPFC of nonhuman primates (Youngren et al. 1999). Enhancing cortical dopaminergic activity may yet provide one mechanism for restoring voluntary behaviour (as in Parkinson's disease).

Interrogating prefrontal cortical dysfunction in schizophrenia

A series of activation studies performed by Weinberger, Berman and colleagues has utilized the Wisconsin Card Sort Test (WCST) (Berman et al. 1986, 1992; Weinberger et al. 1986, 1988). This complex task involves the subject's attempt to follow a rule for card sorting, which is not divulged by the experimenter, and which may change in the course of the experiment. Normal subjects performing this task activate DLPFC, irrespective of practice (Berman et al. 1995). Activation may reflect attention, planning, strategy formation, response-generation, working memory for previous responses or motivation to perform. Thus, the task may probe many of the cognitive functions supporting willed action in 'real life'. What is less transparent is *which* of these functions is/are abnormal in patients performing this task. Those with schizophrenia phenotype have consistently exhibited hypofrontality during WCST performance. The finding seems to be trait-related, being unrelated to concurrent symptomatology. Weinberger's group has also reported deficits in neural integrity (as measured by decreased N-acetylaspartate using magnetic resonance spectroscopy) in DLPFC, which may reverse with antipsychotic medication (Bertolino et al. 2000).

Using different scanning protocols, other groups have demonstrated variability in DLPFC function among single-patient cohorts performing cognitive tasks. Hence, Curtis and colleagues, studying five patients, found them to be hypofrontal (in left DLPFC) on covert verbal fluency but not on a covert semantic-decision task (Curtis et al. 1999). Honey and colleagues, studying an index group of 10 patients performing a verbal working-memory task in an initial context of conventional antipsychotic medication, found enhanced activation of right DLPFC 6 weeks later, after these patients had been changed to risperidone (Honey et al. 1999). Both these studies also revealed SMA dysfunction congruent with that of DLPFC. Spence and colleagues, studying 13 patients, found them to be hypofrontal (in left DLPFC) during free selection of movement in the context of delusional relapse, but not when studied 4–6 weeks later, when recovering (Spence et al. 1998; Figure 11.1). Also relevant are those data from successive UK (Hammersmith Hospital) groups utilizing the (overt) verbal fluency protocol. They did *not* demonstrate hypofrontality in a series of studies of schizophrenia patients with chronic or acute, medicated or unmedicated, symptomatic or asymptomatic profiles (Frith et al. 1995; Fletcher et al. 1996; Dye et al. 1999; Spence et al. 2000). However, in these studies the task was deliberately slowed so that patients could perform satisfactorily. When a graded-memory task was used that varied response demands it was found that prefrontal activation attenuated as those demands increased (cf. normal controls; Fletcher et al. 1998). The implication of the latter may be that the schizophrenic prefrontal cortex 'decouples' at lower response-demands than the 'normal' (which may nevertheless decouple when sufficiently stressed; Goldberg et al. 1998).

Hence, whether a group of patients with schizophrenia exhibits hypofrontality appears to depend upon the cognitive specifications and difficulty of the experimental task; the current symptomatology of the patients; and (possibly) the presence of 'atypical' antipsychotic medication. We may hypothesize that response generation (volition) will be impeded or facilitated in the clinical environment by the presence of similar factors. Does volition decompensate with increasing task or environmental complexity? These data suggest that it 'should'.

Action as a probe of prefrontal function

Action-performance may be used to probe the integrity, the 'functional connectivity', of prefrontal cortex. This form of connectivity refers to the temporal correlation between activities in distributed cerebral regions (Friston 1996). The implication is that brain areas 'wired together, fire together'. We have examined those regions involved in word generation (Spence et al. 2000). Using a quantitative form of voxel-based analysis we have demonstrated a 'functional disconnection' between left DLPFC and ACC in patients who were clinically stable at the time of scanning. These patients were not significantly 'hypofrontal', yet the correlations in activation between DLPFC and ACC were significantly disturbed. These findings await replication but they are congruent with other data suggesting that schizophrenia involves a breakdown in the integration of activity across the prefrontal regions, rather than a simple, focal, hypo- or hyperactivation (Tauscher et al. 1998; Yang et al. 1999). Thus, the necessity to 'act' and to engage these prefrontal regions in the specified task (demanding novel response generation) may reveal an inherent failure of cortical integration (Spence et al. 2000; and see Andreasen 1999).

Formal thought disorder and spontaneous speech

An objective manifestation of disturbed volition is seen in formal thought disorder, which may include: 'looseness (of associations), peculiar word usage, peculiar sentence construction, peculiar logic and distractibility' (McGuire et al. 1998). Such incoherence undermines the performance of meaningful action. In patients performing free monologues, such thought disorder exhibits functional correlations with activity in a range of areas, including ACC (McGuire et al. 1998). This is a region where resting-state blood flow has previously been found to correlate with severity of the 'disorganization' syndrome, a feature of which is formal thought disorder (Liddle et al. 1992).

A cognitive neurobiology of agency

The example of alien control

Phenomenology

Many people with schizophrenia experience subjective abnormalities suggesting a disorder of agency. In the 'made movements' of alien control the movements in question are attributed to an external agent, agency being ceded to that agent. Similar phenomena have occasionally been reported with right-sided parietal lesions, or epileptic foci (Leiguarda et al. 1993; see Spence 2001 for review).

The neuropsychological deficit in alien control

Frith and Done (1989) demonstrated that those experiencing alien control were relatively impaired on tasks requiring them to rely on an 'internal monitoring' of their movements, in the absence of direct visual feedback. In these studies patients had to rely upon their own proprioception to guide their behaviours. Their performance was worse than that of other people with schizophrenia or affective psychoses (who were not experiencing alien control). They seemed 'not [to know] what response they had just made' (Frith and Done 1989). In a subsequent study by Mlakar et al. (1994) the investigators studied patients concurrently experiencing the 'first-rank symptoms' of schizophrenia (including, though not restricted to, those of alien control). They conducted two experiments involving the generation of visual designs, with varying degrees of visual feedback. Patients experiencing first-rank symptoms exhibited increasing deficit as the necessity for reliance upon internal monitoring increased. This deficit was apparent in both the (unguided) copying of an experimenter's visual design and the subsequent identification of their own (the patient's) self-generated design. These deficits were relative to control groups, one of which comprised patients who had previously experienced such symptoms. Therefore, the *current presence* of these symptoms was temporally related to an *impairment of sensory awareness.*

Thus, in two similar studies (and a third by Stirling et al. 1998), patients with alien control have been shown to be impaired on the performance of motor tasks (necessitating 'self-monitoring'). Mlakar et al. (1994) suggest that 'in certain phases of their illness, [these] patients are lacking a clear, distinct and solid representation of internally initiated mental activity' (and congruent findings have been reported by Daprati et al. 1997 and Franck et al. 2001).

It is notable that there is an overlap between these formulations of cognitive impairment underlying alien control and that offered by Angyal (1936), who posited a deficit in proprioception. In terms of their phenomenology, people who experience alien control fail to experience (or to retain a memory of) their motor acts, an abnormality temporally related to the presence of these symptoms.

As outlined in Chapter 10, Frith and colleagues (Blakemore et al. 2000) have shown that those who experience alien control also fail to experience an attenuation in sensory stimulation when they tickle themselves (in contrast to the 'normal' state in which tickling oneself is experienced as being less pleasant than being tickled by someone else!). One possible explanation for such findings (in patients) is the lack of a 'forward model' emerging for the act of tickling (Chapter 10 by Frith).

However, several details require clarification. First, in Blakemore's study the subjects were not reported to be experiencing alien control at the time they were tested. Also, patients who experienced alien control comprised only part of the index study group, the majority of whom did not experience this symptom, but suffered from auditory verbal hallucinations instead. Hence, we need to clarify whether one form of pathophysiology is common to those experiencing alien control and auditory hallucinations. Stirling et al. (1998, see above) combined similar patient groups and summarized their data as referring to 'alien control', although the more robust findings were those specific to auditory hallucinations. Indeed, when IQ and cognitive performance were controlled for, most of the results relating specifically to symptoms of alien control lacked statistical significance.

A subtle difference in the later Frith study (Blakemore et al. 2000) is the move away from the alien control of action (affecting the hand 'doing the tickling'), towards the sensory awareness of the area tickled (elsewhere on the body). Here, the forward model no longer refers to the control of a movement (through feedback) but its anticipated (distal) consequences upon other bodily regions. The problem is not so much that the patient cannot remember their action, but that they cannot predict its consequences.

Since we are primarily interested in why actions are perceived as being under the control of other agents, we will now consider the neural correlates of agency.

The neural correlates of agency

Agency refers to the sense of ownership, experienced by the subject. Hence, the term refers to a subjective experience, rather than an observer's attribution of agency to that subject.

Although patients with alien control may attribute their movements to outside forces, the movements of their limbs generally appear grossly normal. But there is another syndrome in which an affected limb appears objectively 'out of control': the alien or anarchic limb syndrome (the phenomenology is described in detail in Spence 1996a). However, in this case the hand that cannot be controlled is most often still recognized as being part of the subject's own body (Spence and Frith 1999). Hence, failure to control the physical movement of a limb is insufficient to disturb accompanying sense of agency. Two forms of alien hand are seen in which a limb is effectively disinhibited following lesions of the medial premotor cortex or the corpus callosum. In these cases subjects admit to difficulty controlling the affected limb (which seems to perform pseudo-purposeful movements, e.g. grasping objects in the environment) but they do not generally attribute control of that limb to another.

However, with alien limbs seen in the context of a right-sided parietal lesion, the phenomenology may be rather different. Hence, the following report by Leiguarda et al. (1993) of a woman with a right-sided parietal lesion, giving rise to epileptic activity associated with intermittent, abnormal movements of the left arm.

She said: "suddenly I had a strange feeling on my left side; later I could not recognize the left arm as my own; I felt it belonged to someone else and wanted to hurt me because it moved towards me..."

In this case both the intentions and the identity of the alien limb are disturbed. The limb is not only beyond the control of the subject (as it might be in the other forms of alien limb) but is actually perceived to be under the control of another:

'it belonged to someone else'. The limb is also credited with a (conscious) intention to act: it 'wanted to hurt me'.

This disturbance of ownership (and hence agency) of a limb (in the context of a right parietal lesion) was also described by Critchley (1953), and previously by Gerstmann in the 1940s. Critchley described 'somatoparaphrenia', a condition in which limbs were said to 'belong to someone else', where patients might develop erotic feelings for their limbs (which they perceived as those of others), or where family members might mistakenly be identified as the limbs' owners. A similar case has been described by Nightingale (1982), again implicating right-sided parietal dysfunction. Also, Brugger (in press) has provided a compelling account of the deficits in self-recognition, or 'me-ness', which accompany right hemisphere lesions. It seems that the right hemisphere may be particularly involved in recognition of the 'self' and hence, by extrapolation, in recognition of that self's agency. One intriguing finding that has been replicated is that patients with somatoparaphrenia may exhibit temporary remissions in response to vestibular caloric stimulation (where cold water is inserted into the left outer ear). During such stimulation a patient may again experience their left limb as 'their own' but afterwards return to believing that it belongs to someone else (see Bisiach et al. 1991).

The functional anatomy of alien control

In the alien control of movement, 'made movements' are attributed to an external agent; agency being ceded to that 'other'. In our study using positron emission tomography (PET), we found such movements to be associated with hyperactivity in the right inferior parietal cortex and other related areas (Spence et al. 1997). This hyperactivation was relative to other acutely deluded patients, normal controls and the index group themselves as they recovered (4–6 weeks later). The same brain region was hyperactivated whether patients performed freely chosen or stereotypic movements (relative to the resting state).

The right inferior parietal region is an area of heteromodal association cortex implicated in many cognitive functions involved in sensorimotor integration and attention to egocentric space (Eidelberg and Galaburda 1984; Binkofski et al. 1998; Mattingley et al. 1998; Banati et al. 2000). It is also an area engaged in the conscious perception of time (see below) and one where activity is modulated by caloric stimulation (see above, and see Bottini et al. 2001). The parietal cortices are also known to be involved in the programming of unconscious 'intentions' (those cognitive components of motor behaviour of which we are unaware, e.g. the programming of individual muscle transformations necessary to pick up a cup) (Jeannerod 1997; Snyder et al. 1997). Data acquired from nonhuman primates and human patients suggest that these regions engage in the programming of reaching and grasping, adjusting limb responses outside normal human awareness. Only after brain lesions may the expression of such 'intentions' become manifest – as the disinhibited grasping of an 'alien hand' following a medial frontal lesion (above), or the failure of an apraxic hand to grasp an object after a parietal lesion. In the former, the (unconscious) parietal intention is thought to be 'released' from the normal inhibition of the frontal lobe; in the latter this intention is itself disrupted due to parietal damage – the hand cannot grasp (see Spence and Frith 1999 for review).

In a recent study by Ruby and Decety (2001), in which subjects imagined performing actions from a first- and a third-person perspective, it was notable that the third-person perspective was associated with greater activity in the right inferior parietal lobe (as in alien control). This prompts the speculation that overactivity of this region might 'fool' the brain into sensing that a third-person agency was 'in control' of action (as in Leiguarda's patient and those we studied using PET; Spence et al. 1997).

A number of questions remain unanswered. I hypothesized previously that alien control might also involve a misperception of the timing of motor acts (Spence 1996a): that the relationship between unconscious programming and subsequent conscious awareness of action might be disturbed. In this regard it is intriguing that the right inferior parietal cortex is one of the cortical regions involved in subjective perception of time (Harrington et al. 1998). The perception of time in alien control (and schizophrenia generally) deserves further examination. Indeed, a recent study has demonstrated that patients with alien control exhibit abnormalities in the timing of imagined movements: they fail to obey Fitts' law (see Maruff and Currie, in press).

The neuropsychological data obtained by Frith and others (Frith and Done 1989; Mlakar et al. 1994; Stirling et al. 1998) and our own PET data (Spence et al. 1997) support the hypothesis that the cognitive neurobiological substrate of alien control is itself dynamic over time. In other words, both the failure to 'monitor' movements and the hyperactivation of the right parietal cortex accompanying movement appear to come and go. We need to establish the determinants of such intermittent cerebral dysfunction.

Finally, there is an incongruity between the neurological literature cited above and that pertaining to people with schizophrenia. Although right-sided parietal lesions precipitate symptoms in the left side of the body, the symptoms of alien control described in schizophrenia are not so well lateralized. Our patients in the PET study moved their right arms and experienced alien control of these movements. However, the complex functioning of the right parietal cortex may be such that it monitors more than just the left (contralateral) side of the body and space. It is clearly engaged in programming right-sided movements (see Spence et al. 1997). Nevertheless, a number of authors have reported an increased prevalence of left-sided somatic (bodily) symptoms in people with schizophrenia, a finding which might also implicate right parietal dysfunction (Cutting 1989).

Patients complaining of alien control exhibit specific deficits on neuropsychological testing suggesting that there may be a deficit in their awareness of motor performance. These abnormalities appear to be state-specific (absent from those who have recovered). However, the propensity to these symptoms may have a genetic component, shared by relatives who are concordant for psychosis (Loftus et al. 2000).

Conclusions

Although the concepts of volition and the will were 'out of fashion' for much of the twentieth century (Berrios and Gili 1998; O'Shaughnessy 1998), contemporary cognitive neurobiological approaches to neuropsychiatric disorder make it increasingly possible to map these complex phenomena onto neural systems (Spence and Frith 1999). Schizophrenia is not 'just' a disorder of willed action; its effects are seen in a variety of voluntary behaviours and it also affects other cognitive systems. However, schizophrenia manifests itself through action, when the patient performs 'in the world', and action performance may be utilized experimentally as a probe of distributed neural systems. Diffuse deficits in 'functional connectivity' may be revealed (especially in the frontal regions) when the brain attempts 'to act'. In addition, schizophrenia may compromise the sense of agency in ways that implicate parietal lobe dysfunction (as in alien control and somatoparaphrenia). The restitution of autonomy remains one of the central problems for therapies and interventions applied to this disorder. A mechanistic understanding of will, agency and their disturbances will prepare the way for future, principled therapeutic interventions.

REFERENCES

Alexander GE, DeLong MR and Strick PL (1986). Parallel organization of functionally segregated circuits linking basal ganglia and cortex. *Ann Rev Neurosci*, 9, 357–81.

Amin F, Silverman JM, Siever LJ, Smith CJ, Knott PS and Davis KL (1999). Genetic antecedents of dopamine dysfunction in schizophrenia. *Biol Psychiatry*, 45, 1143–50.

Andreasen NC (1999). A unitary model of schizophrenia. Bleuler's 'fragmented phrene' as schizoencephaly. *Arch Gen Psychiatry*, 56, 781–7.

Angyal A (1936). The experience of the body-self in schizophrenia. *Arch Neurol Psychiatry*, 35, 1029–53.

Banati RB, Goerres GW, Tjoa C, Aggleton JP and Grasby P (2000). The functional anatomy of visual-tactile integration in man: a study using positron emission tomography. *Neuropsychologia*, 38, 115–24.

Barnes TRE and Spence SA (2000). Movement disorders associated with antipsychotic drugs: clinical and biological implications. In *The Psychopharmacology of Schizophrenia*, ed. MA Reveley and JFW Deakin, pp. 178–210. London: Hodder.

Barrett K (1999). Treating organic abulia with bromocriptine and lisuride: four case studies. *J Neurol Neurosurg Psychiatry*, 54, 718–21.

Berman KF, Zec RF and Weinberger DR (1986). Physiologic dysfunction of dorsolateral prefrontal cortex in schizophrenia. II. Role of neuroleptic treatment, attention and mental effort. *Arch Gen Psychiatry*, 43, 126–35.

Berman KF, Fuller Torrey E, Daniel DG and Weinberger DR (1992). Regional cerebral blood flow in monozygotic twins discordant and concordant for schizophrenia. *Arch Gen Psychiatry*, 49, 927–34.

Berman KF, Ostrem JL, Randolph C et al. (1995). Physiological activation of a cortical network during performance of the Wisconsin Card Sorting Test: a positron emission tomography study. *Neuropsychologia*, 33, 1027–46.

Berrios GE and Gili M (1998). Disorders of the volition and the will: a conceptual history. In *Disorders of Volition and Action in Psychiatry*, ed. C Williams and A Sims, pp. 9–29. Leeds: Leeds University Press.

Bertolino A, Callicott JH, Elman I et al. (2000). The effects of treatment with antipsychotics on N-acetylaspartate measures in patients with schizophrenia. *Schizophr Res*, 41, 219.

Binkofski F, Dohle C, Posse S et al. (1998). Human anterior intraparietal area subserves prehension. *Neurology*, 50, 1253–9.

Bisiach E, Rusconi ML and Vallar G (1991). Remission of somatoparaphrenic delusion through vestibular stimulation. *Neuropsychologia*, 29, 1029–31.

Blakemore S-J, Smith J, Steel R, Johnstone EC and Frith CD (2000). The perception of self-produced sensory stimuli in patients with auditory hallucinations and passivity experiences: evidence for a breakdown in self-monitoring. *Psychol Med*, 30, 1131–9.

Bottini G, Karnath H-O, Vallar G et al. (2001). Cerebral representations for egocentric space: functional-anatomical evidence from caloric vestibular stimulation and neck vibration. *Brain*, 124, 1182–96.

Brugger P. (in press). From haunted brain to haunted science: a cognitive neuroscience view of paranormal and pseudoscientific thought. In *Spirited Exchanges: Multidisciplinary Perspectives on Hauntings and Poltergeists*, ed. J Houran and R Lange. Jefferson, NC: McFarland.

Bush G, Luu P and Posner MI (2000). Cognitive and emotional influences in anterior cingulate cortex. *Trends Cogn Sci*, 4, 215–22.

Chiarenza GA, Papakostopoulos , Dini M and Cazzullo CL (1985). Neurophysiological correlates of psychomotor activity in chronic schizophrenics. *Electroencephal Clin Neurophysiol*, 61, 218–28.

Chua SE and McKenna PJ (1995). Schizophrenia – a brain disease? A critical review of structural and functional cerebral abnormality in the disorder. *Br J Psychiatry*, 166, 563–82.

Chua SE, Wright IC, Poline J-B et al. (1997). Grey matter correlates of syndromes in schizophrenia. A semi-automated analysis of structural magnetic resonance images. *Br J Psychiatry*, 170, 406–10.

Critchley M (1953). *The Parietal Lobes*. New York: Hafner Press.

Curtis VA, Bullmore ET, Morris RG et al. (1999). Attenuated frontal activation in schizophrenia may be task dependent. *Schizophr Res*, 37, 35–44.

Cutting J (1989). Body image disorders: comparison between unilateral hemisphere damage and schizophrenia. *Behav Neurol*, 2, 201–10.

Daprati E, Franck N, Georgieff N et al. (1997). Looking for the agent: an investigation into consciousness of action and self-consciousness in schizophrenic patients. *Cognition*, 65, 71–86.

Desmond JE, Gabrieli JDE and Glover GH (1998). Dissociation of frontal and cerebellar activity in a cognitive task: evidence for a distinction between selection and search. *Neuroimage*, 7, 368–76.

Dilman I (1999). *Free Will: An Historical and Philosophical Introduction.* London: Routledge.

Dolan RJ, Bench CJ, Liddle PF and Friston KJ (1993). Dorsolateral prefrontal cortex dysfunction in the major psychoses; symptom or disease specificity? *J Neurol Neurosurg Psychiatry*, 56, 1290–4.

Dreher J-C, Trapp W, Banquet J-P, Keil M, Guenther W and Burnod Y (1999). Planning dysfunction in schizophrenia: impairment of potentials preceding fixed/free and single/sequence of self-initiated finger movements. *Exp Brain Res*, 124, 200–14.

Duncan J and Owen AM (2000). Common regions of the human frontal lobe recruited by diverse cognitive demands. *Trends Neurosci*, 23, 475–83.

Dye SM, Spence SA, Bench CJ et al. (1999). No evidence for left superior temporal dysfunction in asymptomatic schizophrenia and bipolar affective disorder. PET study of verbal fluency. *Br J Psychiatry*, 175, 367–74.

Ebmeier KP, Blackwood DHR, Murray C and Souza V (1993). Single photon emission tomography with 99m Tc-exametazine in unmedicated schizophrenic patients. *Biol Psychiatry*, 487–95.

Eidelberg D and Galaburda AM (1984). Inferior parietal lobule: divergent architectonic asymmetries in the human brain. *Arch Neurol*, 41, 843–52.

Fish B, Marcus J, Hans SL, Auerbach JG and Perdue S (1992). Infants at risk for schizophrenia: sequelae of a genetic neurointegrative defect. A review and replication analysis of pandysmaturation in the Jerusalem infant development study. *Arch Gen Psychiatry*, 49, 221–35.

Flashman LA, Flaum M, Gupta S and Andreasen NC (1996). Soft signs and neurophysiological performance in schizophrenia. *Am J Psychiatry*, 153, 526–32.

Fletcher PC, Frith CD, Grasby PM et al (1996). Local and distributed effects of apomorphine upon fronto-temporal function in acute unmedicated schizophrenia. *J Neurosci*, 16, 7055–62.

Fletcher PC, McKenna PJ, Frith CD, Grasby PM, Friston KJ and Dolan RJ (1998). Brain activations in schizophrenia during a graded memory task studied with functional imaging. *Arch Gen Psychiatry*, 55, 1001–8.

Franck N, Farrer C, Georgieff N et al. (2001). Defective recognition of one's own actions in patients with schizophrenia. *Am J Psychiatry*, 158, 454–9.

Friston KJ (1996). Theoretical neurobiology and schizophrenia. *Br Med Bull*, 52, 644–55.

Friston KJ, Herold S, Fletcher P et al. (1995). Abnormal fronto-temporal interactions in schizophrenia. In *Biology of Schizophrenia and Affective Diseases*, ed. SJ Watson, pp. 449–81. New York: Raven Press.

Frith CD (1987). The positive and negative symptoms of schizophrenia reflect impairment in the perception and initiation of action. *Psychol Med*, 17, 631–48.

Frith CD (1996). Commentary on 'Free will in the light of neuropsychiatry'. *Philos Psychiatry Psychol*, 3, 91–4.

Frith CD and Done DJ (1989). Experiences of alien control in schizophrenia reflect a disorder in the central monitoring of action. *Psychol Med*, 19, 359–63.

Frith CD, Friston K, Liddle PF and Frackowiak RSJ (1991*a*). Willed action and the prefrontal cortex in man: a study with PET. *Proc R Soc Lond*, 244, 241–6.

Frith CD, Friston K, Liddle PF and Frackowiak RSJ (1991*b*). A PET study of word finding. *Neuropsychologia*, 29, 1137–48.

Frith CD, Friston KJ, Herold S et al. (1995). Regional brain activity in schizophrenic patients during the performance of a verbal fluency task. *Br J Psychiatry*, 167, 343–9.

Fuster JM (1980). *The Prefrontal Cortex*. New York: Raven Press.

Gehring WJ and Knight RT (2000). Prefrontal-cingulate interactions in action monitoring. *Nat Neurosci*, 3, 516–20.

Goldberg TE, Berman KF, Fleming K et al. (1998). Uncoupling cognitive workload and prefrontal cortical physiology: a PET rCBF study. *Neuroimage*, 7, 296–303.

Goldman-Rakic PS and Selemon LD (1997). Functional and anatomical aspects of prefrontal pathology in schizophrenia. *Schizophr Bull*, 23, 437–58.

Guenther W, Brodie JD, Bartlett EJ and Dewey SL (1994). Diminished cerebral metabolic response to motor stimulation in schizophrenics: a PET study. *Eur Arch Psychiatry Clin Neurosci*, 244, 115–25.

Harrington DL, Haaland KY and Knight RT (1998). Cortical networks underlying mechanisms of time perception. *J Neurosci*, 18, 1085–95.

Honey GD, Bullmore ET, Soni W, Varatheesan M, Williams SC and Sharma T (1999). Differences in frontal cortical activation by a working memory task after substitution of risperidone for typical antipsychotic drugs in patients with schizophrenia. *Proc Natl Acad Sci USA*, 96, 13432–7.

Ingvar DH (1994). The will of the brain: cerebral correlates of wilful acts. *J Theoret Biol*, 171, 7–12.

Jahanshahi M, Dirnberger G, Fuller R and Frith C (1997). The functional anatomy of random number generation studied with PET. *J Cereb Blood Flow Metab*, 17, S643.

Jahanshahi M, Profice P, Brown RG, Riddin MC, Dirnberger G and Rothwell JC (1998). The effects of transcranial magnetic stimulation over the dorsolateral prefrontal cortex on suppression of habitual counting during random number generation. *Brain*, 121, 1533–44.

Jeannerod M (1997). *The Cognitive Neuroscience of Action*. Oxford: Blackwell.

Joyce EM, Collinson SL and Crichton P (1996). Verbal fluency in schizophrenia: relationship with executive function, semantic memory and clinical alogia. *Psychol Med*, 26, 39–49.

Karaman T, Ozkaynak S, Yaltkaya K and Bueyuekberker C (1997). Bereitschaftpotential in schizophrenia. *Br J Psychiatry*, 171, 31–4.

Knight RT, Staines WR, Swick D and Chao LL (1999). Prefrontal cortex regulates inhibition and excitation in distributed neural networks. *Acta Psychol*, 101, 159–78.

Kotrla KJ, Mattay VS, Nawroz S and Van Gelderen P (1995). Primary sensorimotor cortex activation in patients with schizophrenia: a 3-D echo-shifted (ES) flash fMRI study. *J Cereb Blood Flow Metab*, 15, S95.

Kraepelin E (1919). *Dementia Praecox and Paraphrenia*. (Translated by RM Barclay.) Edinburgh: Livingstone.

Leiguarda R, Starkstein S, Nogues M and Berthier M (1993). Paroxysmal alien hand syndrome. *J Neurol Neurosurg Psychiatry*, 56, 788–92.

Libet B (1996). Commentary on 'Free will in the light of neuropsychiatry'. *Philos Psychiatry Psychol*, 3, 95–6.

Libet B, Gleason CA, Wright EW and Pearl DK (1983). Time of conscious intention to act in relation to onset of cerebral activity (readiness potential): the unconscious initiation of a freely voluntary act. *Brain*, 106, 623–42.

Libet B, Freeman A and Sutherland K (ed.) (1999). *The Volitional Brain: Towards a Neuroscience of Free Will*. Exeter: Imprint Academic.

Liddle PF (1993). The psychomotor disorders: disorders of the supervisory mental processes. *Behav Neurol*, 6, 5–14.

Liddle P, Friston KJ, Frith CD, Hirsch SR, Jones T and Frackowiak RSJ (1992). Patterns of cerebral blood flow in schizophrenia. *Br J Psychiatry*, 160, 179–86.

Loftus J, DeLisi LE and Crow TJ (2000). Factor structure and familiality of first-rank symptoms in sibling pairs with schizophrenia and schizoaffective disorder. *Br J Psychiatry*, 177, 15–19.

Luria AR (1966). *Higher Cortical Functions in Man*. London: Tavistock.

Macmurray J (1991). *The Self as Agent*. London: Faber & Faber. (First published 1957.)

Manschreck TC (1986). Motor abnormalities in schizophrenia. In *Handbook of Schizophrenia, Vol.1*, ed. HA Nasrallah and DR Weinberger, pp. 65–96. Amsterdam: Elsevier.

Maruff P and Currie J. (in press). Abnormalities of motor imagery associated with somatic passivity phenomena in schizophrenia. *Schizophr Res*, in press.

Masterman DL and Cummings JL (1997). Frontal-subcortical circuits: the anatomic basis of executive, social and motivated behaviours. *J Psychopharmacol*, 11, 107–14.

Mattingley JB, Husain M, Rorden C, Kennard C and Driver J (1998). Motor role of human inferior parietal lobe revealed in unilateral neglect patients. *Nature*, 392, 179–82.

McGuire PK, Silbersweig DA, Wright I and Murray RM (1995). Abnormal monitoring of inner speech: a physiological basis for auditory hallucinations. *Lancet*, 346, 596–600.

McGuire PK, Quested DJ, Spence SA, Murray RM, Frith CD and Liddle PF (1998). Pathophysiology of 'positive' thought disorder in schizophrenia. *Br J Psychiatry*, 173, 231–5.

McKenna PJ, Thornton A and Turner M (1998). Catatonia inside and outside schizophrenia. In *Disorders of Volition and Action in Psychiatry*, ed. C Williams and A Sims, pp. 105–35. Leeds: Leeds University Press,

Mlakar J, Jensterle J and Frith CD (1994). Central monitoring deficiency and schizophrenic symptoms. *Psychol Med*, 24, 557–64.

Mortimer A and Spence S (2001). *Managing Negative Symptoms of Schizophrenia*. London: Science Press.

Neumann CS and Walker EF (1999). Motor dysfunction in schizotypal personality disorder. *Schizophr Res*, 38, 159–68.

Nightingale S (1982). Somatoparaphrenia: a case report. *Cortex*, 18, 463–7.

O'Shaughnessy B (1998). Contemporary philosophical thinking on the will. In *Disorders of Volition and Action in Psychiatry*, ed. C Williams and A Sims, pp. 40–50. Leeds: Leeds University Press.

Passingham R (1993). *The Frontal Lobes and Voluntary Action*. Oxford: Oxford University Press.

Passingham RE (1997). Functional organization of the motor system. In *Human Brain Function*, ed. RSJ Frackowiak, KJ Friston, CD Frith, RJ Dolan and JC Mazziotta. San Diego: Academic Press.

Perret E (1974). The left frontal lobe of man and the suppression of habitual responses in verbal categorical behaviour. *Neuropsychologia*, 12, 323–30.

Puri BK, Davey NJ, Ellaway PH and Lewis SW (1996). An investigation of motor function in schizophrenia using transcranial magnetic stimulation of the motor cortex. *Br J Psychiatry*, 169, 690–5.

Rogers D (1985). The motor disorders of severe psychiatric illness: a conflict of paradigms. *Br J Psychiatry*, 147, 221–32.

Rogers D (1991). Catatonia: a contemporary approach. *J Neuropsychiatry*, 3, 334–40.

Ruby P and Decety J (2001). Effect of subjective perspective taking during simulation of action: a PET investigation of agency. *Nat Neurosci*, 4, 546–50.

Rypma B, Prabhakaran V, Desmond JE, Glover GH and Gabrieli JDE (1999). Load-dependent roles of frontal lobe regions in the maintenance of working memory. *Neuroimage*, 9, 216–26.

Schroder J, Wenz F, Schad LR, Schroeder and Baudendistel K (1995). Sensorimotor cortex and supplementary motor area changes in schizophrenia. *Br J Psychiatry*, 167, 197–201.

Shallice T and Burgess P (1996). The domain of supervisory processes and temporal organization of behaviour. *Philos Trans R Soc Lond B*, 351, 1405–12.

Snyder LH, Batista AP and Andersen RA (1997). Coding of intention in the posterior parietal cortex. *Nature*, 386, 167–70.

Spence SA (1996*a*). Free will in the light of neuropsychiatry. *Philos Psychiatry Psychol*, 3, 75–90.

Spence SA (1996*b*). Response to the commentaries on 'Free will in the light of neuropsychiatry'. *Philos Psychiatry Psychol*, 3, 99–100.

Spence SA (2001). Alien control: from phenomenology to cognitive neurobiology. *Philos Psychiatry Psychol*, 8, 163–72.

Spence SA and Frith CD (1999). Towards a functional anatomy of volition. *J Consciousness Studies*, 6, 11–28.

Spence SA, Liddle P, Herold S, Fletcher P, Friston K and Frith C (1995). Medial frontal lobe overactivity in reality distortion syndrome during word generation: a PET study. *Schizophr Res*, 15, 99–100.

Spence SA, Brooks DJ, Hirsch SR, Liddle PF, Meehan J and Grasby PM (1997). A PET study of voluntary movement in schizophrenic patients experiencing passivity phenomena (delusions of alien control). *Brain*, 120, 1997–2011.

Spence SA, Hirsch SR, Brooks DJ and Grasby PM (1998). Prefrontal cortex activity in people with schizophrenia and control subjects. Evidence from positron emission tomography for remission of 'hypofrontality' with recovery from acute schizophrenia. *Br J Psychiatry*, 172, 316–23.

Spence SA, Liddle PF, Stefan MD et al. (2000). Functional anatomy of verbal fluency in people with schizophrenia and those at genetic risk. Focal dysfunction and distributed disconnectivity reappraised. *Br J Psychiatry*, 176, 52–60.

Stirling JD, Hellewell JSE and Quraishi N (1998). Self-monitoring dysfunction and the schizophrenic symptoms of alien control. *Psychol Med*, 28, 675–83.

Tauscher J, Fischer P, Neumeister A, Rappelsberger P and Kasper S (1998). Low frontal electroencephalographic coherence in neuroleptic-free schizophrenic patients. *Biol Psychiatry*, 44, 438–47.

Taylor PJ (1998). Disorders of volition: forensic aspects. In *Disorders of Volition and Action in Psychiatry*, ed. C Williams and A Sims, pp. 66–84. Leeds: Leeds University Press.

Walker EF, Savoie T and Davis D (1994). Neuromotor precursors of schizophrenia. *Schizophr Bull*, 20, 441–51.

Weinberger DR and Berman KF (1996). Prefrontal function in schizophrenia: confounds and controversies. *Philos Trans R Soc Lond B*, 351, 1495–503.

Weinberger DR, Berman KF and Zec RF (1986). Physiologic dysfunction of dorsolateral prefrontal cortex in schizophrenia. I. Regional cerebral blood flow evidence. *Arch Gen Psychiatry*, 114–24.

Weinberger DR, Berman KF and Illowsky BP (1988). Physiologic dysfunction of dorsolateral prefrontal cortex in schizophrenia. III. A new cohort and evidence for a monoaminergic mechanism. *Arch Gen Psychiatry*, 45, 609–15.

Yang CR, Seamans JK and Gorelova N (1999). Developing a neuronal model for the pathophysiology of schizophrenia based on the nature of electrophysiological action of dopamine in the prefrontal cortex. *Neuropsychopharmacology*, 21, 161–94.

Youngren KD, Inglis FM, Pivirotto PJ et al. (1999). Clozapine preferentially increases dopamine release in the rhesus monkey prefrontal cortex compared with the caudate nucleus. *Neuropsychopharmacology*, 20, 403–12.

Zec RF (1995). Neuropsychology of schizophrenia according to Kraepelin: disorders of volition and executive functioning. *Eur Arch Psychiatry Clin Neurosci*, 245, 216–23.

de Zubicaray GI, Chalk JB, Rose SE, Rose SE, Semple J and Smith GA (1997). Deficits on self ordered tasks associated with hyperostosis frontalis interna. *J Neurol Neurosurg Psychiatry*, 63, 309–14.

de Zubicaray GI, Williams SCR, Wilson SJ et al. (1998). Prefrontal cortex involvement in selective letter generation: a functional magnetic resonance imaging study. *Cortex*, 34, 389–401.

Part VI

Recent advances in dementia

12

The neurobiology of the tauopathies

Maria Grazia Spillantini[1] and Michel Goedert[2]

[1] Department of Neurology, University of Cambridge, Cambridge, UK
[2] Medical Research Council Laboratory of Molecular Biology, Cambridge, UK

Introduction

Current concepts of neurodegenerative diseases began to develop over a century ago, when the German school of neuropathologists described the salient histological features of what we now know to be the most common of these diseases. In 1907, Alois Alzheimer described the neuritic plaques and neurofibrillary lesions in the disease that was subsequently named after him (Alzheimer 1907). In 1911, Alzheimer also described the presence of Pick bodies as the characteristic neuropathological lesion of Pick's disease, a form of frontotemporal dementia (Alzheimer 1911). In 1912, Friederich Lewy described the inclusions characteristic of Parkinson's disease, the so-called 'Lewy bodies' (Lewy 1912). In the 1960s, electron microscopy was used to show that the above inclusions are made of abnormal filaments (Kidd 1963; Duffy and Tennyson 1965; Rewcastle and Ball 1968). At the time, the identification of these lesions was instrumental in establishing the various diseases as discrete entities. However, this work did not indicate a role for the lesions in the aetiology and pathogenesis of neurodegeneration. Over the past 20 years, a direct correspondence between the formation of the neuropathological lesions and the degenerative process has emerged. Besides the above diseases, this is also true of the prion diseases, of Huntington's disease and the other glutamine repeat diseases, as well as of several other, rarer conditions.

Progress was made possible by the merging of two independent lines of research. On the one hand, the biochemical study of the neuropathological lesions led to the identification of their main molecular components. On the other, the study of familial forms of disease led to the identification of gene defects that cause the inherited variants of the different diseases. Remarkably, in most cases, the defective genes have been found to encode or increase the expression of the main components of the neuropathological lesions. It has therefore been established that the basis of the familial forms of these diseases is a toxic property conferred by mutations in the proteins that make up the filamentous lesions. A corollary of this insight is that a similar toxic property might also underlie the sporadic disease forms.

Alzheimer's disease is the most common neurodegenerative disease. Neuropathologically, it is defined by the presence of abundant extracellular neuritic plaques made of the beta-amyloid protein and intraneuronal neurofibrillary lesions made of the microtubule-associated protein tau (St George-Hyslop et al. 2001). Similar tau lesions, in the absence of beta-amyloid deposits, are also the defining characteristic of a number of other neurodegenerative diseases, the best known of which are progressive supranuclear palsy, corticobasal degeneration and Pick's disease (Lee et al. 2001). Until recently, there was no genetic evidence implicating dysfunction of tau protein in the neurodegenerative process. This changed with the discovery of tau gene mutations in a familial form of frontotemporal dementia and parkinsonism (Hutton et al. 1998; Poorkaj et al. 1998; Spillantini et al. 1998c). Here we review the evidence implicating tau protein in this and other neurodegenerative diseases, and its possible mechanisms of action.

Mutations causing tauopathy

Frontotemporal dementias occur as familial forms and, more commonly, as sporadic diseases. Neuropathologically, they are characterized by a remarkably circumscribed atrophy of the frontal and temporal lobes of the cerebral cortex, often with additional, subcortical changes. In 1994, an autosomal-dominantly inherited form of frontotemporal dementia with parkinsonism was linked to chromosome 17q21.2 (Wilhelmsen et al. 1994). This observation was followed by the identification of other familial forms of frontotemporal dementia that were linked to this region, resulting in the denomination 'frontotemporal dementia and parkinsonism linked to chromosome 17' (FTDP-17) for this class of disease (Foster et al. 1997). All cases of FTDP-17 have so far shown a filamentous pathology made of hyperphosphorylated tau protein. In 1998, the first mutations in *tau* in FTDP-17 patients were identified (Clark et al. 1998; Hutton et al. 1998; Poorkaj et al. 1998; Spillantini et al. 1998c). Currently, 25 different mutations have been described in over 50 families with FTDP-17 (Figure 12.1, colour plate).

Tau is a microtubule-binding protein that is believed to be important in the assembly and stabilization of microtubules (Lee et al. 2001). In nerve cells, it is normally found in axons, but in the tauopathies it is redistributed to the cell body and dendrites. In normal adult human brain, there are six isoforms of tau, produced from a single gene by alternative mRNA splicing (Figure 12.1, colour plate) (Goedert et al. 1988, 1989a, b; Andreadis et al. 1992). They differ from one another by the presence or absence of a 29- or 58-amino-acid insert in the amino-terminal half

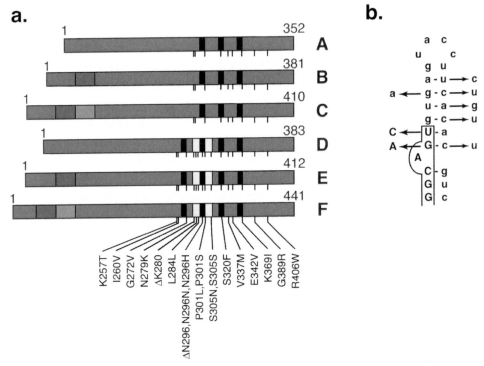

Figure 12.1 Mutations in the *tau* gene in frontotemporal dementia and parkinsonism linked to chromosome 17 (FTDP-17). (a) Schematic diagram of the six tau isoforms (A–F) that are expressed in adult human brain. Alternatively spliced exons are shown in red (exon 2), green (exon 3) and yellow (exon 10); black bars indicate the microtubule-binding repeats. Fourteen missense mutations, two deletion mutations and three silent mutations in the coding region are shown. Amino-acid numbering corresponds to the 441 amino-acid isoform of human brain tau. (b) Stem-loop structure in the pre-mRNA at the boundary between exon 10 and the intron following exon 10. Eight mutations that reduce the stability of the stem-loop structure are shown. Exon sequences are shown in capital and intron sequences in lower-case letters.

of the protein and by the inclusion, or not, of a 31-amino-acid repeat, encoded by exon 10 of *tau*, in the carboxy-terminal half of the protein. The exclusion of exon 10 leads to the production of three isoforms, each containing three repeats, and its inclusion leads to a further three isoforms, each containing four repeats. The repeat region and some flanking sequences constitute the microtubule-binding region of the tau protein. In normal adult human cerebral cortex, there are similar levels of three-repeat and four-repeat isoforms (Goedert and Jakes 1990).

Tau mutations in FTDP-17 are either missense, deletion or silent mutations in the coding region, or intronic mutations located close to the splice-donor site of the intron following the alternatively spliced exon 10 (Figure 12.1, colour plate). Missense mutations have been found in exons 9, 10, 11, 12 and 13 (Clark et al. 1998;

Hutton et al. 1998; Poorkaj et al. 1998; Bugiani et al. 1999; Iijima et al. 1999; Murrell et al. 1999; Lippa et al. 2000; Rizzini et al. 2000; Iseki et al. 2001; Neumann et al. 2001; Rosso et al. 2002). Using the numbering of the 441-amino-acid isoform of tau, these comprise K257T, I260V and G272V (exon 9); N279K, N296H, P301L, P301S and S305N (exon 10); S320F (exon 11); V337M, E342V and K369I (exon 12); and G389R and R406W (exon 13) (Figure 12.1a, colour plate). There are also two mutations with a single amino acid deletion – ∆K280 and ∆N296 – and three silent mutations – L284L, N296N and S305S – all in exon 10 (Figure 12.1a, colour plate) (D'Souza et al. 1999; Rizzu et al. 1999; Spillantini et al. 2000; Stanford et al. 2000; Pastor et al. 2001). The seven reported mutations in exon 10 that change the amino acid sequence will be present only in four-repeat protein isoforms; those lying outside exon 10 will be present in all six tau protein isoforms. Intronic mutations are located at positions +3, +11, +12, +13, +14 and +16 of the intron following exon 10, with the first nucleotide of the splice-donor site taken as +1 (Figure 12.1b, colour plate) (Hutton et al. 1998; Spillantini et al. 1998c; Yasuda et al. 2000; Miyamoto et al. 2001).

Functionally, *tau* mutations fall into two largely nonoverlapping categories – those whose primary effect is at the protein level and those that influence the alternative splicing of tau pre-mRNA. In accordance with their location in the microtubule-binding region of tau, most missense mutations reduce the ability of tau to interact with microtubules, as reflected by a reduction in the ability of mutant tau to promote microtubule assembly (Hasegawa et al. 1998; Hong et al. 1998; Barghorn et al. 2000; De Ture et al. 2000). Similar effects on microtubule function are observed when tau is expressed in a number of cell lines. Expression of a variety of mutations, including G272V, ∆K280, P301L, V337M and R406W, in these cells caused varying degrees of reduced microtubule binding and stability, as well as disorganized microtubule morphology (Dayanandan et al. 1999; Matsumura et al. 1999; Vogelsberg-Ragaglia et al. 2000).

A number of *tau* gene mutations may cause FTDP-17, at least in part, by promoting tau aggregation. Several studies have demonstrated that some of these mutations, including K257T, G272V, ∆K280, P301L, P301S, V337M and R406W, promote heparin- or arachidonic acid-induced tau filament formation in vitro relative to wild-type tau (Goedert et al. 1999a; Nacharaju et al. 1999; Barghorn et al. 2000; Gamblin et al. 2000). This effect is particularly marked for the P301L and P301S mutations. Furthermore, aggregation of mutant tau proteins in intact cells has also been demonstrated in the case of the ∆K280 mutation (Vogelsberg-Ragaglia et al. 2000). Additional mechanisms may also play a role in the case of some coding region mutations. For instance, protein phosphatase 2A is known to be the major tau phosphatase in brain (Goedert et al. 1992a) and to bind to the tandem repeats in tau (Sontag et al. 1999). Accordingly, several FTDP-17 mutations have been found to result in the reduced binding of protein phosphatase 2A to tau (Goedert et al. 2000).

The intronic mutations and some coding region mutations (N279K, L284L, N296N, S305N and S305S) increase the splicing of exon 10, thus changing the ratio between three- and four-repeat isoforms, resulting in an overproduction of four-repeat tau (Clark et al. 1998; Hong et al. 1998; Hutton et al. 1998; Spillantini et al. 1998c, 2000; D'Souza et al. 1999; Goedert et al. 1999b; Hasegawa et al. 1999; Stanford et al. 2000; Yasuda et al. 2000). So far, approximately half of the known *tau* mutations have their primary effect at the RNA level. Thus, to a significant degree, FTDP-17 is a disease of the alternative mRNA splicing of exon 10 of the *tau* gene. It follows that a correct ratio of three-repeat to four-repeat tau isoforms is essential for preventing neurodegeneration and dementia in mid-life. Accordingly, the regulation of the splicing of exon 10 is an area of great current interest. So far, it is known to involve multiple *cis*-acting regulatory elements that either enhance or inhibit the utilization of the 5′-splice site of exon 10 (D'Souza et al. 1999; Grover et al. 1999; D'Souza and Schellenberg 2000; Gao et al. 2000; Jiang et al. 2000). They are located in exon 10 itself and in the intron following exon 10. Splicing regulatory elements within exon 10 appear to include an exon splicing enhancer (ESE) and an exon splicing silencer (ESS). The ESE consists of three domains, a potential SC35-binding element, a purine-rich sequence and an AC-rich sequence. Immediately downstream of the ESE within exon 10 is a purine-rich ESS. Sequences located at the end of exon 10 and at the beginning of the intron following exon 10 inhibit the splicing of exon 10, probably because of the presence of a stem-loop structure that limits access of the splicing machinery to the 5′-splice site. The determination of the three-dimensional structure of a 25-nucleotide-long RNA from the exon 10-5′-intron junction by nuclear magnetic resonance spectroscopy has shown that this sequence forms a stable, folded stem-loop structure (Varani et al. 1999, 2000). The stem consists of a single G-C base pair that is separated from a double helix of six base pairs by an unpaired adenine. As is often the case with single nucleotide purine bulges, the unpaired adenine at position −2 does not extrude into solution but intercalates into the double helix. The apical loop consists of six nucleotides that adopt multiple conformations in rapid exchange.

Pathogenic FTDP-17 mutations in the *tau* gene may alter exon 10 splicing by affecting several of the regulatory elements described above. Thus, the intronic mutations (+3, +11, +12, +13, +14 and +16) and the exonic mutations at codon 305 (S305N and S305S) destabilize the inhibitory stem-loop structure. The S305N mutation and the +3 intronic mutation may also enhance exon 10 splicing by increasing the strength of the 5′-splice site. However, the finding that the S305S mutation that weakens the exon 10 5′-splice site also leads to a predominance of four-repeat tau argues against this as the primary effect of these mutations.

The N279K mutation may improve the function of the ESE by lengthening the purine-rich sequence within this element, thus enhancing exon 10 splicing. The silent L284L mutation that enhances exon 10 splicing may do so by disrupting a potential ESS or by lengthening the AC-rich element within the ESE. The effect of the N296N mutation on splicing of exon 10 is probably due to disruption of an ESS.

In general, the high fidelity of splice-site selection is believed to result from the co-operative binding of transacting factors to *cis*-acting sequences. The heterogeneous nuclear ribonucleoproteins (hnRNPs) and the serine arginine-rich (SR) proteins constitute major classes of proteins involved in splice-site selection. In transfection experiments, several SR proteins have been shown to promote the exclusion of exon 10 of the *tau* gene. Moreover, phosphorylation of SR proteins has also been found to result in the skipping of exon 10 (Hartmann et al. 2001). Exon 10 appears to exhibit a default splicing pattern of inclusion.

Neuropathology of FTDP-17

All cases with *tau* mutations that have been examined to date have shown the presence of a filamentous pathology made of hyperphosphorylated tau (Goedert et al. 1998; Spillantini et al. 1998*a*; Crowther and Goedert 2000) protein. To a large extent, the morphologies of tau filaments and their isoform compositions are determined by whether *tau* mutations affect mRNA splicing of exon 10, or whether they are missense mutations located inside or outside of exon 10 (Figure 12.2, colour plate).

Mutations in *tau* that result in the increased splicing of exon 10 lead to the formation of wide twisted ribbon-like filaments that only contain four-repeat tau isoforms. In all these families, the tau pathology is widespread and present in both nerve cells and glial cells, with an abundant glial component. This has been shown for the +3, +12 and +16 intronic mutations, as well as for mutation N279K in exon 10 (Spillantini et al. 1997; Goedert et al. 1999*b*; Yasuda et al. 1999). Mutation S305S in exon 10 has been found to lead to pathological changes strongly reminiscent of progressive supranuclear palsy (Stanford et al. 2000), whereas mutation N296N in exon 10 resulted in inclusions similar to those of corticobasal degeneration (Spillantini et al. 2000).

Mutations in exon 10 of *tau* that do not affect alternative mRNA splicing lead to the formation of narrow twisted ribbons that contain four-repeat tau isoforms, with a small amount of the most abundant three-repeat isoform. This has been shown for the P301L mutation (Spillantini et al. 1998*b*). Using an antibody specific for mutant tau, biochemical studies have demonstrated that filaments extracted from the brains of patients with the P301L mutation contain predominantly mutant tau

(Rizzu et al. 2000; Miyasaka et al. 2001b). Tau pathology is widespread and present in both nerve cells and glial cells. Compared with mutations that affect the splicing of exon 10, the glial component appears to be less pronounced.

The known coding-region mutations located outside exon 10 lead to a tau pathology that is neuronal, without a significant glial component. Some of these mutations lead to the formation of paired helical and straight filaments that contain all six tau isoforms, like the tau filaments of Alzheimer's disease (Goedert et al. 1992b). This has been shown for the V337M and the R406W mutations (Spillantini et al. 1996; Van Swieten et al. 1999). Using an antibody specific for tau protein with the R406W mutation, both wild-type and mutant proteins were detected in the abnormal filaments (Miyasaka et al. 2001a). The K257T, G272V, S320F, E342V, K369I and G389R mutations lead to a tau pathology similar or identical to that of Pick's disease (Spillantini et al. 1998b; Murrell et al. 1999; Lippa et al. 2000; Rizzini et al. 2000; Neumann et al. 2001; Rosso et al. 2002). These findings indicate that depending on the positions of *tau* mutations in exons 9–13, and perhaps the nature of these mutations, a filamentous tau pathology ensues that resembles either that of progressive supranuclear palsy, corticobasal degeneration, Alzheimer's disease or Pick's disease.

Pathogenesis of FTDP-17

The pathway leading from a mutation in *tau* to neurodegeneration is unknown. The likely primary effect of most missense mutations is a change in the conformation of tau protein that results in its reduced ability to interact with microtubules. It can be overcome by natural osmolytes, such as trimethylamine N-oxide, probably through the promotion of tubulin-induced folding of tau (Smith et al. 2000). The primary effect of these mutations may be equivalent to a partial loss of function, with resultant microtubule destabilization and deleterious effects on cellular processes, such as rapid axonal transport. However, in the case of the intronic mutations and the coding-region mutations whose primary effect is at the RNA level, this appears unlikely. The net effect of these mutations is a simple overproduction of four-repeat tau. It is therefore possible that in cases of FTDP-17 with intronic mutations and those coding region mutations whose primary effect is at the RNA level, microtubules are more stable than in brain from control individuals. Moreover, missense mutations in exon 10 will only affect 20–25% of tau molecules, with 75–80% of tau being normal.

It is possible that a correct ratio of wild-type three-repeat to four-repeat tau is essential for the normal function of tau in human brain. An alternative hypothesis is that a partial loss of function of tau is necessary for setting in motion the mechanisms that will ultimately lead to neurodegeneration. Earlier work has suggested that three-repeat and four-repeat tau isoforms may bind to different sites on microtubules (Goode and Feinstein 1994). Overproduction of tau isoforms with four repeats may result in an excess of tau over available binding sites on microtubules, thus creating a gain of toxic function similar to that of most missense mutations. Validation of this hypothesis will probably require structural information at the atomic level.

From the above, a reduced ability of tau to interact with microtubules emerges as the likely primary effect of the FTDP-17 mutations. It will lead to the accumulation of free tau in the cytoplasm of brain cells and result in its hyperphosphorylation. Over time, hyperphosphorylated tau protein will assemble into abnormal filaments. Although it is clear that the dysfunction of tau protein leads to neuro-degeneration and dementia in FTDP-17, it is at present not known whether the tau filaments themselves cause nerve cell loss, or whether nonassembled, conforma-tionally changed tau protein is toxic.

Relevance of FTDP-17 for the sporadic tauopathies

The study of FTDP-17 has established that dysfunction of tau protein can cause neurodegeneration and dementia. It follows that tau dysfunction is most probably also of central importance in the pathogenesis of other diseases with a filamen-tous tau pathology, such as Alzheimer's disease, progressive supranuclear palsy, corticobasal degeneration and Pick's disease. This is further underlined by the fact that the aforementioned diseases are partially or completely phenocopied by cases of FTDP-17 (Lee et al. 2001).

Several mutations in *tau* give rise to a clinical and neuropathological syndrome that is closely related to Pick's disease. This is the case of mutations K257T and G272V in exon 9 (Spillantini et al. 1998*b*; Rizzini et al. 2000), S320F in exon 11 (Rosso et al. 2002), E342V in exon 12 (Lippa et al. 2000), as well as K369I and G389R in exon 13 (Murrell et al. 1999; Neumann et al. 2001). The finding that overproduction of four-repeat tau leads to its assembly into twisted ribbons and causes disease may shed light on the pathogenesis of progressive supranuclear palsy and corticobasal degeneration. Neuropathologically, both diseases are characterized by a neuronal and glial tau pathology, with the tau filaments comprising only four-repeat tau isoforms (Flament et al. 1991; Ksiezak-Reding et al. 1994; Feany et al. 1996; Sergeant et al. 1999). An association between progressive supranuclear palsy and a dinucleotide repeat polymorphism in the intron between exons 9 and 10 of *tau* has been described (Conrad et al. 1997). The alleles at this locus carry 11–15 repeats. The A0 allele, with 11 repeats, has a frequency of over 90% in patients with progressive supranuclear palsy and about 70% in controls. More recently, two common *tau* haplotypes that differ at the nucleotide level, but not at the level of the protein coding sequence, have been reported (Baker et al. 1999). Homozygosity of the more common allele H1 appears to predispose to progressive supranuclear palsy and corticobasal degeneration, but not to Alzheimer's disease or Pick's disease (Baker et al. 1999, 2000; Di Maria et al. 2000; Houlden et al. 2001; Russ et al. 2001).

This work has led to the suggestion that progressive supranuclear palsy and corticobasal degeneration may be caused by an imbalance between three- and four-repeat tau isoforms, analogous to the FTDP-17 cases with mutations that affect the splicing of exon 10. Interestingly, an individual with a mutation at position 0 of the stem-loop structure at the boundary between exon 10 and the intron following exon 10, and individuals with a homozygous deletion of N296 in exon 10, presented with a clinical picture similar to progressive supranuclear palsy (Stanford et al. 2000; Pastor et al. 2001). Moreover, an individual with the P301S mutation in *tau* presented with a clinical diagnosis of corticobasal degeneration (Bugiani et al. 1999). Finally, the N296N mutation in exon 10 of *tau* gives rise to a neuropathological phenotype that resembles corticobasal degeneration (Spillantini et al. 2000). All in all, this work suggests that dysfunction of tau protein is of central importance in progressive supranuclear palsy and corticobasal degeneration, as it is in Pick's disease.

In the recent past, it has become clear that the tau protein plays a central role, not only in dementing diseases, such as Alzheimer's disease and frontotemporal dementias, but also in movement disorders, such as progressive supranuclear palsy and corticobasal degeneration. In addition, recent studies have described a significant association between the A0 allele of the *tau* gene and Parkinson's disease (Pastor et al. 2000; Golbe et al. 2001). The future will show whether tau protein, which is not found in the filamentous inclusions of Parkinson's disease, is nonetheless involved in the aetiology and pathogenesis of that disease.

Experimental animal models of tauopathies

Animal models of the tauopathies are essential for elucidating the mechanisms by which dysfunction of tau protein leads to neurodegeneration. In addition, they may prove useful for the development and testing of novel therapies.

Several reports have described transgenic mouse lines that express wild-type three-repeat or four-repeat human tau protein in nerve cells (Götz et al. 1995; Brion et al. 1999; Ishihara et al. 1999, 2001; Spittaels et al. 1999; Probst et al. 2000). These mice developed numerous abnormal tau-immunoreactive nerve cell bodies and dendrites and large numbers of pathologically enlarged axons containing tau- and neurofilament-immunoreactive spheroids. The changes were most prominent in spinal cord, but were also seen in the brain. They were accompanied by histological and behavioural signs of amyotrophy. However, abundant tau filaments were not observed. This work has shown that overproduction of nonfilamentous tau is sufficient to lead to axonopathy and amyotrophy. However, unlike the human diseases with tau filaments, there was no sign of nerve cell loss. In contrast, overexpression of wild-type human tau protein in lamprey reticulospinal neurons led to the formation of filamentous tau inclusions and the degeneration of a subset of nerve cells (Hall et al. 1997, 2000).

The discovery of mutations in *tau* in FTDP-17 patients is leading to the production of transgenic mouse lines that express mutant human tau protein in nerve cells and glial cells. In the first published studies, human tau with the P301L mutation in exon 10 was expressed (Lewis et al. 2000; Götz et al. 2001*a*). The mice exhibited an age-dependent and gene-dose-dependent accumulation of filamentous deposits in both brain and spinal cord, with some associated nerve cell loss and reactive gliosis. The filamentous tau deposits contained mostly the mutant human tau protein, in line with in vitro findings showing that the P301L mutation promotes the assembly of recombinant tau protein (Goedert et al. 1999*a*; Nacharaju et al. 1999). In P301L tau mouse lines, co-expression of mutant human amyloid precursor protein or the direct intracerebral injection of beta-amyloid fibrils resulted in an increase in the number of tangle-bearing nerve cells (Götz et al. 2001*b*; Lewis et al. 2001). It thus appears that extracellular beta-amyloid deposits can promote intraneuronal tau pathology. In contrast to these findings with mutant tau protein expression, beta-amyloid deposits failed to induce tangle formation in mice expressing wild-type human tau protein (Götz et al. 2001*a*; Lewis et al. 2001). The existing transgenic mouse models of tauopathies indicate a connection between the development of tau filaments and nerve cell degeneration. This contrasts with *Drosophila melanogaster*, where the overexpression of R406W *tau* or V337M *tau* resulted in massive nerve cell degeneration, in the apparent absence of tau filaments (Wittmann et al. 2001). It suggests that conformationally altered, nonaggregated human tau protein can be neurotoxic, at least in an invertebrate context.

Other approaches have made use of molecules that act on tau. Thus, transgenic mice expressing human p25, an activator of the protein kinase cyclin-dependent kinase 5, developed disturbances in cytoskeletal architecture and behavioural changes (Ahlijanian et al. 2000). Mice expressing human apolipoprotein E4, an allelic risk factor for sporadic Alzheimer's disease, showed an age-dependent increase in tau phosphorylation (Tesseur et al. 2000). Lastly, transgenic mice expressing antibodies to nerve growth factor inside nerve cells developed an extensive age-dependent neurodegeneration, including accumulation of hyperphosphorylated insoluble tau protein and nerve cell loss (Capsoni et al. 2000). However, none of these studies presented any evidence of fibrillary tau pathology.

Conclusion

The discovery of mutations in the tau gene in FTDP-17 has established a central role for tau protein dysfunction in the aetiology and pathogenesis of neurodegeneration. A major implication deriving from this work is that dysfunction of tau protein is also central to the pathogenesis of sporadic diseases characterized by the formation of filamentous tau protein deposits. It follows that an understanding of the detailed mechanisms by which abnormal tau protein causes nerve cell degeneration and dementia is now called for. In due course, this knowledge is likely to lead to the development of mechanism-based therapies for the tauopathies.

REFERENCES

Ahlijanian MK, Barrezueta NX, Williams RD et al. (2000). Hyperphosphorylated tau and neurofilament and cytoskeletal disruptions in mice overexpressing human p25, an activator of cdk5. *Proc Natl Acad Sci USA*, 97, 2910–915.

Alzheimer A (1907). Über eine eigenartige Erkrankung der Hirnrinde. *Allg Z Psychiatrie psychiatrisch-gerichtliche Med*, 64, 146–8.

Alzheimer A (1911). Über eigenartige Krankheitsfälle des späteren Alters. *Z Neurol Psychiatrie*, 4, 356–85.

Andreadis A, Brown MW and Kosik KS (1992). Structure and novel exons of the human tau gene. *Biochemistry*, 31, 10626–33.

Baker M, Litvan I, Houlden H et al. (1999). Association of an extended haplotype in the tau gene with progressive supranuclear palsy. *Hum Mol Genet*, 8, 711–15.

Baker M, Graff-Radford D, Wavrant-DeVrieze F et al. (2000). No association between TAU haplotype and Alzheimer's disease in population or clinic based series or in familial disease. *Neurosci Lett*, 285, 147–9.

Barghorn S, Zheng-Fischhöfer Q, Ackmann M et al. (2000). Structure, microtubule interactions, and paired helical filament aggregation by tau mutants of frontotemporal dementias. *Biochemistry*, 39, 11714–21.

Brion JP, Tremp G and Octave JN (1999). Transgenic expression of the shortest human tau affects its compartmentalization and its phosphorylation as in the pretangle stage of Alzheimer's disease. *Am J Pathol*, 154, 255–70.

Bugiani O, Murrell JR, Giaccone G et al. (1999). Frontotemporal dementia and corticobasal degeneration in a family with a P301S mutation in *tau*. *J Neuropathol Exp Neurol*, 58, 667–77.

Capsoni S, Ugolini G, Comparini A, Ruberti F, Berardi N and Cattaneo A (2000). Alzheimer-like neurodegeneration in aged anti-nerve growth factor transgenic mice. *Proc Natl Acad Sci USA*, 97, 6826–31.

Clark LN, Poorkaj P, Wszolek Z et al. (1998). Pathogenic implications of mutations in the tau gene in pallido-ponto-nigral degeneration and related neurodegenerative disorders linked to chromosome 17. *Proc Natl Acad Sci USA*, 95, 13103–7.

Conrad C, Andreadis A, Trojanowski JQ et al. (1997). Genetic evidence for the involvement of tau in progressive supranuclear palsy. *Ann Neurol*, 41, 277–81.

Crowther RA and Goedert M (2000). Abnormal tau-containing filaments in neurodegenerative diseases. *J Struct Biol*, 130, 271–9.

Dayanandan R, van Slegtenhorst M, Mack TGA et al. (1999). Mutations in tau reduce its microtubule binding properties in intact cells and affect its phosphorylation. *FEBS Lett* 446, 228–32.

De Ture M, Ko LW, Yen S et al. (2000). Missense tau mutations identified in FTDP-17 have a small effect on tau-microtubule interactions. *Brain Res*, 853, 5–14.

Di Maria E, Tabaton M, Vigo T et al. (2000). Corticobasal degeneration shares a common genetic background with progressive supranuclear palsy. *Ann Neurol*, 47, 374–7.

D'Souza I and Schellenberg GD (2000). Determinants of 4-repeat tau expression. Coordination between enhancing and inhibitory splicing sequences for exon 10 inclusion. *J Biol Chem*, 275, 17700–9.

D'Souza I, Poorkaj P, Hong M et al. (1999). Missense and silent tau gene mutations cause frontotemporal dementia with parkinsonism-chromosome 17 type, by affecting multiple alternative RNA splicing regulatory elements. *Proc Natl Acad Sci USA*, 96, 5598–603.

Duffy PE and Tennyson VM (1965). Phase and electron microscopic observations of Lewy bodies and melanin granules in the substantia nigra and locus coeruleus in Parkinson's disease. *J Neuropathol Exp Neurol*, 24, 398–414.

Feany MB, Mattiace LA and Dickson DW (1996). Neuropathologic overlap of progressive supranuclear palsy, Pick's disease and corticobasal degeneration. *J Neuropathol Exp Neurol*, 55, 53–67.

Flament S, Delacourte A, Verny M, Hauw JJ and Javoy-Agid F (1991). Abnormal tau proteins in progressive supranuclear palsy. Similarities and differences with the neurofibrillary degeneration of the Alzheimer type. *Acta Neuropathol*, 81, 591–6.

Foster NL, Wilhelmsen KC, Sima AAF et al. (1997). Frontotemporal dementia and parkinsonism linked to chromosome 17: a consensus statement. *Ann Neurol*, 41, 706–15.

Gamblin TC, King ME, Dawson H et al. (2000). *In vitro* polymerization of tau protein monitored by laser light scattering: method and application to the study of FTDP-17 mutants. *Biochemistry*, 39, 6136–44.

Gao QS, Memmott J, Lafyatis R, Stamm S, Screaton G and Andreadis A (2000). Complex regulation of tau exon 10, whose missplicing causes frontotemporal dementia. *J Neurochem*, 74, 490–500.

Goedert M and Jakes R (1990). Expression of separate isoforms of human tau protein: correlation with the tau pattern in brain and effects on tubulin polymerization. *EMBO J*, 9, 4225–30.

Goedert M, Wischik CM, Crowther RA, Walker JE and Klug A (1988). Cloning and sequencing of the cDNA encoding a core protein of the paired helical filament of Alzheimer disease. *Proc Natl Acad Sci USA*, 85, 4051–5.

Goedert M, Spillantini MG, Jakes R, Rutherford D and Crowther RA (1989a). Multiple isoforms of human microtubule-associated protein tau: sequences and localization in neurofibrillary tangles of Alzheimer's disease. *Neuron*, 3, 519–26.

Goedert M, Spillantini MG, Potier MC, Ulrich J and Crowther RA (1989*b*). Cloning and sequencing of the cDNA encoding an isoform of microtubule-associated protein tau containing four tandem repeats: differential expression of tau protein mRNAs in human brain. *EMBO J*, 8, 393–9.

Goedert M, Cohen ES, Jakes R and Cohen P (1992*a*). MAP kinase phosphorylation sites in microtubule-associated protein tau are dephosphorylated by protein phosphatase 2A$_1$. Implications for Alzheimer's disease. *FEBS Lett*, 312, 95–9.

Goedert M, Spillantini MG, Cairns NJ and Crowther RA (1992*b*). Tau proteins of Alzheimer paired helical filaments: abnormal phosphorylation of all six brain isoforms. *Neuron*, 8, 159–68.

Goedert M, Crowther RA and Spillantini MG (1998). Tau mutations cause frontotemporal dementias. *Neuron*, 21, 955–8.

Goedert M, Jakes R and Crowther RA (1999*a*). Effects of frontotemporal dementia FTDP-17 mutations on heparin-induced assembly of tau filaments. *FEBS Lett*, 450, 306–11.

Goedert M, Spillantini MG, Crowther RA et al. (1999*b*). Tau gene mutation in familial progressive subcortical gliosis. *Nat Med*, 5, 454–7.

Goedert M, Satumtira S, Jakes R, Smith MJ, Kamibayashi C, White CL and Sontag E (2000). Reduced binding of protein phosphatase 2A to tau protein with frontotemporal dementia and parkinsonism linked to chromosome 17 mutations. *J Neurochem*, 75, 2155–62.

Goode BL and Feinstein SC (1994). Identification of a novel microtubule binding and assembly domain in the developmentally regulated interrepeat region of tau. *J Cell Biol*, 124, 769–82.

Golbe LI, Lazzarini AM, Spychala JR et al. (2001). The tau A0 allele in Parkinson's disease. *Mov Disord*, 16, 442–7.

Götz J, Probst A, Spillantini MG, Schäfer T, Jakes R, Bürki, K and Goedert M (1995). Somatodendritic localization and hyperphosphorylation of tau protein in transgenic mice overexpressing the longest human brain tau isoform. *EMBO J*, 14, 1304–13.

Götz J, Chen F, Barmettler R and Nitsch RM (2001*a*). Tau filament formation in transgenic mice expressing P301L tau. *J Biol Chem*, 276, 529–34.

Götz J, Chen F, van Dorpe J and Nitsch RM (2001*b*). Formation of neurofibrillary tangles in P301L tau transgenic mice induced by Aβ42 fibrils. *Science*, 293, 1491–4.

Grover A, Houlden H, Baker M et al. (1999). 5′-Splice site mutations in *tau* associated with the inherited dementia FTDP-17 affect a stem-loop structure that regulates alternative splicing of exon 10. *J Biol Chem*, 274, 15134–43.

Hall GF, Yao J and Lee G (1997). Tau overexpressed in identified lamprey neurons in situ is spatially segregated by phosphorylation state, forms hyperphosphorylated, dense aggregates and induces neurodegeneration. *Proc Natl Acad Sci USA*, 94, 4733–8.

Hall GF, Chu B, Lee G and Yao J (2000). Human tau filaments induce microtubule and synapse loss in an in vivo model of neurofibrillary degenerative disease. *J Cell Sci*, 113, 1373–87.

Hartmann AM, Rujesku D, Giannakouros T et al. (2001). Regulation of alternative splicing of human tau exon 10 by phosphorylation of splicing factors. *Mol Cell Neurosci*, 18, 80–90.

Hasegawa M, Smith MJ and Goedert M (1998). Tau proteins with FTDP-17 mutations have a reduced ability to promote microtubule assembly. *FEBS Lett*, 437, 207–10.

Spillantini MG, Crowther RA and Goedert M (1996). Comparison of the neurofibrillary pathology in Alzheimer's disease and familial presenile dementia with tangles. *Acta Neuropathol*, 92, 42–8.

Spillantini MG, Goedert M, Crowther RA, Murrell JR, Farlow MJ and Ghetti B (1997). Familial multiple system tauopathy with presenile dementia: a disease with abundant neuronal and glial tau filaments. *Proc Natl Acad Sci USA*, 94, 4113–18.

Spillantini MG, Bird TD and Ghetti B (1998a). Frontotemporal dementia and parkinsonism linked to chromosome 17: a new group of tauopathies. *Brain Pathol*, 8, 387–402.

Spillantini MG, Crowther RA, Kamphorst W, Heutink P and van Swieten JC (1998b). Tau pathology in two Dutch families with mutations in the microtubule-binding region of tau. *Am J Pathol* 153, 1359–63.

Spillantini MG, Murrell JR, Goedert M, Farlow MR, Klug A and Ghetti B (1998c). Mutation in the tau gene in familial multiple system tauopathy with presenile dementia. *Proc Natl Acad Sci USA*, 95, 7737–41.

Spillantini MG, Yoshida H, Rizzini C et al. (2000). A novel *tau* mutation (N296N) in familial dementia with swollen achromatic neurons and corticobasal inclusion bodies. *Ann Neurol*, 48, 939–93.

Spittaels K, van den Haute C, van Dorpe J et al. (1999). Prominent axonopathy in the brain and spinal cord of transgenic mice overexpressing four-repeat human tau protein. *Am J Pathol*, 155, 2153–65.

St George-Hyslop PH, Farrer LA and Goedert M (2001). Alzheimer disease and the frontotemporal dementias: diseases with cerebral deposition of fibrillar proteins. In *The Metabolic and Molecular Bases of Inherited Disease*, 8th edn, ed. CR Scriver, AL Beaudet, WS Sly and D Valle, pp. 5875–99. New York: McGraw-Hill.

Stanford PM, Halliday GM, Brooks WS et al. (2000). Progressive supranuclear palsy pathology caused by a novel silent mutation in exon 10 of the tau gene. *Brain*, 123, 880–93.

Tesseur I, van Dorpe J, Spittaels K, van den Haute C, Moechars D and van Leuven F (2000). Expression of human apolipoprotein E4 in neurons causes hyperphosphorylation of protein tau in the brains of transgenic mice. *Am J Pathol*, 156, 951–64.

Van Swieten JC, Stevens M, Rosso SM et al. (1999). Phenotypic variation in hereditary frontotemporal dementia with tau mutations. *Ann Neurol*, 46, 617–26.

Varani L, Hasegawa M, Spillantini MG et al. (1999). Structure of tau exon 10 splicing regulatory element RNA and destabilization by mutations of frontotemporal dementia and parkinsonism linked to chromosome 17. *Proc Natl Acad Sci USA*, 96, 8229–34.

Varani L, Spillantini MG, Goedert M and Varani G (2000). Structural basis for recognition of the RNA major groove in the tau exon 10 splicing regulatory element by aminoglycoside antibiotics. *Nucleic Acids Res*, 28, 710–19.

Vogelsberg-Ragaglia V, Bruce J, Richter-Landsberg C et al. (2000). Distinct FTDP-17 missense mutations in tau produce tau aggregates and other pathological phenotypes in transfected CHO cells. *Mol Biol Cell*, 11, 4093–104.

Wilhelmsen KC, Lynch T, Pavlou E, Higgins M and Nygaard TG (1994). Localization of disinhibition-dementia-Parkinsonism-amyotrophy complex to 17q21-22. *Am J Hum Genet*, 55, 1159–65.

Wittmann CW, Wszolek MF, Shulman JM et al. (2001). Tauopathy in *Drosophila*: neurodegeneration without neurofibrillary tangles. *Science*, 293, 711–14.

Yasuda M, Kawamata T, Komure O et al. (1999). A mutation in the microtubule-associated protein tau in pallido-nigro-luysian degeneration. *Neurology*, 53, 864–8.

Yasuda M, Takamatsu J, D'Souza I et al. (2000). A novel mutation at position +12 in the intron following exon 10 of the tau gene in familial frontotemporal dementia (FTD-Kumamoto). *Ann Neurol*, 47, 422–9.

13

Advances in early diagnosis and differentiation of the dementias

Siân A Thompson[1], Peter J Nestor[1] and John R Hodges[1,2]

[1] Addenbrooke's Hospital, Cambridge, UK; [2] MRC Cognition and Brain Sciences Unit, Cambridge, UK

Introduction

Over the past decades the concept of dementia has evolved from one of progressive global intellectual deterioration, to a syndrome of progressive impairment in memory and at least one other cognitive deficit (aphasia, apraxia, agnosia, or disturbance in executive function) in the absence of another explanatory central nervous system disorder, depression or delirium (DSM-IV). Furthermore, within this broad definition, the delineation of particular patterns of focal cognitive deficit associated with different dementia syndromes has greatly advanced over recent years. In epidemiological terms, dementia presents a significant problem; Alzheimer's disease alone affects 15 million people worldwide at present (Evans et al. 1989), and with the current demographic trend, this number will certainly increase.

With the advent of new and potentially disease-modifying therapies, attention has been focused on the need for reliable and early markers of dementia. In pursuit of this, a major expansion in dementia research has occurred, directed towards both identifying subjects in the preclinical phase of illness and differentiating between dementia syndromes of varying aetiologies. A number of approaches have been followed, encompassing the disciplines of neuropsychology, neuropsychiatry, structural and functional neuro-imaging and neurobiology (the search for biological markers of disease).

In this chapter we will discuss some of the advances that have occurred within the specialities of neuropsychology, neuropsychiatry and neuro-imaging. A comprehensive review of this rapidly expanding field would not be possible in this brief overview of the subject. We have, therefore, concentrated on a number of key topics related to early diagnosis and differential diagnosis.

Neuropsychological studies

The major aims of neuropsychological studies of recent years have been one of the following: (i) to accurately characterize the cognitive profiles of the different dementia syndromes (Alzheimer's disease (AD), frontotemporal dementia (FTD), dementia with Lewy bodies (DLB), vascular dementia (VaD)); (ii) to identify tests with a high predictive value in the predementia phase of the illness; and (iii) to establish neuropsychological tests with high sensitivity and specificity in the differential diagnosis of the dementias.

Early diagnosis of Alzheimer's disease

Not surprisingly, Alzheimer's disease (AD) has attracted the most attention in neuropsychological research. Group studies have shown that memory impairment is both an early and predominant manifestation of AD in the majority of cases. Tests of delayed recall of verbal or visual material are consistently the most sensitive markers of AD, indicating an early and severe impairment in episodic memory (Welsh et al. 1991; Locascio et al. 1995; Greene et al. 1996a). This deficit is considered to reflect the distribution of pathology in the transentorhinal cortex, which functionally deprives the hippocampus of major input and output (Braak and Braak 1991).

With progression of disease, patients with AD show significant disruption to semantic memory, the term applied to knowledge of objects, facts and concepts, as well as word meaning (Tulving 1987). Hodges and Patterson (1995) found that even in subjects with minimal disease (MMSE > 23), performance was impaired on a battery of semantic tests. This and other similar studies have revealed a significant degree of item consistency across different semantic tasks, suggesting that the impairment reflects primarily a breakdown in central semantic knowledge (Chertkow and Bub 1990; Hodges and Patterson 1995; Chan et al. 1997; Lambon et al. 1997). Involvement of attentional and executive processes, praxis and visuoperceptual abilities also follow (Grady et al. 1988; Mendez et al. 1990; Locascio et al. 1995; Binetti et al. 1998; Perry and Hodges 2000b), showing a pattern of progression consistent with current views regarding the pathological advancement of disease (Hyman et al. 1986; Braak and Braak 1991; Van Hoesen et al. 1991; Van Hoesen 1997).

Despite this widely held view of an orderly progression of cognitive changes which parallel the spread of pathology, there is increasing evidence of considerable heterogeneity (Galton et al. 2000). Patients may present with focal non-mnestic deficits. The best documented are progressive aphasia (which may be fluent or nonfluent) (Pogacar and Williams 1984; Green et al. 1990; Benson and Zaias 1991; Greene et al. 1996b) and progressive visuospatial or perceptual impairments, sometimes referred to as posterior cortical atrophy (Cogan 1985; De Renzi 1986; Benson et al. 1988; Berthier et al. 1991; Victoroff et al. 1994; Ross et al. 1996). The prevalence of 'atypical' presentations is unknown. Current criteria for AD emphasize the central role of memory impairment and hence atypical cases are often excluded. Our experience suggests that atypical aphasic patients may be more common than is currently believed.

Mild cognitive impairment

Although the cognitive profile of established AD has been well characterized in recent years, there is still considerable controversy regarding the sensitivity and specificity of tests applied for the diagnosis of disease in the early stages and, importantly, in the predictive value of neuropsychological tests in preclinical cases. The terminology in this area of 'predementia memory impairment' remains confusing and controversial. A number of different labels have been applied, including MCI (mild cognitive impairment), questionable Alzheimer's disease, minimal Alzheimer's disease or Clinical Dementia Rating (an informant and patient-based semi-structured interview for the assessment of dementia) grade 0.5 (Berg 1988) (see Perry and Hodges 2000*b*; Swainson et al. 2001). These patients present with memory complaints but do not fulfil research criteria for AD, in that activities of daily living and cognitive abilities apart from memory are well preserved (Petersen et al. 1997; Ritchie and Touchon 2000). It has recently been proposed that the label MCI be applied only to patients with memory complaints insufficient to interfere with everyday function with evidence of impairment on memory tests (> 1.5 SD below normal) (Petersen et al. 1997). The introduction of more specific criteria is to be welcomed, but the lack of specification of which tests should be used to define impairment is a serious flaw. As discussed below, tests of cross-modal associative learning or free recall are likely to be considerably more sensitive than tests which depend on item recognition. Importantly, this clinical state may represent a transitional period prior to the development of AD in some individuals, whereas in others, MCI appears to be a more benign condition. The conversion rate of MCI to dementia, although differing widely in some studies, converges to a value of about 12% per year, about 10 times higher than the incidence of dementia in the general population (Celsis 2000). The importance of predicting the subgroup of individuals within the spectrum of MCI who will convert to AD is of ever-increasing interest and significance with the possibility that early intervention before clinical dementia may allow us the greatest opportunities of arresting or slowing the course of disease (Hodges 1998).

Two main approaches have been taken to investigate the neuropsychological profile of the predementia syndrome: longitudinal community-based studies and longitudinal studies of asymptomatic individuals at risk of autosomal-dominant familial AD. These studies have not produced entirely consistent results, but do concur that deficits on neuropsychological tests can be detected in patients several years before they reach criteria for a diagnosis of dementia. The cohort of individuals followed up longitudinally as part of the Framingham study (Linn et al. 1995) who subsequently developed dementia ($n = 55$) showed significant deficits on measures of verbal memory and immediate auditory attention span 7 years or more prior to the onset of clinical disease. Similarly, the Bronx Aging Study (Masur et al. 1994) also found that two measures of memory, together with a category fluency task and complex visuomotor test, were able to identify a subgroup of individuals ($n = 64$) with an 85% probability of developing dementia over 4 years before the onset of clinical disease.

Although these studies have established that a preclinical phase of cognitive decline can be identified in predementia subjects there remains little agreement concerning which aspects of cognitive function, and hence neuropsychological measures, are most helpful as predictors of subsequent dementia. Rubin et al. (1998), in a prospective study of healthy elders (n $= 82$) identified only one test of verbal memory on which a decline in performance preceded any detectable clinical changes or global psychometric deterioration. In contrast, the North Manhattan Aging Project (Jacobs et al. 1995) identified three tasks at baseline with high positive predictive value of subsequent dementia, including a confrontation naming test and an abstract reasoning task. Fabrigoule et al. (1998), in their assessment of the results from the Bordeaux (PAQUID) longitudinal study, attempted to define the underlying cognitive disorder responsible for impaired performance on a number of predictive tests of seemingly diverse areas. They concluded that the earliest preclinical deficit in dementia and AD reflects a disturbance of central control processes.

Longitudinal studies of at-risk individuals from autosomal-dominant familial AD, by virtue of the younger age of the study cohort, are less confounded by comorbidity with vascular disease and unpredictability of age-related cognitive decline, than the prospective community-based studies of healthy elderly. Fox et al. (1998) studied 63 'at-risk' subjects over a 6-year period, during which time ten individuals became clinically affected. This subgroup of converters already had significantly lower verbal memory scores and performance IQ measures at their baseline assessment than those who did not convert. This and other studies reviewed above suggest that, in addition to the well-established deficits in episodic memory, there may be more widespread pathology (perhaps synaptic loss) in addition to the medial temporal tangle formation early in AD.

Although these studies have identified a number of neuropsychological measures which appear to be sensitive in defining groups of subjects who will convert to dementia, the search continues for tasks which have predictive and diagnostic sensitivity and specificity for individual case assessment. An ongoing longitudinal study in Cambridge (Swainson et al. 2001) has been following up groups of subjects

Table 13.1. Global cognitive function and memory results (mean (SEM)) from a neuropsychological study of early detection and differential diagnosis of Alzheimer's disease (Swainson et al. 2001). Four study groups were included: mild Alzheimer's disease (AD, n = 26); questionable Alzheimer's disease (QAD, n = 43); depressed subjects (Dep, n = 37) and normal healthy controls (n = 39). The paired-associates learning test (PAL) from the CANTAB computed battery was able to distinguish both the probable AD group and the QAD group from the normal controls and depressed subjects, with equivalent performance by the controls and depressed subjects

Task	AD	QAD	Dep	Control
Global cognitive function				
ADAS-cog	22.4 (1.1)*†‡	11.1 (0.9)*†	9.3 (0.6)*	6.7 (0.4)
Recognition memory				
WRMT words	17.3 (0.6)*†‡	22.3 (0.5)	23.1 (0.5)	24.2 (0.2)
WRMT faces	19.3 (0.5)*†‡	22.0 (0.5)	22.6 (0.5)	23.6 (0.2)
Cued recall				
PAL stages passed	4.8 (0.3)*†‡	7.3 (0.2)*†	7.7 (0.1)	7.9 (0.1)
PAL 6-pattern errors	42.8 (2.8)*†‡	12.8 (2.4)*†	9.4 (1.4)	7.8 (1.1)
Logical memory 30 min	2.0 (0.7)*†‡	12.4 (1.4)*†	16.1 (1.2)*	19.9 (1.0)
Semantic memory				
GNT	14.2 (1.3)*†‡	23.3 (0.7)	22.4 (0.7)	24.1 (0.7)
Category fluency	28.5 (1.8)*†‡	48.6 (2.0)*†	50.4 (2.0)*	61.1 (2.1)

Mann–Whitney U test / Student's t-test; *$P < 0.05$ differs from control; †$P < 0.05$ differs from depressed subjects; ‡$P < 0.05$ differs from QAD.

ADAS-cog, Alzheimer's Disease Assessment Scale, cognitive section (Rosen et al. 1984); WRMT, Warrington short recognition memory tests (Warrington 1996); PAL, CANTAB Paired Associates Learning (Sahakian et al. 1988); logical memory, Wechsler Logical Memory delayed recall (Wechsler 1987); GNT, Graded Naming Test (McKenna and Warrington 1980).

with mild AD, questionable AD and depression. Questionable AD has been defined on the basis of subject complaints of poor memory sufficient to lead to assessment in the memory clinic, in the absence of depression or any identifiable brain disease. The paired associative learning test from the CANTAB computed battery, which combines pattern and spatial components, not only accurately distinguishes AD from depressed and control subjects (Table 13.1), but also reveals an apparent subgroup of questionable patients who perform like AD patients, their scores correlating with the degree of subsequent global cognitive decline. If, as predicted, this subgroup of questionable AD patients progress to dementia during the study time, the associative learning test may be shown to be a useful predictive neuropsychological tool on a case-by-case basis.

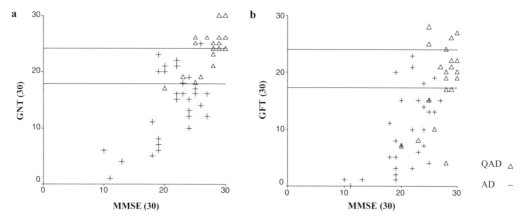

Figure 13.1   Scatterplots showing individual scores from (a) the Graded Naming Test (GNT) (McKenna and Warrington 1980) and (b) the Graded Faces Test (GFT), a graded difficulty test of famous-people naming, for a group of AD patients and questionable AD (QAD) subjects included in a longitudinal study in Cambridge. Seventy-one per cent of the QAD subjects who performed below 2 standard deviations of the control mean on the GFT went on to fulfil research criteria for dementia within the 2-year longitudinal study, compared with 0% of the QAD subjects who performed within the normal range. MMSE, Mini-Mental State Examination.

Results from a parallel longitudinal study in Cambridge suggest that a test examining naming and knowledge of famous people may also provide a useful tool for the early diagnosis of individual subjects with AD. A graded difficulty test of famous-people naming (the Graded Faces Test) was shown to have predictive value in determining which subjects within the questionable AD group would go on to fulfil the criteria for dementia. Seventy-one per cent of subjects who showed a significant impairment on the Graded Faces Test (greater than two standard deviations below the control mean) were subsequently found to have deteriorated cognitively, whilst none of the questionable AD subjects who performed within the normal range on this test moved into the dementia group within the 24-month study period. Scores on this naming test in both the probable AD and questionable AD groups were significantly correlated with the degree of dementia as determined by the Mini-Mental State Examination (MMSE) (Figure 13.1). Although numbers within this study were small, results do suggest that assessment of this domain of knowledge may also be both sensitive in early diagnosis and useful in tracking disease progression.

Differential diagnosis

In addition to the ever-increasing need for early diagnosis and predementia identification of cognitively impaired subjects, differentiating disease entities within the spectrum of dementia is also of utmost importance in terms of both potential treatment and advising family members with regard to prognosis, predicted pattern of decline and genetic implications. There have been substantial advances in the neuropsychological characterization of different dementia syndromes in recent years and attention has focused on which tasks or patient profiles, in terms of neuropsychology and neuropsychiatry, may enable the differentiation of easily confusable disease entities.

Vascular dementia versus Alzheimer's disease

In Western countries vascular dementia (VaD) is the second most common type of dementia after AD (Desmond 1996), and yet considerable controversy surrounds the concept of VaD and its diagnosis (Loeb and Meyer 2000). As a potentially preventable form of dementia, its diagnosis and differentiation from AD is of great importance. There has been a large number of studies that have attempted to compare the performance of patients fulfilling the research criteria for VaD with patients with probable AD in terms of both neuropsychology and neuropsychiatry (Almkvist 1994). Several limitations arise from the nature of this research, particularly the utilization of different diagnostic criteria for VaD by different research groups and the possible circularity problems, common to the majority of studies, owing to the inclusion criteria being clinical rather than neuropathological. Despite these shortcomings, in a recent review of the comparative studies to date (Looi and Sachdev 1999), a number of group differences in neuropsychological deficits in AD and VaD have emerged. For similar levels of overall cognitive decline, VaD patients were more likely to show relative preservation of episodic memory and greater deficits in frontal executive and attentional function than AD patients. The two groups did not differ significantly on tests of language, constructional abilities, working memory or conceptual function. These differences are consistent with the present understanding of the neuropathological basis of these diseases; the relative excess of deficits in faculties ascribed to the prefrontal lobe function in VaD related to the frequent presence of lesions in structures that comprise the frontal subcortical circuits.

Recent studies have also suggested that affective behavioural disturbances in dementia may vary according to the underlying aetiology. Although many similarities exist between the profiles of behavioural changes in AD and VaD, a substantial number of differences have been identified. The cognitive changes in AD are commonly accompanied by anxiety, agitation, psychosis and personality change (Petry et al. 1988; Cummings et al. 1990; Tariot et al. 1995; Cummings 1997), whereas, in contrast, VaD is frequently associated with irritability, apathy and blunted affect (Cummings et al. 1990; Sultzer et al. 1992; Krasuski and Gaviria 1994). In a recent study of 195 patients with AD and 36 patients with ischaemic vascular disease fitting standard research criteria, Hargrave et al. (2000) assessed 16 different affect and behavioural variables. Significant group differences emerged for two variables: decreased affect and withdrawal, and psychomotor slowing, both characteristics present to a greater degree in patients with ischaemic VaD. Further studies are required to assess the utility and reproducibility of such behavioural assessment tools in assisting diagnostic accuracy, but in combination with neuropsychological tests, they may assist in discriminating between these two dementia syndromes.

Frontotemporal dementia versus Alzheimer's disease

Frontotemporal dementia (FTD), the term currently used to describe a range of non-Alzheimer dementias producing focal lobar atrophy involving the frontal lobes and/or the temporal lobes, has received growing interest over the last two decades. The exact prevalence of FTD is uncertain, but growing evidence suggests that it represents the second commonest dementia in the presenium, and may represent up to a fifth of cases (Knopman et al. 1990). The cognitive deficits in patients with frontal pathology are fundamentally different from those with predominantly temporal lobe pathology. The latter presentation, also known as semantic dementia (SD), is characterized by a profound loss of conceptual knowledge, which underlies a progressive anomia with loss of verbal and nonverbal comprehension (Hodges et al. 1992). In contrast, the frontal variant of FTD (fvFTD) is more typically described in terms of the pervasive changes in personality, behaviour and social conduct (Miller et al. 1991). The pathological changes in fvFTD involve predominantly the orbitomedial frontal lobe, which explains the often normal performance on standard neuropsychological tests, which tend to be sensitive to dorsolateral rather than orbitofrontal pathology. A recent comparison of eight patients with relatively mild fvFTD and IQ-matched control volunteers, however, was able to distinguish patients on the basis of two cognitive tasks: a visual-discrimination learning paradigm and a decision-making paradigm, on which patients showed an increase in risk-taking behaviour. Notably, the patients did not differ from controls on a number of computerized tests from the CANTAB battery previously shown to be sensitive to dorsolateral frontal lobe dysfunction, such as planning tasks and spatial working memory (Rahman et al. 1999).

Previous attempts to identify neuropsychological differences between AD and FTD have been largely unsuccessful, probably partly reflecting the variation in patient selection and particular choice of neuropsychological tests (Miller et al. 1991; Elfgren et al. 1994; Frisoni et al. 1995). Gregory et al. (1997) studied 12 patients with frontal variant FTD and 12 AD patients, matched for overall level of dementia on the MMSE, using a number of traditional cognitive tests and rating scales. Tests of memory, attention, language comprehension and executive function failed to separate the groups. Hodges et al. (1999) compared the performance of controls with three patient groups, AD, fvFTD and SD patients, on a comprehensive battery of neuropsychological tasks, including the semantic test battery (Hodges and Patterson 1995). A distinct profile emerged for each group: AD subjects showed a severe deficit in episodic memory with mild but significant impairments on tests of semantic memory and visuospatial function; SD patients showed a profound breakdown in semantic memory, as previously documented, with anomia and surface dyslexia; and the fvFTD group, who were the least impaired overall on the battery, showed mild deficits in episodic memory and verbal fluency, with preserved semantic memory. In a further study (Perry and Hodges 2000a) examining these three patient groups, tests of attention and executive function were found to positively discriminate the fvFTD patients from the SD and AD patients. SD subjects showed preservation of attention and executive function with severe deficits in semantic memory, whereas the fvFTD subjects showed the reverse pattern. The AD subjects, who were densely amnesic, could also be distinguished from the fvFTD patients on the basis of their performance on the executive and attention tasks. More recently, Mathuranath et al. (2000) described results from a simple bedside test battery, the Addenbrooke's Cognitive Examination, designed to both detect early dementia and also differentiate AD from FTD. The 100-point test, which incorporated the MMSE, tested key cognitive areas of orientation, attention, memory, verbal fluency, language and visuospatial abilities. The battery had high construct validity, reliability and sensitivity for the diagnosis of dementia, and using derived component scores (verbal fluency and language/orientation and memory) was highly discriminating for AD and FTD.

A further approach in differentiating FTD and AD has been to focus on the behavioural profiles of these diseases. Using a questionnaire design to assess a wide range of neuropsychiatric features, Bozeat et al. (2000) found that patients with FTD and AD had strikingly different behavioural profiles and were reliably separated into diagnostic groups by incidence of stereotypic behaviours, changes in eating preference, disinhibition and poor social awareness, all being higher in the FTD group. Further characterization of the FTD group into frontal and temporal variants, however, was not reliable using this tool, reflecting the involvement of a common network (the orbitomedial frontal lobe, temporal pole and amygdala). Higher rates of mental rigidity and depression were, however, noted within the SD group compared with the fvFTD patients. In a similar recent study, Snowden et al. (2001) administered a semistructured informant-based interview in SD and fvFTD patients. Logistic regression analysis was able to identify two key areas of discrimination between the temporal and frontal variants: emotion and repetitive compulsive behaviours. The SD group showed less fear in everyday life, as assessed by the questionnaire, than the fvFTD group, whereas the fvFTD patients showed decreased anger, disgust and sadness in comparison. The SD patients also had a higher rate of complex stereotypical behaviours.

Dementia with Lewy bodies versus Alzheimer's disease

Recent clinical and neuropathological studies suggest that dementia with Lewy bodies (DLB) is a common cause of dementia in elderly people (Perry et al. 1990; McKeith et al. 1996). Clinically, DLB is characterized by a cortical dementia with fluctuating confusion, spontaneous parkinsonism with sensitivity to neuroleptic drugs, and psychiatric symptoms, particularly well-formed visual hallucinations early in the course of the disease (McKeith 1988; Hansen et al. 1990; Ballard et al. 1997). In contrast to AD, there have been relatively few neuropsychological studies of patients with DLB. A number of reports of clinical DLB have suggested that the performance of patients on visuospatial tasks may be more severely impaired than in AD. In addition, it has been proposed that cholinergic depletion resulting from pathology in the basal forebrain cholinergic system in DLB produces a deficit in attentional and executive function. Results of studies to address this area of cognition, however, have been controversial (Hansen et al. 1990; Sahgal et al. 1992; Gnanalingham et al. 1997). Little has previously been known about semantic memory status in DLB.

Two recent studies motivated by the questions raised above have compared the performance of DLB and AD patients matched for age and dementia severity (as assessed by their MMSE score) on neuropsychological batteries. Calderon et al. (2001) found that patients with DLB were significantly impaired relative to both AD patients and controls on three subtests of the visual object and space perception battery (VOSP: Warrington and James 1991), the fragmented letters, object decision and cube analysis, considered together to be sensitive to deficits in both the dorsal (where) and ventral (what) visual processing streams. The AD subjects, at the same stage of disease, were only impaired on the silhouette subtest of the VOSP, a task which draws more heavily on semantic knowledge, and therefore, a 'less pure' test of visual or spatial function. The DLB patients also showed pervasive deficits on attentional and executive tasks, over and above those demonstrated in AD. Although the AD subjects were impaired on a test of selective attention, they performed normally on a divided attention task, unlike the DLB patients. These findings are consistent with the hypothesis that severe cholinergic depletion may underlie the attention deficit in DLB. In contrast, AD patients were significantly more impaired than those with DLB on tests of episodic memory.

Lambon Ralph et al. (2001), in addition to assessing visuoperceptual and attentional deficits in DLB and AD patients as part of a comprehensive battery, also studied semantic memory. Both patient groups were significantly impaired compared with controls on an array of semantic tasks using both verbal and visual modalities. However, unlike AD patients, the DLB subjects showed a greater deficit on tests presented in the visual modality than the verbal modality. This modality effect in the DLB group could be explained by their additional visuoperceptual deficit, as demonstrated on other tasks. Both groups were impaired on tests of recognition memory, and in agreement with the study of Calderon et al. (2001), the AD group was more impaired on prose recall than the DLB patients. Together, these two studies provide a cognitive profile of DLB, characterized by a generalized dementia, with profound attentional and visuoperceptual deficits compared with AD, but relatively preserved episodic memory for a similar disease stage.

In summary, significant advances have been made in knowledge concerning the neuropsychology and neuropsychiatry of the dementia syndromes, but despite this, ideal cognitive and behavioural diagnostic tests, with the aims of high specificity, sensitivity and simplicity of application, have not, as yet, been identified. The combination of neuropsychological measures with new imaging techniques (see below) may provide greater diagnostic accuracy.

Neuroimaging in the dementias

In the absence of in vivo noninvasive techniques for the direct measurement of neuropathology (the gold standard for diagnosis in dementia), neuro-imaging provides a means of assessing and monitoring surrogate markers of disease, including cerebral atrophy, decreased cerebral metabolism and regional blood flow changes. In common with neuropsychological studies, neuro-imaging research has been directed towards means of early diagnosis, particularly in AD and MCI, and differential diagnosis of the dementias.

Structural imaging

The spatial resolution and wide availability of magnetic resonance imaging (MRI) has ensured that it has become an important research tool. Based on the neuropathological findings of early involvement of medial temporal lobe structures in AD (Braak and Braak 1991), methods of assessing the degree of atrophy in this region, as a surrogate of cell loss, have received a great deal of attention. The major impetus for the development of methods of temporal lobe assessment has been to improve the accuracy of early diagnosis, but it is also clearly of both practical and theoretical importance to define whether changes are specific to AD or common to a number of dementia syndromes. MRI techniques range from simple visual rating of hippocampal atrophy (Scheltens et al. 1992; Frisoni et al. 1999; Galton et al. 2001) to segmentation and volumetric measures of temporal lobe structures (Convit et al. 1997; Hashimoto et al. 1998; Barber et al. 1999; Frisoni et al. 1999; Jack et al. 1999; Pruessner et al. 2000) (Figure 13.2, colour plate). The former has the advantage of being a relatively fast method of assessment, and can be performed on large numbers of scans in a clinical setting. In contrast, volumetric measurement of regions of interest is both slow and labour intensive, but does provide accurate and detailed measurements of predetermined circumscribed areas.

A number of studies have attempted to identify medial temporal lobe volume changes in at-risk populations for AD, to establish if such measures have a predictive role. Convit et al. (1997) found that measures of hippocampal volume were able to separate a group of MCI subjects from normal, age-matched controls, whereas other temporal lobe measures did not differ between groups. The MCI group could be distinguished from patients with established AD by both degree of medial temporal lobe atrophy and, in addition, by the volume of the fusiform gyrus. Hippocampal volumes also correlated with a measure of delayed memory function. Furthermore, in a recent longitudinal study of neuropsychological measures and neuro-imaging in MCI patients, Jack et al. (1999) found that the rate of conversion from MCI to AD (27 out of 80 subjects followed up) was greater in MCI patients who had smaller hippocampi at baseline, as assessed by volumetric measurements from a three-dimensional MRI data set. Only hippocampal volume, Dementia Rating Scale Score and a test of immediate recall were statistically significant predictor variables of conversion to AD. With the reservation that the true endpoint of such studies can only be ascertained at autopsy, these studies may suggest the utility of medial temporal lobe measurements as a useful research tool in early diagnosis. However, as mentioned, the labour-intensity of this methodology makes its clinical application limited.

But what of differentiating AD from other dementias? A number of structural-imaging studies have attempted to discriminate between dementias of different aetiologies. Galton et al. (2001), using a visual rating scale of temporal lobe struc-tures validated by volumetric measures, showed that hippocampal atrophy was not specific for AD. Fifty per cent of the patients with AD were found to have bilateral hippocampal atrophy, but contrary to expectations, patients with SD also had hippocampal atrophy, which exceeded that seen in AD on the left side. Patients with fvFTD were also indistinguishable from AD using these measures. The SD and AD groups could, however, be distinguished on a number of other parameters: the presence of severe bilateral atrophy of the temporal pole, parahippocampal and lateral temporal lobe regions was specific to SD. Barber et al. (1999) attempted to differentiate between AD, DLB, VaD and controls using structural MRI. Standard clinical criteria were used for the diagnosis of DLB, requiring two out of three of fluctuations in cognitive function, recurrent visual hallucinations or spontaneous parkinsonism for a possible diagnosis, and all dementia groups were matched for length of history. A visual rating scale (Scheltens et al. 1992) was used to esti-mate degree of medial temporal lobe atrophy. It was found that the DLB patient group had less medial temporal lobe atrophy than the AD patients, and patients with VaD showed a similar, though nonsignificant, trend. On an individual case basis, however, they concluded that MRI rating was good at confirming the presence of AD but not specific, and that although the absence of medial temporal lobe atrophy on a scan might be suggestive of DLB, it was not sensitive for the diagnosis.

Studies using detailed volumetric measures of medial temporal lobe structures have produced very similar results. Hashimoto et al. (1998) made volumetric measurements of the hippocampus, amygdala and whole brain on MRI scans acquired from 27 patients with DLB, 27 AD patients and an equal number of normal controls. The mean hippocampal volume of the AD group was significantly less than that of the DLB group. A model using volumetric parameters to predict group membership of individual cases, however, correctly predicted 66.7% of the DLB group and 70.4% of the AD patients only. Frisoni et al. (1999) used quantitative MRI to investigate regional differences in atrophy in FTD and AD patients compared with controls. In agreement with the visual rating study described above (Miller et al. 1991), they found that medial temporal atrophy was present in both groups, and was therefore not useful in discriminating between the two dementia syndromes. Measures of anterior frontal and temporal atrophy did separate the two groups, being significantly greater in the FTD group.

Techniques that measure brain substructures, either by visual rating or manual segmentation and volume analysis, are subject to a number of problems. In particular, these methods introduce both intraobserver and interobserver variability, with increasing measurement error for smaller and less easily defined neuroanatomical structures. Furthermore, a priori decisions are required concerning which anatomical regions are of particular interest. Fox et al. (1996) developed a MRI coregistration technique, which provided a measure of total brain atrophy, and avoided a number of these problems. Registration involved positional matching of a later T1-weighted volumetric scan onto a baseline scan, with visualization and subsequent quantification of the differences between the two scans. Volume loss could then be expressed as a percentage of the initial brain volume, and converted into a rate of atrophy per year. This method was found to be extremely sensitive for differentiating between AD patients and normal ageing, even early in the course of disease (Fox et al. 1996, 1999b). Furthermore, unlike findings from volumetric studies, the serial coregistration showed evidence of global brain atrophy in AD, perhaps suggesting much more diffuse neuronal or synaptic loss than has been commonly appreciated. Results from a longitudinal study of 29 patients with probable AD showed that brain atrophy correlated highly with rate of cognitive decline, assessed by the MMSE (Fox et al. 1999a). This latter finding suggests that this methodology might be of particular use in tracking disease progression, a measure

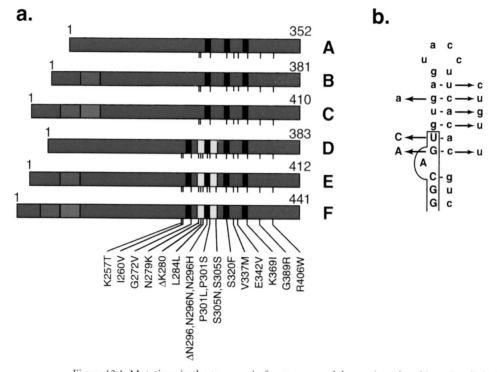

Figure 12.1 Mutations in the *tau* gene in frontotemporal dementia and parkinsonism linked to chromosome 17 (FTDP-17). (a) Schematic diagram of the six tau isoforms (A–F) that are expressed in adult human brain. Alternatively spliced exons are shown in red (exon 2), green (exon 3) and yellow (exon 10); black bars indicate the microtubule-binding repeats. Fourteen missense mutations, two deletion mutations and three silent mutations in the coding region are shown. Amino-acid numbering corresponds to the 441 amino-acid isoform of human brain tau. (b) Stem-loop structure in the pre-mRNA at the boundary between exon 10 and the intron following exon 10. Eight mutations that reduce the stability of the stem-loop structure are shown. Exon sequences are shown in capital and intron sequences in lower-case letters.

FTDP-17 Pathologies

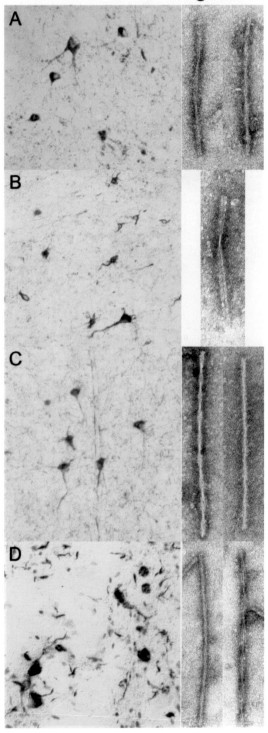

Figure 12.2 Representative pathologies of FTDP-17, as revealed by immunohistochemistry for hyperphosphorylated tau protein and the morphologies of isolated tau filaments. (A) The P301L mutation in exon 10 gives rise to a neuronal and glial tau pathology. Tau filaments consist of narrow twisted ribbons (left) as the majority species and rope-like filaments (right) as the minority species. They are predominantly made of four-repeat tau isoforms. The P301S mutation in exon 10 gives rise to a similar pathology. (B) Mutations in the intron following exon 10 give rise to a neuronal and glial tau pathology. Tau filaments consist of wide twisted ribbons made of four-repeat tau isoforms. The glial pathology is more extensive than in (A). (C) The V337M mutation in exon 12 gives rise to a neuronal tau pathology. Tau filaments consist of paired helical (left) and straight (right) filaments, like the tau filaments of Alzheimer's disease. They contain all six human brain tau isoforms. Paired helical filaments constitute the majority species. The R406W mutation in exon 13 gives rise to a similar pathology. (D) The G389R mutation in exon 13 gives rise to a neuronal tau pathology. Tau filaments consist of straight filaments (left) as the majority species and twisted filaments (right) as the minority species. The tau pathology resembles that of Pick's disease. Filaments consist of three-repeat and four-repeat tau isoforms. The K257T and G272V mutations in exon 9, the S320F mutation in exon 11 and the E342V and K369I mutations in exon 12 give rise to a similar pathology.

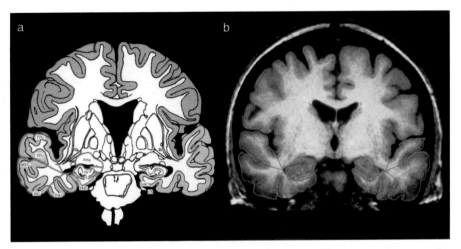

Figure 13.2 Illustration of the volumetric measures and corresponding anatomy (courtesy of Galton et al. 2001). EntC, Entorhinal cortex; CS, collateral sulcus; Amg, amygdala; Hi, hippocampus; S, subiculum; PHG, parahippocampal gyrus; FuG, fusiform gyrus; ITG, inferior temporal gyrus; MTG, middle temporal gyrus; STG, superior temporal gyrus; TTG, transverse temporal gyrus.

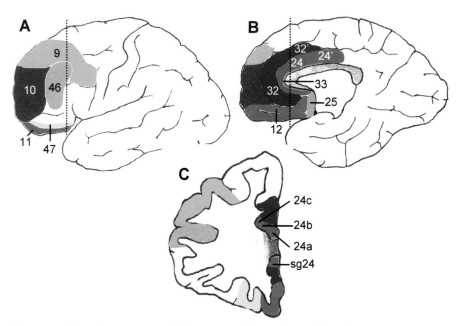

Figure 14.1 Frontal cortex areas and the neuropathology of mood disorder. (A) Lateral, (B) medial and (C) coronal (at the level of the dashed line) views of the cerebral cortex showing Brodmann areas of the frontal cortex implicated in the neuropathology of mood disorder. Some of the subdivisions of area 24 are also shown (Vogt et al. 1995). Note that all markings are approximate, and to an extent arbitrary, because (a) area boundaries are defined by cytoarchitecture not surface anatomy, and (b) there is considerable individual variability in location of a given area (Rajkowska and Goldman-Rakic 1995). Based upon Perry (1994).

which will be of increasing importance with the need to assess the efficacy of potential disease-modifying drugs. This technique, though not labour intensive, does require patients to be scanned on the same machine with exactly the same acquisition protocol, and for this reason is likely to remain confined to use as a research tool for the foreseeable future.

Returning once more to the overall aim of such diagnostic imaging studies, some progress has been made towards the ultimate goal of noninvasive in vivo measurement of dementia neuropathology using neuro-imaging techniques (Fox and Rossor 2000). Recent work by Beneviste et al. (1999) has applied MRI to the detection of microscopic plaques in AD. Although successful in imaging amyloid plaques, the work was performed using postmortem specimens and necessitated over 20 hours of scanning, using a 7 T machine. Clinical MRI at present uses field strengths ranging from 0.5–3 T. Higher-field-strength machines carry potential hazards such as arrhythmia induction, making such a paradigm unfeasible in a clinical setting. Furthermore, movement artefact in vivo is likely to present a significant problem, with arterial pulsation obscuring signals from plaques. Despite these major reservations, this work represents an exciting advance in structural neuro-imaging.

Functional imaging

Functional neuro-imaging, as suggested by its name, has the advantage over structural imaging of providing a measure of cerebral function, which can be either qualitative or quantitative. This must be tempered, however, by its significantly lower spatial resolution. There have been a number of developments in this field including single photon emission computed tomography (SPECT), positron emission tomography (PET) and, most recently, functional magnetic resonance imaging (fMRI).

SPECT is relatively widely available in the clinical setting, unlike PET, and therefore has potentially greater application for clinical diagnosis. The technique is dependent on certain tracers being irreversibly taken up into the brain in a regional pattern that reflects local differences in blood flow. This in turn can disclose changes that reflect the pattern of neuropsychological deficit in different dementia syndromes. Asymmetric bitemporoparietal hypoperfusion has frequently been reported in established AD patients (Neary et al. 1987; Burns et al. 1989; Montaldi et al. 1990; McKeith et al. 1993; Talbot et al. 1995) and anterior changes in cerebral blood flow have been described in patients with FTD (Neary et al. 1987; Miller et al. 1991; Starkstein et al. 1994; Talbot et al. 1995). The usefulness of SPECT scanning as a diagnostic test has, however, been questioned. Greene et al. (1996a) found that SPECT was insensitive in a group of 33 patients with mild AD, with 39% of the AD patients having normal SPECT scans. Neuropsychological tests were far more sensitive in differentiating the AD patients from controls. Furthermore, there was very little association between SPECT data and severity of dementia as assessed by the MMSE. A recent study by Nebu et al. (2001) questioned the poor discriminatory power of SPECT in studies of AD and controls, and suggested that methodological differences between centres may account for these results. In a study of ten patients with very early AD (CDR 0.5), compared with healthy controls, using temporal-lobe-orientated HMPAO-SPECT scanning and high-quality image analysis, they found that the regional cerebral blood-flow ratio of the bilateral medial temporal lobe region was significantly lower in the AD patients than controls, although no other differences were observed. They suggested that SPECT scans using images parallel to the long axis of the hippocampus might be sensitive tools for the diagnosis of AD even in the very early amnesic stage of disease.

A number of studies have investigated the use of SPECT in distinguishing between different dementia syndromes. Results in these studies have again been rather inconsistent. By calculating a ratio of anterior to posterior cerebral blood flow on SPECT (mesial superior frontal gyrus / medial temporal lobes) patients with FTD were separable from other dementia groups and controls with a sensitivity of 87.5% and a specificity of 78.6% (Sjogren et al. 2000). Typical hypoperfusion of the biparietal region and medial temporal lobes was seen in the AD group, but although this pattern of regional blood flow was able to discriminate AD from FTD and controls, it was extremely similar to the changes seen in the patient group with subcortical white matter disease. Talbot et al. (1998) investigated the use of SPECT in the diagnosis of individual subjects rather than groups of dementia patients, in order to assess its true clinical application. They carried out a longitudinal study of 363 consecutive patient referrals over a 6-year period with SPECT scans at baseline. They found that on an individual case basis, SPECT scanning was most useful for distinguishing between AD vs. VaD and FTD, and least useful for differentiating between AD vs. DLB or VaD vs. FTD and progressive aphasia. In conclusion, they suggested that the role of SPECT was confirmatory rather than diagnostic, and provided support for a diagnosis of, for example, AD, only when a particular differential diagnosis was considered.

PET studies, in contrast to SPECT, are capable of providing quantitative measures of brain function. A variety of positron-emitting tracers have been developed, enabling researchers to examine parameters such as glucose metabolism, oxygen consumption, cerebral blood flow or neurotransmitter activity. Although PET (specifically, that which utilizes fluorodeoxyglucose as a marker of glucose metabolism) has been shown to be the most sensitive imaging technique in AD, availability of PET is extremely limited in the UK, and it remains a research tool rather than a clinical test. A large number of PET studies have documented typical regional deficits in AD, with asymmetric biparietotemporal hypometabolism similar to changes seen in regional blood flow with SPECT (Frackowiak et al. 1981; Foster et al. 1983; de Leon et al. 1983; Duara et al. 1986). It has been clarified subsequently that these deficits are due to genuine hypometabolism in brain tissue and not merely an artefact of atrophy. For instance, Ibanez et al. (1998) applied a correction for the partial volume effect of atrophy and demonstrated that regional hypometabolism in AD remained significant. The study did find that in more severely affected subjects the correction had a greater impact on results (suggesting that atrophy does contribute to reductions in regional metabolic rate) but that even in those circumstances true reductions in metabolism per gram of tissue were the most important factor.

Rather surprisingly, medial temporal lobe hypometabolism has not generally been shown in AD patients, even though this region is known to be affected early in the course of disease and functional imaging of this region might be presumed to be of greatest predictive value in patients with MCI. This may reflect the low spatial resolution of PET when attempting to image small structures such as the hippocampus, although work by Minoshima et al. (1997) has offered insights into this apparent paradox. They showed that the earliest region of cortical hypometabolism in subjects with very early AD is the posterior cingulate cortex. As this region is heavily connected with the mesial temporal lobe through the network known as the circuit of Papez (1995) it may be that the posterior cingulate abnormality is, at least in part, a manifestation of deafferentation due to pathology in the mesial temporal region. It should be noted that metabolic activity in the brain, as measured by PET, is thought to largely represent activity at synapses rather than cell bodies. In support of this hypothesis, Minoshima et al. (1999) have subsequently conducted a study using ^{15}O-water as a marker of cerebral perfusion in patients before and after left mesial temporal lobectomy for the treatment of epilepsy. They found that postsurgery, there was a significant reduction of activity in the posterior cingulate and thalamus consistent with the notion that diminished synaptic activity can occur when cell bodies remote from their own synapses are lesioned. Nevertheless, these findings fail to explain the abnormalities in association cortex seen with PET. Given that AD is also known to be associated with a significant loss of synaptic density in the neocortex (DeKosky and Scheff 1990; Terry et al. 1991) it may be that this contributes more to the association cortex dysfunction than the classic histopathological changes of plaques and tangles. Although PET's greatest contribution has been in neocortical imaging, the fact remains that the mesial temporal lobes are the site of the earliest histopathological change and that a vast body of neuropsychological evidence suggests the key role of this region in memory – the very cognitive domain first to malfunction in AD. To this end recent work with high-resolution FDG–PET in AD has yielded very interesting results: in a study by Eustache et al. (2001) a correlation was found between hypometabolism in the left entorhinal cortex and poor performance on a verbal episodic memory task.

The role of PET in the investigation of 'at-risk' cases has been the topic of a considerable number of studies. Kennedy et al. (1995) studied asymptomatic individuals (family members of patients with known genetic mutation for familial AD). In this group of 24 subjects, parietotemporal hypometabolism was noted, which was similar, though less extensive, than that seen in patients with established AD. It has also been shown that measures of cerebral metabolism in subjects with MCI or questionable AD are closely correlated with progression of clinical symptoms (Small et al. 1995; Herholz et al. 1999). In a recent longitudinal study by Jelic and Nordberg (2000), PET patterns of hypometabolism were shown to be highly predictive for conversion from MCI to AD. Using a ratio of parietal association cortex / frontal association cortex glucose metabolism at baseline, corrected for MMSE, clinical outcome in 27 subjects, 26% of whom converted to AD during the 24-month follow-up period, was correctly predicted in 93% of cases.

Patients with DLB have also been found to have a pattern of decreased metabolism in the fronto-temporo-parietal association and limbic cortex (Imamura et al. 1997; Ishii et al. 1998a), suggesting that there is considerable overlap between AD and DLB in terms of patterns of regional metabolism, although DLB may be distinguished by greater occipital hypometabolism (Vander Borght et al. 1997). This pattern has also been found in patients with Parkinson's disease and dementia and is consistent with a number of other functional-imaging studies in DLB (Albin et al. 1996; Vander Borght et al. 1997). PET studies in FTD, in line with findings from SPECT, have typically shown changes in cerebral metabolism, or perfusion, in frontal and temporal regions, often evident before MRI findings of atrophy (Neary et al. 1987; Miller et al. 1991; Ishii et al. 1998b). Frontal hypometabolism has, however, been demonstrated in normal healthy elderly (Kuhl et al. 1982; Leenders et al. 1990; Salmon et al. 1991; Petit-Taboue et al. 1998). A recent study by Garraux et al. (1999) attempted to distinguish between the changes of normal ageing, and patterns of hypometabolism in FTD and progressive supranuclear palsy (PSP) patients: frontal metabolism was noted in the elderly controls compared with the young controls, but quantitative measures of metabolism in this region were able to discriminate the FTD patients from age-matched controls.

Distinguishing dementia of vascular aetiology from other forms of dementia remains difficult. This is largely because a significant proportion of patients with apparently pure AD also shows high signal intensities on T2 MRI of the type seen in patients with cerebrovascular disease. A number of investigators have, therefore, explored whether PET may be a useful tool in distinguishing AD from VaD, and indeed, whether VaD patients, as a group, show a characteristic pattern of metabolic changes (Jellinger 1998). De Reuck et al. (1998) described temporal and parietal changes in regional cerebral blood flow and oxygen metabolism in patients with 'pure' vascular dementia, but these changes were very similar to those described in AD. Furthermore, the total volume of hypometabolic regions related to the severity of dementia has not been found to differ between AD and VaD (Mielke and Heiss 1998). Mendez et al. (1999) studied 30 patients with insidious progression of cognitive decline meeting dementia criteria, all of whom had evidence of moderate to severe subcortical white matter lesions on MRI. They used PET to assign subjects to two groups: those with a pattern of temporoparietal hypometabolism, typical of AD, and those without this pattern. There was no difference in incidence of vascular risk factors between the two groups, but the latter group was significantly worse on tasks of sustained attention, and better on tests of recognition memory than the former group, a neuropsychological pattern more typical of VaD. They concluded that PET might help to distinguish those patients with leukoaraiosis and predominant AD from those who have a greater contribution from VaD. Although interesting, these results clearly require neuropathological confirmation.

Overall, both structural and functional imaging have provided new insights into the pattern and progression of regional cortical changes in these disorders, providing results of great theoretical interest. The practical application of these neuro-imaging techniques, however, remains relatively limited. SPECT can be viewed at present as a confirmatory tool in the diagnosis of different dementia syndromes, but its role in early diagnosis requires further investigation. PET has provided many useful windows into the understanding of regional cerebral metabolism in different dementia aetiologies, but remains very much a research methodology.

Conclusions

In this review we have only touched on two areas of progress in dementia research. There have in addition been very significant advances in the study of epidemiology, neuropathology and pathophysiology of the dementias. As research progressively unravels the neurobiology of these degenerative diseases, through all avenues of investigation, we come closer to finding effective symptomatic and hopefully curative treatments. As we have demonstrated, this has been a very fertile area of study over recent years and we now have within our grasp methods of early and discriminatory diagnosis of different dementia syndromes, using both neuropsychology and neuro-imaging. There is clearly room for refinement of these techniques, and the wealth of ongoing investigation in these areas continues to address the problems of specificity and sensitivity of diagnostic tools. In practical terms, these advances may allow earlier intervention with disease-modifying therapies, and thus achieve the goal of arresting disease progression before the development of significant cognitive disability.

REFERENCES

Albin RL, Minoshima S, D'Amato CJ, Frey KA, Kuhl DA and Sima AA (1996). Fluoro-deoxyglucose positron emission tomography in diffuse Lewy body disease. *Neurology*, 47, 462–6.

Almkvist O (1994). Neuropsychological deficits in vascular dementia in relation to Alzheimer's disease: reviewing evidence for functional similarity or divergence. *Dementia*, 5, 203–9.

Ballard C, McKeith I, Harrison R et al. (1997). A detailed phenomenological comparison of complex visual hallucinations in dementia with Lewy bodies and Alzheimer's disease. *Int Psychogeriatr*, 9, 381–8.

Barber R, Gholkar A, Scheltens P, Ballard C, McKeith IG and O'Brien JT (1999). Medial temporal lobe atrophy on MRI in dementia with Lewy bodies. *Neurology*, 52, 1153–8.

Benson DF and Zaias BW (1991). Progressive aphasia: a case with a postmortem correlation. *Neuropsychiatry Neuropsychol Behav Neurol*, 4, 215–23.

Benson DF, Davis RJ and Snyder BD (1988). Posterior cortical atrophy. *Arch Neurol*, 45, 789–93.

Benveniste H, Einstein G, Kim KR, Hulette C and Johnson GA (1999). Detection of neuritic plaques in Alzheimer's disease by magnetic resonance microscopy. *Proc Natl Acad Sci USA*, 96, 14079–84.

Berg L (1988). Clinical Dementia Rating (CDR). *Psychopharmacol Bull*, 24, 637–9.

Berthier ML, Leiguarda R, Starkstein SE, Sevlever G and Taratuto AL (1991). Alzheimer's disease in a patient with posterior cortical atrophy. *J Neurol Neurosurg Psychiatry*, 54, 1110–11.

Binetti G, Cappa SF, Magni E, Padovani A, Bianchetti A and Trabucchi M (1998). Visual and spatial perception in the early phase of Alzheimer's disease. *Neuropsychology*, 12, 29–33.

Bozeat S, Gregory CA, Ralph MA and Hodges JR (2000). Which neuropsychiatric and be-havioural features distinguish frontal and temporal variants of frontotemporal dementia from Alzheimer's disease? *J Neurol Neurosurg Psychiatry*, 69, 178–86.

Braak H and Braak E (1991). Neuropathological staging of Alzheimer-related changes. *Acta Neuropathol*, 82, 239–59.

Burns A, Philpot MP, Costa DC, Ell PJ and Levy R (1989). The investigation of Alzheimer's disease with single photon emission tomography. *J Neurol Neurosurg Psychiatry*, 52, 248–53.

Calderon J, Perry RJ, Erzinclioglu SW, Berrios GE, Dening TR and Hodges JR (2001). Perception, attention, and working memory are disproportionately impaired in dementia with Lewy bodies compared with Alzheimer's disease. *J Neurol Neurosurg Psychiatry*, 70, 157–64.

Celsis P (2000). Age-related cognitive decline, mild cognitive impairment or preclinical Alzheimer's disease? *Ann Med*, 32, 6–14.

Chan AS, Butters N and Salmon DP (1997). The deterioration of semantic networks in patients with Alzheimer's disease: a cross-sectional study. *Neuropsychologia*, 35, 241–8.

Chertkow H and Bub D (1990). Semantic memory loss in dementia of Alzheimer's type. What do various measures measure? *Brain*, 113, 397–417.

Cogan DG (1985). Visual disturbances with focal progressive dementing disease. *Am J Ophthalmol*, 100, 68–72.

Convit A, De Leon MJ, Tarshish C et al. (1997). Specific hippocampal volume reductions in individuals at risk for Alzheimer's disease. *Neurobiol Aging*, 18, 131–8.

Cummings JL (1997). The Neuropsychiatric Inventory: assessing psychopathology in dementia patients. *Neurology*, 48 (Suppl. 6), S10–16.

Cummings JL, Petry S, Dian L, Shapira J and Hill MA (1990). Organic personality disorder in dementia syndromes: an inventory approach. *J Neuropsychiatry Clin Neurosci*, 2, 261–7.

DeKosky ST and Scheff SW (1990). Synapse loss in frontal cortex biopsies in Alzheimer's disease: correlation with cognitive severity. *Ann Neurol*, 27, 457–64.

Desmond DW (1996). Vascular dementia: a construct in evolution. *Cerebrovasc Brain Metab Rev*, 8, 296–325.

Duara R, Grady C, Haxby J et al. (1986). Positron emission tomography in Alzheimer's disease. *Neurology*, 36, 879–87.

Elfgren C, Brun A, Gustafson L et al. (1994). Neuropsychological tests as discriminators between dementia of Alzheimer's type and frontotemporal dementia. *Int J Geriatr Psychiatry*, 9, 635–42.

Eustache F, Desgranges B, Giffard B, de la Sayette V and Baron JC (2001). Entorhinal cortex disruption causes memory deficit in early Alzheimer's disease as shown by PET. *Neuroreport*, 12, 683–5.

Evans DA, Funkenstein HH, Albert MS et al. (1989). Prevalence of Alzheimer's disease in a community population of older persons. Higher than previously reported. *J Am Med Assoc*, 262, 2551–6.

Fabrigoule C, Rouch I, Taberly A et al. (1998). Cognitive process in preclinical phase of dementia. *Brain*, 121, 135–41.

Foster NL, Chase TN, Fedio P, Patronas NJ, Brooks RA and Di Chiro G (1983). Alzheimer's disease: focal cortical changes shown by positron emission tomography. *Neurology*, 33, 961–5.

Fox NC and Rossor MN (2000). Seeing what Alzheimer saw – with magnetic resonance microscopy. *Nat Med*, 6, 20–1.

Fox NC, Freeborough PA and Rossor MN (1996). Visualisation and quantification of rates of atrophy in Alzheimer's disease. *Lancet*, 348, 94–7.

Fox NC, Warrington EK, Seiffer AL, Agnew SK and Rossor MN (1998). Presymptomatic cognitive deficits in individuals at risk of familial Alzheimer's disease. A longitudinal prospective study. *Brain*, 121, 1631–9.

Fox NC, Scahill RI, Crum WR and Rossor MN (1999*a*). Correlation between rates of brain atrophy and cognitive decline in AD. *Neurology*, 52, 1687–9.

Fox NC, Warrington EK and Rossor MN (1999*b*). Serial magnetic resonance imaging of cerebral atrophy in preclinical Alzheimer's disease. *Lancet*, 353, 2125.

Frackowiak RS, Pozzilli C, Legg NJ et al. (1981). Regional cerebral oxygen supply and utilization in dementia. A clinical and physiological study with oxygen-15 and positron tomography. *Brain*, 104, 753–78.

Frisoni GB, Pizzolato G, Geroldi C, Rossato A, Bianchetti A and Trabucchi M (1995). Dementia of the frontal type: neuropsychological and [99Tc]-HM-PAO SPET features. *J Geriatr Psychiatry Neurol*, 8, 42–8.

Frisoni GB, Laakso MP, Beltramello A et al. (1999). Hippocampal and entorhinal cortex atrophy in frontotemporal dementia and Alzheimer's disease. *Neurology*, 52, 91–100.

Galton CJ, Patterson K, Xuereb JH and Hodges JR (2000). Atypical and typical presentations of Alzheimer's disease: a clinical, neuropsychological, neuroimaging and pathological study of 13 cases. *Brain*, 123, 484–98.

Galton CJ, Gomez-Anson B, Antoun N et al. (2001). Temporal lobe rating scale: application to Alzheimer's disease and frontotemporal dementia. *J Neurol Neurosurg Psychiatry*, 70, 165–73.

Garraux G, Salmon E, Degueldre C, Lemaire C, Laureys S and Franck G (1999). Comparison of impaired subcortico-frontal metabolic networks in normal aging, subcortico-frontal dementia, and cortical frontal dementia. *Neuroimage*, 10, 149–62.

Gnanalingham KK, Byrne EJ, Thornton A, Sambrook MA and Bannister P (1997). Motor and cognitive function in Lewy body dementia: comparison with Alzheimer's and Parkinson's diseases. *J Neurol Neurosurg Psychiatry*, 62, 243–52.

Grady CL, Haxby JV, Horwitz B et al. (1988). Longitudinal study of the early neuropsychological and cerebral metabolic changes in dementia of the Alzheimer type. *J Clin Exp Neuropsychol*, 10, 576–96.

Green J, Morris JC, Sandson J, McKeel DW Jr and Miller JW (1990). Progressive aphasia: a precursor of global dementia? *Neurology*, 40, 423–9.

Greene JD, Miles K and Hodges JR (1996*a*). Neuropsychology of memory and SPECT in the diagnosis and staging of dementia of Alzheimer type. *J Neurol*, 243, 175–90.

Greene JD, Patterson K, Xuereb J and Hodges JR (1996*b*). Alzheimer disease and nonfluent progressive aphasia. *Arch Neurol*, 53, 1072–8.

Gregory CA, Orrel M, Sahakian B and Hodges JR (1997). Can fronto-temporal dementia and Alzheimer's disease be differentiated using a brief battery of tests? *Int J Geriatr Psychiatry*, 12, 375–83.

Hansen L, Salmon D, Galasko D et al. (1990). The Lewy body variant of Alzheimer's disease: a clinical and pathologic entity. *Neurology*, 40, 1–8.

Hargrave R, Geck LC, Reed B and Mungas D (2000). Affective behavioural disturbances in Alzheimer's disease and ischaemic vascular disease. *J Neurol Neurosurg Psychiatry*, 68, 41–6.

Hashimoto M, Kitagaki H, Imamura T et al. (1998). Medial temporal and whole-brain atrophy in dementia with Lewy bodies: a volumetric MRI study. *Neurology*, 51, 357–62.

Herholz K, Nordberg A, Salmon E et al. (1999). Impairment of neocortical metabolism predicts progression in Alzheimer's disease. *Dement Geriatr Cogn Disord*, 10, 494–504.

Hodges J (1998). The amnestic prodrome of Alzheimer's disease. *Brain*, 121, 1601–2.

Hodges JR and Patterson K (1995). Is semantic memory consistently impaired early in the course of Alzheimer's disease? Neuroanatomical and diagnostic implications. *Neuropsychologia*, 33, 441–59.

Hodges JR, Patterson K, Oxbury S and Funnell E (1992). Semantic dementia: progressive fluent aphasia with temporal lobe atrophy. *Brain*, 115, 1783–806.

Hodges JR, Patterson K, Ward R et al. (1999). The differentiation of semantic dementia and frontal lobe dementia (temporal and frontal variants of frontotemporal dementia) from early Alzheimer's disease: a comparative neuropsychological study. *Neuropsychology*, 13, 31–40.

Hyman BT, Van Hoesen GW, Kromer LJ and Damasio AR (1986). Perforant pathway changes and the memory impairment of Alzheimer's disease. *Ann Neurol*, 20, 472–81.

Ibanez V, Pietrini P, Alexander GE et al. (1998). Regional glucose metabolic abnormalities are not the result of atrophy in Alzheimer's disease. *Neurology*, 50, 1585–93.

Imamura T, Ishii K, Sasaki M et al. (1997). Regional cerebral glucose metabolism in dementia with Lewy bodies and Alzheimer's disease: a comparative study using positron emission tomography. *Neurosci Lett*, 235, 49–52.

Ishii K, Imamura T, Sasaki M et al. (1998*a*). Regional cerebral glucose metabolism in dementia with Lewy bodies and Alzheimer's disease. *Neurology*, 51, 125–30.

Ishii K, Sakamoto S, Sasaki M et al. (1998*b*). Cerebral glucose metabolism in patients with frontotemporal dementia. *J Nucl Med*, 39, 1875–8.

Jack CR, Jr, Petersen RC, Xu YC et al. (1999). Prediction of AD with MRI-based hippocampal volume in mild cognitive impairment. *Neurology*, 52, 1397–403.

Jacobs DM, Sano M, Dooneief G, Marder K, Bell KL and Stern Y (1995). Neuropsychological detection and characterization of preclinical Alzheimer's disease. *Neurology*, 45, 957–62.

Jelic V and Nordberg A (2000). Early diagnosis of Alzheimer disease with positron emission tomography. *Alzheimer Dis Assoc Disord*, 14 (Suppl. 1), S109–13.

Jellinger KA (1998). Positron emission tomography in vascular dementia. *J Neurol Sci*, 160, 190–1.

Kennedy AM, Frackowiak RS, Newman SK et al. (1995). Deficits in cerebral glucose metabolism demonstrated by positron emission tomography in individuals at risk of familial Alzheimer's disease. *Neurosci Lett*, 186, 17–20.

Knopman DS, Mastri AR, Frey WH 2nd, Sung JH and Rustan T (1990). Dementia lacking distinctive histologic features: a common non-Alzheimer degenerative dementia. *Neurology*, 40, 251–6.

Krasuski JS and Gaviria M (1994). Neuropsychiatric sequelae of ischaemic cerebrovascular disease: clinical and neuroanatomic correlates and implications for the concept of dementia. *Neurol Res*, 16, 241–50.

Kuhl DE, Metter EJ, Riege WH and Phelps ME (1982). Effects of human aging on patterns of local cerebral glucose utilization determined by the [18F]fluorodeoxyglucose method. *J Cereb Blood Flow Metab*, 2, 163–71.

Lambon Ralph MA, Patterson K and Hodges JR (1997). The relationship between naming and semantic knowledge for different categories in dementia of Alzheimer's type. *Neuropsychologia*, 35, 1251–60.

Lambon Ralph MA, Powell J, Howard D, Whitworth AB, Garrard P and Hodges JR (2001). Semantic memory is impaired in both dementia with Lewy bodies and dementia of Alzheimer's type: a comparative neuropsychological study and literature review. *J Neurol Neurosurg Psychiatry*, 70, 149–56.

Leenders KL, Perani D, Lammertsma AA et al. (1990). Cerebral blood flow, blood volume and oxygen utilization. Normal values and effect of age. *Brain*, 113, 27–47.

de Leon MJ, Ferris SH, George AE et al. (1983). Computed tomography and positron emission transaxial tomography evaluations of normal aging and Alzheimer's disease. *J Cereb Blood Flow Metab*, 3, 391–4.

Linn RT, Wolf PA, Bachman DL et al. (1995). The 'preclinical phase' of probable Alzheimer's disease. A 13-year prospective study of the Framingham cohort. *Arch Neurol*, 52, 485–90.

Locascio JJ, Growdon JH and Corkin S (1995). Cognitive test performance in detecting, staging, and tracking Alzheimer's disease. *Arch Neurol*, 52, 1087–99.

Loeb C and Meyer JS (2000). Criteria for diagnosis of vascular dementia. *Arch Neurol*, 57, 1382–3.

Looi JC and Sachdev PS (1999). Differentiation of vascular dementia from AD on neuropsychological tests. *Neurology*, 53, 670–8.

Masur DM, Sliwinski M, Lipton RB, Blau AD and Crystal HA (1994). Neuropsychological prediction of dementia and the absence of dementia in healthy elderly persons. *Neurology*, 44, 1427–32.

Mathuranath PS, Nestor PJ, Berrios GE, Rakowicz W and Hodges JR (2000). A brief cognitive test battery to differentiate Alzheimer's disease and frontotemporal dementia. *Neurology*, 55, 1613–20.

McKeith IG (1988). Dementia with Lewy bodies: clinical and pathological diagnosis. *Alzheimer's Rep*, 1, 83–7.

McKeith IG, Bartholomew PH, Irvine EM, Cook J, Adams R and Simpson AE (1993). Single photon emission computerised tomography in elderly patients with Alzheimer's disease and multi-infarct dementia. Regional uptake of technetium-labelled HMPAO related to clinical measurements. *Br J Psychiatry*, 163, 597–603.

McKeith IG, Galasko D, Kosaka K et al. (1996). Consensus guidelines for the clinical and pathologic diagnosis of dementia with Lewy bodies (DLB): report of the consortium on DLB international workshop. *Neurology*, 47, 1113–24.

McKenna P and Warrington EK (1980). Testing for nominal dysphasia. *J Neurol Neurosurg Psychiatry*, 43, 781–8.

Mendez MF, Mendez MA, Martin R, Smyth KA and Whitehouse PJ (1990). Complex visual disturbances in Alzheimer's disease. *Neurology*, 40, 439–43.

Mendez MF, Ottowitz W, Brown CV, Cummings JL, Perryman KM and Mandelkern MA (1999). Dementia with leukoaraiosis: clinical differentiation by temporoparietal hypometabolism on (18)FDG-PET imaging. *Dement Geriatr Cogn Disord*, 10, 518–25.

Mielke R and Heiss WD (1998). Positron emission tomography for diagnosis of Alzheimer's disease and vascular dementia. *J Neural Transm Suppl*, 53, 237–50.

Miller BL, Cummings JL, Villanueva-Meyer J et al. (1991). Frontal lobe degeneration: clinical, neuropsychological, and SPECT characteristics. *Neurology*, 41, 1374–82.

Minoshima S, Giordani B, Berent S, Frey KA, Foster NL and Kuhl DE (1997). Metabolic reduction in the posterior cingulate cortex in very early Alzheimer's disease. *Ann Neurol*, 42, 85–94.

Minoshima S, Cross DJ, Foster NL, Henry TR and Kuhl DE (1999). Discordance between traditional pathologic and energy metabolic changes in very early Alzheimer's disease. Pathophysiological implications. *Ann NY Acad Sci*, 893, 350–2.

Montaldi D, Brooks DN, McColl JH et al. (1990). Measurements of regional cerebral blood flow and cognitive performance in Alzheimer's disease. *J Neurol Neurosurg Psychiatry*, 53, 33–8.

Neary D, Snowden JS, Shields RA et al. (1987). Single photon emission tomography using 99mTc-HM-PAO in the investigation of dementia. *J Neurol Neurosurg Psychiatry*, 50, 1101–9.

Nebu A, Ikeda M, Fukuhara R et al. (2001). Utility of (99m)Tc-HM-PAO SPECT hippocampal image to diagnose early stages of Alzheimer's disease using semiquantitative analysis. *Dement Geriatr Cogn Disord*, 12, 153–7.

Papez JW (1995). A proposed mechanism of emotion. 1937. *J Neuropsychiatry Clin Neurosci*, 7, 103–12.

Perry RJ and Hodges JR (2000*a*). Differentiating frontal and temporal variant frontotemporal dementia from Alzheimer's disease. *Neurology*, 54, 2277–84.

Perry RJ and Hodges JR (2000*b*). Fate of patients with questionable (very mild) Alzheimer's disease: longitudinal profiles of individual subjects' decline. *Dement Geriatr Cogn Disord*, 11, 342–9.

Perry RH, Irving D, Blessed G, Fairbairn A and Perry EK (1990). Senile dementia of Lewy body type. A clinically and neuropathologically distinct form of Lewy body dementia in the elderly. *J Neurol Sci*, 95, 119–39.

Petersen RC, Smith GE, Waring SC, Ivnik RJ, Kokmen E and Tangelos EG (1997). Aging, memory, and mild cognitive impairment. *Int Psychogeriatr*, 9 (Suppl. 1), 65–9.

Petit-Taboue MC, Landeau B, Desson JF, Desgranges B and Baron JC (1998). Effects of healthy aging on the regional cerebral metabolic rate of glucose assessed with statistical parametric mapping. *Neuroimage*, 7, 176–84.

Petry S, Cummings JL, Hill MA and Shapira J (1988). Personality alterations in dementia of the Alzheimer type. *Arch Neurol*, 45, 1187–90.

Pogacar S and Williams RS (1984). Alzheimer's disease presenting as slowly progressive aphasia. *R I Med J*, 67, 181–5.

Pruessner JC, Li LM, Serles W et al. (2000). Volumetry of hippocampus and amygdala with high-resolution MRI and three-dimensional analysis software: minimizing the discrepancies between laboratories. *Cereb Cortex*, 10, 433–42.

Rahman S, Sahakian BJ, Hodges JR, Rogers RD and Robbins TW (1999). Specific cognitive deficits in mild frontal variant frontotemporal dementia. *Brain*, 122, 1469–93.

de Renzi E (1986). Slowly progressive visual agnosia or apraxia without dementia. *Cortex*, 22, 171–80.

de Reuck J, Decoo D, Marchau M, Santens P, Lemahieu I and Strijckmans K (1998). Positron emission tomography in vascular dementia. *J Neurol Sci*, 154, 55–61.

Ritchie K and Touchon J (2000). Mild cognitive impairment: conceptual basis and current nosological status. *Lancet*, 355, 225–8.

Rosen WG, Mohs RC and Davis KL (1984). A new rating scale for Alzheimer's disease. *Am J Psychiatry*, 141, 1356–64.

Ross SJ, Graham N, Stuart-Green L et al. (1996). Progressive biparietal atrophy: an atypical presentation of Alzheimer's disease. *J Neurol Neurosurg Psychiatry*, 61, 388–95.

Rubin EH, Storandt M, Miller JP et al. (1998). A prospective study of cognitive function and onset of dementia in cognitively healthy elders. *Arch Neurol*, 55, 395–401.

Sahakian BJ, Morris RG, Evenden JL et al. (1988). A comparative study of visuospatial memory and learning in Alzheimer-type dementia and Parkinson's disease. *Brain*, 111, 695–718.

Sahgal A, Galloway PH, McKeith IG and Edwardson AJ (1992). A comparative study of attentional deficits in senile dementias of Alzheimer and Lewy body types. *Dementia*, 3, 350–4.

Salmon E, Maquet P, Sadzot B, Degueldre C, Lemaire C and Franck G (1991). Decrease of frontal metabolism demonstrated by positron emission tomography in a population of healthy elderly volunteers. *Acta Neurol Belg*, 91, 288–95.

Scheltens P, Leys D, Barkhof F et al. (1992). Atrophy of medial temporal lobes on MRI in Alzheimer's disease and normal ageing: diagnostic value and neuropsychological correlates. *J Neurol Neurosurg Psychiatry*, 55, 967–72.

Sjogren M, Gustafson L, Wikkelso C and Wallin A (2000). Frontotemporal dementia can be distinguished from Alzheimer's disease and subcortical white matter dementia by an anterior-to-posterior rCBF-SPET ratio. *Dement Geriatr Cogn Disord*, 11, 275–85.

Small GW, La Rue A, Komo S, Kaplan A and Mandelkern MA (1995). Predictors of cognitive change in middle-aged and older adults with memory loss. *Am J Psychiatry*, 152, 1757–64.

Snowden JS, Bathgate D, Varma A, Blackshaw A, Gibbons ZC and Neary D (2001). Distinct behavioural profiles in frontotemporal dementia and semantic dementia. *J Neurol Neurosurg Psychiatry*, 70, 323–32.

Starkstein SE, Migliorelli R, Teson A et al. (1994). Specificity of changes in cerebral blood flow in patients with frontal lobe dementia. *J Neurol Neurosurg Psychiatry*, 57, 790–6.

Sultzer DL, Levin HS, Mahler ME, High WM and Cummings JL (1992). Assessment of cognitive, psychiatric, and behavioural disturbances in patients with dementia: the Neurobehavioural Rating Scale. *J Am Geriatr Soc*, 40, 549–55.

Swainson R, Hodges JR, Galton CJ et al. (2001). Early detection and differential diagnosis of Alzheimer's disease and depression with neuropsychological tasks. *Dement Geriatr Cogn Disord*, 12, 265–80.

Talbot PR, Snowden JS, Lloyd JJ, Neary D and Testa HJ (1995). The contribution of single photon emission tomography to the clinical differentiation of degenerative cortical brain disorders. *J Neurol*, 242, 579–86.

Talbot PR, Lloyd JJ, Snowden JS, Neary D and Testa HJ (1998). A clinical role for 99mTc-HMPAO SPECT in the investigation of dementia? *J Neurol Neurosurg Psychiatry*, 64, 306–13.

Tariot PN, Mack JL, Patterson MB et al. (1995). The Behavior Rating Scale for Dementia of the Consortium to Establish a Registry for Alzheimer's Disease. The Behavioural Pathology Committee of the Consortium to Establish a Registry for Alzheimer's Disease. *Am J Psychiatry*, 152, 1349–57.

Terry RD, Masliah E, Salmon DP et al. (1991). Physical basis of cognitive alterations in Alzheimer's disease: synapse loss is the major correlate of cognitive impairment. *Ann Neurol*, 30, 572–80.

Tulving E (1987). Multiple memory systems and consciousness. *Hum Neurobiol*, 6, 67–80.

Vander Borght T, Minoshima S, Giordani B et al. (1997). Cerebral metabolic differences in Parkinson's and Alzheimer's diseases matched for dementia severity. *J Nucl Med*, 38, 797–802.

Van Hoesen GW (1997). Ventromedial temporal lobe anatomy, with comments on Alzheimer's disease and temporal injury. *J Neuropsychiatry Clin Neurosci*, 9, 331–41.

Van Hoesen GW, Hyman BT and Damasio AR (1991). Entorhinal cortex pathology in Alzheimer's disease. *Hippocampus*, 1, 1–8.

Victoroff J, Ross GW, Benson DF, Verity MA and Vinters HV (1994). Posterior cortical atrophy. Neuropathologic correlations. *Arch Neurol*, 51, 269–74.

Warrington EK (1996). *Camden Memory Tests.* Hove: Psychological Press.

Warrington EK and James M (1991). *The Visual Object and Space Perception Battery.* Bury St Edmunds: Thames Valley Test Company.

Wechsler D (1987). *Wechsler Memory Scale–Revised.* San Antonio, TX: Psychological Corporation.

Welsh K, Butters N, Hughes J, Mohs R and Heyman A (1991). Detection of abnormal memory decline in mild cases of Alzheimer's disease using CERAD neuropsychological measures. *Arch Neurol*, 48, 278–81.

Part VII

Affective illness

14

The neuropathology of mood disorders

Paul J Harrison[1,2] and Rebecca Gittins[2]

[1]Warneford Hospital, Oxford, UK; [2]Radcliffe Infirmary, Oxford, UK

Introduction

Mood (affective) disorders exemplify the distinction made in psychiatric classifications between organic and functional. Hence, in ICD–10, organic mood disorders are those with a 'presumed direct causation by a cerebral or other physical disorder'. As such, the category includes mood disorders associated with overt neuropathology, e.g. a meningioma, cerebral vasculitis or Huntington's disease. Although ICD–10 emphasizes that functional disorders are not lacking an organic component, they are defined by an absence of demonstrable, established features of this kind. From a neuropathological perspective, until recently there has been no reason to question this basic assumption as it applies to mood disorders: there were few studies, and no convincing data (Jeste et al. 1988). Whilst the neuropathological understanding of mood disorders is still rudimentary, and far from contributing in any diagnostic or clinical sense, structural correlates are beginning to emerge. The focus here is upon the recent postmortem studies of mood disorder, followed by discussion of the methodological and conceptual issues affecting their interpretation.

Anterior cingulate cortex

The anterior cingulate cortex surrounds the corpus callosum on the medial surface of the frontal lobe. It consists mainly of Brodmann area 24 (Figure 14.1, colour plate). It has long been implicated in affective and emotional processing and their disorders because of neuropsychological, anatomical and functional imaging data (Bench et al. 1992; Devinsky et al. 1995; Ebert and Ebmeier 1996; Price 1999). The main stimulus to histological studies was an MRI report that a specific part of the anterior cingulate cortex, the subgenual region (sg24, also called subgenual (prefrontal) cortex), was 40% smaller in a group of 38 subjects with familial mood disorder compared with 21 controls (Drevets et al. 1997). The sg24 volume decrease was left-sided, and seen in both unipolar and bipolar disorder. The results were extended by Hirayasu et al. (1999), who found left subgenual cortex volume reductions of 25% in 14 patients with first-episode affective psychosis and a family history of mood disorder in first- or second-degree relatives, compared with 20 controls. Lesser and nonsignificant trends were seen in the right hemisphere, in first-episode schizophrenia (n = 17), and in affective-psychosis patients with no family history (n = 10).

Drevets and colleagues proceeded to investigate the cellular correlates of the subgenual volume reduction, in what is likely to become a landmark paper (Öngür et al. 1998), being the first reasonably large and well-conducted neuropathological study of mood disorder and also because of the striking results (Table 14.1). First, in a pilot study, Öngür et al. (1998) identified decreased left sg24 volume and a decreased density and number of glia, though neither finding was conclusive due to the small sample size. To rectify this, the authors carried out a follow-on study using tissue from the Stanley Foundation Neuropathology Consortium, which comprises 15 brains from individuals in each of four groups: major depression, bipolar disorder, schizophrenia and controls (Torrey et al. 2000). The groups are matched for age (mean ~45 years), sex, postmortem interval and brain pH (a marker of agonal hypoxia), and have unusually good documentation, including family, medication and substance misuse histories. In this series, the decrease of glial density and number in sg24 in major depression and bipolar disorder was confirmed, with equivocally larger deficits in familial cases. The decrease was 20–40%. It was also seen in orbitofrontal cortex (though these data were not presented). There were no changes in glial size, or in neuronal density, number or size, no alterations in primary somatosensory cortex (area 3b), and no glial deficits in schizophrenia. No analyses of possible hemispheric differences were presented. Neither medication nor substance abuse seemed to explain the results. A reduction of glia therefore provided the main cellular correlate of the sg24 volume reductions seen previously though, as the authors point out, it is unclear what proportion of the volume decrease the glial reduction explains. The possible origins and consequences of the glial alterations are discussed below.

Two studies of the cingulate cortex are attempts at replication of this work. Cotter et al. (2001) also used the Stanley Foundation tissue, but their study differed from that of Öngür and colleagues in several ways: Cotter et al. studied the supragenual anterior cingulate cortex (area 24b; Figure 14.1, colour plate), and used a somewhat different morphometric method and a more sophisticated statistical analysis. The price of the latter is a complex data set, and difficulty drawing direct comparisons with the results of Öngür et al. (1998), especially as the later authors decided not to analyse results according to family history because of the small subgroups which would result. The main positive findings were in major depression: a decreased glial

Table 14.1. Histological studies of the frontal cortex in mood disorder

Study and area	Cases/controls	Methods and parameters	Main findings in mood disorder[a]
Öngür et al. (1998) BA24 (subgenual), BA3b	a. 4BD, 4MD / 5 CON; b. 14 BD, 9MD / 14 CON[b]	a. Nissl stain; volume, neuron and glia density and number; optical dissector; b. Nissl stain; volume, neuron and glia density and number, optical dissector and rotator	a. Trend for decreased volume. Decreased glial number and density in MD and familial BD. b. Trend for decreased volume. Decreased glial number and density in MD (mainly due to fMD). Decreased glial number and density in fBD. No differences in BA3b.
Rajkowska et al. (1999) Left BA9, 10-47, 47	12 MD / 12 CON	Nissl stain; cortical thickness, neuron density and size; glial density and glial nuclear size	BA9: Decreased neuron size in III and IV (−5% and −7%). Decreased density of large neurons in II, III and IV (by 20–60%), with more small neurons (+40%). 20–30% lower glial density in III and IV. More glia with large nuclei in III. BA47: Decreased neuron size in II; decreased density of large neurons in IIIa and Va. Overall glial density reduced (−15%). Decreased density of glia with medium and large nuclei in V and VI. BA10-47: Reduced cortical thickness (−12%). Decreased neuron size in II and III. Decreased neuron density in II, III and IV (20–60%). Increase in density of small neurons in II (+30–70%). Trend for lower glial density, and fewer glia with medium or large nuclei in IIIa and IV.
Miguel-Hidalgo et al. (2000) Left BA9	14 MD / 15 CON	GFAP immunoreactivity; areal fraction and density of GFAP +ve cells.	No overall differences. Reduced area fraction in III–V in young cases. Trend decreases in density of medium and large glia.
Benes et al. (2000) BA24	5 BD / 12 CON[b]	Nissl stain; neuronal size	No differences.
Cotter et al. (2001) BA24 (supragenual)	15MD, 15BD / 15 CON[b]	Nissl stain; glial and neuron density by optical dissector; neuronal size by nucleator	In MD, decreased glial density (−22%), and decreased neuron size (−18%) in VI, with same trend in V. Neuron density unchanged. No changes in BD.
Benes et al. (2001) BA24	10 BD[c] / 12 CON[b]	Nissl stain; neuronal density and size; glial density	Reduced density of nonpyramidal neurons in II. Trend for lower density of pyramidal neurons in deeper laminae. Pyramidal neurons larger in II; nonpyramidal neurons larger in II and III. No change in glia.
Rajkowska et al. (2001) Left BA9	10 BD / 11 CON	Nissl stain; cortical and laminar thickness; neuronal density and size; glial density and nuclear size	Cortical thickness unchanged. Pyramidal and total neuron density reduced in II, III and V by 9–30%; no change in nonpyramidal neuron density. Neuron size unchanged. Glial density decreased in IIIc and Vb. Larger glia in I and IIIc.

BA, Brodmann area; BD, bipolar disorder; CON, control; f, familial; GFAP, glial fibrillary acidic protein; ICC, immunocytochemistry; MD, major depression.

[a] Roman numerals refer to cortical laminae.

[b] Schizophrenia comparison group included as well (data not shown).

[c] Includes the five subjects studied in Benes et al. (2000).

density in lamina VI, as well as a reduced neuronal size. In bipolar disorder, neuronal size showed the same trend, but glial density was unaltered. Neuronal density did not differ in either mood-disorder group. In addition, significant effects of brain pH and hemisphere were found: neuronal and glial density were higher in the left than the right hemisphere (by 7.5% and 14% respectively), and a hemisphere-by-diagnosis interaction for glial density in major depression was seen in lamina III. Glial density was also affected by pH, with each 0.1 pH unit associated with a 4% increase in glial density. Brain pH, as well as postmortem interval and age, were covariates in the analyses. The study is an extension and partial replication of Öngür and colleagues' (1998) results, providing some additional support for glial pathology, as well as for the neuronal size reductions seen in some studies in other prefrontal regions to be described below. It is unknown whether the nonreplication of other aspects of the results, notably in bipolar disorder, is due to the methodological differences, or to pathological heterogeneity between subgenual and supragenual cingulate cortex.

The other morphometric study of sg24 has only been reported in preliminary form (Kövari et al. 1999). These authors measured neuronal density in 10 patients with (sporadic) bipolar disorder, 10 with (sporadic) major depression and 55 controls. The subjects were older than those in the above investigations, being 65–75 years old. The grey matter was thinner in the patient groups; correcting for this, neuronal density was decreased by 15–20% in laminae III and V in bipolar disorder. No differences were seen in major depression. No glial data are mentioned.

The remaining morphometric studies of anterior cingulate gyrus in mood disorder are by Benes' group (Table 14.1). In five subjects with bipolar disorder, no differences in neuronal size were seen (Benes et al. 2000), but in an expanded group a decreased density of interneurons in lamina II, and a trend towards a lower density of pyramidal neurons, was found (Benes et al. 2001). In contrast, there were no differences in glial density. Consideration of these data together with equivalent studies of schizophrenia and schizoaffective disorder led to the conclusion that mood disorders are associated with involvement of local circuits in lamina II, whereas projection neurons in deeper laminae are more affected in schizophrenia (Benes et al. 2001).

Studies of synapses and dendrites complement investigations of the neuronal cell body. Direct visualization of these structures is problematic in postmortem tissue and so most studies measure gene products localized to these neuronal compartments. The approach has become widely used in other disorders (Masliah and Terry 1993; Harrison and Eastwood 2001). It is now being applied to mood disorders, in part to inform about possible alterations in synaptic connectivity, which are plausible given the nature of the morphometric data. For example, the size of a neuronal cell body is related to the extent of axonal and dendritic arborization, and thereby the synaptic organization, which the neuron must support (Esiri and Pearson 2000). There are also close and multifaceted relationships between synapses and glia (see below). We have observed decrements in three synaptic proteins in area 24 of bipolar disorder in the Stanley Consortium brains (adjacent to the sections studied by Cotter et al. 2001): synaptophysin, complexin II and growth-associated protein 43 (GAP-43; Eastwood and Harrison 2001). Lesser and nonsignificant reductions were seen in the major depression group and in schizophrenia. The findings are consistent with a synaptic pathology to accompany the neuronal and glial alterations in this region; given the roles and locations of the three proteins, the data suggest that there may be a lower density and plasticity of synapses. The identity and neuronal source of the affected synapses is unknown.

Other frontal lobe studies

Ventromedial/orbital and dorsolateral prefrontal cortex have also been implicated in the pathophysiology and neuropsychology of mood disorder (Goodwin 1997; Merriam et al. 1999), and studies are emerging which are suggestive of neuropathological involvement.

Rajkowska and colleagues have performed the main morphometric studies in these areas. The initial report (Rajkowska et al. 1999) was of major depression, with morphometric measurements of neurons and glia in dorsolateral and orbital (rostral and caudal) prefrontal cortices (see Figure 14.1, colour plate). In all three areas, in one or more laminae, there was a decreased glial density and a reduced size of neurons, as well as some other changes (Table 14.1). Subsequently, glial fibrillary acidic protein (GFAP) was used as an immunocytochemical marker of astrocytes, in area 9 of the same subjects, to investigate whether this glial type was affected (Miguel-Hidalgo et al. 2000). The results were equivocal, in that GFAP staining and GFAP-positive cell counts were unaltered, but there was a decrease in the younger (30–45 years) cases of major depression compared with controls. Similar morphometric findings have now been described in bipolar disorder in area 9, with lamina-specific reductions in glial density and pyramidal neuron density, as well as alterations in glial shape and enlargement of glial nuclei (Rajkowska et al. 2001).

There has been only one synaptic protein study, and none of dendritic markers, in the prefrontal cortex in mood disorder. Honer et al. (1999) found a decrease in myelin basic protein, but not synaptophysin or GAP-43, in anterolateral frontal cortex (mainly area 10) in 11 patients with major depression, all of whom died by suicide. The reduced myelin basic protein may indicate alterations in myelination, and hence of connectivity.

In summary, in all areas of the prefrontal cortex yet examined, independent groups have reported decreases in the density of glia, and the density and size of some neurons, in bipolar disorder and major depression. In this respect there is a consistency and robustness to the observations. However, as careful perusal of Table 14.1 shows, there remain notable discrepancies. First, Öngür et al. (1998) found glial pathology but no neuronal changes; Benes et al. (2001) found the opposite; and Rajkowksa et al. (1999, 2001) found both. Second, the laminar distribution of significant differences also varies between studies. Third, Öngür et al. (1998) found differences in bipolar disorder and major depression, whereas Cotter et al. (2001), studying the same brains, found them only in the latter. It is unclear whether the variability in results reflects anatomical, demographic or methodological differences (see below).

Hippocampal formation

The hippocampal formation (dentate gyrus, hippocampus proper, subiculum and parahippocampal cortex) has been implicated in mood disorder for two main reasons. First, several, though not all, imaging studies have reported hippocampal volume to be decreased in major depression (Sheline et al. 1996; Shah et al. 1998; Bremner et al. 2000), possibly related to duration of illness (Sheline et al. 1999). Hippocampal volume may also be reduced, but amygdalar volume increased, in bipolar disorder (Strakowski et al. 1999; Altshuler et al. 2000). Second, there is an influential model of depression linking it to the atrophic effects of glucocorticoids and stress on hippocampal neurons and their dendrites (Brown et al. 1999; Sapolsky 2000) perhaps mediated via specific neuronal second messengers and neurotrophic factors (Duman et al. 1997). Despite these considerations, there have been very few neuropathological studies of the hippocampal formation in mood disorder.

Beckmann and Jakob (1991) described dysplasia and heterotopias in the entorhinal cortex in four cases of bipolar disorder, similar to findings they had reported previously in schizophrenia. A similar though less dramatic finding was reported by Bernstein et al. (1998). If confirmed, such an alteration would have major aetiological implications since it is strongly suggestive of an early developmental anomaly. However, entorhinal abnormalities have not been well replicated in schizophrenia, and so their occurrence in mood disorder must be viewed as highly speculative.

Glucocorticoid-related hippocampal neurotoxicity is likely to be apoptotic rather than necrotic. Hence, in the first direct investigation of the hypothesis, Lucassen et al. (2001) measured several markers of apoptosis and neural injury in 15 major-depression subjects. They found only a minor and inconsistent increase in neuronal apoptosis, and it was not in the hippocampal subfields at risk for glucocorticoid damage (notably CA3). The results cast some neuropathological doubt over the validity of the stress/atrophy model of major depression, and the authors propose that other mechanisms, including glial pathology, mediate the hippocampal volume deficits.

Synaptic and dendritic studies of the hippocampus in mood disorder are in their infancy. Rosoklija et al. (2000) found decreased arborization of apical dendrites, and a lower density of dendritic spines, on subicular pyramidal neurons in six subjects with mood (mainly bipolar) disorder, especially those with a family history. As these dendritic changes are suggestive of decreased or otherwise aberrant afferent synaptic connectivity, these findings are consistent with the reduced expression of synaptic protein genes in the hippocampus, especially the subiculum, in bipolar disorder (Eastwood and Harrison 2000). No hippocampal synaptic pathology has been found in major depression (Eastwood and Harrison 2000; Lucassen et al. 2001).

Focal white matter pathology

Many MRI studies have shown an association between mood disorder and focal signal hyperintensities, occurring particularly in the deep white matter and subcortical nuclei. These white matter hyperintensities (WMHs) are seen in excess both in bipolar disorder and in unipolar depression, the latter especially in elderly subjects (O'Brien et al. 1996; Videbech 1997). In late-life depression, WMHs are linked to risk factors for, and presence of, vascular disease; there is also a related and robust epidemiological association between late-life depression and vascular disease (Alexopoulos et al. 1997), though this was only partially confirmed in a recent postmortem study (O'Brien et al. 2001).

It is generally assumed that the MRI lesions in mood-disorder patients reflect focal white matter damage, especially ischaemia and infarction, as they do in other diseases (O'Brien et al. 1996). The clinical consequences for the symptoms of mood disorder (notably the cognitive slowing seen in elderly subjects with depression) are thought to arise from the consequent interruption of axonal pathways, especially frontosubcortical connections (Greenwald et al. 1998). However, to date there have been no postmortem studies of white matter lesions in mood disorder, and so their neuropathological nature and implications remain unknown.

Monoaminergic nuclei

There is no loss or atrophy of neurons in the locus coeruleus (Klimek et al. 1997; Baumann et al. 1999) or raphe nuclei (Underwood et al. 1999) in mood disorder;

indeed, Baumann et al. (1999) reported increased locus coeruleus neuronal number and size in bipolar disorder. These morphometric data, though preliminary, are important, since they suggest that the monoaminergic deficiencies proposed in the predominant neurochemical hypotheses of depression (Maes and Meltzer 1995; Ressler and Nemeroff 1999) are not due to pathology of the cell bodies of origin – though clearly there may be other alterations yet to be investigated, such as decreased innervation of target regions.

Interpretational issues

Neuropathological studies of psychiatric disorders are complicated by many factors and potential confounds, including medication (see below), mode of death, postmortem interval, hemisphere studied and so on (Harrison and Kleinman 2000). Overcoming, or at least minimizing, these problems requires careful experimental and statistical design, replications and relevant parallel animal studies. To date, none of the reported positive findings in mood disorder meets all these criteria. One problem is alcohol abuse, which is common in mood disorder: 30–50% in epidemiological studies of bipolar disorder. This is relevant because alcoholics have fewer glia (Korbo 1999) and show neuronal morphometric differences (Kril and Halliday 1999). For example, five of the cases studied by Rajkowska et al. (1999) had a history of alcohol or substance abuse. A separate problem for mood-disorder research is the overlap with suicide, since many individuals in postmortem studies of one also meet criteria for the other. Suicide complicates matters for several reasons: it may indicate a more severe or otherwise atypical subtype of mood disorder; it may produce artefacts secondary to the lethality of the method (e.g. many suicides are rapid and are associated with a less acidotic brain than are deaths due to natural causes, which tend to have longer agonal states); and it may even have its own neuropathology. Somewhat similar issues pertain to the overlap between stress and mood disorder (Sheline 2000). A final concern is that of the morphometric methodology. There is much controversy as to the pros and cons of different approaches (Benes and Lange 2001), but it is clear that this factor introduces the potential for considerable error and bias which could mask, or be mistaken for, the neuropathological signal being sought.

Treatment influences

Most patients with a history of major depression have been treated with one or more antidepressants. Some will also have received electroconvulsive therapy (ECT), lithium, antipsychotics or benzodiazepines. Subjects with a history of bipolar disorder will usually have received these drugs too, or other mood stabilizers such as valproate and carbamazepine. The potential therefore exists for these treatments to have caused, or to have ameliorated, the neuropathological alterations described above.

A comprehensive review concluded that electroconvulsive shock produces no demonstrable effects on brain structure (Devenand et al. 1994), and certainly there is no evidence for 'brain damage' (e.g. evidence of inflammation, neurotoxicity). Whilst reassuring, there are small caveats. In rats, electroconvulsive shock can affect dendritic and synaptic markers (Pei et al. 1998; Vaidya et al. 1999), serotonergic axons (Madhav et al. 2000) and GFAP levels (Steward 1994). Recently, electroconvulsive shock has been reported to increase hippocampal neurogenesis (Madsen et al. 2000). The clinical relevance of all these experiments is questionable, since a higher stimulus intensity and frequency has generally been used and only short-term effects measured, but it would be prudent to bear the data in mind if a subject included in postmortem studies had received ECT in the weeks prior to death.

Fatal lithium overdose is associated with findings indicative of acute neurotoxicity (Schneider and Mirra 1994). However, there are no human neuropathological studies of the effects of chronic lithium treatment, nor indeed of other mood stabilizers, or of antidepressants. There are data showing a variety of alterations in neuronal and glial markers in rodents treated with each of these classes of drug (Rocha et al. 1998), but it is unclear whether these are relevant to the clinical situation. Intriguingly, recent data indicate that, like ECT, psychotropic drugs may enhance hippocampal neurogenesis (Chen et al. 2000; Malberg et al. 2000), leading to speculation that this property may be therapeutically beneficial (Manji et al. 2000); again, it is unknown whether any such effects translate into measurable morphological – let alone functional – consequences in patients.

There are more data, both postmortem and experimental, concerning the neuropathological effects of antipsychotics (Harrison 1999). Conventional antipsychotics have many effects on neuronal and synaptic organization, especially in the striatum and less so in the prefrontal cortex; atypical antipsychotics seem to cause fewer and less marked alterations. One study has reported increased glial density in the frontal cortex of monkeys treated chronically with antipsychotics (Selemon et al. 1999). With regard to the glial deficits reported in mood disorder, this finding emphasizes that medication (and other confounders) have the potential to mask as well as produce positive findings.

Conceptual issues

A key question concerns the timing of the neuropathological alterations and whether they are static, progressive or reversible. To be causally important, at least some of the findings should be present at first episode, if not sooner. This is in practice impossible to investigate directly postmortem, and one must rely on inferences from imaging data that this is the case. For example, the occurrence of subgenual abnormalities in first-episode cases (Hirayasu et al. 1999) suggests that the volume decrements, and therefore the histological changes which putatively underlie them, are not merely the consequence of chronic illness or its treatment. Moreover, N-acetylaspartate (a marker of neuronal volume and/or density) may be decreased in the prefrontal cortex in euthymic, medication-free subjects with bipolar disorder (Winsberg et al. 2000, but not Hamakawa et al. 1999). These data suggest that at least part of the neuropathology of mood disorder is present early in the illness and is not secondary to its treatment. Whether the alterations are progressive has not been investigated, though we found that the decreases of synaptic proteins in the cingulate gyrus correlated significantly with the duration of the mood disorder (after the effect of increasing age at death had been partialled out; Eastwood and Harrison 2001). However, establishing the causal sequence and progression of morphological changes in mood disorder will be very difficult, and this is probably best left until the changes themselves are more clearly demonstrated.

Mood disorders are syndromes of unknown aetiology and validity. Whilst neuropathology has the potential to help advance this understanding, equally the current uncertainties cause difficulties interpreting findings. For example, are bipolar and unipolar disorders (or any other mood-disorder category) distinct at a pathological level? To date, the similarities appear greater than the differences, but this may just reflect the inadequacies of the available data – and the fact that few if any studies have been powered to address the question. The same tentative conclusion and caveats also apply to comparison with schizophrenia, although some potentially noteworthy differences, especially concerning the glial changes, require further evaluation (Baumann and Bogerts 1999; Rajkowska et al. 2001). The finding of greater pathology in familial than apparently nonfamilial mood-disorder subjects is a theme from several recent studies, but it would be premature to argue that this is yet established beyond reasonable doubt. Finally, the suggestion that early- and late-onset mood disorder have different pathophysiologies, the latter being more 'vascular' in origin, has considerable support from MRI studies, but as yet no good neuropathological corroboration.

Mood disorders include neuropsychological (cognitive) symptoms as well as affective and somatic symptoms; some of these neuropsychological features are mood related and some persist during remission (Kessing 1998; Ferrier et al. 1999; Sweeney et al. 2000). Which of these are the principal clinical correlates of the reported pathological alterations is unknown, since samples have been far too small (and clinical documentation inadequate) for meaningful subgroup or correlational analyses. Nevertheless, since postmortem samples include patients dying at all phases of illness, it is more likely that the observed alterations are trait- rather than state-related and, as such, may be connected more to the enduring neuropsychological characteristics than to the fluctuating mood symptoms.

Finally, what is the explanation for the unexpected finding of glial deficits in mood disorder? This will depend largely on the glial subtype involved. Glia comprise astrocytes, oligodendrocytes and microglia. Given the predominance of astrocytes in the grey matter, it is likely that they are the glial population primarily affected in mood disorder (though the results of Miguel-Hidalgo et al. (2000) provide only partial support for this), and microglia should not be neglected (Bayer et al. 1999). Astrocytes are now realized to have many functions in addition to their classical one of scar formation and response to degenerative and other insults. Indeed, they appear to have central roles in neuronal migration, synaptogenesis, neurotransmission and synaptic plasticity (Coyle and Schwarcz 2000; Ullian et al. 2001; see also Chapter 3 by Götz). It is speculated that the glial changes are primary, with downstream effects on neurons (Rajkowska 2000), though there many ways by which they might be involved in the pathogenesis and pathophysiology of mood disorder. For example, astrocytes express many serotonergic and adrenergic receptors, and pathological involvement of these cells might contribute to the deficits in these monoamine systems. Furthermore, glia are the main origin of functional imaging signals (both PET and fMR), and hence glial pathology could contribute to differences observed in mood-disorder subjects (Magistretti 2000).

Conclusions

A range of cytoarchitectural abnormalities have been reported in neuropathological studies of mood disorder, especially in medial prefrontal cortex. The prominent findings are decreases in the number or density of glia, together with reduced size and density of some neurons. There is preliminary evidence for accompanying dendritic and synaptic alterations, and some indication that the results are more striking in cases with a family history of mood disorder. At this stage there is no clear evidence for a distinction between bipolar and unipolar disorders. Together the changes are suggestive of an alteration in the cellular composition and neural circuitry in mood disorder which are likely to be developmental or plasticity-related in origin rather than degenerative.

The data provide sufficient reason to investigate the field further, but leave many more questions than answers. Most importantly there is a pressing need for replication, preferably in larger and better-characterized samples, to establish which findings are robust and which are not. Ideally the studies will cross diagnostic boundaries (which may well be unhelpful) and allow variables implicated by the recent work – such as family history, age at onset and anatomical heterogeneity – to be investigated more critically. They will also need to assess the neuropathology of the white matter lesions which MRI studies indicate are common correlates of mood disorders in the elderly. By extrapolation from other diseases, the implied pathology seems likely to be hypoxic/ischaemic in origin, and thus rather different in nature to the cytoarchitectural alterations. The key conceptual and practical issues at this point are very reminiscent of those which corresponding studies of schizophrenia have had to address (Harrison and Roberts 2000; Harrison and Lewis in press), and, as such, awareness of the latter may facilitate progress in this area. Finally, returning to the organic/functional distinction, the neuropathological correlates of mood disorder in neurological diseases may give valuable clues to the brain areas and cellular processes relevant to all mood disorders (Förstl et al. 1992; Hoogendijk et al. 1999; Ballard et al. 2000).

Acknowledgements

We thank the Stanley Foundation for support. RG holds an MRC Studentship.

REFERENCES

Alexopoulos GS, Meyers BS, Young RC, Campbell S, Silbersweig D and Charlson M (1997). 'Vascular depression' hypothesis. *Arch Gen Psychiatry*, 54, 915–22.

Altshuler LL, Bartzokis G, Grieder T et al. (2000). An MRI study of temporal lobe structures in men with bipolar disorder or schizophrenia. *Biol Psychiatry*, 48, 147–62.

Ballard C, McKeith I, O'Brien J et al. (2000). Neuropathological substrates of dementia and depression in vascular dementia, with a particular focus on cases with small infarct volumes. *Dementia*, 11, 59–65.

Baumann B and Bogerts B (1999). The pathomorphology of schizophrenia and mood disorders: similarities and differences. *Schizophr Res*, 39, 141–8.

Baumann B, Danos P, Krell D et al. (1999). Unipolar-bipolar dichotomy of mood disorders is supported by noradrenergic brainstem system morphology. *J Affect Disord*, 54, 217–24.

Bayer TA, Buslei R, Havas L and Falkai P (1999). Evidence for activation of microglia in patients with psychiatric illnesses. *Neurosci Lett*, 271, 126–128.

Beckmann H and Jakob H (1991). Prenatal disturbances of nerve cell migration in the entorhinal region: a common vulnerability factor in functional psychoses. *J Neural Transm*, 84, 155–64.

Bench CJ, Friston KJ, Brown RG, Scott LC, Frackowiak RSJ and Dolan RJ (1992). The anatomy of melancholia – focal abnormalities of cerebral blood flow in major depression. *Psychol Med*, 22, 607–15.

Benes FM and Lange N (2001). Two-dimensional versus three-dimensional cell counting: a practical perspective. *Trends Neurosci*, 24, 11–17.

Benes FM, Todtenkopf MS, Logiotatos P and Williams M (2000). Glutamate decarboxylase$_{65}$-immunoreactive terminals in cingulate and prefrontal cortices of schizophrenic and bipolar brain. *J Chem Neuroanat*, 20, 259–69.

Benes FM, Vincent SL and Todtenkopf M (2001). The density of pyramidal and non-pyramidal neurons in anterior cingulate cortex of schizophrenic and bipolar subjects. *Biol Psychiatry*, 50, 395–406.

Bernstein H-G, Krell D, Baumann B et al. (1998). Morphometric studies of the entorhinal cortex in neuropsychiatric patients and controls: clusters of heterotopically displaced lamina II neurons are not indicative of schizophrenia. *Schizophr Res*, 33, 125–32.

Bremner JD, Narayan M, Anderson ER, Staib LH, Miller HL and Charney DS (2000). Hippocampal volume reduction in major depression. *Am J Psychiatry*, 157, 115–17.

Brown ES, Rush AJ and McEwen BS (1999). Hippocampal remodeling and damage by corticosteroids: implications for mood disorders. *Neuropsychopharmacology*, 21, 474–84.

Chen G, Rajkowksa G, Du F, Seraji-Bozorgzad N and Manji HK (2000). Enhancement of hippocampal neurogenesis by lithium. *J Neurochem*, 75, 1729–34.

Cotter D, Mackay D, Landau S, Kerwin R and Everall I (2001). Glial cell loss and reduced neuronal size in the anterior cingulate cortex in major depressive disorder. *Arch Gen Psychiatry*, 58, 545–53.

Coyle JT and Schwarcz R (2000). Mind glue – implications of glial cell biology for psychiatry. *Arch Gen Psychiatry*, 57, 90–3.

Devenand DP, Dwork AJ, Hutchinson ER, Bolwig TG and Sackeim HA (1994). Does ECT alter brain structure? *Am J Psychiatry*, 151, 957–70.

Devinsky O, Morrell MJ and Vogt BA (1995). Contributions of anterior cingulate cortex to behaviour. *Brain*, 118, 279–306.

Drevets WC, Price JL, Simpson JR Jr et al. (1997). Subgenual prefrontal cortex abnormalities in mood disorders. *Nature*, 386, 824–7.

Duman RS, Heninger GR and Nestler EJ (1997). A molecular and cellular theory of depression. *Arch Gen Psychiatry*, 54, 597–606.

Eastwood SL and Harrison PJ (2000). Hippocampal synaptic pathology in schizophrenia, bipolar disorder and major depression: a study of complexin mRNAs. *Mol Psychiatry*, 5, 425–32.

Eastwood SL and Harrison PJ (2001). Synaptic pathology in the anterior cingulate cortex in schizophrenia and mood disorders. A review and a western blot study of synaptophysin, GAP-43 and the complexins. *Brain Res Bull*, 55, 569–78.

Ebert D and Ebmeier KP (1996). The role of the cingulate gyrus in depression: from functional anatomy to neurochemistry. *Biol Psychiatry*, 39, 1044–50.

Esiri MM and Pearson RCA (2000). Perspectives from other diseases and lesions. In *The Neuropathology of Schizophrenia. Progress and Interpretation*, ed. PJ Harrison and GW Roberts, pp. 257–76. Oxford: Oxford University Press.

Ferrier IN, Stanton BR, Kelly TP and Scott J (1999). Neuropsychological function in euthymic patients with bipolar disorder. *Br J Psychiatry*, 175, 246–51.

Förstl H, Burns A, Luthert P, Cairns N, Lantos P and Levy R (1992). Clinical and neuropathological correlates of depression in Alzheimer's disease. *Psychol Med*, 22, 877–84.

Goodwin GM (1997). Neuropsychological and neuroimaging evidence for the involvement of the frontal lobes in depression. *J Psychopharmacol*, 11, 115–22.

Greenwald BS, Kramer-Ginsberg E, Krishnan KR, Ashtari M, Auerbach C and Patel M (1998). Neuroanatomic localization of magnetic resonance imaging signal hyperintensities in geriatric depression. *Stroke*, 29, 613–17.

Hamakawa H, Kato T, Shiori T, Inubushi T and Kato N (1999). Quantitative proton magnetic resonance spectroscopy of the bilateral frontal lobes in patients with bipolar disorder. *Psychol Med*, 29, 639–44.

Harrison PJ (1999). The neuropathological effects of antipsychotic drugs. *Schizophr Res*, 40, 87–99.

Harrison PJ and Eastwood SL (2001). Neuropathological studies of synaptic connectivity in the hippocampal formation in schizophrenia. *Hippocampus*, 11, 508–19.

Harrison PJ and Kleinman JE (2000). Methodological issues. In *The Neuropathology of Schizophrenia. Progress and Interpretation*, ed. PJ Harrison and GW Roberts, pp. 339–50. Oxford: Oxford University Press.

Harrison PJ and Lewis DA (in press). The neuropathology of schizophrenia. In *Schizophrenia*, 2nd edn, ed. S Hirsch and DR Weinberger. Oxford: Blackwell Science.

Harrison PJ and Roberts GW (2000). *The Neuropathology of Schizophrenia: Progress and Interpretation*. Oxford: Oxford University Press.

Hirayasu Y, Shenton ME, Salisbury DF et al. (1999). Subgenual cingulate cortex volume in first-episode psychosis. *Am J Psychiatry*, 156, 1091–3.

Honer WG, Falkal P, Chen C, Arango V, Mann JJ and Dwork AJ (1999). Synaptic and plasticity-associated proteins in anterior frontal cortex in severe mental illness. *Neuroscience*, 91, 1247–55.

Hoogendijk WJG, Sommer IEC, Pool CW et al. (1999). Lack of association between depression and loss of neurons in the locus coeruleus in Alzheimer disease. *Arch Gen Psychiatry*, 56, 45–51.

Jeste DV, Lohr JB and Goodwin FK (1988). Neuroanatomical studies of major affective disorders. A review and suggestions for future research. *Br J Psychiatry*, 153, 444–59.

Kessing LV (1998). Cognitive impairment in the euthymic phase of affective disorder. *Psychol Med*, 28, 1027–38.

Klimek V, Stockmeier C, Overholser J et al. (1997). Reduced levels of norepinephrine transporters in the locus coeruleus in major depression. *J Neurosci*, 17, 8451–8.

Korbo L (1999). Glial cell loss in the hippocampus of alcoholics. *Alcohol Clin Exp Res*, 23, 164–8.

Kövari E, Giannakopoulos P, Hof PR and Bouras C (1999). Structural changes in the subgenual prefrontal cortex in schizophrenia and mood disorders. *Soc Neurosci Abstr*, 25, 817.

Kril JJ and Halliday GM (1999). Brain shrinkage in alcoholics: a decade on and what have we learned? *Prog Neurobiol*, 58, 381–7.

Lucassen PJ, Müller MB, Holsboer F et al. (2001). Hippocampal apoptosis in major depression is a minor event and absent from subareas at risk for glucocorticoid overexposure. *Am J Pathol*, 158, 453–68.

Madhav TR, Pei Q, Grahame-Smith DG and Zetterström TSC (2000). Repeated electroconvulsive shock promotes the sprouting of serotonergic axons in the lesioned rat hippocampus. *Neuroscience*, 97, 677–83.

Madsen TM, Treschow A, Bengzon J, Bolwig TG, Lindvall O and Tingström A (2000). Increased neurogenesis in a model of electroconvulsive therapy. *Biol Psychiatry*, 47, 1043–9.

Maes M and Meltzer HY (1995). The serotonin hypothesis of major depression. In *Psychopharmacology: the Fourth Generation of Progress*, ed. FE Bloom and DJ Kupfer, pp. 933–44. New York: Raven Press.

Magistretti PJ (2000). Cellular bases of functional brain imaging: insights from neuron-glia metabolic coupling. *Brain Res*, 886, 108–12.

Malberg JE, Eisch AJ, Nestler EJ and Duman RS (2000). Chronic antidepressant treatment increases neurogenesis in adult rat hippocampus. *J Neurosci*, 20, 9104–10.

Manji HK, Moore GJ and Chen G (2000). Clinical and preclinical evidence for the neurotrophic effects of mood stabilizers: implications for the pathophysiology and treatment of manic-depressive illness. *Biol Psychiatry*, 48, 740–54.

Masliah E and Terry RD (1993). The role of synaptic proteins in the pathogenesis of disorders of the central nervous system. *Brain Pathol*, 3, 77–86.

Merriam EP, Thase ME, Haas GL, Keshavan MS and Sweeney JA (1999). Prefrontal cortical dysfunction in depression determined by Wisconsin Card Sorting Test performance. *Am J Psychiatry*, 156, 780–2.

Miguel-Hidalgo JJ, Baucom C, Dilley G et al. (2000). Glial fibrillary acidic protein immunoreactivity in the prefrontal cortex distinguishes younger from older adults in major depressive disorder. *Biol Psychiatry*, 48, 861–73.

O'Brien JT, Ames D and Schweitzer I (1996). White matter changes in depression and Alzheimer's disease: a review of magnetic resonance imaging studies. *Int J Geriatr Psychiatry*, 11, 681–94.

O'Brien J, Thomas A, Ballard C et al. (2001). Cognitive impairment in depression is not associated with neuropathologic evidence of increased vascular or Alzheimer-type pathology. *Biol Psychiatry*, 49, 130–6.

Öngür D, Drevets WC and Price JL (1998). Glial reduction in the subgenual prefrontal cortex in mood disorders. *Proc Natl Acad Sci USA*, 95, 13290–5.

Pei Q, Burnet PJW and Zetterström TSC (1998). Changes in mRNA abundance of microtubule-associated proteins in the rat brain following electroconvulsive shock. *Neuroreport*, 9, 391–4.

Perry RH (1994). A guide to the cortical regions. In *Neuropsychiatric Disorders*, ed. GW Roberts, PN Leigh and DR Weinberger, pp. 1.1–1.10. London: Wolfe.

Price JL (1999). Prefrontal cortical networks related to visceral function and mood. *Ann N Y Acad Sci*, 877, 383–96.

Rajkowska G (2000). Postmortem studies in mood disorders indicate altered numbers of neurons and glial cells. *Biol Psychiatry*, 48, 766–77.

Rajkowska G and Goldman-Rakic PS (1995). Cytoarchitectonic definition of prefrontal areas in the normal human cortex. II. Variability in locations of areas 9 and 46 and relationship to the Talairach coordinate system. *Cereb Cortex*, 5, 323–37.

Rajkowska G, Miguel-Hidalgo JJ, Wei JR et al. (1999). Morphometric evidence for neuronal and glial prefrontal cell pathology in major depression. *Biol Psychiatry*, 45, 1085–98.

Rajkowska G, Halaris A and Selemon LD (2001). Reductions in neuronal and glial density characterize the dorsolateral prefrontal cortex in bipolar disorder. *Biol Psychiatry*, 49, 741–52.

Ressler KJ and Nemeroff CB (1999). Role of norepinephrine in the pathophysiology and treatment of mood disorder. *Biol Psychiatry*, 46, 1219–33.

Rocha E, Achaval M, Santos P and Rodnight R (1998). Lithium treatment causes gliosis and modifies the morphology of hippocampal astrocytes in rats. *Neuroreport*, 9, 3971–4.

Rosoklija G, Toomayan G, Ellis SP et al. (2000). Structural abnormalities of subicular dendrites in subjects with schizophrenia and mood disorders – preliminary findings. *Arch Gen Psychiatry*, 57, 349–56.

Sapolsky RM (2000). Glucocorticoids and hippocampal atrophy in neuropsychiatric disorders. *Arch Gen Psychiatry*, 57, 925–35.

Schneider JA and Mirra SS (1994). Neuropathologic correlates of persistent neurologic deficit in lithium intoxication. *Ann Neurol*, 36, 928–31.

Selemon LD, Lidow MS and Goldman-Rakic PS (1999). Increased volume and glial density in primate prefrontal cortex associated with chronic antipsychotic drug exposure. *Biol Psychiatry*, 46, 161–72.

Shah PJ, Ebmeier KP, Glabus MF and Goodwin GM (1998). Cortical grey matter reductions associated with treatment-resistant chronic unipolar depression – controlled magnetic resonance imaging study. *Br J Psychiatry*, 172, 527–32.

Sheline YI (2000). 3D MRI studies of neuroanatomic changes in unipolar major depression: the role of stress and medical comorbidity. *Biol Psychiatry*, 48, 791–800.

Sheline YI, Wang PW, Gado MH, Csernansky JG and Vannier MW (1996). Hippocampal atrophy in recurrent major depression. *Proc Natl Acad Sci USA*, 93, 3908–13.

Sheline YI, Sanghavi M, Mintun MA and Gado MH (1999). Depression duration but not age predicts hippocampal volume loss in medically healthy women with recurrent major depression. *J Neurosci*, 19, 5034–43.

Steward O (1994). Electroconvulsive seizures upregulate astroglial gene expression selectively in the dentate gyrus. *Mol Brain Res*, 25, 217–24.

Strakowski SM, DelBello MP, Sax KW et al. (1999). Brain magnetic resonance imaging of structural abnormalities in bipolar disorder. *Arch Gen Psychiatry*, 56, 254–60.

Sweeney JA, Kmiec JA and Kupfer DJ (2000). Neuropsychologic impairments in bipolar and unipolar mood disorders on the CANTAB neurocognitive battery. *Biol Psychiatry*, 48, 674–84.

Torrey EF, Webster M, Knable M, Johnston N and Yolken RH (2000). The Stanley Foundation brain collection and Neuropathology Consortium. *Schizophr Res*, 44, 151–5.

Ullian EM, Sapperstein S, Christopherson K and Barres BA (2001). Control of synapse number by glia. *Science*, 291, 657–61.

Underwood MD, Khaibulina AA, Ellis SP et al. (1999). Morphometry of the dorsal raphe nucleus serotonergic neurons in suicide victims. *Biol Psychiatry*, 46, 473–83.

Vaidya VA, Siuciak JA, Du F and Duman RS (1999). Hippocampal mossy fiber sprouting induced by chronic electroconvulsive seizures. *Neuroscience*, 89, 157–66.

Videbech P (1997). MRI findings in patients with affective disorder: a meta-analysis. *Acta Psychiatr Scand*, 96, 157–68.

Vogt BA, Nimchinsky EA, Vogt LJ and Hof PR (1995). Human cingulate cortex: surface features, flat maps, and cytoarchitecture. *J Comp Neurol*, 359, 490–506.

Winsberg ME, Sachs N, Tate DL, Adalsteinsson E, Spielman D and Ketter TA (2000). Decreased dorsolateral prefrontal *N*-acetyl aspartate in bipolar disorder. *Biol Psychiatry*, 47, 475–81.

15

The neural substrates of anxiety

Simon Killcross

Cardiff University, Cardiff, UK

Introduction

The aim of this chapter is to try to bring together some of the recent advances in the study of the neural substrates of fear and anxiety in laboratory animals to form a coherent overview that will facilitate comparisons between these basic studies and clinical investigations. The advances made in the study of animal models of anxiety over the past decade are little short of remarkable, especially in the field of conditioned fear. We may now with some confidence map out likely neural mechanisms from the level of functional systems to the cellular and molecular details. We know much of which neuroanatomical areas, neural projections, neurotransmitter systems and receptors are involved in the acquisition and expression of a number of fear-related behaviours.

This is fine progress indeed, but often begs the question of direct relevance to clinical applications. To what extent is the study of conditioned fear and anxiety in animals easily translated into the neuropsychiatric domain? There are several approaches to answering this question. One might suggest that clinical anxiety does indeed reflect a specific neuropathology in a specific behavioural system that is well described at the neurobiological and behavioural level (e.g. patterns of defensive behaviour; Rodgers 1997). This approach values certain forms of animal model over others (e.g. ethological vs. conditioning-based models), and to a certain degree adheres to the suggestion that anxiety reflects a pathological state of a perfectly normal fear system. A second approach is to accept that just as there is diversity in the clinical diagnosis of anxiety (e.g. generalized anxiety disorder, specific phobias, social phobias, panic disorder, posttraumatic stress disorder, and obsessive–compulsive disorder), so there are multiple tests of anxiety in animal models. This is a pragmatic approach, but care must surely be taken to ensure that one has sufficient knowledge of the behaviours being studied to ensure that one knows to which aspects of anxiety they may be related. An excellent example of this approach is seen in recent work by Mineka and colleagues (Bouton et al. 2001; Ohman and Mineka 2001) in which perspectives from modern learning theory are applied with some success to anxiety disorders in general and to panic disorder and the notion of preparedness in phobias in particular. A similar excellent example, this time in the field of depression, is represented by the work on repeated maternal separation by Matthews (Chapter 16 in this volume). Here a single early manipulation in rats produces a well-characterized neuropathology, as well as disrupted performance across a range of animal models of depression including responses to novelty and reinforcement and hedonic processing. A third approach is to take a middle road between these two. One assumes that there is some commonality between emotions and emotional responding in humans and laboratory animals, that clinical anxiety reflects a disordered state of emotional processing, and that a variety of animal models may be used to examine these systems of emotional processing. This approach does not seek to suggest that any individual behaviour in animals is related to clinical anxiety as it may be manifest in this or that patient group. It is not an explicit attempt to produce a complete model of human anxiety disorders. Nor does it seek necessarily to provide an easy and simple route for identifying novel anxiolytics as part of a behavioural screening programme. What it does intend to do is to use cognitive and behavioural neuroscience techniques to elucidate the neurobiological substrates of brain systems that are involved in the sorts of emotional behaviour that are abnormal in different aspects of clinical anxiety.

The following discussion will attempt to follow this middle road, presenting recent evidence that highlights a wide range of behavioural and neuroscientific studies concerned with fear- and anxiety-related behaviours in laboratory animals. This will be a broad-brush approach, not seeking to elucidate the precise neurochemical or cellular mechanisms involved – others may achieve that with greater depth and detail than are possible here (Quirk et al. 1997; Davis 2000). Rather, the intention is to describe connected systems that are likely to be involved in anxiety-related behaviours. Many of these systems, individually or in combination, have been associated with a variety of fear-related behaviours in animals, and often also with the effectiveness of established anxiolytic agents. Other systems have simply not been examined in sufficient detail, and the following discussion will try to highlight these. Finally, the areas discussed will be concentrated on the amygdala, a structure long implicated in emotional processing. This is not to suggest that the amygdala is the seat of anxiety in humans or laboratory animals, nor to suggest that to understand the minutiae of amygdala function is fully to understand fear or anxiety. The reason for focusing on the amygdala is because the functional neuroanatomy of this structure provides a useful framework around which to conceptualize the neural systems that appear most intimately concerned with anxiety; it appears to have direct connections to or from (or both) almost every other structure considered to have a role in anxiety. This of course is no accident. We have known the importance of the amygdala in emotional processing for many years. However, what is becoming evident is that we are now able to go beyond this rather general conceptualization and attempt to understand the ways in which the many various inputs and outputs of the amygdala may contribute to discrete, dissociable aspects of fear- and anxiety-related behaviours, and also to coordinated responses across several behavioural or psychological systems. The basic research reviewed below examines a wide variety of individual paradigms that selectively explore the many different components of fear-related behaviour, and reviews multiple sources of evidence to emphasize the particular relevance of different neuroanatomical projection systems.

Dissociable systems of the amygdala in anxiety

There are, to judge by recent research, two clearly dissociable subsystems within the amygdala that may be divided functionally and neuroanatomically, and that are intimately involved in fear-related behaviours. The basis of this division lies in the dissociable projections of the basolateral complex (including both lateral and basal nuclei of the amygdala) and the central nucleus. These projections are summarized in Figure 15.1.

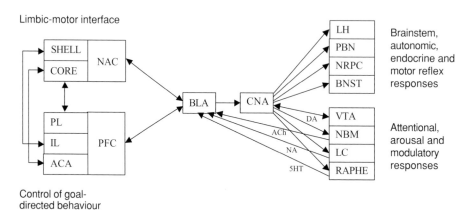

Figure 15.1   Output pathways from the rat amygdala in the control and coordination of fear and anxiety. See text for full details. Abbreviations: BLA, basolateral amygdala; CNA, central nucleus of the amygdala; NAC, nucleus accumbens; PFC, prefrontal cortex; PL, prelimbic cortex; IL, infralimbic cortex; ACA, anterior cingulate area; LH, lateral hypothalamus; PBN, parabrachial nucleus; NRPC, nucleus reticularis pontis caudalis; BNST, bed nucleus of the stria terminalis; VTA, ventrotegmental area NBM, nucleus basalis magnocellularis; LC, locus coeruleus; RAPHE, dorsal raphé nucleus; DA, dopamine; NA, noradrenaline; ACh, acetylcholine; 5-HT, serotonin.

For complete details of this connectivity, readers are referred to Pitkänen (2000). First, to consider in brief the differential outputs of these regions, at the one extreme the lateral nucleus and basal nuclei project to the medial temporal lobe system, striatum, hippocampal formation, hypothalamus and cortical (especially prefrontal) regions. In contrast, the central nucleus projects predominantly to the midbrain, pons, medulla, bed nucleus of the stria terminalis, hypothalamus and to cholinergic and monoaminergic neurons of the locus coeruleus, ventral tegmental area, substantia nigra, raphé and nucleus basalis magnocellularis (see also Swanson and Petrovitch 1998). Hence, targets of the basolateral complex are largely to areas of premotor and prefrontal cortex, as well as areas of forebrain output such as the striatum, providing routes to the control of complex behaviour at many levels. The central nucleus has contact with hypothalamic and brainstem sites that control autonomic, endocrine and somatomotor reflex responses, as well as general arousal and attentional functions. At an output level the distinction is clear: the basolateral complex projects to regions that allow control of complex actions, whereas the central nucleus is perhaps able to marshal the coordinated reflexive responses to fear-related stimuli. As we shall see, both of these systems are crucial to the control of varied aspects of fear-related behaviour observed in animals.

Details of the inputs to the basolateral and central nuclei of the amygdala are rather more complicated, and perhaps more controversial. Various researchers have suggested the lateral nucleus of the amygdala serves as the primary focus of both higher-order and thalamic sensory input to the entire amygdala structure, with this information then being distributed to other nuclei within the formation by a complex array of intra-amygdala connections. In this model, the predominant output in the control of learned fear is suggested to be via the central nucleus projections to hypothalamic and brainstem sites (Davis 1992; LeDoux 1996). However, recent research has challenged this view (see below; Killcross et al. 1997a) providing behavioural evidence of independent input–output streams through the basolateral and central regions. This work has since been supported by similar studies from other laboratories (Vazdarjanova and McGaugh 1998; Amorapanth et al. 2000), and also has the backing of more recent neuroanatomical data demonstrating that higher-order sensory information projects directly to the capsular and lateral subdivisions of the central nucleus in a manner that parallels input to the lateral nucleus (McDonald 1998; Pitkänen 2000). The central nucleus also receives highly processed information from the entorhinal cortex to the capsular subdivision. These converging lines of evidence suggest that, although the input to the lateral amygdala is by far the most pronounced, there are likely to be parallel streams of highly processed sensory input to other amygdala nuclei, including the central nucleus.

With these two systems mapped out, it is now possible to examine the ways in which they might come to influence dissociable aspects of anxiety-related

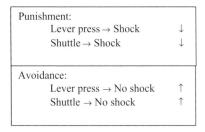

Involuntary, reflexive

Pavlovian conditioning

Pairings of stimulus with aversive
event e.g. tone with footshock:

   Tone (CS) $\Rightarrow$ Footshock (US)

Tone presentation evokes changes in
involuntary systems:

Skeleto-muscular:	
Freezing	$\uparrow$
Fear potentiated startle	$\uparrow$
Conditioned suppression	$\uparrow$

Autonomic:	
Blood pressure	$\uparrow\downarrow$
Heart rate	$\uparrow\downarrow$
Galvanic skin responses	$\uparrow$

Endocrine:	
Stress hormones	
via alterations in HPA axis	$\uparrow$

Voluntary, goal-directed

Instrumental learning

Establishment of a relationship between a
response and occurrence of an aversive event:

   Response $\Rightarrow$ Footshock
   Response $\Rightarrow$ Avoid footshock

Changes in propensity to perform responses:

Punishment:	
Lever press $\rightarrow$ Shock	$\downarrow$
Shuttle $\rightarrow$ Shock	$\downarrow$

Avoidance:	
Lever press $\rightarrow$ No shock	$\uparrow$
Shuttle $\rightarrow$ No shock	$\uparrow$

Figure 15.2 Dissociable behavioural systems in fear conditioning. $\downarrow$, decreased response; $\uparrow$, increased response; $\downarrow\uparrow$, variable effects on response rate. See text for further details.

behaviours, from reflexive responses evoked by fear-related cues, changes in attentional bias, alterations in arousal and autonomic function, through to variation in voluntary, goal-directed behaviours and avoidance discriminations. The difference in these types of behaviour, and the terminology frequently used in animal studies, are illustrated in Figure 15.2. This schematic places different forms of behaviour (reflexive vs. voluntary) in the context of generic assessments of fear learning that have been used to quantify conditioned fear and anxiety. It should be noted that although a binary division is suggested here, there are a number of procedures used which involve aspects of different behavioural systems and are therefore indeterminate with respect to this simple division. For example, passive avoidance procedures in which an animal must remain in a given location to avoid shock might nominally be regarded as a punishment procedure, as any movement to an alternative location (shuttle response) is punished. However, at the same time it is clear that there are elements of Pavlovian conditioning in which the alternative chamber becomes a conditioned stimulus or signal for footshock and this in itself will tend to inhibit any natural tendency to approach this chamber. For a more in-depth discussion of the issues surrounding the possible nature and status of different response systems, readers are referred to Killcross and Blundell (2002).

The individual neural systems involved in fear and anxiety in relation to particular, highly selective behaviours such as freezing or fear-potentiated startle are dealt with in admirable detail elsewhere. The intention is not to rehearse well-tested arguments but rather to provide an overview of some of the evidence supporting the various roles of the amygdala and related structures in different behavioural manifestations of fear and anxiety. This will begin by consideration of the brainstem and hypothalamic outputs of the central nucleus of the amygdala.

Brainstem and hypothalamic projections of the central nucleus of the amygdala

The central nucleus of the amygdala projects to a wide range of brainstem and hypothalamic nuclei, each of which is implicated in a variety of forms of fear-related behaviour (Davis 1992). Projections to the lateral hypothalamus are involved in the control of heart rate, galvanic skin responses, and changes in blood-flow patterns and blood pressure by activation of the sympathetic autonomic nervous system. Projections to the dorsal motor nucleus of the vagus also influence heart rate, as well as gastric secretion and bowel and bladder control. Projections to the central grey control reflexive immobility or freezing, whereas projections to the nucleus reticularis pontis caudalis produced heightened startle responding (see below). Projections to the parabrachial nucleus are likely to be involved in the regulation of respiration. Finally, projections to the bed nucleus of the stria terminalis and then to the paraventricular nucleus are able to influence neuroendocrine stress responses such as corticosterone release.

The majority of work supporting these findings has come from studies of conditioned fear in laboratory animals (predominantly rats, but also rabbits and mice), together with linking anecdotal evidence from the evocation of fear and fear responses during temporal lobe epilepsy in humans. There are two dominant methods of assessment of learned fear in animals, both based on simple Pavlovian conditioning. Conditioned freezing examines the changes in levels of rigid immobility in the presence of a conditioned stimulus (CS) such as a light or tone, following pairings of that CS with an aversive unconditioned stimulus (US) such as mild footshock. If a novel CS is presented to an unrestrained animal prior to fear conditioning, it frequently elicits orienting responses and a moderate increase in general activity. However, if the animal receives, for example, two pairings of the CS with mild footshock US, subsequent presentation of the CS alone will produce high levels of freezing – characteristic rigid immobility, with no movement other than respiration. This is a species-specific defence response to signals for danger. The benefits of this means of assessment of learned fear are that it is quick, simple and easily determined. The second form of commonly assessed Pavlovian fear conditioning examines fear-potentiated startle. Here, following similar pairings of CS and US to those outlined above, one examines the influence of presentation of the CS on the level of startle response produced by brief presentation of an intense acoustic stimulus such as a 100dB burst of white noise. This noise burst will normally elicit a startle or jump response in animals, and this response is enhanced if the burst of white noise coincides with presentation of a fear-conditioned (but not neutral) CS such as a light. Once again, this measure has a number of advantages in terms of ease of use, reliability and simplicity, and may also be observed under certain circumstances in humans.

Using these two procedures, researchers have been able to demonstrate that damage to, or chemical inactivation of, the central nucleus of the amygdala produces deficits in conditioned fear. A recent review (Davis 2000) lists some dozen or so studies demonstrating this finding using freezing or startle measures (as well as a number of other assessments of Pavlovian conditioned fear) and employing electrolytic and neurotoxic lesions as well as reversible inactivation by lidocaine or muscimol. There now seems little doubt as to the role of the central nucleus of the amygdala in Pavlovian conditioned fear as measured by changes in behavioural activation, presumably dependent on outputs to the central grey and nucleus reticularis pontis caudalis. Further work demonstrates that similar lesion manipulations of the central nucleus will also reduce neuroendocrine and autonomic measures of conditioned fear, particularly changes in heart rate during a fear-eliciting CS as well as alterations in blood pressure and stress hormone release. A far smaller number of studies also show that similar lesions can also block or blunt unconditioned hormonal, neuroendocrine and behavioural measures of fear in response to stressful events such as immobilization, footshock alone, exposure to cats and to novel open spaces. In each instance, it appears that both learned and innate reflexive responses to fear-eliciting stimuli are influenced by manipulation of the central nucleus. Furthermore, other evidence points to these specific output pathways as the neuroanatomical basis of each particular form of behavioural, neuroendocrine or autonomic response. That is, manipulation of individual output mechanisms by lesioning or pharmacological means produces orderly effects that reflect the specific function of individual targets of the central nucleus. In this sense, the amygdala is seen as part of a highly organized system for coordinating responses to threat (Graeff et al. 1997).

Cholinergic system projections of the central nucleus of the amygdala

In addition to these subcortical output systems directly involved in the production of specific emotional responses, the central nucleus of the amygdala also projects to regions of the brain that are known to be involved in the modulation of higher-order control processes such as attentional function and memory. Some of these functions are summarized in Figure 15.3.

The importance of attentional bias and changes in patterns of orienting in anxiety scarcely needs to be stressed here. However, the emergence of research linking

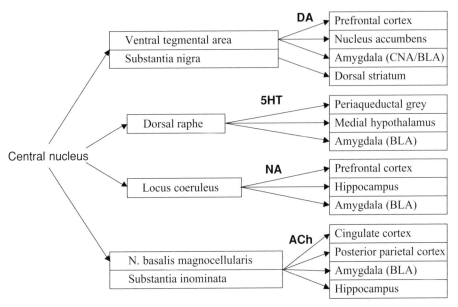

Figure 15.3   Output connections from the central nucleus of the amygdala to modulatory neurotransmitter systems influencing attention, arousal, memory consolidation and stress responses. Abbreviations as for Figure 15.1.

various brain regions to the top-down control of stimulus processing and selective attention potentially provides a link between the more cognitive aspects of anxiety (Eysenck 1992, 1997) that emphasize hypervigilance, selective attentional bias and appraisal processes, and basic studies of behavioural neuroscience in laboratory animals. One example of a system that influences the modulation of stimulus processing by top-down cognitive factors is the forebrain cholinergic system (Everitt and Robbins 1997). Although it appears that the role played by central cholinergic systems depends upon their precise connectivity, recent evidence suggests that the cholinergic projection from the nucleus basalis magnocellularis in the basal forebrain to the neocortex is intimately involved in attentional function (Muir et al. 1992, 1993, 1994; Sarter and Bruno 1997). In the context of the amygdala, the central nucleus projects directly to the nucleus basalis, and the role of this projection in attentional function has been studied in rats using a variety of tasks that assess behaviour and learning directed towards novel stimuli or cues with uncertain outcomes. Hence lesions of the central nucleus abolish spontaneous orienting responses to novel cues (Gallagher et al. 1990), a response thought to reflect an overt component of attentional processing, as well as cortical desynchronization thought to reflect widespread changes in stimulus processing (Kapp et al. 1992).

Damage to the central nucleus also brings about changes in attentional function that occur as a direct result of learning and experience. Stimuli that consistently predict the same outcome come, over time, to elicit less and less orienting in animals

(Pearce and Hall 1980). However, orienting responses are restored as soon as a given stimulus is followed by an unexpected outcome rather than the previously trained event, and this increase in orienting is reflected in the amount of attention directed towards, and learning produced by, the new sequence of events. Once again, lesions of the central-nucleus abolish this increase in attentional processing and reduce learning about new consequences of old stimuli (Holland and Gallagher 1993a, b). Using this same test of attentional function, other research has shown that this central-nucleus-induced deficit is dependent upon the modulation of basal forebrain cholinergic systems projecting to the posterior parietal cortex. Hence, similar disruptions in attention are seen following lesions of the nucleus basalis magnocellularis and substantia innominata (Chiba et al. 1995) and removal of the cholinergic input to the posterior parietal cortex by the immunotoxin 192 IgG saporin (Bucci et al. 1998). Most compellingly, crossed lesions of the central nucleus and its output targets of nucleus basalis magnocellularis and substantia innominata also reproduce attentional deficits (Han et al. 1999).

This research would seem to indicate that the outputs of the central nucleus do not simply modulate downstream fear-output systems at a behavioural level, but can also change the way in which top-down and bottom-up influences alter selective attentional processing of relevant stimuli. Although the vast majority of these lesion studies of attentional function were conducted using appetitive tasks, the conclusions are very likely to remain the same when considering learning about aversive cues (especially in view of the fact that the underlying theoretical view of attentional change was developed in aversive procedures; Hall and Pearce 1979). A valuable future contribution would be to investigate the effects of manipulation of these systems in aversive procedures. Similarly, the precise nature of central nucleus attentional modulation has yet to be fully described – when is it evoked? Which inputs to the amygdala are crucial in determining attentional change? Is it possible to artificially alter these specific attentional processes neurochemically? There are intriguing hints that begin to address some of these points; for example, electrical stimulation of the central nucleus produces cortical desynchronization, an effect blocked by cholinergic antagonists (Kapp et al. 1994), as well as increasing pupil dilation and pinna-orienting responses (Applegate et al. 1982).

Monoaminergic projections of the central nucleus of the amygdala

The central nucleus provides the main source of amygdala projections to the midbrain, pons and medulla. Within these regions, the central nucleus projects to the whole of the substantia nigra, the ventral tegmental area, the locus coeruleus and the dorsal raphé. Hence, the central nucleus is in a position to modulate dopaminergic (DA), noradrenergic (NA) and serotonergic (5-hydroxytryptamine; 5HT) systems.

In each case, though to differing degrees, these neurotransmitter systems have been associated with changes occurring in fear, stress and anxiety. For example, much recent work has suggested that the serotonergic systems of the brain play a central role in the control of behaviour by aversive events (Deakin and Graeff 1991; Wilkinson et al. 1996). 5HT projections form an important part of an integrated system for the control and elaboration of innate and learned responses to anxiety- or fear-provoking stimuli in the environment. The efficacy of 5HT-active drugs such as the $5HT_{1A}$ partial agonist buspirone in the treatment of clinical anxiety has been demonstrated (Taylor et al. 1985), and in some cases has been shown to be more effective than treatment with classic benzodiazepine anxiolytics such as diazepam and midazolam. However, it is apparent that the precise effect of alterations in 5HT activity on anxiety- and fear-related behaviours is likely to depend crucially on the specific site of action of the drug, and also on the precise model of anxiety employed. Hence, the effects of $5HT_{1A}$ ligands in animal models of anxiety is rather variable, regardless of whether the model employs conditioned or unconditioned behaviour. Overall, it has been suggested that increases in 5HT activity are anxiogenic in models dependent on behavioural inhibition for their measure of fear reduction, but anxiolytic in situations where the aversive stimulus produces an active response (Handley et al. 1993; Graeff et al. 1997). Such paradoxical findings are also observed clinically, with the $5HT_{2A/2C}$ receptor antagonist ritanserin alleviating generalized anxiety disorder, but increasing panic attacks (Den Boer and Westenberg 1990). As 5HT pathways in the brain involve not only postsynaptic receptors but also somatodendritic inhibitory autoreceptors, it is clear that systemic treatment with specific receptor agonists or antagonists might therefore produce variable results depending on the predominant mode of action (File et al. 1996). Nevertheless, anxiolytic activity of $5HT_{1A}$ ligands has been demonstrated (albeit rather inconsistently) in a variety of conditioned-fear models, including conditioned suppression (Stanhope and Dourish 1996), conflict models (Sanger 1992; Barrett and Vanover 1993) and fear-potentiated startle (Mansbach and Geyer 1988; Melia and Davis 1991).

It has been suggested that 5HT neurons in the dorsal raphé operate by activating danger-evaluation processes in the amygdala in response to learned threat stimuli, whilst at the same time inhibiting neurons in the dorsal periaqueductal grey (PAG) that produce flight and fight responses in situations of extreme proximal danger (Deakin and Graeff 1991; Graeff et al. 1997). The 5HT innervation of the dorsal PAG, running from the dorsal raphé nucleus via the periventricular tract, appears to be responsible for the control of innate flight and fight responses that most closely resemble panic in man. Within this system, increased 5HT activity is inhibitory, leading to a reduction of fear responding. Hence, increasing activity in 5HT pathways from the dorsal raphé reduces one-way escape behaviour in an elevated T-maze. Similarly, infusion of the $5HT_{1A}$ full agonist 8-hydroxy-(2-di-*n*-propylamino)-tetralin (8-OH-DPAT) into the PAG attenuates escape behaviours elicited by excitatory amino-acid stimulation of the PAG, an effect reversed by systemic treatment with the $5HT_{1A}$ receptor antagonist WAY100635. However, systemic administration of 8-OH-DPAT enhanced PAG-stimulated escape, indicative of differential effects of pre- and postsynaptic receptor agonism (Beckett and Marsden 1997). In humans, selective release of 5HT from dorsal raphé pathways by D-fenfluramine reduced unconditioned anxiety evoked by simulated public speaking, but enhanced conditioned fear measured by changes in skin conductance to an aversive CS (Graeff et al. 1996). In contrast, the serotonergic innervation of the amygdala, also originating in the dorsal raphé nucleus but traversing the dorsal raphé–forebrain tract, appears to be involved in anticipatory responses to Pavlovian conditioned fear stimuli, most frequently producing an inhibition of responding. In this situation it is likely that the influence of increasing 5HT activity is to increase anxiety. Hence, activation of the dorsal raphé 5HT system by systemic administration of D-fenfluramine in the rat enhanced inhibitory avoidance whilst reducing one-way escape in the elevated T-maze (Graeff et al. 1997). Similarly, systemic treatment with 8-OH-DPAT enhanced rates of punished responding in a conflict schedule (an anxiolytic profile in this test), whereas intra-amygdala infusion of 8-OH-DPAT or 5HT itself reduced punished responding (Hodges et al. 1987). This is likely to reflect the ability of systemic treatment with 8-OH-DPAT to activate somatodendritic inhibitory autoreceptors at the level of the raphé, thereby *reducing* 5HT activity on the amygdala and producing a reduction in fear and anxiety. In support of this, recent research has used in vivo dialysis to demonstrate that systemic 8-OH-DPAT does indeed reduce levels of 5HT in the central nucleus (Bosker et al. 1997). In addition, it has been suggested that activity in the central nucleus, which projects to the dorsal raphé nucleus, has a facilitatory influence on 5HT release that decreases activity in the dorsal PAG flight system and increases activity in the amygdala anticipatory fear system (Graeff et al. 1997). This activity appears to be tonically inhibited by GABA activation in the amygdala, producing a dynamic balance of anticipatory fear and flight responding (Graeff 1994). In this way the dorsal raphé 5HT system forms yet a further part of a coordinated system controlling various aspects of fear and anxiety, directing responding away from innate flight and fight responses and towards more controlled, learned responses.

As suggested above, one potential difficulty in the study of 5HT-related anxiolytic function in animals is that manipulations of serotonergic function influence not only anxiety- and fear-related behaviours, but also produce robust disinhibition of responding that is not necessarily restricted to aversive stimuli or events (Harrison et al. 1997). As many behavioural tasks examining anxiolytic potential depend upon release of a response that is unusually inhibited in normal animals (e.g. conditioned suppression, Geller–Seifter conflict tasks etc.), the potential confound is clear. In one approach that discriminates between these possible effects in serotonergic agents, we have examined the effects of the $5HT_{1A}$ partial agonist buspirone on the conditioned elevation of avoidance responding. In this procedure, rats are trained to respond on a Sidman avoidance lever-press schedule in which responding on a lever delays the presentation of a mild footshock that would normally occur at fixed time intervals. Responding is therefore maintained by the anticipation and avoidance of an aversive event. Using this procedure we have demonstrated (Killcross, unpublished observations) that normal animals show an *enhancement* of responding during presentation of a fear-evoking CS that has been separately paired with mild footshock, and hence an anxiolytic effect is manifest by a *reduction* of lever pressing during CS presentation. In contrast, a disinhibitory effect would appear as a general increase in responding during the CS. Systemic administration of low doses of buspirone produce an anxiolytic profile, reducing the fear-induced increase in responding during an aversive CS. In contrast, higher doses of buspirone (likely to be less selective for $5HT_{1A}$ receptors than lower doses, and to influence differentially postsynaptic receptors and somatodendritic inhibitory autoreceptors) produce an increase in responding, indicative of a general disinhibitory effect.

In contrast to 5HT, there is little evidence that the DA systems of the brain are directly involved in anxiety. However, exposure to mildly stressful situations clearly leads to an enhancement of dopamine release and metabolism in the medial prefrontal cortex (Thierry et al. 1976) and this has been linked to aspects of posttraumatic stress disorder (Deutch and Young 1995). Furthermore, there is evidence that DA within both the medial prefrontal cortex and nucleus accumbens is altered during the course of simple Pavlovian fear conditioning (Wilkinson et al. 1998), and may be related to the observed level of freezing and degree of habituation to the CS. The indirect DA agonist amphetamine can increase the punishing impact of stimuli that have been paired with aversive footshock (Killcross et al. 1997b), an effect that is reversed by the DA D1/2 receptor antagonist alpha-flupenthixol. However, the ability of this DA antagonist to reduce the impact of punishing stimuli appears to be qualitatively (but not quantitatively) different to similar anxiolytic effects produced by the benzodiazepine midazolam (Killcross et al. 1997b). On the basis of these results we suggested that the effect of enhancing DA release was to increase the salience and behavioural impact of all stimuli, be they aversive or appetitive in nature. This effect is also observed in response to aversive events (e.g. footshock) themselves (Killcross and Robbins 1993; Killcross et al. 1994). Further research is needed to determine the central site of action of the influence of DA systems on the salience and behavioural impact of aversive stimuli and events, and based on work examining appetitive learning (Hitchcott and Phillips 1998), the DA projection to the amygdala remains a possible candidate.

Stressful situations also produce increases in brain NA function, with increases most marked in amygdala, hippocampus and cortex. In addition to these effects of acute stressors, chronic exposure to stress leads to enhanced responsiveness of NA neurons to normal stimulation, and to enhanced NA release in the medial prefrontal cortex (Finlay and Abercrombie 1991) and hippocampus (Nisenbaum et al. 1991). Furthermore, there is evidence that lesions of the dorsal and ventral NA systems influence fear conditioning in rats (Cole and Robbins 1987), although it is not clear whether this effect is due to effects on mechanisms of learning per se or due to the influence of NA manipulations on stimulus processing. Clear evidence supports a role for NA systems in the enhanced acquisition of fear conditioning brought about by natural or artificial increases in brain levels of glucocorticoid stress hormones at the time of learning (McGaugh et al. 2000). Further evidence suggests that the critical site for this modulation is the basolateral nucleus of the amygdala (Roozendaal and McGaugh 1996). Hence, lesions of the basolateral, but not central, nucleus of the amygdala block the memory-enhancing effects of systemic injection of the synthetic glucocorticoid dexamethasone. This effect is likely to be mediated via NA β-receptor activation in the basolateral nucleus, as posttraining systemic administration of β-adrenoreceptor antagonists block memory-enhancing effects of glucocorticoid activation. Similarly, posttraining infusions of NA into the basolateral amygdala enhance, and of propranolol into the same region impair, spatial memory in rats (Hatfield and McGaugh 1999). In turn, stressful events such as footshock cause an increase in NA release in the amygdala, with release increasing in relation to the level of aversive stimulation (Quirarte et al. 1998). At least one possibility that suggests itself is that, in the intact animal, NA activation is caused in part by descending projections from the central nucleus of the amygdala, causing a feedback increase in NA levels in the basolateral region and a consequent increase in memory consolidation for emotionally arousing events. A similar overall pattern of NA influence on memory formation is suggested in humans, where administration of propranolol impairs memory for an emotionally arousing story, but not a neutral story (Cahill et al. 1994). Hence the suggestion is that the emotional impact of stimuli can, via NA-dependent mechanisms in the amygdala, lead to an increase in the strength of consolidation and subsequent retrieval of emotionally charged, or traumatic, memories. Perturbations of this system have been linked to the development of posttraumatic stress disorder (Cahill 1997), creating a scenario in which chronic exposure to stressful events leads to a sensitization of NA systems, which in turn produces a heightened NA release in response to further stressful episodes, promoting enhanced memory for emotionally significant events, and ultimately leading to clinical psychopathology. There is also evidence suggesting that NA function may be disrupted in some patients with panic disorder (Charney et al. 1987), and indications that there is elevated NA release in phobic patients in response to phobia-salient stimuli.

Each of the major output systems of the central nucleus of the amygdala, whether they are to specific brainstem nuclei controlling discrete autonomic, endocrine or behavioural responses, or to regions that lead to the modulation of diffuse systems, appear to be involved in the development of fear- and anxiety-related behaviours. In both unconditioned and conditioned animal models, manipulations of these target regions and systems leads to alterations in fear responding, and these findings are frequently supported by clinical evidence. Several points should be highlighted at this stage. First, the nature of the change in fear-related behaviours produced by a given manipulation depends upon the target system being manipulated. Although lesions of the central nucleus itself produce wide-ranging alterations in fear-related behaviours, lesions of the individual target systems can produce more behaviourally selective effects (for example, manipulation of individual serotonergic systems). In some instances, the precise psychological relevance of these individual effects is well described and well understood, both at a neural and psychological level, facilitating comparison with clinical conditions. However, there are a number of effects that remain unexplored – for example, the possible role of cholinergic control of attentional function towards aversive events, or the role of dopaminergic mechanisms in fear conditioning and modulation of salience of fear-related cues. These avenues deserve further exploration. Second, the central nucleus rarely, if ever, functions as an isolated system. It is part of a coordinated system for controlling responding to emotionally significant stimuli. To understand the importance of the central nucleus in anxiety, one will need to understand this interactive system. Third, at a general level it appears that the central nucleus is more directly important in coordinating reflexive responses to fear- and anxiety-related cues than in the co-ordination and direction of complex behavioural response patterns in the face of threat situations. To understand these reflexive systems is no small undertaking, but will provide only a partial answer to questions that derive from clinical observations in humans. Finally, as the role of NA in emotional memory suggests, the production of coordinated psychological and behavioural responses to emotionally salient stimuli frequently requires the involvement of both the central and basolateral nuclei of the amygdala, and output systems controlled by both structures. It is to the basolateral nucleus of the amygdala this discussion now turns.

Cortical, striatal and hippocampal connections of the basolateral complex of the amygdala

To reiterate briefly, the basolateral nucleus of the amygdala, in contrast to the central nucleus, is directly connected to a variety of cortical and striatal sites associated with higher-order cognitive functions and motor-output circuits. The importance of this feature is perhaps most obviously demonstrated with reference to dissociations in fear-related behaviours in the rat. As mentioned briefly above, recent evidence has

analysis of acquisition of reflexive suppression in these animals. Analysis of the first block of five training trials in sham- and basolateral-lesioned animals revealed that, despite a numerical difference (mean suppression ratios (where 0.5 means no learning and 0 means good learning): sham = 0.22; basolateral = 0.31) there was no significant effect of lesion (Student's t-test, $P = 0.26$). Analysis of further blocks of five trials failed at any point to reveal an effect of lesion or an interaction of trial blocks and lesion. In contrast, the deficit observed in animals with lesions of the central nucleus was present on the first block of training trials (means: sham = 0.22; central = 0.42; Student's t-test, $P < 0.02$) and persisted across all levels of training examined. Therefore, learning in animals with lesions of the basolateral amygdala cannot be a consequence of extended training and was statistically equivalent to that seen in controls within five trials. These results demonstrate beyond any doubt that there are parallel systems of information flow through the amygdala in relation to different aspects of fear-related behaviours. Indeed, following these findings, there have been a number of reports indicating that there are a variety of possible routes involving the amygdala by which information relating to threat stimuli can come to control behaviour, including ventral striatum, prefrontal cortex, hippocampus and anterior cingulate cortex. These are detailed in the following section.

Interactions of the basolateral complex of the amygdala with corticostriatal systems

The basolateral region of the amygdala projects to a number of systems that are implicated in anxiety- or fear-related behaviours (Pitkänen 2000). For example, there are projections from the entorhinal cortex and subfield CA1 of the hippocampus to the lateral and basal nuclei, as well as from regions of ventral subiculum. Further, reciprocal connections exist between the lateral nucleus and the prelimbic and infralimbic medial prefrontal cortex, whilst the basal nucleus has even heavier interactions with these regions as well as the anterior cingulate cortex, and the ventral and lateral aspects of the frontal cortex (including lateral and medial orbital and agranular areas). Finally, the lateral amygdala projects to the nucleus accumbens (particularly lateral shell subregion) and the basal nucleus to the rostromedial nucleus accumbens (shell and medial core regions) as well as caudate–putamen (in a topographical manner). In many cases these connections are reciprocal, and in some instances it is the same amygdala neuron that projects to several regions (e.g. from basal nucleus to both prefrontal cortex and striatum; McDonald 1991). Furthermore, many of these target regions are also closely linked – for example there are links between the shell region of the nucleus accumbens and the infralimbic region of the prefrontal cortex, and from the core region of the nucleus accumbens to the anterior cingulate and prelimbic areas of medial prefrontal cortex. These systems are connected to pallidal output systems as part of the limbic motor interface (Mogenson et al. 1984). Overall, the basolateral amygdala appears to be involved in a cortico-striato-pallido-thalamo-cortical loop (Alexander et al. 1990) controlling the complex motor output of limbic–prefrontal interactions.

That these anatomical relationships are of functional, as well as theoretical, note is readily demonstrated. Hence, using the conditioned punishment task outlined above in the study dissociating central and basolateral regions of the amygdala, we have pursued the role of the various output targets of the basolateral amygdala in the control of dissociable voluntary and reflexive aspects of responding to conditioned fear stimuli. As predicted in our original paper (Killcross et al. 1997a) we have found that connected regions of prefrontal cortex and ventral striatum are crucial to the control of voluntary, but not reflexive, components of conditioned fear responding. We have shown that lesions of the infralimbic (Coutureau et al. 2001) and anterior cingulate regions (Killcross, Bussey and Robbins, unpublished observations) of the prefrontal cortex, but not the prelimbic (Coutureau et al. 2001) region of the prefrontal cortex, produce selective deficits in the voluntary control of aversively motivated behaviours, but have no impact on the acquisition reflexive suppression of responding. Similarly, the shell, but not core, subregion of the nucleus accumbens appears to be intimately involved in voluntary, but not reflexive, components of fear responding (Dix et al. 2001). Further, we have demonstrated that crossed unilateral lesions of the basolateral amygdala and medial prefrontal cortex abolish voluntary, but not reflexive, fear responses, emphasizing the importance of these regions as part of a functional circuit controlling and coordinating instrumental actions related to fear and anxiety (Coutureau et al. 2000). Finally, there is also evidence demonstrating that, at least at the prefrontal level, this involvement appears to be selective to aversive, fear-related stimuli and does not generalize to equivalent appetitive situations. Hence, lesions of the medial prefrontal cortex that included both prelimbic and infralimbic regions did not influence a conditioned reinforcement procedure in which behaviour was controlled by stimuli associated with rewarding outcomes (Burns et al. 1993). Similarly, lesions of the anterior cingulate cortex failed to disrupt performance in an alternative conditioned reinforcement task that directly paralleled the conditioned punishment task described above (Killcross, Bussey and Robbins, unpublished observations). In contrast, lesions of the prelimbic prefrontal cortex, which did not disrupt conditioned punishment, have been shown to alter performance in appetitively motivated instrumental tasks (Balleine and Dickinson 1998; Killcross and Coutureau, unpublished manuscript). Within the ventral striatum it appears that there may be more commonality across appetitively and aversively motivated behaviours, as both core and shell subregions of the nucleus accumbens have been implicated in varied aspects of reward-related instrumental performance (Balleine and Killcross 1994; Kelley et al. 1997; Parkinson et al. 1999).

Other researchers have also reported similar dissociations of fear-related behaviours at the level of the amygdala. Selden et al. (1991) reported that excitotoxic lesions of the basolateral amygdala abolished conditioning to a discrete cue but left intact aversive learning about contextual or environment cues based on a place preference measure. Similarly, Cahill et al. (2000) reported the acquisition of conditioned freezing in rats with excitotoxic lesions of the basolateral amygdala that was not impaired relative to sham-operated controls but nevertheless demonstrated substantial evidence of conditioned fear. Vazdarjanova and McGaugh (1998) reported that lesions of the basolateral complex influenced both unconditioned and conditioned aspects of freezing behaviour, but also permitted significant acquisition of conditioned fear as assessed by performance in a Y-maze in which rats had to avoid a maze-arm previously paired with mild footshock. Finally, in a study very similar to that reported earlier (Killcross et al. 1997a), Amorapanth et al. (2000) reported that damage to the central nucleus interfered with freezing to a tone, but left intact performance in a task in which animals had to perform a response to turn off the aversive CS in a novel context. In contrast, lesions of the basal region of the amygdala produced the reverse pattern of results, whereas damage to the lateral nucleus produced deficits in both tasks. Each of these experiments adds to the strong conclusion that different amygdala output mechanisms are crucially involved in the control and coordination of fear- and anxiety-related responding.

These revealing results nevertheless represent only the beginning of an investigation into this basolateral output system of the amygdala and its role in anxiety and anxiety-related behaviours. There is much still to find out. For example, the infralimbic region of the prefrontal cortex, in addition to its connections to the basolateral amygdala and shell of the nucleus accumbens, also shares many of its outputs with the brainstem and hypothalamic targets of the central nucleus of the amygdala (Hurley et al. 1991). Recent work has highlighted a selective role for this region in the extinction of conditioned fear (Quirk et al. 2000) and the control of inhibitory responding in aversive situations (Frysztak and Neafsey 1994; Jinks and McGregor 1997). Although the role of the cingulate cortex in voluntary action appears to be selective to aversively motivated procedures, this region is also known to be involved in certain aspects of appetitively motivated responding (Bussey et al. 1997). How might these roles be related? Similarly, exposure to the acute stress of escapable footshock has been shown to enhance rates of acquisition of self-stimulation in the medial prefrontal cortex (Balleine 1991), emphasizing this region's role in interactions of appetitive and aversive systems. We might ask to what extent these regions are involved in representing the aversive nature of cues. What is their function in representing the (appetitive or aversive) outcome of a voluntary instrumental response, or in the inhibition of ongoing appetitive behaviour in the face of alternative contingencies that predict the likely occurrence of aversive events?

A more complete understanding of the interactions of these various different amygdaloid output targets, both with the amygdala and with each other, will be central to our full understanding of fear and anxiety.

Future directions and genetic approaches

There is little doubt that the evidence reviewed in this chapter strongly suggests that multiple neural systems are involved in anxiety, and that these systems interact to different qualitative and quantitative degrees in the manifestation of individual anxiety disorders. What does the future hold with respect to the possibility of disentangling these interactive systems, and in the production of highly selective and efficacious anxiolytics? As mentioned in the introduction to this piece, great strides have been made over the last decade in our understanding of the neural substrates of learned fear (albeit narrowly defined as learning processes that produce conditioned freezing or fear-potentiated startle). It is to be hoped that similar advances may now be made in our understanding of the interaction of these systems with neural mechanisms that underpin the control of controlled, voluntary responding. After all, these systems are those most likely to be responsible for the avoidance behaviour and feelings of anticipatory anxiety that are common to many anxiety disorders. This progress may be achieved by the combination of skilled application of neuroanatomical and neuropharmacological techniques with a sophisticated understanding of the psychological basis of associative learning and the control of reflexive and voluntary responding. As has been the case for Pavlovian fear conditioning, it is this approach that will allow us insight into the systems, cells and molecules involved in the control of instrumental fear responding. What is equally clear is that the use of extremely simple behavioural screening tests to identify putative anxiolytic agents is unlikely to provide levels of face, construct and predictive validity (see Chapter 16 by Matthews) that will be required for the development of the next generation of clinically useful drugs. A more selective approach to the development of pharmaceuticals for the treatment of dissociable anxiety disorders demands an equally sensitive and selective approach to the understanding of behaviours that are used to investigate and model these disorders. But how are we to approach the broader picture, to identify which combinations of fear-learning systems are involved in different forms of anxiety in the clinic? And how might we identify individuals who are at risk for anxiety disorders? It is here that emerging genetic and transgenic technologies are likely to play an increasingly important role. Recent work by Flint and colleagues (Flint et al. 1995; Turri et al. 2001; see also Gora-Maslak et al. 1995) has started to attempt to identify common sets of genes that influence anxiety-related behaviours. Using mostly ethologically based tests of anxiety in mice (such as the elevated plus-maze, open-field test and the light–dark box) they have attempted to identify quantitative trait loci (QTLs) on individual chromosomes that control behavioural responding in specific anxiety-provoking situations. This approach offers two possible insights that may prove beneficial to our understanding of the neural basis of anxiety. The first is that the identification of QTLs may lead to the more selective identification of individual gene products that control anxiety-related behaviour. For example, recent targeted mutations have identified (or perhaps confirmed) a role for the $5HT_{1A}$ receptor in anxiety (Heisler et al. 1998). Second, the use of QTL analysis following behavioural screening on tests of anxiety allows one to determine whether or not individual tests of anxiety do indeed reflect some underlying specific phenotype related to anxiety. Unfortunately, the success or failure of this approach again lies with the choice of measure for anxiety. Recent work producing a QTL analysis across five different ethological tests of anxiety has demonstrated that the genetic influences in the tests were far more complicated that anticipated, and that many of the identified genetically controlled behavioural effects were unrelated to anxiety (Turri et al. 2001). Different loci were found that reflected general effects in the tests such as locomotor activity and exploration. This emphasizes once again the point made throughout this chapter. Anxiety is not a unitary disorder and cannot be modelled or elucidated by using a restricted set of behavioural analyses. A related problem is the stability of behavioural assessments of anxiety across generations in selective breeding programmes. If the behavioural variability is too large, due to either the test itself or the possible environmental variability, then attempts to generate a particular phenotype are doomed to failure. This is not to undervalue the genetic approach – indeed, the study above (Turri et al. 2001) identified a QTL on chromosome 15 in mice that appeared highly selective for avoidance behaviours across all five tests. It would be of interest to determine the role of such QTLs in measures of avoidance in learned fear procedures.

The examination of animals with targeted gene mutations such as transgenic mice (which have a new gene added to the genome) and knockout mice (which have a selective gene deletion) may also provide insight into the neural substrates of anxiety. (see also Chapter 19 by Stephens et al.). As genes are added or deleted from the genome, behavioural phenotyping allows the identification of individual genes that contribute to selective aspects of fear- and anxiety-related behaviours. However, once again this technology comes with its own problems. It is obviously the case that many of the problems associated with QTL analysis also apply to the use of single-gene mutations. Indeed, recent work identified the elevated plus-maze, the light–dark box and the open-field test as appropriate animal models of anxiety for use in phenotypic screening of transgenic and knockout mice – exactly those tests which revealed multiply-determined QTLs, many of which were unrelated to anxiolytic profiles. The use of novel genetic techniques in the study of anxiety is all too frequently limited by the poorly specified behavioural phenotyping that accompanies targeted genetic mutation. Furthermore, as Crawley (1999) points out, except in the rare case in which a knockout is being used to examine a human disorder that itself results from a single-point mutation, there are additional problems. Any mutation that is imposed on the organism exists in all cells in the body for the entire duration of development and ageing. Not only is this very unlike the disorders that the models seek to mimic, but it may well be unfeasible to determine the central or peripheral site of action of the mutation that controls behavioural phenotype. This is not only because of uncertainty about the crucial locus of effect, but also because of developmental adaptations that may cause other genes or gene products to be adjusted to take over the role of, or compensate for the effect of the original targeted mutation. One possible solution to some of these problems is the use of conditional knockouts (or, more generally, conditional mutations). This allows specific mutations to be induced only at specific times in development, allowing one to examine the effect of the mutation on behavioural phenotype independently of any possible effect of the mutation during developmental processes. In essence, genes may be turned 'on' or 'off' on demand. Although this technology is at a relatively early stage, further improvements will allow genetic manipulation to become a genuinely useful tool in the study of the neural basis of anxiety.

Summary and relationship to studies in humans

So far, this discussion has concentrated almost exclusively on studies examining the role of different systems in controlling anxiety-related behaviours in animals. Recent work has suggested that the amygdala is a structure of central importance in the neural architecture supporting the coordinated response systems brought into play by conditioned fear stimuli. The review above has also attempted to emphasize that these systems go far beyond the reflexive output systems of the central nucleus to brainstem and hypothalamic regions controlling neuroendocrine, autonomic and reflexive behavioural responses. The levels of analysis available to researchers examining animals' responses to stressful situations extend considerably beyond a simple examination of reflexive responses evoked by cues associated with mild footshock. The increasingly cognitive nature of associative learning theory in animals has made for ever-more-detailed and explicit comparisons and correlations between behaviour in humans and nonhuman animals. For example, models of the mechanisms within the prefrontal cortex devoted to performance of conditional tasks that require the reconciliation of conflicting information and demands are general to rats (Honey and Ward-Robinson 2001), nonhuman primates (Miller and Cohen 2001) and humans (Botvinik et al. 1999). With this progression of theoretical insight as a backdrop, we now know that the multiple layers of neural architecture surrounding the amygdala involve projections to diffuse neurotransmitter systems involved in a variety of higher-order cognitive functions. Cholinergic systems clearly play a role in the attentional resources directed towards stimuli. Dopaminergic systems influence the salience of appetitive and aversive cues, modulating the behavioural impact of such cues. Noradrenergic systems are involved not only in diffuse arousal processes and heightened cortical signal-to-noise ratios, but are also explicitly involved in the modulation of memory for emotionally significant events. Finally, in addition to their involvement in inhibition and impulsivity, serotonergic systems are also more specifically concerned with the coordination of varied aspects of defensive responding. The outputs of the basolateral amygdala to cortex and striatum also play a crucial role in performance of a wide variety of high-level behaviours in response to fear-evoking cues. Prelimbic, infralimbic and anterior cingulate cortices all appear involved to some degree in the control of responding to aversive cues, perhaps with specific reference to the inhibition of ongoing behaviours in the face of aversive cues or changed contingencies. The core and shell subregions of the nucleus accumbens are also implicated, both in terms of interaction of the behavioural effects of appetitive and aversive cues and the continued development of output systems for the influence of emotionally salient cues on voluntary actions. Analysis of dopaminergic function suggests that these striatal systems may in turn be modulated by activation of DA projections from the ventral tegmental area to the striatum by the central nucleus of the amygdala (Robledo et al. 1996). Recent evidence (Setlow et al. 2000) also implicates the basolateral amygdala–nucleus accumbens projection in the corticosteroid and NA-based modulation of memory in the presence of emotionally significant events. Finally, we have also found intriguing results demonstrating that the $5HT_{1A}$ partial agonist buspirone is far more potent as an anxiolytic in a conditioned punishment test of voluntary control of fear-related behaviour than in a test of reflexive suppression of responding, emphasizing the multiple roles played by 5HT in anxiety. In each of these cases, evidence points towards modulation of the target regions of basolateral amygdala outputs by systems which are themselves target structures of output from the central nucleus. This multilevel interaction emphasizes the central role of the amygdala in the coordination of behaviour, at the same time as making clear the importance of dissociable influences on behaviour of different nuclei of the amygdala.

Many questions remain to be answered concerning these interacting neural systems. Although it has been proposed that this amygdaloid framework is most profitably viewed as part of some response hierarchy, it is not clear that the evidence for this is strong. Although one might choose to suggest that there is a continuum of responding from reflexive, involuntary visceral reactions through to highly developed, voluntary, flexible responses, it does not seem that response systems are necessarily organized in a hierarchical manner. In fact, different response systems appear to operate in parallel, with coordination and competition between different behavioural outputs via multiple mechanisms. For example, in the serotonergic system, flight is inhibited to allow for more flexible response modes. In the prefrontal cortex, ongoing behaviour is inhibited in response to changing contingencies, perhaps allowing new behavioural plans or schema to be adopted. In the striatum, there is evidence to suggest both aversive and appetitive mechanisms coexist, under the influence of separate systems that are in turn controlled by dissociable amygdala outputs. Each of these factors must obviously be reconciled to produce coherent behavioural responses. Important issues that remain revolve around the nature of many of these interactive systems and how they integrate or compete to produce responses to fear- and anxiety-related cues.

Finally, it is important to mention the way in which the systems identified above relate to clinical findings and issues. Anxiety in human subjects may be characterized as a negative affective state represented at cognitive, behavioural and somatic levels. In many cases, clinical evidence supports the role of different neurotransmitter systems (e.g. 5HT, NA) in various aspects of anxiety disorders, and the previous discussion has highlighted some of these where relevant. Similarly, the importance of somatic changes in the determination of affective state and behaviour has recently been highlighted (Damasio 1998). In terms of the various higher-order regions identified above in connection with the basolateral amygdala, a recent discussion of functional neuro-imaging data (Chua and Dolan 2000; see also Chapter 7 by Dolan) identified key structures in the control of fear and anxiety in humans (as assessed by studies of patients suffering from generalized anxiety disorders, phobic disorders, obsessive–compulsive disorders and posttraumatic stress disorders). These comprised the amygdala, insular cortex, anterior cingulate cortex and orbitofrontal cortex. There is a very clear parallel between these structures and those highlighted above in our studies of circuitry underlying the control of voluntary responding by rats in the face of aversive stimuli. This emphasizes the value of an integrative approach examining a wide variety of behaviours thought to be important in anxiety. As is the case for research examining the rat, little is known of the way in which these regions interact in humans to produce coordinated responses to anxiety-provoking stimuli, or how these regions may function differently in patients suffering from anxiety relative to control populations. What is the nature of the information processing in each of these areas? How might fear-related cues be represented differently? Is there a role for these regions in the conscious, subjective aspects of anxiety? It seems likely that approaches seeking to combine research findings from multiple models, across different species, are going to begin to provide solutions to some of these puzzles in the very near future.

Acknowledgements

Preparation of this chapter was supported by a UK Medical Research Council Career Establishment Grant to SK.

REFERENCES

Alexander GE, Crutcher MD and DeLong MR (1990). Basal ganglia–thalamocortical circuits: parallel substrates for motor, oculomotor, 'prefrontal', and 'limbic' functions. *Prog Brain Res*, 85, 119–46.

Amorapanth P, LeDoux JE and Nader K (2000). Different lateral amygdala outputs mediate reactions and actions elicited by a fear-arousing stimulus. *Nat Neurosci*, 3, 74–9.

Applegate CD, Frysinger RC, Kapp BS and Gallagher M (1982). Multiple unit activity recorded from amygdala central nucleus during Pavlovian heart rate conditioning. *Brain Res*, 238, 457–62.

Balleine BW (1991). The acquisition of self-stimulation of the medial prefrontal cortex following exposure to escapable or inescapable footshock. *Behav Brain Res*, 43, 167–74.

Balleine BW and Dickinson A (1998). Goal-directed instrumental action: contingency and incentive learning and their cortical substrates. *Neuropsychopharmacology*, 37, 407–19.

Balleine BW and Killcross AS (1994). Effects of ibotenic acid lesions of the nucleus accumbens on instrumental action. *Behav Brain Res*, 65, 181–93.

Barrett JE and Vanover K (1993). 5-HT receptors as targets for the development of novel anxiolytic drugs: models, mechanisms and future directions. *Psychopharmacology*, 112, 1–12.

Beckett S and Marsden CA (1997). The effect of central and systemic injection of the 5HT1A receptor agonist 8-OH-DPAT and the 5HT1A receptor antagonist WAY 100635 on periaqueductal grey-induced defence behaviour. *J Psychopharmacol*, 11, 35–40.

Bosker F, Vrinten D, Klompmakers A and Westenberg H (1997). The effects of a 5-HT1A receptor agonist and antagonist on the 5-hydroxytryptamine release in the central nucleus of the amygdala: a microdialysis study with flesinoxan and WAY100635. *N-S Arch Pharmacol*, 355, 347–53.

Botvinik M, Nystrom LE, Fissell K, Carter CS and Cohen JD (1999). Conflict monitoring versus selection-for-action in anterior cingulate cortex. *Nature*, 402, 179–81.

Bouton ME, Mineka S and Barlow DH (2001). A modern learning theory perspective on the etiology of panic disorder. *Psychol Rev*, 108, 4–32.

Bucci DJ, Holland PC and Gallagher M (1998). Removal of cholinergic input to rat posterior parietal cortex disrupts incremental processing of conditioned stimuli. *J Neurosci*, 18, 8038–46.

Burns LH, Robbins TW and Everitt BJ (1993). Differential effects of excitotoxic lesions of the basolateral amygdala, ventral subiculum and medial prefrontal cortex on responding with conditioned reinforcement and locomotor activity potentiated by intra-accumbens infusions of d-amphetamine. *Behav Brain Res*, 55, 167–83.

Bussey TJ, Everitt BJ and Robbins TW (1997). Dissociable effects of cingulate and medial prefrontal cortex lesions on stimulus-reward learning using a novel Pavlovian autoshaping procedure in the rat: implications for the neurobiology of emotion. *Behav Neurosci*, 111, 908–19.

Cahill L (1997). The neurobiology of emotionally influenced memory – implications for the treatment of traumatic memory. *Ann NY Acad Sci*, 821, 238–46.

Cahill L, Prins B, Weber M and McGaugh JL (1994). β-adrenergic activation and memory for emotional events. *Nature*, 371, 702–3.

Cahill L, Vazdarjanova A and Setlow B (2000). The basolateral amygdala complex is involved with, but is not necessary for, rapid acquisition of Pavlovian 'fear' conditioning. *Eur J Neurosci*, 12, 3044–50.

Charney DS, Woods SW, Goodman WK and Heninger GR (1987). Neurobiological mechanisms of panic anxiety: biochemical and behavioural correlates of yohimbine-induced panic attacks. *Am J Psychiatry*, 144, 1030–6.

Chiba AA, Bucci DJ, Holland PC and Gallagher M (1995). Basal forebrain cholinergic lesions disrupt increments but not decrements in conditioned-stimulus processing. *J Neurosci*, 15, 7315–22.

Chua P and Dolan RJ (2000). The neurobiology of anxiety and anxiety-related disorders: a functional neuroimaging perspective. In *Brain Mapping: The Disorders*, ed. JC Mazziotta, AT Toga and RSJ Frackowiak, pp. 509–22. San Diego: Academic Press.

Cole BJ and Robbins TW (1987). Dissociable effects of lesions to dorsal and ventral noradrenergic bundle on the acquisition, performance, and extinction of aversive conditioning. *Behav Neurosci*, 101, 476–88.

Coutureau E, Dix SL and Killcross AS (2000). Involvement of the medial prefrontal cortex-basolateral amygdala pathway in fear related behaviour in rats. *Eur J Neurosci*, 12, 156.

Coutureau E, Dix SL and Killcross AS (2001). Functional heterogeneity of the medial prefrontal cortex in fear-related behaviour. *Behav Pharmacol*, 12, 24.

Crawley JN (1999). Behavioral phenotyping of transgenic and knockout mice: experimental design and evaluation of general health, sensory functions, motor abilities, and specific behavioural tests. *Brain Res*, 835, 18–26.

Damasio AR (1998). The somatic marker hypothesis and the possible functions of the prefrontal cortex. In *The Prefrontal Cortex: Executive and Cognitive Functions*, ed. AC Roberts, TW Robbins and L Weiskrantz, pp. 36–50. Oxford: Oxford University Press.

Davis M (1992). The role of the amygdala in conditioned fear. In *The Amygdala: Neurobiological Aspects of Emotion, Memory and Mental Dysfunction*, ed. JP Aggleton, pp. 255–306. New York: Wiley-Liss.

Davis M (2000). The role of the amygdala in unconditioned and conditioned fear and anxiety. In *The Amygdala: A Functional Analysis*, ed. JP Aggleton, pp. 213–88. New York: Oxford University Press.

Deakin JFW and Graeff FG (1991). 5HT and mechanisms of defence. *J Psychopharmacol*, 5, 301–15.

Den Boer JA and Westenberg HGM (1990). Serotonin function in panic disorder: a double blind placebo controlled study with fluvoxamine and ritanserin. *Psychopharmacology*, 102, 85–94.

Deutch AY and Young CD (1995). A model of the stress-induced activation of the prefrontal dopamine system: coping and the development of post-traumatic stress disorder.

In *Neurobiological and Clinical Consequences of Stress*, ed. MJ Friedman, DS Charney and AY Duetch, pp. 163–75. Philadelphia: Lippincott-Raven.

Dix SL, Coutureau E and Killcross AS (2001). Dissociable roles of the nucleus accumbens core and shell in fear-related behaviour in rats. *Behav Pharmacol*, 12, 30.

Everitt BJ and Robbins TW (1997). Central cholinergic systems and cognition. *Annu Rev Psychol*, 48, 649–84.

Eysenck MW (1992). *Anxiety: The Cognitive Perspective.* London: Lawrence Erlbaum Associates.

Eysenck MW (1997). *Anxiety and Cognition: A Unified Theory.* Hove: Psychology Press.

File SE, Gonzalez LE and Andrews N (1996). Comparative study of pre- and post-synaptic 5-HT1A receptor modulation of anxiety in two ethological animal tests. *J Neurosci*, 16, 4810–15.

Finlay JM and Abercrombie ED (1991). Stress induced sensitisation of norepinephrine release in the medial prefrontal cortex. *Soc Neurosci Abstr*, 17, 151.

Flint J, Corley R, DeFries JC et al. (1995). A simple genetic basis for a complex psychological trait in laboratory mice. *Science*, 269, 1432–5.

Frysztak RJ and Neafsey EJ (1994). The effect of medial prefrontal cortex lesions on cardiovascular conditioned emotional responses in the rat. *Brain Res*, 643, 181–93.

Gallagher M, Graham PW and Holland PC (1990). The amygdala central nucleus and appetitive Pavlovian conditioning – lesions impair one class of conditioned behavior. *J Neurosci*, 10, 1906–11.

Gora-Maslak G, McClearn GE, Crabbe JC, Phillips TJ Belknap JK and Plomin R (1995). Use of recombinant inbred strains to identify quantitative trait loci in psychopharmacology. *Psychopharmacology*, 104, 413–24.

Graeff FG (1994). Neuroanatomy and neurotransmitter regulation of defensive behaviours and related emotions in mammals. *Brazil J Med Biol Res*, 27, 811–29.

Graeff FG, Guimaraes FS, De Andrade TGCS and Deakin JFW (1996). Role of 5HT in stress, anxiety and depression. *Pharmacol Biochem Behav*, 54, 129–49.

Graeff FG, Viana MB and Mora PO (1997). Dual role of 5-HT in defence and anxiety. *Neurosci Biobehav Rev*, 21, 791–9.

Hall G and Pearce JM (1979). Latent inhibition of CS during CS-US pairings. *J Exp Psychol Anim Behav Process*, 5, 31–42.

Han JS, Holland PC and Gallagher M (1999). Disconnection of the amygdala central nucleus and substantia innominata/nucleus basalis disrupts increments in conditioned stimulus processing in rats. *Behav Neurosci*, 113, 143–51.

Handley SL, McBlane JW, Critchley MAE and Njunge K (1993). Multiple serotonin mechanisms in animal models of anxiety – environmental, emotional and cognitive factors. *Behav Brain Res*, 58, 203–10.

Harrison AA, Everitt BJ and Robbins TW (1997). Central 5-HT depletion enhances impulsive responding without affecting the accuracy of attentional performance: interactions with dopaminergic mechanisms. *Psychopharmacology*, 133, 329–42.

Hatfield T and McGaugh JL (1999). Norepinephrine infused into the basolateral amygdala posttraining enhances retention in a spatial water maze task. *Neurobiol Learn Memory*, 71, 232–9.

Heisler LK, Chu HM, Brennan TJ et al. (1998). Elevated anxiety and anti-depressant-like responses in serotonin 5-HT1A receptor mutant mice. *Proc Natl Acad Sci USA*, 95, 15049–54.

Hitchcott PK and Phillips GD (1998). Double dissociation of the behavioural effects of R(+) 7-OH-DPAT infusions in the central and basolateral amygdala nuclei upon Pavlovian and instrumental conditioned appetitive behaviours. *Psychopharmacology*, 140, 458–69.

Hodges H, Green S and Glenn B (1987). Evidence that the amygdala is involved in benzodiazepine and serotonergic effects on conditioned responding but not on discrimination. *Psychopharmacology*, 92, 491–504.

Holland PC and Gallagher M (1993*a*). Effects of amygdala central nucleus lesions on blocking and unblocking. *Behav Neurosci*, 107, 235–45.

Holland PC and Gallagher M (1993*b*). Amygdala central nucleus lesions disrupt increments, but not decrements, in conditioned-stimulus processing. *Behav Neurosci*, 107, 246–53.

Honey RC and Ward-Robinson J (2001). Transfer between contextual conditional discriminations: an examination of how stimulus conjunctions are represented. *J Exp Psychol Anim Behav Process*, 27, 196–205.

Hurley KM, Hernert H, Moga MM and Saper CB (1991). Efferent projections of the infralimbic cortex of the rat. *J Comp Neurol*, 308, 249–76.

Jinks AL and McGregor IS (1997). Modulation of anxiety-related behaviors following lesions of the prelimbic or infralimbic cortex in the rat. *Brain Res*, 772, 181–90.

Kapp BS, Whalen PJ, Supple WF and Pascoe JP (1992). Amygdaloid contributions to conditioned arousal and sensory information processing. In *The Amygdala: Neurobiological Aspects of Emotion, Memory and Mental Dysfunction*, ed. JP Aggleton, pp. 229–54. New York: Wiley-Liss.

Kapp BS, Supple WF and Whalen PJ (1994). Effects of electrical-stimulation of the amygdaloid central nucleus on neocortical arousal in the rabbit. *Behav Neurosci*, 108, 81–93.

Kelley AE, SmithRoe SL and Holahan MR (1997). Response-reinforcement learning is dependent on N-methyl-D-aspartate receptor activation in the nucleus accumbens core. *Proc Natl Acad Sci USA*, 94, 12174–9.

Killcross AS and Blundell P (2002). Associative representations of emotionally significant outcomes. In *Emotional Cognition (Advances in Consciousness Research)*, ed. S Moore and M Oaksford. John Benjamins: Amsterdam.

Killcross AS and Robbins TW (1993). Differential effects of intra-accumbens and systemic amphetamine on latent inhibition using an on-baseline, within-subject conditioned suppression paradigm. *Psychopharmacology*, 110, 449–59.

Killcross AS, Dickinson A and Robbins TW (1994). Amphetamine-induced disruptions of latent inhibition are reinforcer mediated: Implications for animal models of schizophrenic attentional dysfunction. *Psychopharmacology*, 115, 185–95.

Killcross AS, Everitt BJ and Robbins TW (1997*a*). Different types of fear-conditioned behaviour mediated by separate nuclei within the amygdala. *Nature*, 388, 377–80.

Killcross AS, Everitt BJ and Robbins TW (1997*b*). Symmetrical effects of amphetamine and alpha-flupenthixol on conditioned punishment and reinforcement: contrasts with midazolam. *Psychopharmacology*, 129, 141–52.

LeDoux JE (1992). Emotion and the amygdala. In *The Amygdala: Neurobiological Aspects of Emotion, Memory, and Mental Dysfunction*, ed. JP Aggleton, pp. 339–52. New York: Wiley-Liss.

LeDoux JE (1996). *The Emotional Brain: The Mysterious Underpinnings of Emotional Life*. New York: Touchstone.

Mansbach RS and Geyer MA (1988). Blockage of potentiated startle responding in rats by 5-hydroxytryptamine1A receptor ligands. *Eur J Pharmacol*, 156, 375–83.

McDonald AJ (1991). Organisation of amygdaloid projections to the prefrontal cortex and associated striatum in the rat. *Neuroscience*, 44, 1–14.

McDonald AJ (1998). Cortical pathways to the mammalian amygdala. *Prog Neurobiol*, 55, 257–332.

McGaugh JL, Ferry B, Vazdarjanova A and Roozendaal B (2000). Amygdala: role in modulation of memory storage. In *The Amygdala: A Functional Analysis*, ed. JP Aggleton, pp. 391–423. New York: Oxford University Press.

Melia KR and Davis M (1991). Effects of septal lesions on fear potentiated startle, and on the anxiolytic effects of buspirone and diazepam. *Physiol Behav*, 49, 603–11.

Miller EK and Cohen JD (2001). An integrative theory of prefrontal cortex function. *Annu Rev Neurosci*, 24, 167–202.

Mogenson G, Jones DL and Yim CY (1984). From motivation to action: functional interface between the limbic system and the motor system. *Prog Neurobiol*, 14, 69–97.

Muir JL, Dunnett SB, Robbins TW and Everitt BJ (1992). Attentional functions of the forebrain cholinergic systems – effects of intraventricular hemicholinium, physostigmine, basal forebrain lesions and intracortical grafts on a multiple-choice serial reaction-time-task. *Exp Brain Res*, 89, 611–22.

Muir JL, Page KJ, Sirinathsinghji DJS, Robbins TW and Everitt BJ (1993). Excitotoxic lesions of basal forebrain cholinergic neurons – effects on learning, memory and attention. *Behav Brain Res*, 57, 123–31.

Muir JL, Everitt BJ and Robbins TW (1994). AMPA-induced excitotoxic lesions of the basal forebrain – a significant role for the cortical cholinergic system in attentional function. *J Neurosci*, 14, 2313–26.

Nisenbaum LK, Zigmund MJ, Sved AF and Abercrombie ED (1991). Prior exposure to chronic stress results in enhanced synthesis and release of hippocampal norepinephrine in response to a novel stressor. *J Neurosci*, 11, 1473–84.

Ohman A and Mineka S (2001). Fears, phobias and preparedness: toward an evolved module of fear and fear learning. *Psychol Rev*, 108, 483–522.

Parkinson JA, Olmstead MC, Burns LH, Robbins TW and Everitt BJ (1999). Dissociation of effects of lesions of the nucleus accumbens core and shell on appetitive Pavlovian approach behaviour and the potentiation of conditioned reinforcement and locomotor activity by d-amphetamine. *J Neurosci*, 19, 2401–11.

Pearce JM and Hall G (1980). A model for Pavlovian learning: variations in the effectiveness of conditioned but not of unconditioned stimuli. *Psychol Rev*, 87, 532–52.

Pitkänen A (2000). Connectivity of the rat amygdaloid complex. In *The Amygdala: A Functional Analysis*, ed. JP Aggleton, pp. 31–115. New York: Oxford University Press.

Quirarte GL, Galvez R, Roozendaal, B and McGaugh JL (1998). Norepinephrine release in the amygdala in response to footshock and opioid peptodergic drugs. *Brain Res*, 808, 134–40.

Quirk GJ, Armony JL and LeDoux JE (1997). Fear conditioning enhances different temporal components of tone-evoked spike trains in auditory cortex and lateral amygdala. *Neuron*, 19, 613–24.

Quirk GJ, Russo GK, Barron JL and Lebron K (2000). The role of the ventromedial prefrontal cortex in the recovery of extinguished fear. *J Neurosci*, 20, 6225–31.

Robledo P, Robbins TW and Everitt BJ (1996). Effects of excitotoxic lesions of the central amygdaloid nucleus on the potentiation of reward-related stimuli by intra-accumbens amphetamine. *Behav Neurosci*, 110, 981–90.

Rodgers RJ (1997). Animal models of 'anxiety': where next? *Behav Pharmacol*, 8, 477–96.

Roozendaal B and McGaugh JL (1996). Amygdaloid nuclei lesions differentially affect glucocorticoid-induced memory enhancement in an inhibitory avoidance task. *Neurobiol Learn Memory*, 65, 1–8.

Sanger DJ (1992). Increased rates of punished responding produced by buspirone-like compounds in rats. *J Pharmacol Exp Therapeut*, 254, 420–6.

Sarter M and Bruno JP (1997). Cognitive functions of cortical acetylcholine: toward a unifying hypothesis. *Brain Res Rev*, 23, 28–46.

Selden NRW, Everitt BJ, Jarrard LE and Robbins TW (1991). Complementary roles for the amygdala and hippocampus in aversive conditioning to explicit and contextual cues. *Neuroscience*, 42, 335–50.

Setlow B, Roozendaal B and McGaugh JL (2000). Involvement of a basolateral amygdala complex-nucleus accumbens pathway in glucocorticoid-induced modulation of memory consolidation. *Eur J Neurosci*, 12, 367–75.

Stanhope KJ and Dourish CT (1996). Effects of 5-HT1A receptor agonists, partial agonists and a silent antagonist on the performance of the conditioned emotional response test in the rat. *Psychopharmacology*, 128, 293–303.

Swanson L and Petrovich G (1998). What is the amygdala? *Trends Neurosci*, 21, 323–31.

Taylor DP, Eison MS, Riblet LA and Vandermaelen CP (1985). Pharmacological and clinical effects of buspirone. *Pharmacol Biochem Behav*, 23, 687–94.

Thierry AM, Tassin JP, Blanc G and Glowinski J (1976). Selective activation of mesocortical dopaminergic system by stress. *Nature*, 263, 242–4.

Turri MG, Datta SR, DeFries J, Henderson ND and Flint J (2001). QTL analysis identifies multiple behavioural dimensions in ethological tests of anxiety in laboratory mice. *Curr Biol*, 11, 725–34.

Vazdarjanova A and McGaugh JL (1998). Basolateral amygdala is not critical for cognitive memory of contextual fear conditioning. *Proc Natl Acad Sci USA*, 95, 15003–7.

Wilkinson LS, Humby T, Killcross AS, Everitt BJ and Robbins TW (1996). Dissociations in hippocampal 5HT release following Pavlovian aversive conditioning to discrete and contextual stimuli. *Eur J Neurosci*, 8, 1479–87.

Wilkinson LS, Humby T, Killcross AS, Torres EM, Everitt BJ and Robbins TW (1998). Dissociations in dopamine release in medial prefrontal cortex and ventral striatum during the acquisition and extinction of classical aversive conditioning in the rat. *Eur J Neurosci*, 10, 1019–26.

16

Social separation models of depression

Keith Matthews

Ninewells Medical School, Dundee, UK

Introduction

The clinical presentations that attract the label 'depression' represent a major public health concern because of their high prevalence, stigma, morbidity and mortality. Despite best efforts, research has, thus far, failed to illuminate a plausible pathophysiology of depression, to explain why some individuals are more at risk than others or to explain the efficacy of available treatments. Modelling pathophysiological states in experimental animals has proven an effective strategy in improving our understanding of many other major medical conditions and has led to the development of better treatments. In this chapter, I shall review a range of work with experimental animals that may contribute to our eventual understanding of some aspects of depression. This review focuses on the manipulation of social environment as a means of perturbing physiology and behaviour and attempts to relate findings from animal studies to core clinical concepts.

What is depression?

Depression is a common, complex and poorly understood condition. Perhaps because the same word is used to describe the brief periods of unhappiness and disappointment that everyone experiences in response to minor life upsets, there is a popular view that depression is a relatively trivial and self-limiting problem. The reality is very different.

It (depression) was the worst experience of my life. More terrible even than watching my wife die of cancer . . . I was in a state that bears no resemblance to anything I had experienced before, I was not just feeling low . . . I was seriously ill. (Wolpert 1999)

I was feeling in my mind a sensation close to, but indescribably different from pain . . . for myself, the pain is most closely connected to drowning or suffocation – but even these images are off the mark. (Styron 1992)

Depression can be a lifelong illness with persistent, overwhelming feelings of sadness and grief. There can be profound impairment of the ability to experience pleasure, to feel, to eat, to concentrate and think, to sleep and to make decisions. The more severe forms of depressive disorder afflict 1 in 20 of the general population at some point in their lives, with less severe manifestations afflicting around 1 in 5 (Smith and Weissman 1992). In its more dramatic manifestations, it is life threatening, either as a result of suicide or through a dramatic failure to maintain food and fluid intake. Indeed, death by dehydration and emaciation was a frequent clinical observation in the era before the introduction of effective treatments. Such presentations are now rare, at least in the developed world, although there has been an apparent increase in the prevalence of milder forms of illness during the latter half of the last century (Smith and Weissman 1992). Over the past two decades, much emphasis has been placed on improving public awareness and diagnostic practice in primary care. However, even with successful treatment and full recovery from an episode of depression, there remains a high risk of recurrence (Judd 1997). Furthermore, available treatments remain inadequate. Up to 40% of depressed patients fail to demonstrate a response to first-line antidepressant drug treatment and of those that do respond, only a modest proportion will achieve full recovery. Between 5 and 15% of depressive episodes last longer than 24 months and as many as 1.5% of the general population suffer from chronic (>24 months), severe depression (Judd 1997). The degree of treatment-unresponsiveness increases with the duration of illness and the number of previous episodes of depression. Hence, there are many individuals with depression for whom no drug treatments or psychological therapies alleviate symptoms. For many (between 4–15%) with such chronic, refractory depression, after years of marked loss of social and occupational function, suicide is the eventual outcome (Judd 1997). For these reasons, the identification of new treatment strategies is a public health priority.

Clinical concepts

Depression is widely considered a spectrum disorder, reflecting an apparent continuity between the normal emotional responses of transient sadness and dysphoria in response to adverse events, through a range of disabling mood disorders that vary in their persistence and severity, to the severe, episodic, behavioural and cognitive disturbance of bipolar disorder. An individual who suffers from bipolar disorder will also experience episodes of what often appears quite the reverse of depression, so-called mania or, if less severe, hypomania. During a period of mania, sufferers can appear euphoric, grandiose, full of energy and ideas, to have a diminished requirement for sleep and to be socially disinhibited. Within the major classification systems, depressive episodes are distinguished from the 'normal' experience of sadness and adjustment to adversity by their persistence (>2 weeks), their pervasiveness and the degree of functional disturbance that accompanies them. A typical depressive episode will be defined by the presence of core symptoms: low or sad mood, loss of interest or the capacity to experience pleasure, and an array of associated features that include reduced energy, enhanced fatigue, sleep impairment, loss of appetite, weight change, persistent thoughts of guilt, worthlessness and/or suicide (ICD–10, World Health Organization 1992; DSM–IV, American Psychiatric Association 1994). In the absence of specific diagnostic tests or the identification of a defining neuropathological/neurophysiological abnormality, there is a continuing reliance upon the temporal aggregation of diverse clinical factors for diagnosis. Here lies the first major impediment to the development of valid models of depression. Although present in some other psychiatric conditions, the altered capacity to experience pleasure, or anhedonia, is currently considered the defining feature of depressive disorder. Hence, this has represented a legitimate focus for many animal models over the past 20 years (Willner 1984).

What is the pathophysiology of depression?

The risk of developing depression is not equally distributed. Epidemiological research has identified several potent risk factors that increase the probability of developing depression, notably female gender, a history of depressive disorder in the immediate family, early childhood adversity and stressful life events in adulthood (Smith and Weissman 1992). Indeed, the role of early stress as a mediator of vulnerability and of adult stress as a precipitant of depression is acknowledged as influential by current psychological (Beck et al. 1979) and neurobiological (Nemeroff 1998) explanatory models. This predisposition, or vulnerability, to depression is a poorly understood and complex product of genetic and environmental factors that somehow influences the psychological perception of, and response to, social and environmental events, translating them into neurophysiological changes.

Structural and functional changes in the brain associated with depression

Converging evidence from structural brain imaging (Drevets et al. 1997), functional brain imaging (Drevets 1998) and from postmortem histopathological studies (see Chapter 14 by Harrison and Gittins) suggests that depression is associated with regionally specific changes in brain structure and function, both at the cellular and systems levels. The earliest reports of significant structural changes were based on X-ray computerized tomography (CT scanning). Jacoby and Levy (1980) reported that 9 of 41 elderly depressed subjects had enlarged cerebral ventricles and reduced brain substance. Subsequent studies have tended to confirm that cortical atrophy and ventricular enlargement are associated with depression of late onset, particularly where cognitive impairment is prominent. Such subjects are also more likely to show imaging correlates of cerebrovascular disease (Krishnan et al. 1993).

Correspondingly, such general brain shrinkage is thought to be associated with a nonspecific ischaemic process that has an uncertain relationship with depression. With improved technologies, however, recent studies have delineated more anatomically specific changes. A number of independently conducted studies have identified localized reductions in metabolic activity in the dorsolateral prefrontal cortex of depressed subjects whilst in the resting state (Sackeim 2001). Reports of changes in activity of medial and orbital prefrontal cortex have been less consistent. However, in familial major depressive disorder (MDD) and bipolar disorder (BD), the medial, orbital and dorsolateral subregions of the prefrontal cortex (PFC) have been shown to have reduced grey matter densities that appear to be associated with decreased numbers of glial cells and an increased neuronal density (Ongur et al. 1998; Rajkowska et al. 1999). Similarly, there have also been changes identified in some of the subcortical structures that are functionally linked with relevant PFC subregions by an intricate network of corticostriatal thalamic loop circuitry (Alexander et al. 1986). Specifically, the volumes of the head of the caudate and of the ventral striatum (including the nucleus accumbens) appear reduced in MDD (Baumann et al. 1999). There have also been reports of volume changes in medial temporal lobe structures. Magnetic resonance imaging (MRI) studies have identified reductions in hippocampal volume in euthymic female subjects with a previous history of recurrent depression, the magnitude of which correlate with duration of depressive episodes (Sheline et al. 1996). Despite these investigations, we have no clear understanding of the significance of these changes. Do they reflect state (illness) or trait (vulnerability) phenomena? We do not know whether these changes reflect the causes or the consequences of depression. We also do not know if, or how, these changes might relate to symptom profile, response to treatment or natural course of illness.

Why attempt to model in experimental animals?

It will be clear from the above that we remain profoundly ignorant of the detailed pathophysiology of a major public health problem – depressive disorder. One approach adopted to tackle this problem has been to attempt to model some of the neurobiological and behavioural alterations associated with human depression in experimental animals. This has proven a controversial strategy. Many have argued that human emotional experience can neither be induced, recorded nor manipulated in nonhuman species. However, such arguments have diminished with the anatomical and functional brain-imaging studies cited above. These recent findings challenge long-held assumptions that mental disorders, such as depression, are somehow expressions of psychological distress, divorced from the neurophysiological processes in the brain that regulate and generate emotion and thought. Much antipathy from clinicians has arisen through exaggerated and premature clinical labelling of potentially interesting behavioural and neurochemical findings in experimental animals. However, many of the questions raised by epidemiology, by pathophysiological studies and by the observation of clinical populations are simply not amenable to direct study. Fortunately, studies with experimental animals permit the design of prospective, hypothesis-driven manipulations of independent variables in precisely the manner that is impossible in human subjects for ethical and logistical reasons. Thus, animal models offer an opportunity to exert control over many of the variables which clinical and epidemiological research suggests may be influential in the aetiology of depression, for example, genotype, early social experience, and magnitude, timing, type and duration of environmental stresses (Smith and Weissman 1992). Certain species also offer a sufficiently rapid development and short life span to permit developmental studies within a reasonable timescale.

The disadvantages of the approach are equally obvious. The brain, behaviour and biology of laboratory animals are very different from those of humans. Indeed, there is no compelling evidence that any experimental animal exhibits, or is even capable of experiencing, any mental state or physiological condition that resembles human affective disorder. However, much of the core psychopathology of depressive illness is believed to involve neural processes that are subserved by the so-called 'limbic brain'; structures and systems that demonstrate considerable homology with those of laboratory animals such as the rat. Ultimately, the single most potent argument in favour of animal behavioural studies of psychopathology may be the continuing paucity of neurobiological detail gathered from humans with affective illness.

Overview of animal models of depression and their validity

Interested readers are directed towards the influential and detailed reviews of animal models of depression authored by McKinney and Bunney (1969), Katz (1981) and Willner (1984). Within each review, a range of models is categorized and explicit criteria for their validation are defined. Key concepts addressed by these authors include that of *predictive validity* – a model's ability to correctly identify effective antidepressant treatments, usually drugs. Also known as 'assay models', the best performers within this category are capable of discriminating pharmacologically diverse antidepressant drug treatments with a minimum of false positive or negative results. Face validity of a model refers to whether or not specific attributes of the model resemble specific aspects of the clinical disorder, that is, whether a phenomenological similarity exists. The construct validity of a model refers to the accuracy with which the model can replicate the key abnormalities or changes under study within the clinical condition. This concept addresses the critical consideration of whether or not the observations in the model 'stand in an established empirical or theoretical relationship' (Willner 1984) to those in the clinical disorder.

An important related concept is that of aetiological validity, whereby the circumstances that lead to development of the target phenomenon in the model are the same as those which generate the same phenomenon in the clinical disorder. Yet another related concept is that of convergent/discriminant validity. These terms refer to the degree to which the measurements from a model appear to measure the same construct as other models. Specifically, discriminant validity would permit a test to examine different aspects of a phenomenon from those measured by other related models of the same phenomenon, thus enhancing overall understanding of the phenomenon. The establishment of overall construct validity of a model requires parallel studies to determine degrees of discriminant and convergent validity. It will be clear from the preceding discussion that uncertainty with respect to core aetiological and pathophysiological constructs within clinical populations offers fertile ground for the development of spurious and unhelpful animal models.

Types of model

The extensive array of animal models of depression that have been proposed can be categorized according to almost any number of criteria (Willner 1984). It is crucial to note that different models subserve different purposes. Hence, the inherent value of any single model can only be judged according to its specific aims and utility. In this chapter, to set in context the potential value of models that focus on the manipulation of social stimuli, I have adopted the simple categorization of models as either empirical or theoretical in nature. Within the first category are those models that have been developed primarily for the detection of drug treatments with antidepressant efficacy, e.g. the forced swim test (Porsolt et al. 1977). These can be considered 'assay' or 'empirical' models. The strength of such models lies in their predictive value and reliability. Hence, they are commonly used within the pharmaceutical industry as a method of screening novel compounds for potential antidepressant efficacy. It is equally true to state that such models tend to have little, or no, face, aetiological or construct validity. Nevertheless, these models can be of considerable use as behavioural 'assays' of drug action, provided the effect is reliable. These models are distinguished from those of greater behavioural and psychological sophistication that can be termed the 'theoretical' or 'analogue' group of models. As mentioned above, there are many excellent reviews of the relative strengths and validity of assay models (Katz 1981; Willner 1984). In this chapter, I shall focus on one of the major 'theoretical' approaches that have been revisited in recent years – social separation models of depression.

Social separation and loss – an historical perspective

Separation and loss have long been thought to lead to serious affective disorder. Losses of sexual partner, lifelong companionship, a child, or stable employment are considered to be amongst the most powerful stressors that have to be endured in human society. Loss, particularly of a significant interpersonal relationship – a social separation – has been linked aetiologically with severe depression from the earliest clinical descriptions of the disorder. In his treatise published in 1621, Burton described losses as a central factor in the production of 'melancholia', extending the concept of loss to include loss of social status and personal circumstances as well as of persons and material possessions (see Burton 1989). One of the outstanding research questions for basic and clinical neuroscience is how the absence of something (or someone) can lead to such significant bodily dysfunction and ill health? Another, is why one individual, or group of individuals, ought to be more sensitive or vulnerable to the adverse effects of separation and loss? Whereas there are well-developed psychological explanatory models for the effects of loss (Bowlby 1969), neurobiological aspects of these phenomena remain poorly understood.

Prior to the influential writings of Sigmund Freud (Freud 1963), western culture placed little emphasis on the significance of early environmental and emotional experience on subsequent behavioural development. Freud's theories of personality development, particularly those concerning the role of early maternal and paternal influences, had a profound and pervasive impact upon twentieth century culture as well as upon clinical practice. Arguably, the cornerstone of his theories was the hypothesis that specific parental behaviours (mainly maternal) were responsible for the direction and suppression of infant physiological drives, a process that shaped not only infant behaviour, but also adult personality and behavioural development. However, outwith a relatively small group of enthusiastic converts, it was more generally accepted that the provision of nutrition and protection from adverse environment and infection was all that was necessary for normal early human development. This assumption was challenged when Ribble (1944) described what were believed to be the consequences of 'inadequate mothering' in 600 newborn children. Coining the term 'marasmus', Ribble described a syndrome of impaired appetite, hypersomnia, muscular weakness and wasting as 'a general disorganisation of functions and a deterioration of primary body reflexes due in large measure to a lack of mothering or stimulation'. This hypothesis was a controversial one; it was widely dismissed, yet the concept of early social environment as a determinant of development began to influence others. Spitz (1945) reported an extraordinarily high infant mortality rate (90% within the first 12 months) in a cohort of institutionalized infants in the city of Baltimore. Spitz also conducted a direct comparison of the cognitive, behavioural and physiological development of infants reared either in a nursery or in a foundling home (Spitz 1945; Spitz and Wolf 1946). Although the children came from similar socio-economic backgrounds, those reared in the foundling home exhibited a profound retardation in gross development (indices of growth, acquisition of developmental milestones) and a much higher mortality from infection. The main difference between the two institutions, at least as reported by Spitz, was a reduced interaction with adult caregivers and a lack of environmental stimulation. Although, methodologically, there were numerous problems with these studies, the notion that early rearing conditions and social interaction, particularly maternal contact, were exerting a significant influence over infant development became established.

Attachment theory

Drawing together theoretical perspectives from both ethology and psychoanalysis, and combining them with data from extensive clinical observation and from animal studies, the psychotherapist John Bowlby was the first to systematize the way in which early mother–infant relationships might influence adult health and behaviour (Bowlby 1969). His research interest in the role of early environment as a determinant of adult behaviour began with a retrospective study of 44 juvenile delinquents referred to a 'child guidance' clinic (Bowlby 1944). He identified an excess of maternal separations of more than 6 months' duration, during the first 5 years of life, in the delinquents who had a history of stealing. Similarly, he identified a high prevalence of such separations in those deemed to have difficulties in forming adult relationships. These observations led him to speculate that early separation from mother had an injurious impact upon subsequent emotional and moral development. Subsequently, he conducted experimental studies to test his hypotheses (Bowlby et al. 1956) and he published a highly influential monograph for the World Health Organization (Bowlby 1951) that radically changed the way in which children were looked after in hospitals and other institutions. Although his earliest attempts to explain the mechanisms of enduring separation-induced pathology required the invocation of untestable psychodynamic concepts, the evolution of his theories was accompanied by an increasing awareness of empirical data from animal studies (Bowlby 1969). Indeed, he spent considerable time discussing his ideas with preeminent ethologists of the day (e.g. Konrad Lorenz, Robert Hinde), a testimony to his own evaluation of the worth of animal studies.

In its most simplified form, Bowlby's attachment theory (Bowlby 1969) infers the presence of infantile motivational systems that respond to physical separation from the primary attachment figure (usually the mother) by the activation of a predictable, biphasic response, with the earliest phase characterized by an array of 'protest' behaviours such as vocalization and increased locomotion. If reunion does not occur, these responses persist until the neonate enters a stage of hyporesponsivity to external stimuli, locomotor hypoactivity, hypothermia and reduced cardiovascular tone, the 'despair' phase (Bowlby 1969). In some species, including humans, Bowlby held that there was a third phase following reunion, that of 'detachment'. During this third phase, the infant would appear uninterested in the returned mother and would fail to exhibit the robust 'attachment' behaviours evident prior to separation. Although there are species-specific differences, the basic biphasic response to early separation appears common to most mammals, including humans, as well as some ovine species (reviewed by Katz 1981). The 'detachment' response following reunion has proven much more difficult to identify in nonhuman species. Attachment theory further postulates that separation experiences and the nature of social 'attachments' during early development determine responses to separation and loss in adulthood (Bowlby 1969). A number of clinical studies conducted during the 1960s appeared to confirm Bowlby's primary hypothesis. For example, Munro (1966) reported a significant association between severe depressive illness and early loss of mother through bereavement, relative to mildly depressed and nondepressed control subjects. Likewise, Beck et al. (1963) reported a stronger association between early maternal loss and severe depression than with mild depression. Hill (1969) reported that females who lost their fathers through bereavement between the ages of 10 and 14 years were at increased risk of developing depression and of committing suicide in adulthood. However, as with the clinical studies upon which Bowlby had based his original hypotheses (for review see Ainsworth 1962), numerous methodological problems confounded the interpretation of these data. Indeed, the lack of sophistication of these studies of early loss was highlighted by the influential work of George Brown and colleagues (Brown and Harris 1978). In a series of studies designed to define the magnitude of the influence of environmental circumstances and life events on the development of depression in women, Brown and colleagues introduced several concepts that remain influential today. For example, Brown and Harris (1978) highlighted the now rather obvious fact that not all 'losses' have equivalent emotional impact, or have equivalent meaning for different individuals. This research group popularized the concepts of there being 'vulnerability' factors for depression and an 'additivity' of effect for acute stresses and more chronic 'difficulties'. Specifically, they emphasized the role of early loss in conferring a subsequent lifelong vulnerability to develop depression in response to provoking events in adulthood, typically a further loss (Brown and Harris 1978). With subsequent refinements in methodology and with increasing explanatory sophistication, these concepts have become as pervasive and influential in clinical practice as Bowlby's attachment concepts. Indeed, they are frequently brought together as different aspects of the same unitary process, with disordered childhood 'attachment' leading to both relationship difficulties and to an enhanced 'vulnerability' to depression in later life.

The biology of attachment

A major criticism that could be aimed at much of the sociologically grounded research outlined above is the absence of a biological perspective. At much the same time as Bowlby and others were investigating the relationships between early social environment and subsequent development, Harlow and colleagues (Harlow 1958; Harlow and Harlow 1962; Seay et al. 1962) and Hinde (Hinde et al. 1966; Hinde and Spencer-Booth 1971) were asking similar questions in monkeys. In the light of their phylogenetic proximity to man, their advanced cognitive capacity and their complex social structures, studies in monkeys have provided the bulk of the behavioural and neurobiological data in support of social separation models of depression. To determine if the phasic protest–despair–detachment syndrome could be demonstrated in monkeys as well as in humans, Seay et al. (1962) separated four infant rhesus monkeys from their mothers for 3 weeks. This study supported their hypothesis, with the exception of only demonstrating a 'detachment' response in one of the four infants when reunited with their mothers. A subsequent study with eight mother–infant pairs, this time depriving the infants of olfactory, auditory and visual cues from their mothers as well, had a similar effect (Seay and Harlow 1965), again eliciting a robust 'protest' response followed by 'despair'. The impact of shorter periods of separation were reported by Hinde et al. (1966), who went on to demonstrate enduring effects of brief separation during infancy on subsequent behavioural development when tested at 12 and 24 months (Hinde and Spencer-Booth 1971). After only 6 days of separation when aged 6 months, alterations were observed with respect to the separated monkeys' responses to novelty and their independent exploration of the immediate environment. Thus, even very brief periods of maternal separation appeared capable of inducing enduring alterations in behaviour.

Not all studies of maternal separation in monkeys resulted in a demonstration of the anticipated (desired) response, however. The existence of marked species differences in the response to separation was confirmed by Rosenblum and Kaufman (1968). Whereas protest and despair responses had been reliably elicited from rhesus (*Macaca mulatta*) and pigtail (*M. nemestrina*) macaque monkeys, bonnet macaques (*M. radiata*) exhibited no 'behavioural depression' after an initial protest phase. Interestingly, in the light of the developing literature on social support and vulnerability to depression in humans, this was interpreted as being due to the differences in social structures between the different species (Rosenblum and Kaufman 1968).

What is the long-term significance of 'attachment'?

A reasonable conclusion from the wealth of studies of mother–infant separation in nonhuman primates might be that the optimal development of social attachment behaviour (and the mediating neurobiological mechanisms) requires maternal contact during early development and peer contact during later life (n.b. social attachment behaviour in this context can be defined as the repertoire of adult behaviours that promote and maintain adaptive and beneficial social relationships with other adults, permitting integration within the social group). Further, the nature of the mother–infant contact during the early neonatal period has a profound influence over subsequent behavioural development. For example, by rearing monkeys with inanimate surrogate mothers with the capacity to repel the infant (Rosenblum and Kaufman 1968), or by rearing monkeys in peer groups with no mother (Mineka and Suomi 1978), the infants were much more prone to develop separation-induced 'despair' responses in later life. Similarly, repeated separations during early development appeared to lead to an attenuation of the initial 'protest' response to social separation at a later stage, but to an augmentation of the 'despair' response (Suomi et al. 1970, 1973). The variability in responsivity to separation and subsequent reunion seemed to be determined, at least in part, by the nature of the mother–infant relationship before separation. This opinion seems entirely consonant with prevailing clinical theories of early experience and subsequent 'vulnerability' to depression (Brown and Harris 1978).

Primate separation responses as models of depression

The organismic response to maternal separation during infancy appears to generalize, perhaps even to be homologous, across primate species, including humans (Bowlby 1969). However, there is no evidence that an infant 'despair' response bears other than a superficial relationship with adult depression. In accord with the developing sophistication of sociological research into depression in humans (Brown and Harris 1978), primate 'despair' reactions to separation are also influenced by genetic and environmental variables, particularly by early social environment. The nature of early 'attachments' exerts a powerful influence over subsequent responses to changes in social environment, specifically to social separation. In naturally occurring adverse social circumstances, such as falling in rank, monkeys can exhibit an obvious and prolonged withdrawal from social interaction and a suppression of aggression (Everitt and Keverne 1979). Thus, some nonhuman primate analogues of the common precipitants of human depressive episodes ('exit events'; Paykel and Hollyman 1984) can reliably induce 'despair' reactions and behavioural changes reminiscent of human depression, thus conferring a degree of face validity. In turn, these responses are strongly influenced by genes (species differences), early social experience, social 'support' networks and other physical aspects of environment. In addition, the 'despair' responses are associated with physiological changes. Perhaps of greatest interest are the observations of:

1. A phase delay in circadian rhythmicity (Reite and Short 1983), despite maintenance of other potent zeitgebers such as the light/dark cycle and feeding times and,
2. the alteration of sleep architecture with increased REM latency, a decreased amount of REM sleep and increased wakefulness (Reite and Short 1983).

Depressive episodes in humans are frequently accompanied by a circadian phase shift and by altered sleep architecture. However, whereas the separated monkeys show a phase delay in circadian rhythmicity, clinical studies have generally implicated a phase advance (Wehr et al. 1980). Similarly, depression is associated with a decreased latency to enter REM sleep and increased density of REM sleep (Kupfer and Foster 1972), changes that are opposite in direction to those described in the separated monkeys. It is worth bearing in mind, however, that the changes in sleep and circadian rhythmicity in depression are heterogeneous and vary with symptom profile and with treatment. The fact that separation can influence these biological rhythms per se may yet have value as information about the biological regulatory functions of social relationships.

Mindful of the need for predictive validity in any valuable animal model of depression, the effects of psychotropic drugs have been tested in separated monkeys. Suomi et al. (1978) reported more interest in the environment and less 'self-directed' behaviour in peer-separated infant rhesus monkeys following chronic treatment with the prototypical tricyclic antidepressant drug imipramine. Similarly, Hrdina et al. (1979) have claimed less behavioural disruption in maternally separated infant monkeys following treatment with desmethylimipramine. However, the pharmacological specificity of these effects is questionable, since chlorpromazine (an antipsychotic drug with very weak, if any, clinical antidepressant activity), alcohol and diazepam have been reported to have similar effects, depending on dose administered and actual measures recorded (reviewed by Kraemer 1988). However, repeated electroconvulsive stimulation, an analogue of the highly effective antidepressant treatment electroconvulsive therapy (ECT), has also been shown to have an 'anti-despair' profile of effects (Kraemer 1988). Chemically induced lesions of central monoamine and indoleamine systems have been attempted to augment the 'despair' responses (Kraemer and McKinney 1979). Whereas there was some evidence of an augmented 'despair' response following interference with noradrenaline synthesis, there was no apparent effect following disruption of serotonin synthesis. However, these pharmacological manipulations were relatively nonselective chemically, regionally nonspecific and probably inconclusive. Examination of biogenic amines and their metabolites in the cerebrospinal fluid (CSF) of separated monkeys has suggested that those monkeys with the lowest basal levels of CSF noradrenaline were more prone to develop a 'despair' reaction (Kraemer et al. 1984a) and the same authors have reported that socially isolated monkeys developed a behavioural hypersensitivity to systemic d-amphetamine (Kraemer et al. 1984b). However, such indirect measures of central transmitter function have very limited power of persuasion. Attempts to examine more direct indices of neurochemical function in separated monkeys have been rare. The reasons for this are obvious. Even where scientific justification for such studies is very strong, primate work is expensive, can be conducted in very few centres and takes a very long time (Martin et al. 1991). Furthermore, the climate of public opinion has become very hostile towards experimentation with all animals, particularly monkeys, rendering such work even more difficult to resource. Nevertheless, some information on the neurobiological consequences of social separation is available from primate studies.

Rhesus macaque monkeys reared in social isolation during the first year of life (taken away from mothers within hours of birth and reared in separate stainless-steel chambers with only intermittent experimenter contact to facilitate feeding in the first 20 weeks), then reared in social groups, displayed increased 'self-directed' behaviours, social withdrawal, apathy to external stimuli, increased aggression and enhanced responsivity to blepharospasm induced by the dopamine receptor ago-nist apomorphine as adults (reviewed by Kraemer et al. 1984*a, b*; Beauchamp and Gluck 1988; Lewis et al. 1990). Postmortem examination of the brains of some of these monkeys (aged 19–24 years) revealed marked alterations in the chemoar-chitecture of the striatum (Martin et al. 1991). There was a regional selectivity to the changes, with calbindin and tyrosine hydroxylase immunoreactivity markedly diminished in the matrix of the caudate/putamen and with substance P and leu-enkephalin immunoreactivity reduced in the patch regions of the caudate. Inter-estingly, the nucleus accumbens appeared relatively unaffected by isolation. These authors concluded that early isolation affected the postnatal maturation of specific neurotransmitter phenotypes in a manner consistent with the behavioural evi-dence for increased sensitivity to direct (apomorphine) and indirect (amphetamine) dopamine receptor agonist drugs. More recently, Coplan et al. (1996) have reported that bonnet macaque monkeys reared under 'variable foraging demand' conditions as infants (meaning that the daily food ration was presented in an unpredictable manner, with differing response requirements for the mother each day) demon-strated persistent elevations in cerebrospinal fluid (CSF) levels of corticotrophin releasing factor (CRF), suggesting that unpredictable and 'less secure' mothering induced enduring changes in central CRF function. Unfortunately, there were no behavioural data presented with the CRF assays and the concept of 'less secure' and unpredictable mothering is clearly different from that of total social isolation. Indeed, this species was previously reported to be relatively resistant to the effects of early social separation (Rosenblum and Kaufman 1968). In addition, it is not known how well CSF levels of CRF might relate to chemoarchitectural changes in these monkeys.

Social separation models in nonprimate species

One of the earliest reports of maternal separation effects in a nonprimate species was that of Seitz (1959), who studied cats. He reported that cats separated from their mothers at 2 weeks of age differed from nonseparated controls (and from a group separated at 6 weeks of age) with respect to their adult responsiveness to novelty. Separated cats were more fearful in novel environments, more aggressive as adults and slower to adapt to environmental change. However, the controls in this study were inadequate. Two-week-old kittens are unable to feed themselves and, therefore, were artificially fed by the experimenter. Thus, there was a difference in the amount of neonatal handling and in the nutritional status of the separated and nonseparated cats, rendering direct comparison problematic. Most nonprimate work on maternal separation, however, has been conducted on rodent species. Whereas human studies of 'attachment' have tended to focus on individual differences in the development of patterns of attachment behaviours and on the mental representations that are inferred from these behaviours, studies in rodents have sought to identify generalities in responding, the underlying physiological mechanisms and opportunities to manipulate responses pharmacologically. Studies in the rat have generated a wealth of data on the complex mechanisms by which infant physiology is regulated by the provision of maternal stimuli. Indeed, the extensive degree of homeostatic control exerted by maternal stimuli has led Hofer (1994*a*, *b*) to propose that separation of a neonatal mammal from its mother leads to a process he has labelled 'the loss of hidden regulators'. Multiple maternally specific stimuli are involved, with each responsible for the homeostatic regulation of discrete aspects of neonatal physiology. Correspondingly, Hofer has proposed that the 'protest' and 'despair' phases of acute neonatal maternal separation are attributable to dysregulation of the homeostatic control normally exerted by maternally generated stimuli. Furthermore, he has proposed (Hofer 1994*b*) that the integrated 'protest–despair' response might best be conceptualized as the withdrawal of multiple 'hidden regulators' that act on different systems, across different time scales.

Maternal separation and the rat

When electing to study the role of the mother in the early development of laboratory rats in the late 1960s, Hofer believed that any responses to neonatal maternal separation would be free from the confounds of complex cognitive concepts such as 'attachment' (Hofer 1994*b*). However, one of his rat mothers escaped from her nest cage one night, leaving her 2-week-old pups unattended for a period of several hours. When examined by Hofer the following day, the rat pups were apathetic, unresponsive and had low heart rates. This serendipitous finding confirmed (at least for Hofer) that maternal separation elicited a very specific phasic response, presumably of adaptive evolutionary value, across diverse species of very different cognitive capacity, 'suggesting deep biological roots and a long evolutionary history' (Hofer 1994*b*). Subsequently, careful study in rats and guinea pigs has permitted the definition of many physiological mechanisms that are specific to the mother–infant unit and may have direct relevance to human 'attachment'.

Acute separation of a rat pup from its dam leads to a constellation of time-dependent changes (Hofer 1994*a*, *b*), with increased locomotion and vocalization the hallmark of the early stages (0–60 min). Thereafter, indices of physiological function alter in the following order: decreased secretion of growth hormone (onset 60 min +), increased sucking movements (120 min +), increased adrenal corticosterone release (120 min +), decreased heat production and heart rate (240 min +). One of Hofer's earliest experiments demonstrated that the ambient temperature in which the separation took place could affect the constellation of responses. For example, the effect of separation upon locomotor activity was dependent upon temperature. Pups kept warm (nest temperature of 32°C) would become very active as separation was prolonged towards 24 hr, whereas pups kept at room temperature would become sluggish and inactive. However, ambient temperature had no effect on cardiac rate, which slowed independent of temperature. Instead, heart rate could be restored to 'normal' by artificial feeding (Hofer 1994*b*), which, in turn, had no effect on behavioural reactivity or on locomotion. Similarly, the switching off of growth-hormone release was relatively independent of ambient temperature and of nutritional status, instead being most affected by restoration of tactile contact (Kuhn et al. 1978, 1990; Hofer 1994*b*). These data established three important points.

First, that multiple maternal stimuli were essential for optimal growth and development in the neonatal rat and that several of the homeostatic mechanisms operated independently of each other. Second, that the effects of separation were dependent upon environmental variables (e.g. temperature). (It is interesting to speculate that an attenuated responsivity to d-amphetamine might have been demonstrated in separated monkeys had they been kept in warmer conditions; see Kraemer et al. 1984*b*). Third, that it seems possible to account for the cross-species 'protest' response to maternal separation as a release from ongoing regulation of arousal, behaviour and physiology by the mother (Hofer 1994*a*, *b*). Given the multisystem physiological disruption associated with even brief neonatal maternal separation, and the sensitivity of the developing mammalian nervous system to insult, it seems plausible that such early 'social' adversity might result in enduring changes in brain function that might act either through effects on gross neural development, or upon synaptic plasticity. Hofer has also speculated that these regulatory interactions exert influence beyond tissue and behavioural development and are responsible for the formation of mental representations and associated 'emotions' (Hofer 1994*b*), ideas that bear obvious comparison with some influential psychological models of depression (Beck et al. 1979). Thus, the study of attachment phenomena in nonhuman species again offers data compatible with the notion of early experience leading to an enduring 'vulnerability' as derived from human study.

Stress, early environment and depression models

A parallel and related line of study in the rat has been that of the influence of early environment on the development of the neuroendocrine systems that mediate responses to stress. With the development of the 'vulnerability' concept in depressive illness and the undisputed epidemiological relationship between 'exit life events' and the precipitation of depression (Paykel and Hollyman 1984), comes the obvious interest in the regulation of the major neurohormonal response to stress, adrenal corticosteroid release. Also, several strands of evidence from clinical studies have implicated abnormalities in the glucocorticoid response to stress in depressives, with a hyperactivity of the hypothalamic–pituitary–adrenal (HPA) axis that is probably driven by hypersecretion of corticotrophin-releasing factor or hormone (CRF/CRH) (Axelson et al. 1993; Nemeroff 1998). In the adult, glucocorticoid hormones play a key role in the regulation of an organism's responses to stress. In man and other animals, the stress response is characterized by an activation of the HPA axis by the release of CRF from the paraventricular nucleus of the hypothalamus into the portal-venous circulation. This peptide hormone acts together with arginine vasopressin (AVP) to release adrenocorticotrophin (ACTH) from the anterior pituitary gland. An increase in circulating ACTH leads to stimulation of the release of cortisol/corticosterone (corticosterone is the rat analogue of the human hormone cortisol) from the cortex of the adrenal glands. Glucocorticoid hormones are released in response to a wide variety of psychological and physical stressors and represent a core component of adaptive responsivity to environmental change and threat. Amongst the many actions of cortisol/corticosterone (CORT) are the promotion of gluconeogenesis and lipolysis, processes that will increase the availability of stored energy resources to facilitate activity, typically the 'flight/fight' response. The degree of HPA axis activity is finely controlled through a series of homeostatic negative-feedback mechanisms, including glucocorticoid receptors sited in the cortex, hippocampus, hypothalamus and pituitary. These functions act over a wide range of inhibitory and permissive mechanisms, usually on a temporary basis. However, the same hormones are involved in quite different processes during early development, exerting *permanent* effects on tissue growth and differentiation – particularly in the central nervous system (De Kloet et al. 1988). In rats, glucocorticoids have been shown to regulate the phenotypic expression of certain types of neuron, affecting the genetic and environmentally influenced processes that sculpt the developing brain (De Kloet et al. 1988). Therefore, it seems intuitively plausible that disruption in the normal development of the glucocorticoid hormone systems could lead both to altered brain development and to altered vulnerability to the effects of stress in adult life.

During ontogeny, the different components of the HPA system demonstrate characteristic patterns of development (Sapolsky and Meaney 1986). Immediately before and after birth, basal levels of CORT are very high in the rat. By postnatal day 2, however, the levels plummet and remain extremely low until postnatal days 12–14. This is known as the 'stress-hyporesponsive period' (SHRP) (Sapolsky and Meaney 1986). Not only do the neonatal rats demonstrate very low basal levels of CORT secretion, they also become profoundly unresponsive to stimuli that evoke robust ACTH and CORT responses in adulthood (Sapolsky and Meaney 1986; De Kloet et al. 1988). This phenomenon has been extensively studied to define the mechanisms by which HPA axis activity is regulated during this period. It is generally believed that the SHRP acts to protect the rapidly developing neonatal brain from the adverse effects of high CORT levels on neuronal development. It is also generally believed that the main regulatory influences over the maintenance of the SHRP are thermal and tactile cues provided by the mother (Cirrulli et al. 1992; Suchecki et al. 1993). However, it is equally clear that some CORT release is essential for optimal development (De Kloet et al. 1988). Intriguingly, the one manipulation which appears to be capable of disrupting the SHRP and provoking the release of significant quantities of ACTH and CORT is physical separation of the neonate from its dam (Suchecki et al. 1993). Maternal separation leads to both an acute CORT response that increases with repeated separation (Hennessy 1997), and chronic effects on HPA responsivity into adulthood, which differ according to the specifics of the separation experience (Ladd et al. 1996; Rots et al. 1996). For example, a single 24-hour separation conducted on postnatal day 3 leads to chronic upregulation of basal ACTH and CORT with increased adrenal gland size (Rots et al. 1996) in the rat. Repeated 6-hour separations between postnatal days 2 and 20 lead to increased basal and evoked ACTH release, with no change in CORT, but a substantial upregulation of median eminence and anterior pituitary CRF receptor binding in the rat (Ladd et al. 1996). There is a wealth of evidence to support the contention that similar processes occur in other species. For example, studies in nonhuman primates have established that mother–infant separation is a potent stimulus for neonatal HPA activation (Hill et al. 1973). HPA activation in response to mother–infant and peer separation has also been demonstrated in guinea pigs (for review see Hennessy 1997). Indeed, Hennessy (1997) has speculated that the magnitude of the CORT response to separation correlates with the degree of 'attachment' demonstrated in guinea pigs before separation (with 'attachment' in this instance defined as the propensity to follow and the propensity to demonstrate behavioural distress on involuntary separation). The importance of the HPA responses to social separation, particularly to maternal separation, lies in the possibility of identifying a mechanism to explain the chronic effects of separation on behavioural development. Hennessy (1997) concluded in his review of this concept, that evidence for HPA activation in response to the disruption of an 'attachment bond' has been found in several different species, yet no responses are seen in others, with no obvious identifying characteristics for distinguishing between those that do and those that do not. Specifically, there is no evidence that cognitive capacity or phylogenetic position are determinants of a positive association between HPA response and social separation. Instead, he concludes (Hennessy 1997) that 'separation of partners exhibiting signs of emotional attachment leads to an immediate and persistent HPA response, whereas separation of partners that are affiliative, but do not exhibit attachment, has little or no effect on HPA activity'. The validity of this hypothesis remains to be tested. However, if social separation can act as a potent stimulus for HPA activation, what then might be the consequences of such a response during early development?

Before detailing some of the known effects of altered glucocorticoid function on brain development, it seems prudent to clarify that very little is known about such effects on the human brain. Almost all of the following mechanisms have been defined in the rat. Comparing rat brain development with that of the human is problematic, with much of rat brain development taking place later than in the human, i.e. postnatally vs. prenatally. Also, the rat brain develops much more rapidly and, as such, is more susceptible to temporary environmental insult. Caution is, therefore, warranted before attempting to extrapolate the following across species.

Glucocorticoids exert predominantly catabolic effects; that is, they inhibit cell division and protein synthesis. Within the brain, they have been shown to inhibit the rate of cell proliferation and to promote a 'precocious cessation' of cell division in some types of stem cell (Bohn 1980). Where cells have ceased dividing, glucocorticoids retard myelination, synaptogenesis and the formation of dendritic spines (Bohn 1980). The neonatal rat hippocampus appears particularly susceptible to high glucocorticoid levels, perhaps because of its role as a critical locus for negative-feedback regulation (along with several other sites). With such a range of disruptive and potentially pathogenic actions on neural development, the biological and evolutionary advantage of the SHRP is obvious. If an extremely adverse early environment, such as maternal separation, overpowers the SHRP, it is possible that high circulating levels of glucocorticoids penetrate the developing brain, irreversibly altering the 'optimal' neuronal and dendritic sculpting processes. These neonatal manipulations certainly lead to altered HPA function in adulthood (see above) and may impact on other developing systems and structures.

Maternal separation as a model of depression

If manipulations of social environment, particularly early in life, can exert influence over adult responsivity to stressors, can they also impact upon other key behavioural constructs that might be relevant to depression, for example, responsivity to reward? A model capable of encompassing developmental influences that lead to an adult hyperresponsivity to stress alongside changes in behavioural responses to reward could represent a major advance – particularly if these changes were associated with regionally specific changes in brain structure and function similar to those reported in depression.

Repeated maternal separation (RMS) and the neonatal rat

We have conducted a series of studies describing the adult behavioural effects of a specific repeated maternal separation procedure conducted during the neonatal period (Matthews et al. 1996a, b, 1999, 2001). We have focused on the study of behavioural responses to appetitive stimuli under different experimental conditions. The timing and duration of the neonatal separations (6 hours) were selected to maximize the potential for disruption of normal mother–pup interactions without overt morbidity (see above and Hofer 1994a, b). Each cohort of rats was derived from separate batches of time-mated, out-bred Lister-Hooded dams obtained at 13 days' gestation. Dams were permitted to habituate to the novel surroundings for a week before parturition. Dams and pups were housed, by litter, in plastic breeding cages with food and water available ad libitum. Solid-bottomed cages measuring $56 \times 38 \times 18$ cm with a sawdust floor covering and shredded paper bedding were used. All animals were housed in the same temperature and humidity-controlled holding facility ($21\,^\circ$C) on a 12-hour light/dark cycle (lights on at 07.30). With day of parturition designated as postnatal day 0, rat pups were left undisturbed until day 5, with the exception of brief handling on day 2 to permit sexing and culling of each litter to 8–10. On 10 occasions spaced randomly between days 5 and 20, litters allocated to the separation procedure were removed from the nest cages and placed in wire baskets, by litter, inside a temperature and humidity-controlled incubator for a period of 6 hours. The wire baskets were lined with paper towels and a small quantity of home cage shavings to maintain nest odours. Temperature inside the incubator was maintained at $33\,^\circ$C for the first five separations and $32\,^\circ$C for the final five. Relative humidity remained constant throughout at 45%. Control litters were removed from home cages and placed into identical wire baskets, with paper towel and nest shavings, for 2 minutes on each separation day as a control for the effects of handling. The use of the paper towel and nest shavings minimized any temperature drop and maintained familiar nest odours in the immediate environment. Each pup was lifted individually, very gently, from one location to the

Table 16.1. Effects of RMS on physical and behavioural development

	Enhanced	Attenuated	No effect
Gross physical development			X
Weight gain	X		
Locomotor response to novelty		X	
Locomotor response to systemic d-amphetamine		X	
Pavlovian appetitive conditioning		X	
Behavioural sensitivity to dopamine D_2 receptor antagonist	X		
Behavioural sensitivity to dopamine D_1 receptor antagonist			X
Sucrose preference			X
Incentive contrast sensitivity		X	
Cocaine self-administration – 'high dose'	X		
Cocaine self-administration – 'low dose'		X	

other. Pups were not subjected to stroking or any other manipulation. All animals were weaned by removing the dams from the home cages on postnatal day 21. Two weeks postweaning, pups were group housed by gender and then left entirely undisturbed until adulthood. Throughout each study, all subjects were allowed access to food and water ad libitum, except where dictated by individual experimental design.

Adult behavioural effects of repeated neonatal maternal separation (RMS)

The major behavioural effects of RMS are summarized in Table 16.1. Although basic tests of consummatory behaviour (e.g. food consumption, sucrose preference) indicated no differences from control-reared animals (Matthews et al. 1996a), RMS resulted in a profound, developmentally specific attenuation of adult behavioural responses to primary and conditioned reward stimuli (Matthews et al. 1996a, b), including those to artificial reinforcers such as intravenous cocaine (Matthews et al. 1999). The RMS procedure appeared to have relatively little impact upon gross development. For example, RMS had no effect on the timing of eye opening (Matthews, unpublished observations), a commonly used measure of developmental delay. Similarly, there was no detrimental impact upon body weight gain; indeed, separated rat pups tended to be heavier than their controls (Matthews et al. 1996a, b).

Spontaneous response to novelty

Although habituated baseline locomotor activity levels were unaltered, the initial locomotor response to novelty was attenuated in adult RMS rats (Matthews et al. 1996a, b). With mild novelty representing an appetitive stimulus for the rat, these data are suggestive of a deficit in responsivity to at least one category of 'rewarding' stimulus.

Pavlovian appetitive conditioning

Exposure to a simple Pavlovian food-conditioned locomotion procedure revealed that adult RMS rats showed a delayed acquisition and an attenuated maximal expression of response (Matthews et al. 1996a, b), i.e. an attenuated acquisition and expression of Pavlovian appetitive conditioning of preparatory responses to contextual cues. By placing hungry rats in a distinctive environment (in this case wire-mesh locomotor-activity cages), at the same time each day, shortly before they receive their daily ration of food, a Pavlovian association forms between the compound environmental stimuli and anticipation of the delivery of food. Consequently, the rats display enhanced locomotor activity in anticipation of food delivery – an exhibition of biologically significant 'preparatory' behaviours. Indeed, locomotion represents only one component of the conditioned response, with salivation also prominent. Since the delivery of the reinforcer was independent of any action on behalf of the animal, this represents a form of classical, or Pavlovian, conditioning (Mackintosh 1974)· The process by which stimuli acquire affective properties as a consequence of their predictive association with a primary reinforcer in this manner is known to be dependent upon the functional integrity of the basolateral amygdala (Cador et al. 1991). A deficit in the acquisition of the conditioned locomotor response to food presentation is compatible with altered function of the amygdala as a consequence of the RMS procedure. Indeed, Kaneko et al. (1994) have reported electrophysiological evidence of altered function in both the amygdala and the hippocampus of rats that were subjected to a maternal separation regimen broadly comparable to that employed in our studies. In addition to the above effects of RMS on food-conditioned locomotion, there was also a differential sensitivity to the conditioned activity-enhancing effects of the indirect dopamine agonist d-amphetamine, the activity-attenuating effects of the selective dopamine D_2 receptor antagonist sulpiride and the mixed α_1-α_2-adrenoceptor agonist clonidine (Matthews et al. 1996b). RMS rats of both sexes were less responsive to the activity-enhancing effects of low-dose d-amphetamine in the fasted state and their conditioned locomotor activity was suppressed markedly by prefeeding. Administration of the selective dopamine D_1 receptor antagonist SCH 23390 caused a reduction in the expression of conditioned activity across both rearing conditions, but with a significantly greater effect on male animals and a trend towards a greater effect in separated animals. Taken together, these data suggest that RMS animals show behavioural evidence consistent with reduced central dopaminergic function and possibly also of reduced noradrenergic function (Matthews et al. 1996b).

Sucrose as a reinforcer

There is ample evidence that sweet solutions of sucrose or saccharin are capable of acting as potent reinforcers for behavioural experimental work with laboratory rodents (Katz 1982; Phillips et al. 1991). In addition to their use as simple reinforcers when training rats to perform specific tasks, the relative responsivity to sucrose or saccharin solutions, usually quantified as the consumption thereof, has been used as a measure of hedonic state (Katz 1982; Willner et al. 1987). For example, it can readily be demonstrated that the consumption of sucrose solutions of rising concentration will generate a typical 'inverted-U-shaped' dose–response function with peak responding, at least with respect to consumption, around the 7–15% w/v (weight per unit volume) range (Phillips et al. 1991). With increasing concentration beyond this point, total consumption will fall, often assumed attributable to the appearance of some aversive sensory properties of the solution. However, concentrations of solution selected from this portion of the dose–response function, the 'descending limb', can be demonstrated to have intense reinforcing value according to other behavioural measures, for example progressive ratio responding to break point, and resistance to extinction when previously acting to reinforce an operant response. However, provided that solution concentrations are selected from the ascending limb of the function (< 7–15% w/v), a rat will demonstrate an incremental preference for, consumption of, lick rate response to and latency to approach, rising solution concentration in a monotonic fashion (Phillips et al. 1991).

The degree to which a rat will exhibit a preference for a sucrose solution over plain drinking water can be quantified in simple two-bottle tests where free access to each is permitted. Typically, a rat will show a strong preference for the sucrose solution, even at low concentrations ($< 1\%$). Such sucrose preference scores have been used as the dependent variable in a number of behavioural studies (see Willner et al. 1987), often where there is manipulation of mesolimbic dopaminergic function as the independent variable (Phillips et al. 1991). However, the history of such studies has ably demonstrated the limitations of the technique, particularly if primary motivation and alterations in metabolic state are not controlled meticulously (Matthews et al. 1995; Forbes et al. 1996). Nevertheless, the sucrose preference technique seems to provide a reasonably reliable and valid method for the gross assessment of motivation.

RMS and sucrose preference

To assess responding for sucrose solutions sited at different points on the concentration–response function (1, 15 and 34%), we tested subjects with some in a food-deprived state and the others a nondeprived state. RMS had no effect on measures of sucrose preference taken from three points on the concentration–response function in either the fasted or sated state (Matthews et al. 1996a).

RMS and incentive contrast

As a more sophisticated extension of the assessment of motivation with sucrose preference measures, it is also possible to use sucrose solutions of differing concentrations as reinforcers in experimental designs that examine incentive contrast effects. The term 'contrast' generally refers to demonstrations of an exaggeration of the perception of differences between reinforcing stimuli, particularly when two rewards of differing magnitude are juxtaposed in close temporal proximity. The most influential studies of the behavioural effects of such 'reward-shifts' were conducted by Crespi (1944), who demonstrated that when rats were trained to run along an alley to receive a reward and then were shifted from their usual reward to one of a lesser value, the speed achieved in the runway would diminish to a level below that which was achieved by rats who only ever experienced the lower value of reward. Crespi (1944) also reported the opposite effect, i.e. an enhancement of extrapolated runway speed following a shift from a lower-value reward to a larger one. Such downward and upward shifts in reward magnitude reliably induced behavioural changes that were deemed to reflect emotional responses in the rats, often characterized as 'frustration' and 'elation' respectively. Similar contrast phenomena have also been demonstrated by varying the concentration of sucrose solution rewards and measuring the lick rate response (Ashton and Trowill 1970). Correspondingly, the behavioural effects of both positive and negative successive contrast shifts with sucrose solutions were examined in RMS and control-reared subjects (Matthews et al. 1996a). The procedures directly evaluated the 'suppressant' effect of pre-exposure to 15% sucrose on the consumption of 2.1% sucrose. Similarly, the 'excitatory' influence of pre-exposure to a 5% sucrose solution on the responding for a 15% solution was measured. Controlling for the potential caloric and metabolic influences of the quantity of solution consumed during the preshift test sessions, RMS animals altered their lick rate to a significantly lesser degree than the controls, under conditions of both positive and negative contrast. Since lick rate during such a brief period varies monotonically with reward magnitude (at least until the concentration increases to a level at which it assumes aversive properties), a blunted shift in lick rate can be interpreted as evidence of disturbed comparative appreciation of reward.

Although numerous theoretical constructs have been invoked to explain incentive contrast, evidence to support a motivational/emotional interpretation is available (Flaherty 1982). The influences of privation and of previous experience of reward implicate both motivational and cognitive mechanisms respectively. In addition, downward shifts in reward strength activate the HPA-axis stress response with release of adrenal corticosteroids (Goldman et al. 1973) and it is generally observed that successive negative contrast effects can be ameliorated or abolished by drugs with anxiolytic properties such as ethanol, barbiturates and benzo-diazepines. In fact, numerous pharmacological studies have consistently shown that different drugs with anxiolytic properties can ameliorate negative contrast effects when given systemically (Flaherty and Driscoll 1980). The fact that negative contrast elicits a robust neuroendocrine stress response raises the possibility that the effects of RMS on negative contrast may be attributable to the well-documented stress-response-reducing effects of neonatal handling (O'Donnell et al. 1994) and the stress-response-enhancing effects of periodic maternal separation (Ladd et al. 1996). However, there are no comparable data available to speculate on the role for such a mechanism in positive contrast. Furthermore, a candidate mechanism to mediate the altered behavioural effects as a consequence of raised or lowered corticosterone levels is lacking, although both the amygdala and the hippocampus are known to be involved in the mediation of stress responses.

RMS and responding for intravenous cocaine

We have also studied the impact of RMS on adult responses to psychostimu-lant drugs. Although there are some data suggesting that RMS adult rats are less responsive to the unconditioned locomotor effects of systemic d-amphetamine (Matthews et al. 1996b), the most intriguing data relate to the effects of RMS on vulnerability to acquire self-administration of cocaine. Using standard drug self-administration techniques, we have demonstrated a rightward shift in the acquisi-tion dose–effect function in RMS rats, although the effects are dose- and gender-dependent (Matthews et al. 1999). Furthermore, determination of the dose–effect function following a period of stable cocaine self-administration revealed a right-ward shift for females and a downward shift for males. The significance of these data are that RMS alters adult vulnerability to acquire cocaine self-administration such that acquisition is enhanced at moderate to high doses and attenuated at lower doses. This pattern of responding can be considered broadly opposite to that de-scribed following neonatal handling or chronic stress where acquisition is generally facilitated and the dose–effect function elevated (Altman et al. 1996).

What are the neural substrates of RMS?

The behavioural effects listed above (summarized in Table 16.1) invite a series of hypotheses concerning the mediating neural substrates for RMS. However, it is likely that small procedural differences during neonatal separation may lead to major differences in the adult behavioural and neurochemical effects. Consequently, there is a compelling need to study behaviour and neurochemistry in the same experimental subjects. We have recently reported data from a postmortem study

Table 16.2. Effects of RMS on neurochemical development – regional monoamine neurotransmitter levels in adult postmortem tissue

	Increased	Reduced
Dorsal striatum dopamine	X	
Ventral striatum dopamine	X	
Turnover of dopamine in medial prefrontal cortex		X
Hippocampal noradrenaline (females only)	X	
Hippocampal serotonin		X
Medial prefrontal cortex serotonin (males only)		X

of tissue neurochemical measures, comparing adult RMS rats with control-reared animals (Matthews et al. 2001). We have identified a series of potentially interesting regional changes, affecting the mesolimbic and mesoprefrontal dopamine systems and other key limbic cortical structures. These changes are summarized in Table 16.2. Adult RMS rats had increased tissue levels of dopamine in both dorsal and ventral striatum. The turnover of dopamine, as determined by the ratio of the metabolite DOPAC to its parent transmitter, was decreased in the medial prefrontal cortex of RMS subjects. Levels of serotonin were reduced in the dorsal hippocampus of RMS rats of both sexes and in the medial prefrontal cortex of male RMS rats. Noradrenaline levels were increased in the dorsal hippocampus in female, but not in male, RMS rats. These data provide preliminary evidence that, in addition to the adult behavioural consequences, RMS leads to profound, region- and potentially gender-specific changes in brain monoamine content.

RMS as a model of depression

Since no 'therapeutic' manipulations have been attempted, there are no data on which to assess the 'predictive' validity of RMS as a model of depression. Thus, it is reasonable to consider RMS with respect to the degree to which it confers 'face', 'aetiological' and 'construct' validity as a model of depression.

Face validity of RMS

Adult rats exposed to the RMS procedure demonstrated an enhanced weight gain, a decreased behavioural responsivity to novelty and a reduced sensitivity to the psychostimulant drugs AMPH and cocaine. Responding to a range of primary and conditioned appetitive stimuli was attenuated. RMS rats showed a blunting of the behavioural response to incentive contrast when drinking sucrose solutions. Pavlovian conditioning to primary appetitive reinforcers was attenuated. The key clinical features of major depressive disorder according to the DSM–IV classification system are either a persistent depressed mood or a blunting of the capacity to experience pleasure. Both may be, but need not be, present at the same time. Loss of interest in food with altered perception of taste is common. Depressed patients tend not to be heavier than nondepressed controls, indeed weight loss is a characteristic feature of major depression, although certain subpopulations of depressed patients do experience weight gain. Sleep tends to be disturbed, most often manifesting as severe insomnia. Sleep parameters have not been assessed in the RMS rat and thus cannot be commented upon. Reduced locomotor activity and a sense of profound fatigue are often described, as is the opposing symptom cluster of motor restlessness or 'agitation'. No changes in general locomotor functions were observed in the RMS rats. The other major clinical features relate to aspects of higher cognitive function, for example, recurrent thoughts of guilt, pessimism and suicide, many of which are untestable and unrecordable in nonhuman species. Setting aside measures of responsivity to appetitive reinforcement (considered below) and taking these other clinical features (which determine diagnostic classification), RMS has poor immediate face validity as a model for depression.

Comorbidity between depression and psychostimulant drug use, for example nicotine and cocaine, is common (Altman et al. 1996). There are several hypotheses that attempt to explain this association (Markou et al. 1998). First, the vulnerability to depression and the vulnerability to self-administer psychostimulants may be conferred by the same genetic and environmental factors, perhaps even sharing common neural substrates. Second, depression may modify psychostimulant drug experience rendering repeated use more likely or may even render some aspects of drug use 'therapeutic'. Third, repeated psychostimulant use may lead to brain changes that lead to depression. Clinical pharmacological data on the treatment of depression are broadly compatible with the hypothesis that increased dopamine transmission is associated with the elevation of mood and reduced transmission with lowering of mood (Willner 1995). Thus, one might reasonably expect that any change in sensitivity to psychostimulant drugs in depressed populations might be in the direction of an *enhanced* effect and not a reduced one as seen with RMS. However, there are circumstances (female gender, mid-range dose of cocaine) where acquisition was greatly facilitated. If this test had been conducted in isolation, it would have been easy to conclude that RMS *enhanced* the acquisition of cocaine self-administration and thus enjoyed a degree of face validity as a model of the comorbidity between depression and substance misuse. However, the effects of RMS (in the broadest sense) were to shift the acquisition dose–response function to the right, an effect analogous to that of treating rats with neuroleptic drugs. To this writer's knowledge, there are no demonstrations that depressed humans are less sensitive per se to the psychostimulant properties of AMPH (De Wit et al. 1987) or cocaine, although the mood-elevating response to AMPH and the related stimulant drug methylphenidate has been used to predict likelihood of responding to antidepressant drug treatment (Fawcett and Siomopoulos 1971; Gwirtsman and Guze 1989). There is reputed to be a correlation between acute psychostimulant response and subsequent antidepressant drug response, implying that 'treatment-resistant' or 'treatment nonresponsive' depressed patients may be *insensitive* to the euphoriant effects of psychostimulants. Thus, the RMS rat may actually enjoy substantial face and construct validity as a model of a specific subgroup of depressed patients, arguably those who present the greatest problems in the clinical arena. Again, there is no evidence that depressed patients are more sensitive to the psychological or behavioural effects of dopamine antagonists (with the possible exception of an increased risk of developing tardive dyskinesia; see Yassa et al. 1987). Indeed, rather than showing an enhanced sensitivity to the negative hedonic effects of dopamine antagonists, such as chlorpromazine and thioridazine, there have been demonstrations of mild antidepressant effects in clinical trials (Robertson and Trimble 1981), although the effects tend to be seen only at lower doses.

RMS and anhedonia

As mentioned previously, the blunting of the capacity to experience pleasure (anhedonia) is regarded as one of the core psychopathological changes in depression (American Psychiatric Association 1994), and might reasonably be expected to manifest as a reduction in the vigour of responding for primary and conditioned reinforcers in the rat. In this respect, the RMS model does appear to enjoy a degree of face and construct validity. Demonstrations of behavioural phenomena in experimental animals that do seem to model anhedonia are relatively rare. However, the RMS rats do show a significantly reduced motivation for sucrose, a blunted response to changes in reward magnitude and an impaired acquisition of conditioned appetitive reinforcement (see Table 16.1).

Neurochemistry of RMS as a model of depression

Recent in vivo studies in clinical populations have identified alterations in indices of dopamine transmission in the striatum of depressed patients (D'Haenen and Bossuyt 1994; Ebert et al. 1996; Shah et al. 1997). Specifically, these have suggested that striatal dopamine (DA) release may be reduced in depression (Ebert et al. 1996), particularly where associated with psychomotor retardation, with evidence of an increased density of postsynaptic DA D_2 receptors (D'Haenen and Bossuyt 1994). Further, Laasonen-Balk et al. (1999) have reported increased DA transporter binding in the striatum of drug-naïve depressed subjects. Collectively, these data suggest that depressed subjects may exhibit changes in striatal DA function that bear some similarities with those seen in adult rats following RMS. Similarly, reduced serotonergic function in the frontal and prefrontal cortex has been implicated in the pathogenesis of depression, particularly in those instances where behavioural control over impulsive acts is compromised, i.e. suicide (Arango et al. 1997), although direct evidence from human studies for this low-serotonin-induced impulsivity is sparse (Mann and Stoff 1997). However, dynamic imaging studies conducted in recovered depressives following acute tryptophan depletion (a procedure believed to deprive the brain of its reserves of the precursor of serotonin and thus to reduce serotonin transmission) have demonstrated reduced cerebral metabolism in the dorsolateral prefrontal and orbitofrontal cortical areas in depressives in parallel with the reappearance of depressive symptomatology (Bremner et al. 1997). The magnitude of the change in blood flow correlated with severity of symptoms. In general support of these data, using the technique of cerebral microdialysis, chronic administration of the so-called selective serotonin reuptake inhibitor antidepressants has been shown to lead to enhanced serotonin transmission in the medial prefrontal cortex of rats (Tanda et al. 1997). It is, therefore, of some interest that male RMS rats had lowered levels of serotonin in tissue samples taken from the medial prefrontal cortex (Matthews et al. 2001 and Table 16.2).

Conclusions

In this chapter, I have attempted to relate current clinical concepts to data derived from social-separation-based animal models of depression. With advances in our understanding of the neurobiological changes that are associated with depression, we now have a range of possible targets for the development of depression models that do not rely on simple behavioural changes or on neurochemical changes with tenuous connections to those thought to be induced by antidepressant drugs. Derived from a variety of species, we have consistent data to support the general contention that neural and behavioural development is profoundly influenced by early social environment. Some of the main effects of early social adversity can be demonstrated in the dysregulation of neurohormonal responses to stress and altered behavioural responses to reward. Interestingly, some of these effects may not be apparent until triggered by specific stimuli in adult life. The prospects for neuroscience to illuminate the pathophysiology of a complex mental disorder and to reconcile diverse and theoretically antagonistic epidemiology, sociology and psychology with neurobiology are encouraging.

REFERENCES

Ainsworth MD (1962). *The Effects of Maternal Deprivation: A Review of Findings and Controversy in the Context of Research Strategy*. Geneva: World Health Organization.

Alexander GE, DeLong MR and Strick PL (1986). Parallel organisation of functionally segregated circuits linking basal ganglia and cortex. *Annu Rev Neurosci*, 9, 357–81.

Altman J, Everitt BJ, Glautier S et al. (1996). The biological, social and clinical bases of drug addiction: commentary and debate. *Psychopharmacology*, 125, 285–345.

American Psychiatric Association (1994). *Diagnostic and Statistical Manual of Mental Disorders*, 4th edn. Washington, DC: APA.

Arango V, Underwood MD and Mann JJ (1997). Biologic alterations in the brainstem of suicides. *Psychiatric Clin N Am*, 20, 581–93.

Ashton AB and Trowill JA (1970). Effects of reinforcement shifts upon lick rate. *Psychonom Sci*, 21, 7–8.

Axelson DA, Doraiswamy PM, McDonald WM et al. (1993). Hypercortisolemia and hippocampal changes in depression. *Psychiatry Res*, 47, 163–73.

Baumann B, Danos P, Krell D et al. (1999). Reduced volume of limbic system-affiliated basal ganglia in mood disorders: preliminary data from a postmortem study. *J Neuropsychiatry Clin Neurosci*, 11, 71–8.

Beck AT, Sethi BB and Tuthill RW (1963). Childhood bereavement and adult depression. *Arch Gen Psychiatry*, 9, 295–302.

Beck AT, Rush AJ, Shaw B and Emery G (1979). *Cognitive Therapy of Depression*. New York: Guilford.

Bernstein H and Bogerts B (1999). Reduced volume of limbic system-affiliated basal ganglia in mood disorders: preliminary data from a post-mortem study. *J Neuropsych Clin Neurosci*, 11, 71–8.

Bohn MC (1980). Granule cell genesis in the hippocampus of rats treated neonatally with hydrocortisone. *Neuroscience*, 5, 2003–12.

Bowlby J (1944). Forty-four juvenile thieves: their characters and home life (II). *Int J Psychoanal*, 25, 107–27.

Bowlby J (1951). *Maternal Care and Mental Health*. Geneva: World Health Organization.

Bowlby J (1969). *Attachment and Loss: Volume 1 – Attachment*. London: Hogarth Press.

Bowlby J, Ainsworth M, Boston M and Rosenbluth D (1956). The effects of mother-child separation: a follow-up study. *Br J Med Psychol*, 29, 211–44.

Bremner JD, Innis RB, Salomon RM et al. (1997). Positron emission tomography measurement of cerebral metabolic correlates of tryptophan depletion-induced depressive relapse. *Arch Gen Psychiatry*, 54, 364–74.

Brown GW and Harris TO (1978). *Social Origins of Depression: A Study of Psychiatric Disorder in Women*. London: Tavistock Publications.

Burton R (1989). *The Anatomy of Melancholy*, ed. NC Faulkner, TC Faulkner and RL Blair. Oxford: Oxford University Press.

Cador M, Taylor JR and Robbins TW (1991). Potentiation of the effects of reward-related stimuli by dopaminergic mechanisms in the nucleus accumbens. *Psychopharmacology*, 104, 377–85.

Cirruli F, Gottlieb SL, Rosenfeld P and Levine S (1992). Maternal factors regulate stress responsiveness in the neonatal rat. *Psychobiology*, 20, 143–52.

Coplan JD, Andrews MW, Rosenblum LA et al. (1996). Persistent elevations of cerebrospinal fluid concentrations of corticotrophin-releasing factor in adult non-human primates exposed to early life stressors: implications for the pathophysiology of mood and anxiety disorders. *Proc Natl Acad Sci USA*, 93, 1619–23.

Crespi LP (1944). Amount of reinforcement and level of performance. *Psychol Rev*, 51, 341–57.

D'Haenen HA and Bossuyt A (1994). Dopamine D2 receptors in depression measured with single photon emission computed tomography. *Biol Psychiatry*, 35, 128–32.

Drevets WC (1998). Functional neuroimaging studies of depression: the anatomy of melancholia. *Ann Rev Med*, 49, 341–61.

Drevets WC, Price JL, Simpson JR et al. (1997) Subgenual prefrontal cortex abnormalities in mood disorders. *Nature*, 386, 824–7.

Ebert D, Feistel H, Loew T and Pirner A (1996). Dopamine and depression-striatal dopamine D2 receptor SPECT before and after antidepressant therapy. *Psychopharmacology*, 126, 91–4.

Everitt BJ and Keverne EB (1979). Models of depression based on behavioural observations of experimental animals. In *Psychopharmacology of Affective Disorders*, ed. ES Paykel and A Coppen, pp. 41–59. Oxford: Oxford University Press.

Fawcett J and Siomopoulos V (1971). Dextroamphetamine response as a possible predictor of improvement with tricyclic therapy in depression. *Arch Gen Psychiatry*, 25, 247–55.

Flaherty CF (1982). Incentive contrast: a review of behavioral changes following shifts in reward. *Anim Learn Behav*, 10, 409–40.

Flaherty CF and Driscoll C (1980). Amylobarbitone sodium reduces successive negative gustatory contrast. *Psychopharmacology*, 69, 161–2.

Forbes N, Stewart CA, Matthews K and Reid IC (1996). Chronic mild stress and sucrose consumption: validity as a model of depression. *Physiol Behav*, 60, 1481–4.

Freud S (1963). *The Standard Edition of the Complete Psychological Works of Sigmund Freud.* (Translated by J Strachey.) London: Hogarth Press.

Goldman L, Coover GD and Levine S (1973). Bidirectional effects of reinforcement shifts on pituitary adrenal activity. *Physiol Behav*, 10, 209–14.

Gwirtsman HE and Guze BH (1989). Amphetamine, but not methylphenidate, predicts antidepressant response. *J Clin Psychopharmacol*, 9, 453–4.

Harlow H (1958). The nature of love. *Am Psychol*, 13, 673–85.

Harlow H and Harlow M (1962). Social deprivation in monkeys. *Sci Am*, 207, 137–46.

Hennessy MB (1997). Hypothalamic-pituitary-adrenal responses to brief social separation. *Neurosci Biobehav Rev*, 21, 11–29.

Hill OW (1969). The association of childhood bereavement with suicidal attempt in depressive illness. *Br J Psychiatry*, 115, 301–4.

Hill SD, McCormack SA and Mason WA (1973). Effects of artificial mothers and visual experience on adrenal responsiveness of infant monkeys. *Dev Psychobiol*, 6, 421–9.

Hinde RA and Spencer-Booth Y (1971). Effects of brief separation from mothers on rhesus monkeys. *Science*, 173, 117–18.

Hinde RA, Spencer-Booth Y and Bruce M (1966). Effects of 6-day maternal deprivation on rhesus monkey infants. *Nature*, 210, 1021–33.

Hofer MA (1994a). Early relationships as regulators of infant physiology and behavior. *Acta Paediatr*, 397 (Suppl. 1), S9–18.

Hofer MA (1994b). Hidden regulators in attachment, separation, and loss. In *The Development of Emotion Regulation: Biological and Behavioral Considerations*, ed. NA Fox. *Monogr Soc Res Child Dev*, 59, 192–283.

Hrdina PD, von Kulmiz P and Stretch R (1979). Pharmacological modification of experimental depression in infant macaques. *Psychopharmacology*, 64, 89–93.

Jacoby RJ and Levy R (1980). Computed tomography in the elderly: affective disorder. *Br J Psychiatry*, 136, 270–5.

Judd LL (1997). The clinical course of unipolar major depressive disorders. *Arch Gen Psychiatry*, 54, 989–91.

Kaneko WM, Riley EP and Ehlers CL (1994). Behavioral and electrophysiological effects of early repeated maternal separation. *Depression*, 2, 43–53.

Katz RJ (1981). Animal models and human depressive disorders. *Neurosci Biobehav Rev*, 5, 231–46.

Katz RJ (1982). Animal model of depression: pharmacological sensitivity of a hedonic deficit. *Pharmacol Biochem Behav*, 16, 965–8.

De Kloet ER, Rosenfeld P, Van Eekelen J, Sutanato W and Levine S (1988). Stress, glucocorticoids and development. In *Progress in Brain Research, Vol. 73*, ed. GJ Boer, M Feenstra, M Mirmira, D Swaab and F Van Haaren, pp. 101–20. Amsterdam: Elsevier.

Kraemer GW (1988). Speculations on the developmental neurobiology of protest and despair. *Anim Mod Psychiatr Disord*, 2, 101–39.

Kraemer GW and McKinney WT (1979). Interactions of pharmacological agents which alter biogenic amine metabolism and depression: an analysis of contributing factors within a primate model of depression. *J Affect Disord*, 1, 33–54.

Kraemer GW, Ebert MH, Lake CR and McKinney WT (1984*a*). Cerebrospinal fluid measures of neurotransmitter changes associated with pharmacological alteration of the despair response to social separation in rhesus monkeys. *Psychiatry Res*, 11, 303–15.

Kraemer GW, Ebert MH, Lake CR and McKinney WT (1984*b*). Hypersensitivity to d-amphetamine several years after early social deprivation in rhesus monkeys. *Psychopharmacology*, 82, 266–71.

Krishnan KR, McDonald WM, Doraiswamy PM et al. (1993). Neuroanatomical substrates of depression in the elderly. *Eur Arch Psychiatry Clin Neurosci*, 243, 41–6.

Kuhn CM, Butler SR and Schanberg SM (1978). Selective depression of growth hormone during maternal deprivation in rat pups. *Science*, 201, 1034–6.

Kuhn CM, Pauk J and Schanberg SM (1990). Endocrine responses to mother–infant separation in developing rats. *Dev Psychobiol*, 23, 395–410.

Kupfer DJ and Foster FG (1972). Interval between onset of sleep and rapid eye movement sleep as an indicator of depression. *Lancet*, 2, 684–6.

Laasonen-Balk T, Kuikka J, Viinamaki H, Husso-Saastamoinen M, Lehtonen J and Tiihonen J (1999). Striatal dopamine transporter density in major depression. *Psychopharmacology*, 144, 282–5.

Ladd CO, Owens MJ and Nemeroff CB (1996). Persistent changes in corticotrophin-releasing factor neuronal systems induced by maternal deprivation. *Endocrinology*, 137, 1212–18.

Lewis MH, Gluck JP, Beauchamp AJ, Keresztruy MF and Mailman RB (1990). Long-term effects of early social isolation in *Macaca mulatta*: changes in dopamine receptor function following apomorphine challenge. *Brain Res*, 513, 67–73.

Mackintosh NJ (1974). *The Psychology of Animal Learning*. London: Academic Press.

Mann JJ and Stoff DM (1997). A synthesis of current findings regarding neurobiological correlates and treatment of suicidal behavior. *Ann NY Acad Sci*, 836, 352–63.

Markou A, Kosten TR and Koob GF (1998). Neurobiological similarities in depression and drug dependence: a self-medication hypothesis. *Neuropsychopharmacology*, 18, 135–74.

Martin LJ, Spicer DM, Lewis MH, Gluck JP and Cork LC (1991). Social deprivation of infant rhesus monkeys alters the chemoarchitecture of the brain: I. Subcortical regions. *J Neurosci*, 11, 3344–58.

Matthews K, Forbes N and Reid IC (1995). Sucrose consumption as an hedonic measure following chronic unpredictable mild stress. *Physiol Behav*, 57, 241–8.

Matthews K, Wilkinson LS and Robbins TW (1996*a*). Repeated maternal separation of pre-weanling rats attenuates the behavioural responses to primary and conditioned incentives in adulthood. *Physiol Behav*, 59, 99–107.

Matthews K, Hall FS, Wilkinson LS and Robbins TW (1996*b*). Retarded acquisition and reduced expression of conditioned locomotor activity in adult rats following repeated early maternal separation: effects of prefeeding, d-amphetamine, dopamine antagonists and clonidine. *Psychopharmacology*, 126, 75–84.

Matthews K, Robbins TW, Everitt BJ and Caine SB (1999). Repeated neonatal maternal separation alters intravenous cocaine self-administration in adult rats. *Psychopharmacology*, 141, 123–34.

Matthews K, Dalley JW, Matthews CA, Tsai TH and Robbins TW (2001). Periodic maternal separation of neonatal rats produces region and gender-specific effects on biogenic amine content in post-mortem adult brain. *Synapse*, 40, 1–10.

McKinney WT and Bunney WE (1969). Animal model of depression: review of evidence and implications for research. *Arch Gen Psychiatry*, 21, 240–8.

Mineka S and Suomi SJ (1978). Social separation in monkeys. *Psychol Bull*, 85, 1376–400.

Munro A (1966). Parental deprivation in depressive patients. *Br J Psychiatry*, 112, 443–57.

Nemeroff CB (1998). The neurobiology of depression. *Sci Am*, 278, 42–9.

O'Donnell D, Larocque S, Seckl JR and Meaney MJ (1994). Postnatal handling alters glucocorticoid but not mineralocorticoid mRNA expression in adult rats. *Mol Brain Res*, 26, 242–8.

Ongur D, Drevets WC and Price JL (1998). Glial reduction in the subgenual prefrontal cortex in mood disorders. *Proc Natl Acad Sci USA*, 95, 13290–5.

Paykel ES and Hollyman JA (1984). Life events and depression – a psychiatric view. *Trends Neurosci*, 12, 478–81.

Phillips GD, Willner P and Muscat R (1991). Suppression or facilitation of operant behaviour by raclopride dependent on concentration of sucrose reward. *Psychopharmacology*, 105, 239–46.

Porsolt RD, LePichon M and Jalfre M (1977). Depression: a new animal model sensitive to antidepressant treatment. *Nature*, 266, 730–2.

Rajkowska G, Miguel-Hidalgo JJ, Wei J et al. (1999). Morphometric evidence for neuronal and glial prefrontal cell pathology in major depression. *Biol Psychiatry*, 45, 1085–98.

Reite M and Short R (1983). Maternal separation studies: rationale and methodological considerations. In *Ethopharmacology: Primate Models of Neuropsychiatric Disorders*, ed. KA Miczek, pp. 219–53. New York: Liss.

Ribble MA (1944). Infantile experience in relation to personality development. In *Personality and Behavior Disorders*, ed. JM Hunt, pp. 621–51. New York: Ronald Press.

Robertson MM and Trimble MR (1981). Neuroleptics as antidepressants. *Neuropsychopharmacology*, 21, 1335–6.

Rosenblum L and Kaufman IC (1968). Variations in infant development and response to mother loss in monkeys. *Am J Orthopsychiatr*, 38, 418–26.

Rots N, De Jong J, Workel JO, Levine S, Cools AR and de Kloet ER (1996). Neonatal maternally deprived rats have as adults elevated basal pituitary adrenal activity and enhanced susceptibility to apomorphine. *J Neuroendocrinol*, 8, 501–6.

Sackeim HA (2001). Functional brain circuits in major depression and remission. *Arch Gen Psychiatry*, 58, 649–50.

Sapolsky RM and Meaney MJ (1986). Maturation of the adrenal stress response: neuroendocrine control mechanisms and the stress-hyporesponsive period. *Brain Res Rev*, 11, 65–76.

Seay BM and Harlow H (1965). Maternal separation in the rhesus monkey. *J Nerv Ment Dis*, 140, 434–41.

Seay BM, Hansen EW and Harlow H (1962). Mother–infant separation in monkeys. *J Child Psychol Psychiatry*, 3, 123–32.

Seitz PFD (1959). Infantile experience and adult behaviour in animal subjects: age of separation from the mother and adult behavior in the cat. *Psychosom Med*, 21, 353–78.

Shah PJ, Ogilvie AD, Goodwin GM and Ebmeier KP (1997). Clinical and psychometric correlates of dopamine D2 binding in depression. *Psychol Med*, 27, 1247–56.

Sheline YL, Wang PW, Gado MH, Csernansky JG and Vannier MW (1996). Hippocampal atrophy in recurrent major depression. *Proc Natl Acad Sci USA*, 93, 3908–13.

Smith AL and Weissman MM (1992). Epidemiology. In *Handbook of Affective Disorders*, 2nd edn, ed. ES Paykel, pp. 111–31. London: Churchill Livingstone.

Spitz RA (1945). Hospitalism. *Psychoanal Study Child*, 1, 53–74.

Spitz RA and Wolf KA (1946). Anaclitic depression: an inquiry into the genesis of psychiatric conditions in early childhood. *Psychoanal Study Child*, 2, 313–42.

Styron W (1992). *Darkness Visible*. London: Picador.

Suchecki D, Rosenfeld P and Levine S (1993). Maternal regulation of hypothalamic-pituitary-adrenal axis in the infant rat: the role of feeding and stroking. *Dev Brain Res*, 75, 185–92.

Suomi SJ, Harlow H and Domek CJ (1970). Effect of repetitive mother–infant separation of young monkeys. *J Abnorm Psychol*, 76, 161–72.

Suomi SJ, Mineka S and DeLizio RD (1973). Short and long-term effects of repetitive mother–infant separations on social development in rhesus monkeys. *Dev Psychol*, 19, 770–86.

Suomi SJ, Seaman SF, Lewis JK, DeLizio RD and McKinney WT (1978). Effects of imipramine treatment of separation-induced social disorders in rhesus monkeys. *Arch Gen Psych*, 35, 321–5.

Tanda G, Frau R and Di Chiara G (1997). Chronic desipramine and fluoxetine differentially affect extracellular dopamine in the rat prefrontal cortex. *Psychopharmacology*, 127, 83–7.

Wehr TA, Muscettola G and Goodwin FK (1980). 3-methoxy-4-hydroxyphenolglycol circadian rhythm: early timing (phase advance) in manic depressives compared with normal subjects. *Arch Gen Psychiatry*, 37, 257–63.

Willner P (1984). The validity of animal models of depression. *Psychopharmacology*, 83, 1–16.

Willner P (1995). Dopaminergic machanisms in depression and mania. In *Psychopharmacology: the Fourth Generation of Progress*, ed. FE Bloom and DJ Kupfer, pp. 921–32. New York: Raven Press.

Willner P, Towell A, Sampson D, Sophokleous S and Muscat R (1987). Reduction of sucrose preference by chronic unpredictable mild stress, and its restoration by a tricyclic antidepressant. *Psychopharmacology*, 93, 358–64.

De Wit H, Ulenhath EH and Johanson CE (1987). The reinforcing properties of amphetamine in overweight subjects and subjects with depression. *Clin Pharm Therap*, 42, 127–36.

Wolpert L (1999). *Malignant Sadness: The Anatomy of Depression*. London: Faber and Faber.

World Health Organization (1992). *The ICD-10 Classification of Mental and Behavioural Disorders: Clinical Descriptions and Diagnostic Guidelines*. Geneva: WHO.

Yassa R, Camille Y and Belzile L (1987). Tardive dyskinesia in the course of antidepressant therapy: a prevalence study and review of the literature. *J Clin Psychopharmacol*, 7, 243–6.

Part VIII

Aggression

relationship between aggression and impulsivity and (c) suggest several directions for future research.

Methodological issues and aggression research with humans

Critical to understanding the biology of aggressive behaviour is accurate measurement of this behaviour. Approaches to the study of aggressive responding include epidemiological studies, field studies and field experiments, psychometric approaches and laboratory-based investigations (Gaebelein 1981; Gothelf et al. 1997; Lane and Cherek 2000). Examples of field studies of aggression include observations of children in playgrounds or classroom (Hinshaw et al. 1989; Pepler and Craig 1995), and observations of patients in psychiatric clinics (Crowner et al. 1994). These observations may be recorded using systems developed by individual researchers, or standardized scales, such as the Overt Aggression Scale (Yudofsky et al. 1986, and see Gothelf et al. 1997). Aggressive behaviour often has a low probability of occurrence in the field, however, making it difficult to accurately assess its frequency or severity (Buss 1961; Hinshaw et al. 1989). In field experiments variables may be directly manipulated to increase the probability of aggressive responding, such as blocking the passage of drivers through intersections (Turner et al. 1975).

One disadvantage of field research for studying aggressive behaviour, particularly field studies, is the problem of measurement. In the field, there are many response topographies that may be categorized as aggressive. For example, researchers have argued that aggressive behaviour may either be overt or covert (Quay 1966; Loeber and Schmaling 1985), or reactive or proactive (Dodge and Coie 1987). Without determining whether the outcome of the response is aversive for the recipient, and without determining the variables that control responding in the actor, it is difficult to specify whether a response is aggressive. In addition, in the field many of the variables that can contribute to aggressive responding are uncontrolled.

Due to the infrequent occurrence of aggressive behaviour in the field and the problems of measurement, researchers have developed a variety of questionnaires and rating scales that collect verbal reports of subjects and observers to assess subjects' past aggressive behaviour and current aggressive tendencies (see Campbell et al. 1999; Lane and Cherek 2000). Some of these instruments include the Buss–Perry Aggression Questionnaire (Buss and Perry 1992), the Buss–Durkee Hostility Inventory (Buss and Durkee 1957), Conners Teacher Questionnaire (Conners 1969) and the Child Behavior Checklist (Achenbach 1999). In addition to circumventing some of the problems of field research, these instruments are relatively easy and quick to administer.

Despite these benefits, psychometric approaches have several disadvantages. First, because the frequency and severity of aggressive responding are assessed indirectly (i.e. by verbal reports) rather than directly, the validity of their results is often questioned (Buss 1961). Second, because psychometric instruments do not provide continuous or direct measures of responding, they are not well suited for some types of experimental manipulations (e.g. drug administrations or manipulating consequences of responding). Laboratory-based approaches, however, permit (a) precise control and manipulation of independent variables, (b) measurement of the dynamics of these behaviours (e.g. ongoing assessment of behavioural patterns and changes) and (c) the opportunity for repeated measures (within-subject designs) which allows reliable, dose–response determinations of drug effects.

Several different laboratory procedures have been developed to study aggressive behaviour. Typically, in aggression procedures subjects are told that they are paired with a partner during the experimental session and that they will have the opportunity to deliver an aversive stimulus to this person. One of the first laboratory procedures to study aggression was developed by Buss (1961). In this procedure, sometimes called the 'teacher–learner' paradigm or 'aggression machine', the subject is instructed that he or she will play the role of a teacher in a learning experiment. The subject's task is to shock the learner (an accomplice who does not actually receive any shocks) whenever an incorrect response occurs. The primary measure of aggressive responding is the shock intensity selected by the subject.

Another laboratory task using shock delivery as a measure of aggressive responding was developed by Taylor (1967). In this procedure, called the Taylor Competitive Reaction Time Task, subjects are told that they will be competing against another individual and that the person who responds first during a trial can deliver shock to their opponent. In actuality, the subject works alone and 'wins' on half of the trials. Unlike the Buss (1961) procedure, the subject is provoked during the experiment by increasing the shock intensity that the subject experiences across trials. These provocations are designed to mimic circumstances that motivate aggressive responding outside the laboratory.

These two laboratory procedures, although yielding reliable measures of aggressive responding, have been criticized on several grounds. For example, Tedeschi and Quigley (1996) have argued that in the teacher–learner paradigm shock deliveries are unlike aggressive responses that occur outside the laboratory because the subject is told that shock deliveries help the learner. Second, with few exceptions (see Zeichner et al. (1999) for a recent modification of the Competitive Reaction Time Task) these procedures do not provide nonaggressive response alternatives against which the strength of aggressive responding can be compared.

A third procedure developed to study aggressive responding is the Point Subtraction Aggression Paradigm (PSAP; Cherek 1981). In this task, money is periodically subtracted from the subject's earnings throughout the session and these subtractions are attributed to the responses of a fictitious partner. The subject is presented with three response options. Responses on the aggressive response option ostensibly subtract money from the partner's earnings and also produce a temporary cessation of monetary subtractions directed at the subject. (Because these responses present an aversive stimulus to the other person they are operationally defined as aggressive.) Responses on a monetary-reinforced option produce money. Responses on a third, escape option also produce a temporary cessation of monetary subtractions. The PSAP procedure not only provides multiple response options, but because the subtraction of money rather than shock delivery is used as an aversive stimulus, it can be used to study aggressive responding in a variety of populations, including children, repeatedly over many sessions.

Within the PSAP procedure, the comparison of drug effects on aggressive, monetary-reinforced and escape responding allows an evaluation of the specificity of drug action (Cherek and Steinberg 1987). Nonspecific sedative or stimulant effects would be indicated by proportional decreases or increases in monetary-reinforced responses as well as similar directional changes in either aggressive or escape responses. Previous studies employing the PSAP procedure have shown that the rate of monetary-reinforced responding changes in the expected directions when central nervous system (CNS) stimulants and depressants are administered. For example, monetary-reinforced responding increased following nicotine/tobacco, d-amphetamine and caffeine administrations, and decreased following alcohol, diazepam and secobarbital administrations (Cherek 1981; Cherek et al. 1983, 1985, 1986, 1989, 1990b). These same categories of substances also tended to produce reductions and increases in aggressive responding. Because the effects on monetary-reinforced responding and aggressive responding differed, the changes in aggressive responding cannot be attributed to a nonspecific sedative or stimulant drug action.

The PSAP procedure has been used in numerous studies to show differences between violent and nonviolent individuals (Cherek et al. 1996, 1997b, 2000), and to show changes in aggressive responding following administration of a variety of drug classes (Cherek et al. 1985; Casat et al. 1995; Cherek and Dougherty 1995; Dougherty et al. 1996). Studies using this procedure have also shown that the provocations are important determinants of aggressive responding. Cherek et al. (1990a) showed that when aggressive responding had no effect on the frequency of provocations, aggressive responding was maintained at low levels and eventually ceased. Furthermore, Cherek et al. (1991) showed that rates of aggressive responding varied directly with the provocation frequency.

External validity of laboratory studies

Several researchers have questioned the external (or ecological) validity of results from laboratory studies, stating that aggressive behaviour observed in the laboratory may not be related to the frequency or intensity of aggressive behaviour that occurs under more naturalistic contexts (Tedeschi and Quigley 1996). In response to these types of criticisms, Berkowitz and Donnerstein (1982) argued that laboratory procedures, regardless of their formal similarity to 'real-world' situations, provide important information about variables that influence aggressive responding. They noted that the experimental realism (i.e. internal validity) of aggression experiments should be emphasized over how closely the procedures mimic naturally occurring situations.

Other researchers have explicitly investigated the external validity of laboratory studies by examining the relationship between the frequency of aggressive responding during laboratory tasks and measures of aggression from alternative sources. These studies have shown that laboratory measures of aggressive responding are often positively correlated with measures of aggression obtained from rating scales and questionnaires (Coccaro et al. 1996; Cherek et al. 1997*a*; Dougherty et al. 1999; Zeichner et al. 1999). Studies have also shown that the frequency of aggressive responding in laboratory tasks is correlated with the frequency of subjects' past history of aggressive responding. For example, Wolfe and Baron (1971) showed that in a laboratory task, prison inmates responded aggressively at higher rates than college students. Cherek et al. (1996, 1997*a*) compared rates of aggressive responding across more similar subject populations, male parolees with and without histories of violent behaviour, and showed that rates of aggressive responding were higher in parolees with violent histories. Similar results were shown in a study with female parolees (Cherek et al. 2000).

In summary, laboratory procedures can produce reliable, quantitative measures of aggressive responding, they can be used to investigate a variety of factors that affect behaviour and, as these latter studies show, rates of aggressive responding obtained under laboratory conditions are frequently consistent with measures of aggression obtained from alternative sources.

Serotonin and aggression

Of the many biological correlates of aggressive behaviour that have been investigated, perhaps the most consistent finding is the inverse relationship between aggressive responding and the neurotransmitter serotonin (5-hydroxytryptamine or 5HT) (Linnoila et al. 1983; Depue and Spoont 1986; Kruesi et al. 1990; Olivier et al. 1990; Coccaro and Kavoussi 1996; Tuinier et al. 1996; Berman et al. 1997; Lane and Cherek 2000). Studies have documented that diminished cerebrospinal fluid (CSF) serotonin levels are related to: suicides and violent suicide attempts (Asberg et al. 1987; Modai et al. 1989); a history of criminal violence (Linnoila et al. 1983; Virkkunen et al. 1989); alcohol dependence and corresponding violent behaviour (Virkkunen et al. 1994; Fils-Aime et al. 1996) and diagnosed psychopathologies highlighted by impulse control problems (Brown and Goodwin 1984; Virkkunen et al. 1987; Stein et al. 1993). Alterations of CNS serotonin levels through dietary amino acid intake (i.e. tryptophan depletion or supplementation) found changes in predicted directions in self-reported mood/hostility (Young et al. 1985, 1988; Cleare and Bond 1995).

Further evidence linking serotonin and aggression comes from studies showing that a variety of pharmacological agents that interact with serotonergic systems affect aggressive responding. For example, the drug D,L-fenfluramine, whose principal action is to release and block reuptake of serotonin and dopamine (Feldman et al. 1997) has been reported to suppress footshock-induced aggression in mice and rats (Panksepp 1973; Rolinski and Herbut 1981), as well as aggression in rats induced by apomorphine (McKenzie 1981). D,L-fenfluramine has also been used by clinicians to manage disruptive behaviour in children and adults (Aman et al. 1993a, b; Leventhal et al. 1993; Saletu et al. 1993).

Laboratory research with humans has also played an important role in the investigation of the serotonin–aggression relationship. Several studies have manipulated CNS serotonin levels through dietary amino-acid intake and have shown that decreasing tryptophan levels increased rates of aggressive responding (Moeller et al. 1996; Bjork et al. 1999) and that increasing tryptophan levels decreased rates of aggressive responding (Pihl et al. 1995). A study in our laboratory employing the PSAP procedure showed that the acute administration of D,L-fenfluramine produced significant decreases in aggressive responding among a group of male subjects with childhood conduct disorder (Cherek and Lane 1999b). Serotonin functioning has also been assessed in laboratory studies with a procedure known as a neuro-endocrine challenge. This procedure consists of administering a challenge agent (buspirone, D- and D,L-fenfluramine) that, through its interaction with serotonergic systems, releases hormones such as prolactin (Berman et al. 1997). Prolactin concentrations thus serve as a putative estimate of the reactivity of the serotonergic system. A study by Cherek et al. (1999) with male conduct-disorder subjects showed that blunted serotonergic activity following serotonin challenge was related to baseline levels of aggressive behaviour. Together, these studies suggest that manipulating serotonin levels can influence aggressive responding in laboratory tasks, that individuals who show high rates of aggressive responding may exhibit reduced serotonin functioning and that pharmacological agents that increase serotonin levels in these individuals may decrease the frequency of aggressive responding.

The aggression–impulsivity relationship

A considerable amount of research has shown that aggression is often associated with various types of impulsive behaviour. Like aggressive responding, impulsivity has been studied in the laboratory with several different procedures. One commonly used procedure, a delay-of-gratification task, is designed to measure the ability of subjects to tolerate delays between a response and reward delivery. In this task, subjects are presented with choices between a small reward available after a short delay and a larger reward available after a longer delay (Rachlin and Green 1972; Ainslie 1975; Logue et al. 1986; Logue 1988; Mischel et al. 1989; Rachlin 1995). This methodology has demonstrated sensitivity in detecting impulsiveness in human populations with impulse control difficulties (Logue 1988; Mischel et al. 1989; Sonuga-Barke et al. 1989; Cherek et al. 1997*b*; Allen et al. 1998; Cherek and Lane 1999*a*).

Studies using this procedure have shown a positive relationship between aggressive responding and impulsivity. For example, studies using a delay-of-gratification task known as an adjusting-delay procedure (Mazur 1987) have shown that violent male parolees selected the impulsive option on 59.7% of trials and that violent female parolees chose this option on 65.7% of trials (Cherek et al. 1997*b*; Cherek and Lane 1999*a*). These impulsive choices are much higher than those observed in studies conducted with college students (using slightly different nonadjusting procedures) that have reported an almost exclusive preference for the self-control option (the impulsive option was typically selected on < 5% of trials) (Logue et al. 1986; King and Logue 1990). In a sequence of studies using the adjusting-delay and the PSAP procedure, Cherek et al. (1997*a*, *b*) showed positive correlations between aggressive and impulsive responding.

As with aggressive behaviour, reduced serotonin functioning has been implicated in the aetiology of impulsivity (Depue and Spoont 1986; Soubrié 1986). In nonhumans, naturalistic studies have linked reduced serotonin levels to aggressive and impulsive behaviour (Raleigh et al. 1984; McGuire and Raleigh 1987; Popova et al. 1991; Higley et al. 1992, 1994, 1996*c*; Mehlman et al. 1994). For example, primates with low CSF levels of the serotonin metabolite 5-hydroxyindoleacetic acid (5-HIAA) were much more likely to engage in impulsive, risk-taking behaviour involving leaps of considerable distance at great heights between trees in their compound (Mehlman et al. 1994). Laboratory studies with nonhuman subjects using a delay-of-reward procedure have shown decreases in impulsive behaviour following administration of serotonin reuptake inhibitors (Bizot et al. 1988), serotonin agonists (Soubrié 1986; Poulos et al. 1996) and serotonin-releasing agents (Poulos et al. 1996). Response inhibition procedures with nonhuman subjects (designed to measure the ability of subjects to withhold responding) have also noted decreased impulsive responding following administration of serotonin agonists or reuptake inhibitors (Fletcher 1993; Richards et al. 1993). Conversely, lesioning of serotonin pathways produced impairments in the ability to withhold responding (Soubrié and Bizot 1990; Fletcher 1995; Al-Zahrani et al. 1996; Ho et al. 1998) and deficiencies in waiting for larger, delayed reinforcers (Wogar et al. 1993; Ho et al. 1998).

In humans, neuroendocrine challenge assessments have revealed blunted serotonin response in children with conduct disorder (Stoff et al. 1992); personality-disordered individuals with high levels of violence, aggression and impulsivity (Coccaro et al. 1989; Moss et al. 1990; O'Keane et al. 1992; Cherek et al. 1999); individuals with substance-abuse disorders and high levels of impulsivity (Fishbein et al. 1989); and normal, healthy adults who showed the highest self-reported levels of aggression and impulsiveness (Manuck et al. 1998). In a recent study, Cherek and Lane (2000) found that acute doses of D,L-fenfluramine (releaser of serotonin) decreased impulsive responses in subjects with a history of childhood conduct disorder while the performance of matched controls was unaffected.

Aggression, impulsivity and low serotonergic functioning are also related to substance abuse, including alcohol abuse and dependence (Brady et al. 1998). For example, research suggests that aggressive behaviour, particularly among children, is an excellent predictor of subsequent impulsive and risky behaviour such as drug use, abuse and eventually dependence (Kellam et al. 1998). In a laboratory study employing the PSAP procedure, Allen et al. (1997) showed that individuals with a history of substance abuse showed higher rates of aggressive responding than matched controls. In a subsequent study these subjects also were more impulsive under laboratory conditions (Allen et al. 1998). Moreover, similar to individuals who show high rates of aggressive and impulsive responding, individuals who abuse alcohol also showed reduced serotonergic functioning compared with nonabusers (LeMarquand et al. 1994).

Collectively, the scientific database with both nonhumans and humans strongly suggests that reduced transmission of CNS serotonin plays a role in excessive forms of impulsive and aggressive behaviour. The importance of reduced serotonergic activity in both aggression and impulsivity suggests that serotonin may serve a common inhibitory function which is not specific to any particular type of behaviour such as aggression (Robbins 1997).

Aggression as a form of impulsivity

The term 'impulsive' has been used to modify and thereby identify a particular type of human aggression. That is, several investigators, most notably Ernest Barratt, have suggested that at least two types of human aggression need to be differentiated, i.e. premeditated and impulsive (Barratt and Slaughter 1998; Barratt et al. 1999, 2000). Premeditated aggression, as its name implies, involves planning prior to action. The behaviour typically produces some gain for the aggressor, e.g. financial, and this consequence maintains responding. In contrast, impulsive aggression is a swift reaction to varying levels of provocation and the consequences of this aggressive behaviour are not generally considered by the perpetrator. These distinct types of aggression, although described in different terms (e.g. reactive, affective, etc.), have been identified in normal children and adolescent inpatients in a state hospital (Dodge and Coie 1987; Vitiello et al. 1990).

Impulsive aggression has delayed, negative consequences for the subject and other persons associated with them. Because these delayed outcomes seem to have little influence on behaviour, it is likely that individuals who engage in impulsive aggressive behaviour also exhibit other types of behaviour which could be viewed as impulsive, such as gambling, bouts of drug abuse, and/or risky sexual behaviour (Block et al. 1988; Tremblay et al. 1994; Logue 1995). Because the tendency to engage in impulsive aggression may be indicative of a general lack of sensitivity to delayed, or even relatively immediate, consequences, it may be useful to view it as a form of impulsivity – perhaps an extreme form because of its potentially severe consequences. Thus, the term *aggressive impulsivity*, rather than impulsive aggression, may more accurately depict the relationship between aggressive and impulsive behaviour.

Variables influencing serotonin functioning, aggression and impulsivity

A variety of factors may contribute to individual differences in serotonin functioning. Serotonin functioning may be controlled in part by genetic mechanisms. Studies with nonhumans have shown that parent and offspring 5-HIAA concentrations are positively correlated (Higley et al. 1993), that strains of rats selectively bred for high or low rates of aggressive behaviour show low and high levels of serotonin, respectively (Naumenko et al. 1989), and that domesticated silver foxes have lower levels of serotonin than their wild predecessors (Popova et al. 1991). Twin studies have also suggested that serotonergic functioning, such as platelet serotonin uptake, has a heritable component (Meltzer and Arora 1988).

Diet may also influence serotonin functioning. Malnutrition (reduced dietary protein) in animals can produce reduced reactivity to drugs which interact with all major CNS transmitter systems, including serotonin, demonstrating that diet can alter CNS function (Almeida et al. 1996). In rats, diets low in the serotonin precursor, tryptophan, have been shown to reduce brain serotonin concentrations (Biggio et al. 1974) and a study by Carpenter et al. (1998) showed that consumption of an amino-acid beverage without tryptophan reduced both plasma tryptophan and CSF 5-HIAA levels in normal adult humans. Low-fat diets have also been associated with reduced serotonin responsiveness in monkeys as assessed by fenfluramine challenge (Muldoon et al. 1992). Women consuming low-calorie diets have shown reduced plasma tryptophan levels (Walsh et al. 1995; Wolfe et al. 1997), which suggests that dieting can affect CNS serotonin concentrations.

Social environments have also been shown to influence serotonin functioning in nonhumans. In a series of manipulations with vervet monkeys, Raleigh et al. (1984) showed that social status in males was positively correlated with serotonin concentrations, that changes in social status affected serotonin levels, and that high serotonin concentrations were maintained in dominant males by social interactions. Research also suggests that chronic exposure to social stressors is correlated with decreased serotonergic functioning. Fontenot et al. (1995) reported that cynomolgus macaques who were exposed to frequent changes in the membership of their social group showed decreased concentrations of serotonin and 5-HIAA in their prefrontal cortex compared with subjects living in stable social environments. Similarly, Higley et al. (1996*b*) showed that rhesus macaques, separated from their mothers and reared with peers, had lower CSF 5-HIAA concentrations than subjects reared by their mothers. Notably, these peer-reared individuals also consumed more alcohol and exhibited more aggressive behaviour than mother-reared individuals (Higley et al. 1996*a*). In addition, bonnet macaques reared with mothers exposed to a variable food source exhibited reduced behavioural responsiveness to a serotonin agonist compared with individuals reared with mothers exposed to a constant food source (Rosenblum et al. 1994). It should also be noted that other neurotransmitter systems may be affected by rearing conditions. For example, Kraemer et al. (1989) reported that peer-reared rhesus monkeys showed reduced norepineprine levels compared with mother-reared individuals.

Social and environmental factors may also influence serotonin functioning in humans. Matthews et al. (2000) have argued that individuals with low socio-economic status (SES) may experience more stressful social environments than individuals with high SES, and that this social stress may contribute to decreased serotonergic activity. In support of this hypothesis, studies have shown that low-SES children ages 6–10 years had higher salivary cortisol levels than middle- and high-SES children, indicative of higher levels of environmental stress (Lupien et al. 2000). Studies have also shown that SES is inversely correlated with numbers of aversive life events (McLeod and Kessler 1990), rates of aggressive responding (Kellam et al. 1998) and measures of impulsivity (Matthews et al. 2000). Moreover, Matthews et al. (2000) reported that individuals with low SES show decreased serotonin responsiveness as assessed by neuroendocrine challenge.

Chaotic environments in which noxious stimuli occur unpredictably may be especially conducive to generating stress and contributing to the development of aggressive and impulsive behaviour. Research with humans has shown that subjects exposed to loud noise under uncontrollable-noise conditions evidenced neuro-endocrine, autonomic and mood changes consistent with stress, whereas subjects exposed to noise under subject-controlled conditions produced no changes in these measures (Breier et al. 1987). In humans, the aversiveness of unpredictable noxious stimuli is supported by studies showing that conditions in which unavoidable shock presentations are signalled are preferred to situations in which the shock presentations are unsignalled (Badia et al. 1979; but see Arthur 1986). Exposing pregnant rhesus monkeys to environmental stress generated by unpredictable loud noise also produced neurotransmitter changes in the offspring up to 6 months following birth that were consistent with changes produced by direct exposure to stress (Schneider et al. 1998). Thus, exposure to conditions in which aversive or noxious events occur unpredictably may produce biological changes that are related to aggressive and impulsive behaviour.

Research linking stressful environmental conditions to both serotonergic functioning and aggressive/impulsive behaviour is consistent with arguments made by researchers that certain environments may foster the development of psychopathology in humans (Sroufe 1997). Furthermore, research concerning the role of environmental stressors in early childhood development has led scientists to focus attention on the early stages in the development of antisocial behaviour (Dawson et al. 2000).

Aggressive and impulsive behaviours are not necessarily maladaptive or pathological. For example, impulsive behaviour may be adaptive in unpredictable or chaotic environments if interruptions interfere with the acquisition of delayed outcomes (Kagel et al. 1986). Applied behavioural studies have also shown that aggressive behaviour is often maintained because it produces escape from aversive situations, social attention, food or other important outcomes (Carr and Durand 1985; Hile and Desrochers 1993; Vollmer et al. 1999). Should such aggressive and impulsive behaviours be considered pathological, or predictable outcomes of developmental processes and stressful or chaotic environmental conditions?

In summary, individual differences in serotonergic functioning, aggression and impulsivity are likely determined by genetic factors and multiple social and environmental variables. However, much additional research is needed to clarify these relationships. For example, how environmental factors (i.e. rearing conditions, exposure to unpredictable noxious stimuli, etc.) affect aggressive and impulsive behaviour, and the mechanisms by which these conditions affect serotonin functioning, require further investigation.

Future research

The serotonergic system is only one of many biological systems correlated with aggressive behaviour. Two promising areas of future research include: (a) the relationship between the neurotransmitter γ-aminobutyric acid (GABA) and aggressive behaviour and (b) the use of brain-imaging technology to determine the brain areas in humans that are involved in aggression.

GABA

For some time, aggression researchers have speculated that GABA, in addition to serotonin, plays an inhibitory role in the regulation of aggressive behaviour (Singhal and Telner 1983; Valzelli 1984; Siegel et al. 1999). Research with nonhumans has

episodes had reduced metabolism in the medial temporal and prefrontal cortex compared with control subjects. In another PET study, murderers pleading not guilty by reason of insanity were found to have reduced glucose metabolism in the prefrontal cortex, superior parietal gyrus, left angular gyrus and the corpus callosum compared with matched controls (Raine et al. 1997). Magnetic resonance imaging (MRI) revealed a reduced prefrontal grey matter volume in participants with antisocial personality disorder compared with healthy control subjects and substance-dependent subjects (Raine et al. 2000).

Several brain-imaging studies have also investigated brain activity while subjects imagined that they were involved in aggressive encounters. For example, in a PET study, Pietrini et al. (2000) asked subjects to imagine themselves in nonaggressive and aggressive scenarios and found correlated changes in subjects' prefrontal cortex. Future studies could utilize laboratory methodologies to conduct such studies. Using aggression procedures such as the PSAP during brain imaging would allow researchers to better investigate brain activity during provocations and aggressive responding. Joel L. Steinberg (unpublished), in our research group, has pilot data from a study using fMRI and the PSAP procedure demonstrating increased amygdala and frontal cortex activity in a subject with very frequent aggressive responding compared with a subject with low rates of aggressive responding. Undoubtedly, the combination of sensitive behavioural techniques with brain-imaging technology will advance our understanding of the brain areas involved in human aggression.

Acknowledgements

The authors' research was supported by Grants from the National Institute on Drug Abuse (NIH/NIDA) DA03166-15 and DA 10552-04. The authors wish to acknowledge the technical assistance of Jennifer Sharon and Sheila White. The first author would also like to acknowledge the collaboration of the following investigators over the course of the past several years of PSAP research: Scott D. Lane, Ph.D., Joel L. Steinberg, MD, Gerard Moeller, MD, Donald M. Dougherty, Ph.D., Ralph Spiga, Ph.D. and Thomas H. Kelly, Ph.D.

REFERENCES

Achenbach TM (1999). The Child Behavior Checklist and related instruments. In *The Use of Psychological Testing for Treatment Planning and Outcomes Assessment*, ed. ME Maruish, pp. 429–66. Mahway, NJ: Lawrence Erlbaum Associates.

Ainslie G (1975). Specious reward: a behavioral theory of impulsiveness and impulse control. *Psychol Bull*, 82, 463–96.

Allen TJ, Moeller FG, Rhoades HM and Cherek DR (1997). Subjects with a history of drug dependence are more aggressive than subjects with no drug use history. *Drug Alcohol Depend*, 46, 95–103.

Allen TJ, Moeller FG, Rhoades HM and Cherek DR (1998). Impulsivity and history of drug dependence. *Drug Alcohol Depend*, 50, 137–45.

Almeida SS, Tonkiss J and Galler JR (1996). Malnutrition and reactivity to drugs acting in the central nervous system. *Neurosci Biobehav Rev*, 20, 389–402.

Al-Zahrani SS, Ho MY, Velazquez Martinez DN, Lopez Cabrera M, Bradshaw CM and Szabadi E (1996). Effect of destruction of the 5-hydroxytryptaminergic pathways on the acquisition of temporal discrimination and memory for duration in a delayed conditional discrimination task. *Psychopharmacology (Berlin)*, 123, 103–10.

Aman MG, Kern RA, McGhee DE and Arnold LE (1993a). Fenfluramine and methylphenidate in children with mental retardation and ADHD: clinical and side effects. *J Am Acad Child Adolesc Psychiatry*, 32, 851–9.

Aman MG, Kern RA, McGhee DE and Arnold LE (1993b). Fenfluramine and methylphenidate in children with mental retardation and attention deficit hyperactivity disorder: laboratory effects. *J Autism Dev Disord*, 23, 491–506.

Arthur AZ (1986). Stress of predictable and unpredictable shock. *Psychol Bull*, 100, 379–83.

Asberg M, Schalling D, Traksman-Bendz L and Wagner A (1987). Psychobiology of suicide, impulsivity, and related phenomenon. In *Psychopharmacology: Third Generation of Progress*, ed. HY Meltzer, pp. 655–88. New York: Raven Press.

Badia P, Harsh J and Abbott B (1979). Choosing between predictable and unpredictable shock conditions: data and theory. *Psychol Bull*, 86, 1107–31.

Barratt ES and Slaughter L (1998). Defining, measuring and predicting impulsive aggression: a heuristic model. *Behav Sci Law*, 16, 285–302.

Barratt ES, Stanford MS, Felthous AR and Kent TA (1997). The effects of phenytoin in impulsive and premeditated aggression: a controlled study. *J Clin Psychopharmacol*, 17, 341–9.

Barratt ES, Stanford MS, Dowdy L, Liebman MJ and Kent TA (1999). Impulsive and premeditated aggression: a factor analysis of self-reported acts. *Psychiatry Res*, 86, 163–73.

Barratt ES, Kent T, Liebman MJ and Coates DD (2000). Criterion measures of aggression – impulsive versus premeditated aggression. In *The Science, Treatment and Prevention of Antisocial Behaviors: Application to the Criminal Justice System*, ed. DH Fishbein, pp. 4-1–4-18. Kingston, NJ: Civic Research Institute.

Berkowitz L and Donnerstein E (1982). External validity is more than skin deep. Some answers to criticisms of laboratory experiments. *Am Psychol*, 37, 245–57.

Berman ME, Kavoussi RJ and Coccaro EF (1997). Neurotransmitter correlates of human aggression. In *Handbook of Antisocial Behavior*, ed. DM Stoff, J Breiling and JD Maser, pp. 305–13. New York: John Wiley & Sons.

Biggio G, Fadda F, Fanni P, Tagliamonte A and Gessa GL (1974). Rapid depletion of serum tryptophan, brain tryptophan, serotonin, and 5-hydroxyindoleacetic acid by a tryptophan-free diet. *Life Sci*, 14, 1321–9.

Bizot JC, Thiebot MH, Le Bihan C, Soubrié P and Simon P (1988). Effects of imipramine-like drugs and serotonin uptake blockers on delay of reward in rats: possible implications in the behavioral mechanism of action of antidepressants. *J Pharmacol Exp Therapeut*, 246, 1144–51.

Bjork JM, Dougherty DM, Moeller FG, Cherek DR and Swann AC (1999). The effects of tryptophan depletion and loading on laboratory aggression in men: time course and a food restricted control. *Psychopharmacology*, 142, 24–30.

Block J, Block JH and Keyes S (1988). Longitudinally foretelling drug usage in adolescence: early childhood personality and environmental precursors. *Child Dev* 59, 336–55.

Brady KT, Myrick H and McElroy S (1998). The relationship between substance use and disorders, impulse control disorders, and pathological aggression. *Am J Addictions*, 7, 221–30.

Breier A, Albus M, Pickar D, Zahn TP, Wolkowitz OM and Paul SM (1987). Controllable and uncontrollable stress in humans: alteration in mood and neuroendocrine and psychophysiological function. *Am J Psychiatry*, 144, 1419–25.

Brizer DA (1988). Psychopharmacology and the management of violent patients. *Psychiatr Clin N Am*, 11, 551–68.

Brown GL and Goodwin FK (1984). Diagnostic, clinical and personality characteristics of aggressive men with low CSF 5-HIAA. *Clin Neuropharmacol*, 7, S408–9.

Buss AH (1961). *The Psychology of Aggression*. New York: John Wiley and Sons.

Buss AH and Durkee A (1957). An inventory for assessing different kinds of hostility. *J Consult Psychol*, 21, 343–9.

Buss AH and Perry M (1992). Personality processes and individual differences: the aggression questionnaire. *J Pers Social Psychol*, 63, 452–9.

Campbell M, Cueva JE and Adams PB (1999). Pharmacotherapy of impulsive-aggressive behavior. In *Personality and Psychopathology*, ed. CR Cloninger, pp. 431–55. Washington, DC: American Psychiatric Press.

Carpenter LL, Anderson GM, Pelton GH et al. (1998). Tryptophan depletion during continuous CSF sampling in healthy human subjects. *Neuropsychopharmacology*, 19, 26–35.

Carr EG and Durand MV (1985). Reducing behavior problems through functional communication training. *J Appl Behav Anal*, 18, 111–26.

Casat CD, Pearson DA, Van Davelaar MJ and Cherek DR (1995). Methylphenidate effects on laboratory aggression measure in children with ADHD. *Psychopharmacol Bull*, 31, 353–6.

Cherek DR (1981). Effects of smoking different doses of nicotine on human aggressive behavior. *Psychopharmacology*, 75, 339–45.

Cherek DR and Dougherty DM (1995). Provocation frequency and its role in determining the effects of smoked marijuana on human aggressive responding. *Behav Pharmacol*, 6, 405–12.

Cherek DR and Lane SD (1999a). Laboratory and psychometric measurements of impulsivity among violent and nonviolent female parolees. *Biol Psychiatry*, 46, 273–80.

Cherek DR and Lane SD (1999b). Effects of d,l-fenfluramine on aggressive and impulsive responding in adult males with a history of conduct disorder. *Psychopharmacology*, 146, 473–81.

Cherek DR and Lane SD (2000). Fenfluramine effects on impulsivity in a sample of adults with and without a history of conduct disorder. *Psychopharmacology*, 152, 149–56.

Cherek DR and Steinberg JL (1987). Psychopharmacology of human aggression: laboratory studies. In *Ethopharmacology of Agnostic Behaviour in Animals and Humans*, ed. B Olivier, J Mos and PF Brain, pp. 245–55. Dordrecht: Martinus Nijhoff Publishers.

Cherek DR, Steinberg JL and Brauchi JT (1983). Effects of caffeine on human aggressive behavior. *Psychiatry Res*, 8, 137–45.

Cherek DR, Steinberg JL and Manno BR (1985). Effects of alcohol on human aggressive behavior. *J Studies Alcohol*, 46, 321–8.

Cherek DR, Steinberg JL, Kelly TH and Robinson D (1987). Effects of d-amphetamine on aggressive responding of normal male subjects. *Psychiatry Res*, 21, 257–65.

Cherek DR, Steinberg JL, Kelly TH and Sebastian CS (1989). Effects of d-amphetamine on human aggressive responding maintained by avoidance of provocation. *Pharmacol Biochem Behav*, 34, 65–71.

Cherek DR, Spiga R, Steinberg JL and Kelly TH (1990*a*). Human aggressive responses maintained by avoidance or escape from point loss. *J Exp Anal Behav*, 53, 293–303.

Cherek DR, Steinberg JL, Kelly TH, Robinson DE and Spiga R (1990*b*). Effects of acute administration of diazepam and d-amphetamine on aggressive and escape responding of normal male subjects. *Psychopharmacology*, 100, 173–81.

Cherek DR, Spiga R, Bennett RH and Grabowski J (1991). Human aggression and escape responding effects of provocation frequency. *Psychol Rec*, 41, 3–17.

Cherek DR, Schnapp W, Moeller FG and Dougherty DM (1996). Laboratory measures of aggressive responding in male parolees with violent and nonviolent histories. *Aggress Behav*, 22, 27–36.

Cherek DR, Moeller FG, Dougherty DM and Rhoades H (1997*a*). Studies of violent and nonviolent male parolees: II. Laboratory and psychometric measurements of impulsivity. *Biol Psychiatry*, 41, 523–9.

Cherek DR, Moeller FG, Schnapp W and Dougherty DM (1997*b*). Studies of violent and nonviolent male parolees: I. Laboratory and psychometric measurements of impulsivity. *Biol Psychiatry*, 41, 514–22.

Cherek DR, Moeller FG, Khan-Dawood F, Swann A and Lane SD (1999). Prolactin responses to buspirone was reduced in violent compared to nonviolent parolees. *Psychopharmacology*, 142, 144–8.

Cherek DR, Lane SD, Dougherty DM, Moeller FG and White S (2000). Laboratory and questionnaire measures of aggression among female parolees with violent or nonviolent histories. *Aggress Behav*, 26, 291–307.

Cheu JW and Siegel A (1998). GABA receptor mediated suppression of defensive rage behaviour elicited from the medial hypothalamus in the cat: role of the lateral hypothalamus. *Brain Res*, 783, 293–304.

Cleare AJ and Bond AJ (1995). The effect of tryptophan depletion and enhancement on subjective and behavioural aggression in normal male subjects. *Psychopharmacology*, 118, 72–81.

Clement J, Simler S, Ciesielski L, Mandel P, Cabib S and Puglisi-Allegra S (1987). Age-dependent changes of brain GABA levels, turnover rates and shock-induced aggressive behaviour in inbred strains of mice. *Pharmacol Biochem Behav*, 26, 83–8.

Coccaro EF and Kavoussi RJ (1996). Neurotransmitter correlates of impulsive aggression. In *Aggression and Violence: Genetic, Neurobiological, and Biosocial Perspectives*, ed. DM Stoff and RB Cairns, pp. 67–85. Mahwah, NJ: Lawrence Erlbaum Associates.

Coccaro EF, Siever LJ, Klar HM et al. (1989). Serotonergic studies in patients with affective and personality disorders. *Arch Gen Psychiatry*, 46, 587–99.

Coccaro EF, Berman ME, Kavoussi RJ and Hauger RL (1996). Relationship of prolactin response to d-fenfluramine to behavioural and questionnaire assessments of aggression in personality-disordered men. *Biol Psychiatry*, 40, 157–64.

Conners CK (1969). A teacher rating scale for use in drug studies with children. *Am J Psychiatry*, 126, 884–8.

Crowner ML, Stepcic F, Gordana P and Czobor P (1994). Typology of patient-patient assaults detected by videocameras. *Am J Psychiatry*, 151, 1669–72.

Dawson G, Ashman SB and Carver LJ (2000). The role of early experience in shaping behavioral and brain development and its implications for social policy. *Dev Psychopathol*, 12, 695–712.

Delini-Stula A and Vassout A (1978a). Modulatory effects of baclofen, muscimol and GABA on interspecific aggressive behavior in the rat. *Neuropharmacology*, 17, 1063–5.

Delini-Stula A and Vassout A (1978b). Influence of baclofen and GABA-mimetic agents on spontaneous and olfactory-bulb-ablation-induced muricidal behavior in rats. *Arzneimittelforschung*, 28, 1508–9.

Depue RA and Spoont MR (1986). Conceptualizing a serotonin trait: a behavioral dimension of constraint. In *Psychobiology of Suicidal Behavior. Annals of New York Academy of Sciences, Vol. 487*, ed. JJ Mann and M Stanley, pp. 47–62. New York: New York Academy of Sciences.

Dodge KA and Coie JD (1987). Social-information-processing factors in reactive and proactive aggression in children's peer groups. *J Pers Social Psychol*, 53, 1146–58.

Dougherty DM, Cherek DR and Bennett RH (1996). The effects of alcohol on the aggressive responding of women. *J Studies Alcohol*, 52, 178–86.

Dougherty DM, Bjork JM, Huckabee HCG, Moeller FG and Swann AC (1999). Laboratory measures of aggression and impulsivity in women with borderline personality disorder. *Psychiatry Res*, 85, 315–26.

Dunn RT, Frye MS, Kimbrell TA, Denicoff KD, Leverich GS and Post RM (1998). The efficacy and use of anticonvulsants in mood disorders. *Clin Neuropharmacol*, 21, 215–35.

Feldman, RS, Meyer JS and Quenzer LF (1997). *Principles of Neuropsychopharmacology*. Sunderland, MA: Sinauer Associates.

File SE, Zharkovsky A and Gulati K (1991). Effects of baclofen and nitrendipine on ethanol withdrawal responses in the rat. *Neuropharmacology*, 30, 183–90.

Fils-Aime M, Eckardt MJ, George DT, Brown GL, Mefford I and Linnoila M (1996). Early onset alcoholics have lower cerebrospinal fluid 5-HIAA than late-onset alcoholics. *Arch Gen Psychiatry*, 53, 221–6.

Fishbein DH, Lozovsky D and Jaffe JH (1989). Impulsivity, aggression, and neuroendocrine responses to serotonergic stimulation in substance abusers. *Biol Psychiatry*, 25, 1049–66.

Fletcher PJ (1993). A comparison of the effects of dorsal or median raphe injections of 8-OH-DPAT in three operant tasks measuring response inhibition. *Behav Brain Res*, 54, 187–97.

Fletcher PJ (1995). Effects of combined or separate 5,7-dihydroxytraptamine lesions of the dorsal and median raphe nuclei on responding maintained by a DRL 20s schedule of food reinforcement. *Brain Res*, 675, 45–54.

Fontenot MB, Kaplan JR, Manuck SB, Arango V and Mann JJ (1995). Long-term effects of chronic social stress on sertonergic indices in the prefrontal cortex of adult male cynomolgus macaques. *Brain Res*, 705, 105–8.

Gaebelein J (1981). Naturalistic versus experimental approaches to aggression; theoretical and methodological issues. *Aggress Behav*, 7, 325–39.

Gardner, DL and Cowdry RW (1986). Positive effects of carbamazepine on behavioral dyscontrol in borderline personality disorder. *Am J Psychiatry*, 143, 519–22.

Gedye A (1992). Serotonin-GABA treatment is hypothesized for self-injury in Lesch–Nyhan syndrome. *Med Hypoth*, 38, 325–8.

Giakas WJ, Seibyl JP and Mazure CM (1990). Valproate in the treatment of temper outbursts. *J Clin Psychiatry*, 51, 525.

Gothelf D, Apter A and van Praag HM (1997). Measurement of aggression in psychiatric patients. *Psychiatry Res*, 71, 83–95.

Haas S, Vincent K, Holt J and Lippmann S (1997). Divalproex: a possible treatment alternative for demented, elderly aggressive patients. *Ann Clin Psychiatry*, 9, 145–7.

Higley JD, Mehlman PT, Taub DM et al. (1992). Cerebrospinal fluid monoamine and adrenal correlates of aggression in free-ranging rhesus monkeys. *Arch Gen Psychiatry*, 49, 436–41.

Higley, JD, Thompson WW, Champoux M et al. (1993). Paternal and maternal genetic and environmental contributions to cerebrospinal fluid monoamine metabolites in rhesus monkeys (*Macaca mulatta*). *Arch Gen Psychiatry*, 50, 615–23.

Higley JD, Linnoila M and Suomi SJ (1994). Ethological contributions. In *Handbook of Aggressive and Destructive Behavior in Psychiatric Patients*, ed. M Hersen, RT Ammerman and LA Sission, pp. 17–32. New York: Plenum Press.

Higley JD, Suomi SJ and Linnoila M (1996a). A nonhuman primate model of Type II excessive alcohol consumption? Part 1. Low cerebrospinal fluid 5-hydroxyindoleacetic acid concentrations and diminished social competence correlate with excessive alcohol consumption. *Alcoholism: Clin Exp Res*, 20, 629–42.

Higley, JD, Suomi SJ and Linnoila M (1996b). A nonhuman primate model of type II excessive alcohol consumption? Part 2. Diminished social competence and excessive aggression correlates with low cerebrospinal fluid 5-hydroxyindoleacetic acid concentrations. *Alcoholism: Clin Exp Res*, 20, 643–50.

Higley JD, Mehlman PT, Poland RE et al. (1996c). CSF testosterone and 5-HIAA correlate with different types of aggressive behaviours. *Biol Psychiatry*, 40, 1067–82.

Hile MG and Desrochers MN (1993). The relationship between functional assessment and treatment selection for aggressive behaviors. *Res Dev Disabil*, 14, 265–74.

Hinshaw SP, Henker B, Whalen CK, Erhardt D and Dunnington RE Jr (1989). Aggressive, prosocial, and nonsocial behavior in hyperactive boys: dose effects of methylphenidate in naturalistic settings. *J Consult Clin Psychol*, 57, 636–43.

Ho M-Y, Al-Zahrani SSA, Al-Ruwaitea CM, Bradshaw CM and Szabadi E (1998). 5-Hydroxytryptamine and impulse control: prospects for a behavioural analysis. *J Psychopharmacol*, 12, 68–78.

Kagel JH, Green L and Caraco T (1986). When foragers discount the future: constraint or adaptation? *Anim Behav*, 34, 271–83.

Kastner T, Finesmith R and Walsh K (1993). Long-term administration of valproic acid in the treatment of affective symptoms in people with mental retardation. *J Clin Psychopharmacol*, 13, 448–51.

Kaufmann H (1965). Definitions and methodology in the study of aggression. *Psychol Bull*, 64, 351–64.

Kazdin AE (1987). Treatment of antisocial behavior in children: current status and future directions. *Psychol Bull*, 102, 187–203.

Keck PE Jr, McElroy SL and Nemeroff CB (1992). Anticonvulsants in the treatment of bipolar disorder. *J Neuropsychiatry Clin Neurosci*, 4, 395–405.

Kellam SG, Ling X, Merisca R, Brown CH and Ialongo N (1998). The effect of the level of aggression in the first grade classroom on the course and malleability of aggressive behaviour into middle school. *Dev Psychopathol*, 10, 165–85.

King GR and Logue AW (1990). Humans' sensitivity to variation in reinforcer amount: effects of the method of reinforcer delivery. *J Exp Anal Behav*, 53, 33–45.

Kraemer, GW, Ebert MH, Schmidt, DE and McKinney WT (1989). A longitudinal study of the effect of different social rearing conditions on cerebrospinal fluid norepinephrine and biogenic amine metabolites in rhesus monkeys. *Neuropsychopharmacology*, 2, 175–89.

Kruesi MJP, Rapoport JL, Hamburger S et al. (1990). Cerebrospinal fluid monoamine metabolites, aggression, and impulsivity in disruptive behavior disorders of children and adolescents. *Arch Gen Psychiatry*, 47, 419–26.

Lane SD and Cherek DR (2000). Biological and behavioral investigation of aggression and impulsivity. In *The Science, Treatment, and Prevention of Antisocial Behaviors: Application To the Criminal Justice System*, ed. DH Fishbein, pp. 5-1–5-21. Kingston, NJ: Civic Research Institute.

Lavine R (1997). Psychopharmacological treatment of aggression and violence in the substance abusing population. *J Psychoactive Drug*, 29, 321–9.

LeMarquand D, Pihl RO and Benkelfat C (1994). Serotonin and alcohol intake, abuse, and dependence: clinical evidence. *Biol Psychiatry*, 36, 326–37.

Leventhal, BL, Cook EH Jr, Morford M, Ravitz AJ, Heller W and Freedman DX (1993). Clinical and neurochemical effects of fenfluramine in children with autism. *J Neuropsychiatry Clin Neurosci*, 5, 307–15.

Lindenmayer JP and Kotsaftis A (2000). Use of sodium valproate in violent and aggressive behaviors: a critical review. *J Clin Psychiatry*, 61, 123–8.

Linnoila M, Virkkunen M Scheinin, M, Nuutila R and Goodwin FK (1983). Low cerebrospinal fluid 5-hydroxyindoleacetic acid concentration differentiates impulsive from nonimpulsive violent behaviour. *Life Sci*, 33, 2609–14.

Loeber R and Schmaling KB (1985). Empirical evidence for overt and covert patterns of antisocial conduct problems: a metaanalysis. *J Abnorm Child Psychol*, 13, 337–52.

Logue AW (1988). Research on self-control: an integrated framework. *Behav Brain Sci*, 11, 665–709.

Logue AW (1995). *Self-control*. Englewood Cliffs, NJ: Prentice-Hall.

Logue AW, Pena-Correal TE, Rodriguez ML and Kabela E (1986). Self-control in adult humans: variation in positive reinforcer amount and delay. *J Exp Anal Behav*, 46, 159–73.

Low AR and Brandes M (1999). Gabapentin for the management of agitation. *J Clin Psychopharmacol*, 19, 482–3.

Lupien SJ, King S, Meaney MJ and McEwen BS (2000). Child's stress hormone levels correlate with mother's socioeconomic status and depressive state. *Biol Psychiatry*, 48, 976–80.

Mandel P, Ciesielski L, Maitre M, Simler S, Mack G and Kempf E (1979). Involvement of central GABAergic systems in convulsions and aggressive behavior. *Adv Exp Med Biol*, 123, 475–92.

Manuck SB, Flory JD, McCaffery JM, Mathews KA, Mann JJ and Muldoon MF (1998). Aggression, impulsivity, and central nervous system serotonergic responsivity in a nonpatient sample. *Neuropsychopharmacology*, 19, 287–99.

Mattes JA (1986). Psychopharmacology of temper outbursts: a review. *J Nerv Ment Disord*, 174, 464–70.

Mattes JA (1992). Valproic acid for nonaffective aggression in the mentally retarded. *J Nerv Ment Disord*, 180, 601–2.

Matthews KA, Flory JD, Muldoon MF and Manuck SB (2000). Does socioeconomic status relate to central serotonergic responsivity in healthy adults? *Psychosom Med*, 62, 231–7.

Mazur JE (1987). An adjusting procedure for studying delayed reinforcement. In *Quantitative Analyses of Behavior Vol. 5: The Effect of Delay And Intervening Events*, ed. ML Commons, JE Mazur, JA Nevin and H Rachlin, pp. 55–73. Hillsdale, NJ: Lawrence Erlbaum Associates.

McElroy SL and Keck PE Jr (1995). Antiepileptic drugs. In *Textbook of Psychopharmacology*, ed. AE Schatzberg and CB Nemeroff, pp. 351–75. Washington, DC: American Psychiatric Press.

McElroy SL, Keck PE Jr, Pope HG and Hudson JI (1992). Valproate in bipolar disorder: literature review and treatment guidelines. *J Clin Psychopharmacol*, 12, 42S–52S.

McGuire MT and Raleigh MJ (1987). Serotonin, social behavior, and aggression in vervet monkeys. In *Ethopharmacology of Agonistic Behaviour in Animals and Humans*, ed. B Olivier, J Mos and PF Brain, pp. 207–22. Dordrecht: Martinus Nijhoff Publishers.

McKenzie GM (1981). Dissociation of the antiaggression and serotonin-depleting effects of fenfluramine. *Can J Physiol Pharmacol*, 59, 830–6.

McLeod JD and Kessler RC (1990). Socioeconomic status differences in vulnerability to undesirable life events. *J Health Social Behav*, 31, 162–72.

Mehlman PT, Higley JD, Faucher I et al. (1994). Low CSF 5-HIAA concentrations and severe aggression and impaired impulse control in nonhuman primates. *Am J Psychiatry*, 151, 1485–91.

Meltzer HY and Arora RC (1988). Genetic control of serotonin uptake in blood platelets: a twin study. *Psychiatry Res*, 24, 263–9.

Miczek KA, DeBold JF, van Erp AM and Tornatzky W (1997). Alcohol, GABA A-benzodiazepine receptor complex, and aggression. *Rec Dev Alcoholism*, 13, 139–71.

Mischel W, Shoda Y and Rodriguez ML (1989). Delay of gratification in children. *Science*, 244, 933–8.

Modai I, Apter, A, Meltzer M, Tyano S, Walevski A and Jerushalmy Z (1989). Serotonin uptake by platelets of suicidal and aggressive adolescent psychiatric inpatients. *Neuropsychobiology*, 21, 9–13.

Moeller FG, Dougherty DM, Swann AC, Collins D, Davis CM and Cherek DR (1996). Tryptophan depletion and aggressive responding in healthy males. *Psychopharmacology*, 126, 97–103.

Molina VA, Ciesielski L, Gobaille S and Mandel P (1987). Effects of the potentiation of the GABAergic neurotransmission in the olfactory bulbs on mouse killing behavior. *Pharmacol Biochem Behav*, 24, 657–64.

Moss HB, Yao JK and Panzak GL (1990). Serotonergic responsivity and behavioral dimensions in antisocial personality disorder with substance abuse. *Biol Psychiatry*, 28, 325–38.

Muldoon MF, Kaplan JR, Manuck SB and Mann JJ (1992). Effects of a low-fat diet on brain serotonergic responsivity in cynomolgus monkeys. *Biol Psychiatry*, 31, 739–42.

Naumenko EV, Popova NK, Nikulina EM et al. (1989). Behavior, adrenocortical activity, and brain monoamines in Norway rats selected for reduced aggressiveness towards man. *Pharmacol Biochem Behav*, 33, 85–91.

O'Keane V, Moloney E, O'Neill H et al. (1992). Blunted prolactin response to *d*-fenfluramine in sociopathy. Evidence for subsensitivity of central serotonergic function. *Br J Psychiatry*, 160, 643–6.

Olivier B, Mos J, Tulp M, Schipper J, den Daas S and van Oortmerssen G (1990). Serotonergic involvement in aggressive behavior in animals. In *Violence and Suicidality: Perspectives in Clinical and Psychobiological Research. Clinical and Experimental Psychiatry, Vol. 3*, ed. HM van Praag, R Plutchik and A Apter, pp. 79–137. New York: Brunner/Mazel.

Panksepp J (1973). Fenfluramine: effects on aggression. *Biol Psychiatry*, 6, 181–6.

Paredes RG and Agmo A (1992). GABA and behavior: the role of receptor subtypes. *Neurosci Biobehav Rev*, 16, 145–70.

Pepler DJ and Craig WM (1995). A peek behind the fence: naturalistic observations of children with remote audiovisual recording. *Dev Psychol*, 31, 548–53.

Pietrini P, Guazzelli M, Basso G, Jaffe K and Grafman J (2000). Neural correlates of imaginal aggressive behavior assessed by positron emission tomography in healthy subjects. *Am J Psychiatry*, 157, 1772–81.

Pihl, RO, Young SN, Harden P, Plotnik S, Chamberlain B and Ervin FR (1995). Acute effect of altered tryptophan levels and alcohol on aggression in normal human males. *Psychopharmacology*, 119, 353–60.

Popova NK, Voitenko NN, Kulikov AV and Avgustinovich DF (1991). Evidence for the involvement of central serotonin in mechanism of domestication of Silver Foxes. *Pharmacol Biochem Behav*, 40, 751–6.

Post RM (1990). Non-lithium treatment for bipolar disorder. *J Clin Psychiatry*, 51, 95–165.

Post RM, Denicoff KD, Frye MA et al. (1998). A history of the use of anticonvulsants as mood stabilizers in the last two decades of the 20th century. *Neuropsychobiology*, 38, 152–66.

Potegal M (1987). Differential effects of ethyl (R,S)-nipecotate on the behaviors of highly and minimally aggressive female golden hamsters. *Psychopharmacology*, 89, 444–8.

Potter LB and Mercy JA (1997). Public health perspective on interpersonal violence among youths in the United States. In *Handbook of Antisocial Behavior*, ed. DM Stoff, J Breiling and JD Maser, pp. 3–11. New York: John Wiley and Sons.

Poulos CX, Parker JL and Le AD (1996). Dexfenfluramine and 8-OH-DPAT modulate impulsivity in a delay-of-reward paradigm: implications for a correspondence with alcohol consumption. *Behav Pharmacol*, 7, 395–9.

Primrose DA (1979). Treatment of self-injurious behavior with a GABA analogue. *J Ment Deficiency Res*, 23, 163–73.

Quay HC (1966). Personality patterns in pre-adolescent delinquent boys. *Educ Psychol Measure*, 26, 99–110.

Rachlin H (1995). Self-control: beyond commitment. *Behav Brain Sci*, 18, 109–59.

Rachlin H and Green L (1972). Commitment, choice and self-control. *J Exp Anal Behav*, 17, 15–22.

Raine A, Buchsbaum M and LaCasse L (1997). Brain abnormalities in murderers indicated by positron emission tomography. *Biol Psychiatry*, 42, 495–508.

Raine A, Lencz T, Bihrle S, LaCasse L and Colletti P (2000). Reduced prefrontal gray matter volume and reduced autonomic activity in antisocial personality disorder. *Arch Gen Psychiatry*, 57, 119–27.

Raleigh MJ, McGuire MT, Brammer GL and Yuwiler A (1984). Social and environmental influences on blood serotonin concentrations in monkeys. *Arch Gen Psychiatry*, 41, 405–10.

Richards JB, Sabol KE and Seiden LS (1993). Fluoxetine prevents the disruptive effects of fenfluramine on differential-reinforcement-of-low-rate 72-second schedule performance. *J Pharmacol Exp Therapeut*, 267, 1256–63.

Robbins TW (1997). Arousal systems and attentional processes. *Biol Psychol*, 45, 57–71.

Rodgers RJ and Depaulis A (1982). GABAergic influences on defensive fighting in rats. *Pharmacol Biochem Behav*, 17, 451–6.

Roeling TAP, Kruk MR, Schuurmans R and Veening JG (1994). Behavioral responses of bicuculline methiodide injections into the ventral hypothalamus of freely moving socially interacting rats. *Brain Res*, 615, 121–7.

Rolinski Z and Herbut M (1981). The role of serotonergic system in foot shock-induced behavior in mice. *Psychopharmacology*, 73, 246–51.

Rosenblum, LA, Coplan JD, Friedman S, Bassoff T, Gorman JM and Andrews MW (1994). Adverse early experiences affect noradrenergic and serotonergic functioning in adult primates. *Biol Psychiatry*, 35, 221–7.

Saletu B, Barbanoj MJ, Anderer P, Sieghart W and Grunberger J (1993). Clinical-pharmacological study with the two isomers (d-, l-) of fenfluramine and its comparison with chlorpromazine and d-amphetamine: blood levels, EEG mapping and safety evaluation. *Methods Find Exp Clin Pharmacol*, 15, 291–312.

Schatzberg AF and Nemeroff CB, eds. (1995). *The American Psychiatric Press Textbook of Psychopharmacology*. Washington, DC: American Psychiatric Press.

Schneider ML, Clarke AS, Kraemer GW et al. (1998). Prenatal stress alters brain biogenic amine levels in primates. *Dev Psychopathol*, 10, 427–40.

Siegel A, Roeling TA, Gregg TR and Kruk MR (1999). Neuropharmacology of brain-stimulation-evoked aggression. *Neurosci Biobehav Rev*, 23, 359–89.

Simler S, Puglisi-Allegra S and Mandel P (1983). Effects of n-di-propylacetate on aggressive behavior and brain GABA level in isolated mice. *Pharmacol Biochem Behav*, 18, 717–20.

Singhal, RL and Telner JI (1983). Psychopharmacological aspects of aggression in animals and man. *Psychiatry J Univ Ottawa*, 8, 145–53.

Sonuga-Barke, EJ, Lea SE and Webley P (1989). The development of adaptive choice in a self-control procedure. *J Exp Anal Behav*, 51, 77–85.

Soubrié P (1986) Reconciling the role of central serotonin neurons in human and animal behavior. *Behav Brain Sci*, 9, 319–64.

Soubrié P and Bizot JC (1990). Monoaminergic control of waiting capacity (impulsivity) in animals. In *Violence and Suicidality: Perspectives in Clinical and Psychobiological Research. Clinical and Experimental Psychiatry, Vol. 3*, ed. HM van Praag, R Plutchik and A Apter, pp. 257–72. New York: Brunner/Mazel.

Sroufe LA (1997). Psychopathology as an outcome of development. *Dev Psychopathol*, 9, 251–68.

Stein G (1992). Drug treatment of personality disorders. *Br J Psychiatry*, 161, 167–84.

Stein DJ, Hollander E and Liebowitz MR (1993). Neurobiology of impulsivity and the impulse control disorders. *J Neuropsychiatry Clin Neurosci*, 5, 9–17.

Stoff DM, Pastiempo AP, Yeung JH, Cooper TB, Bridger WH and Rabinovich H (1992). Neuroendocrine responses to challenge with *d,l*-fenfluramine and aggression in disruptive behavior disorders of children and adolescents. *Psychiatry Res*, 43, 263–76.

Sulcova A, Krsiak M and Masek K (1978). Effects of baclofen on agonistic behavior in mice. *Activitas Nervosa Superior*, 20, 241–2.

Taylor SP (1967). Aggressive behavior and physiological arousal of function of provocation and the tendency to inhibit aggression. *J Pers*, 35, 297–310.

Tedeschi JT and Quigley BM (1996). Limitations of laboratory paradigms for studying aggression. *Aggress Viol Behav*, 1, 163–77.

Tremblay, RE, Pihl RO, Vitaro F and Dobkin PL (1994). Predicting early onset of male antisocial behavior from preschool behavior. *Arch Gen Psychiatry*, 51, 732–9.

Tuinier S, Verhoeven WMA and van Praag HM (1996). Serotonin and disruptive behavior: a critical evaluation of the clinical data. *Hum Psychopharmacol*, 11, 469–82.

Turner CW, Layton JF and Simons LS (1975). Naturalistic studies of aggressive behavior: aggressive stimuli, victim visibility and horn honking. *J Pers Social Psychol*, 31, 1098–107.

Valzelli L (1984). Reflections on experimental and human pathology of aggression. *Prog Neuro-Psychopharmacol Biol Psychiatry*, 8, 311–25.

Virkkunen M, Nuutila A, Goodwin FK and Linnoila M (1987). Cerebrospinal fluid metabolites in male arsonists. *Arch Gen Psychiatry*, 44, 241–7.

Virkkunen M, DeJong J, Bartko J and Linnoila M (1989). Psychobiological concomitants of history of suicide attempts among violent offenders and impulsive fire setters. *Arch Gen Psychiatry*, 46, 604–6.

Virkkunen M, Kallio E, Rawlings R et al. (1994). Personality profiles and state aggressiveness in Finnish alcoholic, violent offenders, fire setters, and healthy volunteers. *Arch Gen Psychiatry*, 51, 28–33.

Vitiello B, Behar D, Hunt J, Stoff D and Ricciuti A (1990). Subtyping aggression in children and adolescents. *J Neuropsychiatry Clin Neurosci*, 2, 189–92.

Volkow ND, Tancredi LR, Grant C et al. (1995). Brain glucose metabolism in violent psychiatric patients: a preliminary study. *Psychiatry Res*, 61, 243–53.

Vollmer TR, Borero JC, Lalli JS and Dency D (1999). Evaluating self-control and impulsivity in children with severe behavior disorders. *J Appl Behav Anal*, 32, 451–66.

Walsh AES, Oldman AD, Franklin M, Fairburn CG and Cowen PJ (1995). Dieting decreases plasma tryptophan and increases the prolactin response to *d*-fenfluramine in women but not men. *J Affect Disord*, 33, 89–97.

Wogar MA, Bradshaw CM and Szabadi E (1993). Effects of lesions of the ascending 5-hydroxytryptaminergic pathways on choice between delayed reinforcers. *Psychopharmacology*, 113, 239–43.

Wolfe BM and Baron RA (1971). Laboratory aggression related to aggression in naturalistic social situations: effects of an aggressive model on the behavior of college student and prisoner observers. *Psychonomic Sci*, 24, 193–4.

Wolfe BE, Metzger ED and Stollar C (1997). The effects of dieting on plasma tryptophan concentration and food intake in healthy women. *Physiol Behav*, 61, 537–41.

Young SN, Smith SE, Pihl RO and Erwin FR (1985). Tryptophan depletion causes a rapid lowering of mood in normal males. *Psychopharmacology*, 87, 173–7.

Young SN, Pihl RO and Ervin FR (1988). The effect of altered tryptophan levels on mood and behavior in normal human males. *Clin Neuropharmacol*, 11 (Suppl. 1), S207–15.

Yudofsky SC, Silver JM, Jackson W, Endicott J and Williams D (1986). The overt aggression scale for the objective rating of verbal and physical aggression. *Am J Psychiatry*, 143, 35–9.

Zeichner A, Frey FC, Parrott DJ and Butryn MF (1999). Measurement of laboratory aggression: a new response-choice paradigm. *Psychol Rep*, 85, 1229–37.

18

A neurocognitive model of the psychopathic individual

R J R Blair

University College London, London, UK

Introduction

The goal of this chapter is to consider a neurocognitive model of the psychopathic individual. Psychopathy is not synonymous with a diagnosis of either conduct disorder (CD) or antisocial personality disorder (APD) but rather is an extension of these DSM–IV diagnoses (American Psychiatric Association 1994). Psychopathy, in both children and adults, is currently defined by high scores on clinically based rating scales: for children, the Psychopathy Screening Device (PSD; Frick and Hare, in press) and for adults, the Revised Psychopathy Checklist (PCL–R; Hare 1991). Factor analyses of behaviours rated on both the PSD and PCL reveal two independent factors: (1) an emotion dysfunction factor defined largely by emotional shallowness and lack of guilt and (2) an antisocial behaviour factor defined largely by impulsive aggression and the commission of a wide variety of offence types (Harpur et al. 1989; Hare et al. 1991; Frick et al. 1994). High scores on Factor 2 of the PSD and PCL are closely associated with the diagnosis of CD and APD respectively (Frick et al. 1994). However, high scores on Factor 1, while highly correlated with scores on Factor 2, are less closely associated with the DSM diagnoses. More interestingly, scores on Factor 1 have different correlates from scores on Factor 2. Thus, both socio-economic status and IQ are correlated with Factor 2 scores, but neither is associated with scores on Factor 1 (Hare et al. 1991). Moreover, while Factor 2 score declines with age, Factor 1 score remains constant (Harpur and Hare 1994). This persistence suggests that Factor 1, the emotion dysfunction factor, may more closely reflect the neurocognitive impairment(s) that are thought to result in the development of psychopathy. Factor 2, and by implication the diagnoses of CD and APD, may more accurately reflect the interaction between this neurocognitive impairment and the individual's social environment.

The neurocognitive impairment underlying psychopathy

Within this chapter, two nonemotion-based and two emotion-based models of the neurocognitive impairment underlying psychopathy will be considered. These are: the executive dysfunction model (Moffitt 1993a), the response set modulation hypothesis (Newman 1998), the fear model (Patrick 1994) and the violence inhibition mechanism model (Blair 1995). Two further models, the somatic marker hypothesis (Damasio 1994) and the social response reversal model (Blair and Cipolotti 2000) will not be considered. This is due to considerations of space and the fact that implications of these models for psychopathy are discussed in more detail elsewhere (Blair 2001). In addition, although the somatic marker hypothesis has been suggested as an account of psychopathy (Damasio 1994; Anderson et al. 1999), there are empirical data that are incompatible with the model. Thus, one of the main impairments assumed to follow somatic marker dysfunction is a failure to generate autonomic responses to social and emotional stimuli (Damasio 1994; Tranel and Damasio 1994). Yet, psychopathic individuals do not show generalized hypo-autonomic reactivity to emotional stimuli (Patrick et al. 1993; Blair et al. 1997). As regards the social response reversal model (Blair and Cipolotti 2000), this is a model of the reactive antisocial behaviour shown by patients following orbitofrontal cortex damage. Reactive aggression is elicited in response to frustration/threat while instrumental aggression is more purposeful and goal directed (Berkowitz 1993). Psychopathic individuals present with a marked preponderance for instrumental, rather than reactive, antisocial behaviour (Williamson et al. 1987; Cornell et al. 1996). Moreover, impairments attributed to social response reversal impairment, such as dysfunction in processing angry expressions, are not seen in psychopathic individuals (Blair et al. 1997, 2001a).

Executive function theories

Executive functions refer to the processes that underlie flexible goal-directed behaviour, e.g. inhibiting dominant responses, creating and maintaining goal-related behaviours and temporally sequencing behaviour (Burgess et al. 1998). Impairment of executive functions is associated with damage to prefrontal areas (Luria 1966; Fuster 1980; Baddeley and Della Sala 1998); in particular, dorsolateral prefrontal cortex (Duncan 1986; Shallice 1988). Neuropsychological, functional imaging and animal lesion evidence suggest that different aspects of executive functions are dissociable, and mediated by distinct neural systems subserved by different regions of the prefrontal cortex (Luria 1966; Fuster 1980; Shallice 1988; Baddeley and Della Sala 1998; Roberts et al. 1998).

There have been frequent attempts to relate executive dysfunction to antisocial behaviour (Elliot 1978; Gorenstein 1982; Moffitt 1993a; Barratt 1994; Krakowski et al. 1997). It has been claimed, for example, that antisocial behaviour is due to poor planning or an inability to inhibit violent impulses (Barratt 1994; Krakowski et al. 1997). In line with these models, there is evidence that individuals with antisocial behaviour do show impaired performance on measures of executive functioning, including those of 'inhibitory control' (Seguin et al. 1999); see, for reviews of the literature, Moffitt (1993*b*) and Morgan and Lilienfeld (2000). Moreover, there have been functional and structural neuro-imaging studies that have indicated both impoverished prefrontal cortex functioning or prefrontal structural abnormalities in violent, antisocial adults (Volkow and Tancredi 1987; Raine et al. 1994, 2000). Many of these adults would have met criteria for the DSM–IV diagnosis of antisocial personality disorder.

However, the executive dysfunction models face serious difficulties. First, it appears clear that psychopathic individuals do not present with executive dysfunction; they have been consistently found to present with no impairment in executive functions relying on dorsolateral prefrontal cortex (Hart et al. 1990; LaPierre et al. 1995); see, for a review, Kandel and Freed (1989). Moreover, in the only study that contrasted functioning in predatory murderers and reactively aggressive murderers, it was only the reactively aggressive murderers who showed reductions in prefrontal cortex activity (Raine et al. 1994). As stated above, instrumental, predatory murderers are far more likely to meet criteria for psychopathy than reactively aggressive murderers (Cornell et al. 1996; Hare 1998). Second, there is good reason to believe that the antisocial behaviour shown by individuals with 'acquired sociopathy' following lesions of frontal cortex is due to dysfunction not in executive systems mediated by dorsolateral prefrontal cortex but rather in the executive emotion systems that are reliant on medial and orbitofrontal cortex. Thus, EVR and other patients with acquired sociopathy studied by Damasio and colleagues have shown preserved functioning on classic measures of executive functioning that involve the dorsolateral prefrontal cortex (Eslinger and Damasio 1985; Damasio et al. 1991; Damasio 1994). Moreover, in a large group study, investigating the relationship between aggression and damage to prefrontal cortex, Grafman and colleagues demonstrated that it was lesions to orbitofrontal and medial frontal cortex, rather than dorsolateral prefrontal cortex, that was associated with violence (Grafman et al. 1996).

Thus, in conclusion, it appears that executive dysfunction, at least for those executive systems implicating dorsolateral prefrontal cortex, is not related to psychopathy.

Response set modulation

An influential model of psychopathy is the response modulation hypothesis of Newman and colleagues (Patterson and Newman 1993; Newman 1998). Response modulation involves 'a rapid and relatively automatic (i.e. non-effortful or involuntary) shift of attention from the effortful organization and implementation of goal-directed behaviour to its evaluation' (Newman et al. 1987). The initial physiological basis of the model (Gorenstein and Newman 1980) was based on the work of Gray and others on the implications of septo-hippocampal lesions for emotional learning (Gray 1971). 'In animal studies, deficient response modulation typically involves response perseveration or a tendency to continue some goal-directed behaviour (e.g., running down the arm of a maze) despite punishment or frustrative nonreward (i.e., extinction)' (Newman 1998, p. 85).

There are three studies driven by the response set modulation hypothesis. One set of studies has used the one-pack card-playing task that can be conceptualized as an extinction task under partial reinforcement conditions; initially, all of the participant's card choices are reinforcing but as the number of trials increases, the probability of reward decreases. Consistent with the response set modulation model, both children and adults with psychopathy choose to view significantly more cards than individuals without psychopathy (Newman et al. 1987; Shapiro et al. 1988; O'Brien and Frick 1996; Fisher and Blair 1998). A second set of studies has used a passive avoidance task, where the participant is presented with a series of two-digit numbers. Pressing a response button during the presentation of half of these numbers results in reward. Pressing a response button during the presentation of the other half results in punishment. Using this task, children and adults with psychopathy have been found to show reduced passive avoidance; they are significantly more likely to press the response button during the presentation of numbers that result in punishment (Newman and Kosson 1986; Newman and Schmitt 1998). A third set of studies, as yet unreplicated, involves the participant having to respond according to whether two pictures/words are conceptually related. The participant is informed whether the trial will be a picture or word trial. Then the participant is simultaneously shown a picture and a word. If, for example, it is a picture trial, the picture is irrelevant and the word irrelevant. Then, the participant will see another picture and will have to decide whether the two pictures are conceptually related. However, the relevant stimuli may either be conceptually related or unrelated to the test stimulus that is then presented (i.e. in the above example, the word may be related to the picture or not). Importantly, when the pictures/words are unrelated, participants respond significantly more slowly when the irrelevant stimulus is related to the test stimulus than when it is not (Gernsbacher and Faust 1991). Strikingly, however, this is not the case for psychopathic individuals, who showed no interference by the irrelevant stimuli on deciding that the task stimuli were irrelevant (Newman et al. 1997).

The response set modulation hypothesis thus has a considerable body of literature in its support. However, it faces several difficulties. First, it cannot adequately account for the specific nature of the emotional impairment shown by psychopathic individuals (Williamson et al. 1991; Blair 1995; see below). Second, other accounts would also predict the above results and can also account for the specific nature of the emotional impairment shown by psychopathic individuals (see below).

Emotion-based models

The clinical and empirical picture of the psychopath describes an individual who has some form of emotional deficit (Schalling 1978; Aniskiewicz 1979; Williamson et al. 1991; Patrick et al. 1994). Cleckley (1976) suggested that there was discordance in the linguistic and experiential components of emotion in psychopaths. As Johns and Quay (1962; p. 217) put it, psychopaths 'know the words but not the music'. Hare's (1991) Revised Psychopathy Checklist (PCL–R) suggests that the psychopath lacks remorse or guilt (item 6) and empathy (item 8).

The fear-based models

One of the main positions regarding the emotional impairment shared by psychopathic individuals is that there is impairment in the neurophysiological systems modulating fear behaviour (Hare 1978; Trasler 1978; Fowles 1988; Patrick 1994; Mealey 1995). The lack of emotional responsiveness of psychopaths to threatening stimuli has been demonstrated through several paradigms (Lykken 1957; Hare 1982; Ogloff and Wong 1990; Patrick et al. 1994; Levenston et al. 2000). For example, psychopaths have been shown to be deficient in the acquisition of anxiety responses to threatening stimuli (Lykken 1957). They have also been found, when anticipating aversive shock, to show smaller electrodermal responses that occur later in the warning interval in comparison with nonpsychopaths (Hare 1965, 1982; Hare et al. 1978; Ogloff and Wong 1990). In addition, psychopathic individuals show reduced autonomic reactivity relative to nonpsychopathic controls during the imagery of unpleasant and fearful experiences (Patrick et al. 1994). Only if the threatening stimulus is a picture (e.g. of a snake) have psychopaths been found to show similar responses to nonpsychopaths (Patrick et al. 1993; Levenston et al. 2000). However, this finding has only been found to hold if the skin conductance response indexes responsiveness. If it is indexed by startle reflex, psychopaths have been found to show reduced responsiveness to these stimuli relative to controls (Levenston et al. 2000).

The fear theories have generated a wealth of interesting data. However, they face at least two difficulties. First, they assume that fear is mediated by a unitary system. For example, it is thought that there might be dysfunction within a unitary behavioural inhibition system (BIS) (Gray 1987; Fowles 1988). This BIS is thought to generate autonomic responses to punished stimuli (through classical conditioning) as well as inhibiting responding following punishment (through instrumental conditioning). However, the neural circuitry to achieve aversive classical and instrumental conditioning appears to be doubly dissociable (Killcross et al. 1997). Moreover, Prather et al. (2001) have recently demonstrated that while early amygdala lesions result in reduced neophobia and other object-based anxiety, they do not reduce social phobia to novel conspecifics. This again suggests dissociable fear systems: one for fear of objects and one for fear of conspecifics.

Secondly, and more crucially, it is unclear why the fear theories should predict the antisocial behaviour shown by psychopathic individuals. Psychopathy is a disorder where the afflicted individual engages in instrumental antisocial behaviour including aggression with striking frequency; the psychopathic individual uses antisocial behaviour to achieve his or her goals (Williamson et al. 1987; Cornell et al. 1996). This has usually been taken to indicate that the psychopathic individual has failed to be socialized away from using antisocial behaviour (Eysenck 1964; Trasler 1978; Blair 1995). The fear positions assume that this moral socialization is achieved through the use of punishment (Eysenck 1964; Trasler 1978). The healthy individual is frightened by punishment and associates this fear with the action that resulted in the punishment, thus making the individual less likely to engage in the action in the future. The suggestion is that psychopathic individuals, because they are less aversively aroused by punishment, make weaker associations and thus are more likely to engage in the punished action in the future than healthy individuals.

However, the assumption that conditioned fear responses play a crucial role in moral socialization has been questioned (Blackburn 1988; Blair and Morton 1995). The developmental literature indicates that moral socialization is not achieved through the formation of conditioned fear responses but rather through the induction and fostering of empathy (Hoffman 1994). Studies have shown, for example, that moral socialization is better achieved through the use of induction (reasoning that draws children's attention to the effects of their misdemeanors on others and increases empathy) than through harsh authoritarian or power-assertive parenting practices which rely on the use of punishment (Hoffman and Saltzstein 1967; Baumrind 1971, 1983). Indeed, there have been suggestions that while empathy facilitates moral socialization, fear actually hinders it (Hoffman 1994). In a review of a large number of studies of disciplinary methods, Brody and Shaffer (1982) concluded that punishment-based power assertion had an adverse effect on moral socialization regardless of age. Hoffman (1988) has suggested that the primary utility of power assertion is to prevent the parent from being ignored while the child is transgressing. Thus, in conclusion, while the fear positions have generated a considerable body of data, it remains unclear why fear impairment should result in the development of psychopathy.

Violence inhibition mechanism model

The importance of empathy for moral socialization was one of the reasons for the development of the original violence inhibition mechanism model of psychopathy (Blair 1995; Blair et al. 1997). This model was prompted by work suggesting that most social animals possess mechanisms for the control of aggression (Lorenz 1966; Eibl-Eibesfeldt 1970). They noted that submission cues displayed to a conspecific aggressor terminate attacks; e.g. an aggressor dog will cease fighting if its opponent bares its throat. The violence inhibition mechanism (VIM) is considered to be a functionally similar mechanism in humans, where sad facial affects (i.e. distress cues) function as a human submission response. At its simplest, the VIM is thought to be a system that when activated by distress cues, the sad and fearful expressions of others, results in increased autonomic activity, attention and activation of the brainstem threat response system (usually resulting in freezing) (Blair 1995). It should be noted that the VIM is thought to be activated whenever distress cues are displayed. It is not reliant upon contextual information about ongoing violence for activation. In line with this, the display of distress cues has been found to result in the inhibition of not only aggression (Perry and Perry 1974) but also nonviolent disputes over property ownership (Camras 1977) and sexual activity (Chaplin et al. 1995).

According to the model, moral socialization occurs through the pairing of the activation of the mechanism by distress cues with representations of the acts that caused the distress cues (i.e. moral transgressions; e.g. one person hitting another) (Blair 1995). Through association these representations of moral transgressions become triggers for the mechanism. The appropriately developing child thus initially finds the pain of others aversive and then, through socialization, thoughts of acts that cause pain to others aversive also. It is proposed that psychopathic individuals have had disruption to this system such that representations of acts that cause harm to others do not become triggers for the VIM (Blair 1995).

One early index of appropriate moral socialization, and thus the developmental integrity of the VIM, is the demonstration by the child of the moral/conventional distinction. From the age of 3.5 years, children distinguish in their judgements between moral (victim-based) and conventional (social-disorder-based) transgressions; see Smetana (1993). Crucially for the model (Blair 1995), normally developing children best discriminate in their judgements between two types of transgressions when they are asked to imagine situations where there are no rules prohibiting the transgressions. In contrast, adults with psychopathy and children with psychopathic tendencies are least likely to make a discrimination under these conditions (Blair 1995, 1997; Blair et al. 1995a; see also Nucci and Herman (1982) and Arsenio and Fleiss (1996) for similar work with children with behaviour disorder and conduct

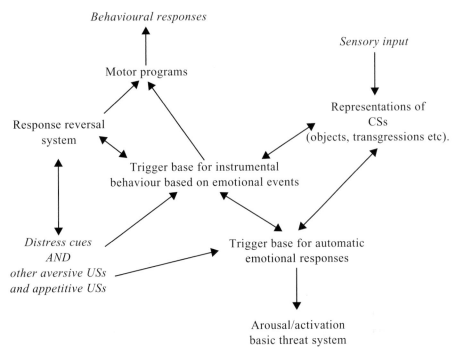

Figure 18.1 The revised violence inhibition mechanism model. CS, conditioned stimulus; US, unconditioned stimulus.

disorder). In addition, and in line with the VIM position, psychopathic adults show reduced comprehension of situations likely to induce guilt although they show appropriate comprehension of happiness, sadness and even complex emotions such as embarrassment (Blair et al. 1995*b*). Finally, and a direct prediction of the model, psychopathic adults and children with psychopathic tendencies show reduced autonomic activity to the sadness and fear of others (House and Milligan 1976; Aniskiewicz 1979; Blair et al. 1997; Blair 1999).

However, while the original VIM model could provide an account of the emergence of instrumental antisocial behaviour in psychopathic individuals and while it did generate a variety of predictions that have been empirically confirmed, it faced a serious difficulty; it could not account for the data associated with the response set modulation and fear hypotheses. This has resulted in an expansion of the model at both the cognitive and neural levels as is illustrated in Figure 18.1.

The first difference between this new model and the previous formulation of the VIM theory is that two trigger databases are specified. The second difference is that the new model makes more reference to a putative anatomical substrate. Following the work of Killcross et al. (1997) (see also Chapter 15 by Killcross), a distinction is made between a trigger base for reflexive, automatic responses to conditioned stimuli and a trigger base for instrumental behaviour based on emotional events. It is this second trigger base that allows the activation of motor programmes. Again following Killcross et al. (1997), these trigger databases are attributed to the central and basolateral nuclei of the amygdala respectively. Through association, pairings of the activation of representations of conditioned stimuli held in temporal cortex with activation by the unconditioned stimuli of aversive and appetitive unconditioned stimuli (including sad faces) will result in the conditioned stimuli activating the autonomic nervous system and a basic threat-response system mediated by the brainstem. In addition, reinforcement/punishment of actions from the trigger base for instrumental behaviour will increase/decrease the probability of these actions occurring in the future.

It is suggested that psychopathy is due to amygdala dysfunction. Certainly, psychopathic individuals show impaired performance on tasks in which the central nucleus of the amygdala is implicated. Thus, animal studies have implicated the central nucleus of the amygdala in aversive conditioning (Killcross et al. 1997; Davis 2000). Patients with amygdala lesions show impaired aversive conditioning (Bechara et al. 1995; LaBar et al. 1995) as do psychopathic individuals (Lykken 1957). Moreover, in a recent neuro-imaging study, amygdala activation has been reported to stimuli that anticipated shock (though no shock was given) (Phelps et al. 2001). Psychopathic individuals have been found to show reduced electrodermal responses when anticipating shock (Hare 1965, 1982; Hare et al. 1978; Ogloff and Wong 1990). Finally, the central nucleus of the amygdala has been implicated in the augmentation of the startle response by threat primes (Davis 2000). Patients with amygdala lesions show reduced augmentation by threat primes (Angrilli et al. 1996) as do psychopathic individuals (Patrick et al. 1993; Levenston et al. 2000).

There is also suggestion that psychopathic individuals show impaired performance on tasks in which the basolateral nucleus of the amygdala is implicated. Thus, the basolateral nucleus of the amygdala has been implicated in instrumental learning (Killcross et al. 1997; Davis 2000) and there is preliminary work with patients with amygdala lesions and psychopathic individuals showing impairments in instrumental learning (Fine 2000). Moreover, there is considerable work implicating the basolateral nucleus of the amygdala in passive avoidance learning (Ambrogi Lorenzini et al. 1999). As noted above, psychopathic individuals show pronounced impairments on passive avoidance tasks (Newman and Kosson 1986; Newman and Schmitt 1998).

The role of the amygdala in processing the expressions of others is currently under debate. It is less frequently believed that the amygdala plays a role in processing only fearful expressions though an impairment in the recognition of fearful expressions is the most common expression-processing abnormality found in patients with amygdala lesions (see, for a review, Fine and Blair 2000; see also Adolphs et al. 1999). Moreover, functional-imaging studies have shown that the amygdala is activated by fearful expressions (Morris et al. 1996; Phillips et al. 1997). Recently, Rapczak et al. (2000) reported that they could find no indications of disproportionate impairments for fearful expressions in their 13 patients with amygdala lesions. However, it is worth noting that of these 13 patients, 11 had had unilateral temporal lobectomy and the other 2 had had herpes encephalitis; i.e. their lesions were extensive and included structures external to the amygdala. It is thus perhaps unsurprising that this study found little evidence of selective impairment.

It has been suggested that the amygdala is part of a general neural system for recognizing emotions that signal potential harm to the organism, i.e. fear and anger (Adolphs et al. 1999). The major problem for this theory is that reports of impairments in processing sad expressions in patients with amygdala lesions are at least as common as reports of patients with amygdala lesions being impaired in processing angry expressions (Fine and Blair 2000). Moreover, and crucially, angry expressions have not been found to activate the amygdala in neuro-imaging studies (Sprengelmeyer et al. 1998; Whalen et al. 1998; Blair et al. 1999).

An alternative position, and the one favoured here, is developed from the work on the amygdala's role in emotional associative learning (Davis 2000; Everitt et al. 2000; LeDoux 2000). The suggestion is that the amygdala is crucially involved in processing those expressions that act as social unconditioned stimuli, i.e. fearful and sad expressions (Blair et al. 1999). In line with this position both fearful and sad expressions have been found to activate the amygdala in neuro-imaging studies (Schneider et al. 1995; Morris et al. 1996; Phillips et al. 1997; Blair et al. 1999). However, it should be noted that patients with amygdala lesions frequently do not show impairment in processing sad expressions. Indeed, in a recent review, only 6 of 13 patients with amygdala lesions presented with impairment for sad expressions while 10 of 13 presented with impairment for fearful expressions (Fine and Blair 2000). Of course, this may be due to the relative ease with which sad expressions can be recognized (Ekman and Friesen 1976).

As regards psychopathy, children with psychopathic tendencies show impairment when processing sadness and fearfulness but not when processing expressions of anger, disgust, happiness or surprise (Blair et al. 2001a; Blair and Coles, in press; Stevens et al., in press). Interestingly, adult psychopathic individuals show a pattern of impairment more similar to patients with amygdala lesions. For adult psychopathic individuals, recognition of sad expressions appears to be too easy and thus while they may show reduced autonomic activity to this expression (House and Milligan 1976; Aniskiewicz 1979; Blair et al. 1997; Blair 1999), they only show an expression recognition impairment for fearful expressions (Blair et al., submitted). In addition, children and adults with psychopathy show selective impairments when processing sad and fearful affect in vocal tones. Neuro-imaging results have implicated the amygdala in the response to, at least, fearful vocal affect (Phillips et al. 1998; Morris et al. 1999) although the neuropsychological literature has been less consistent (Scott et al. 1997; Anderson and Phelps 1998).

In Figure 18.1, the connections from the trigger bases to the representations of the conditioned stimuli are shown as reciprocal, in line with suggestions that amygdala activation strengthens the activity of the representations that have activated the amygdala; i.e. increasing 'attention' to these representations. Thus, the activation of the representations of emotional words (e.g. murder) may be boosted by the reciprocal interactions with the amygdala if these words have become conditioned stimuli for amygdala activity. In lexical decision tasks where the participant has to decide whether a letter string is a word or not, participants are faster to respond that emotional words are words than to respond that neutral words are words (Graves et al. 1981; Strauss 1983). This is potentially because of the emotional words' increased salience due to activation from the amygdala. Interestingly, psychopathic individuals fail to show any reaction-time differential between neutral and emotional words (Williamson et al. 1991).

The third and final difference between this new model and the previous formulation of the VIM position is that connections with other systems are considered; in particular, systems allowing response reversal following changes in contingency. The interconnections between the basolateral nucleus of the amygdala and orbitofrontal cortex have a critical role in encoding and using associative information about the motivational significance of stimuli (Schoenbaum et al. 1998, 2000; Gallagher et al. 1999). Within this circuit, the amygdala has a critical role in forming associations between unconditioned and conditioned stimuli and between conditioned stimuli (Killcross et al. 1997; Schoenbaum et al. 1998; Davis 2000). Orbitofrontal cortex encodes the motivational significance of the cues and the incentive value of expected outcomes (Thorpe et al. 1983; Gallagher et al. 1999; Schoenbaum et al. 2000). Orbitofrontal cortex acts a system for response reversal when the incentive value of expected outcomes differs from actual outcomes and alters behaviour. But both the basolateral amygdala and orbitofrontal cortex are involved in encoding the value of a stimulus, and lesions to either system impair reversals in responding following changes in the value of reinforcement (Hatfield et al. 1996; Rolls 1997; Gallagher et al. 1999). Indeed, both amygdala and orbitofrontal cortex dysfunction have been found to result in poor performance on the gambling task (Bechara et al. 1999). In this task, the participant must reverse their responses away from the two packs giving high reward in favour of the two packs giving lower reward, as the high reward packs also supply higher levels of punishment. In line with the suggestion of amygdala dysfunction in psychopathic individuals, both children with psychopathic tendencies and adult psychopaths show impairment on this task (Blair et al. 2001b); though, it should be noted that Schmitt et al. (1999)

found that adult psychopaths did not show impairment on this task but this may be due to their different task instructions. Failure in this system may also be the reason that children with psychopathic tendencies and adult psychopathic individuals continue to play cards on the one-pack card-playing task despite the escalating increase in punishment levels (Newman et al. 1987; Shapiro et al. 1988; O'Brien and Frick 1996; Fisher and Blair 1998).

It is interesting to note, however, that the impairment shown by adult psychopathic individuals on Bechara's gambling task is considerably greater than that shown by children with psychopathic tendencies. Moreover, on simpler response-reversal tasks, where the contingencies change from always-rewarded for the response to always-punished, although adult psychopathic individuals show impairment (LaPierre et al. 1995), children with psychopathic tendencies do not (Blair et al. 2001*b*). This suggests that the impairment in this system is more pronounced in adult psychopaths than in children with psychopathic tendencies. Children with psychopathic tendencies may be able to weakly represent the incentive value of expected outcomes and thus fail only those tasks where the contingency change is very subtle. In contrast, adult psychopaths may have very limited ability to represent the incentive value of expected outcomes and thus fail even those tasks where the contingency change is abrupt. Why should there be this difference between children with psychopathic tendencies and adult psychopaths? It may reflect gradual degeneration of the circuit connecting the amygdala and orbitofrontal across development as documented by Bachevalier and colleagues (Bachevalier 1994). Alternatively, it may reflect the lifestyle of adult psychopathic individuals, where substance abuse is very common (Hare 1991). Amphetamine drug use has been associated with orbitofrontal cortex dysfunction (Rogers and Robbins 2001) (see also Chapter 20 by Rogers and Robbins).

Conclusions

In this chapter, I have developed a neurocognitive model of psychopathy that is capable of integrating the data obtained from the response set modulation, fear theories and violence inhibition mechanism model. This model assumes a fundamental deficit within the amygdala that is responsible for the individual's failure to be concerned by his or her victims and their lack of moral socialization. In addition, it is assumed that during development increased dysfunction may be seen in related systems.

Acknowledgements

This work was supported by the Medical Research Council (ref. G9716841) and Department of Health (VISPED initiative).

REFERENCES

Adolphs R, Tranel D, Young AW et al. (1999). Recognition of facial emotion in nine individuals with bilateral amygdala damage. *Neuropsychologia*, 37, 1111–17.

Ambrogi Lorenzini CG, Baldi E, Bucherelli C, Sacchetti B and Tassoni G (1999). Neural topography and chronology of memory consolidation: a review of functional inactivation findings. *Neurobiol Learn Mem*, 71, 1–18.

American Psychiatric Association (1994). *Diagnostic and Statistical Manual of Mental Disorders*, 4th edn (DSM–IV). Washington, DC: APA.

Anderson AK and Phelps EA (1998). Intact recognition of vocal expressions of fear following bilateral lesions of the human amygdala. *Neuroreport*, 9, 3607–16.

Anderson SW, Bechara A, Damasio H, Tranel D and Damasio AR (1999). Impairment of social and moral behavior related to early damage in human prefrontal cortex. *Nat Neurosci*, 2, 1032–7.

Angrilli A, Mauri A, Palomba D et al. (1996). Startle reflex and emotion modulation impairment after a right amygdala lesion. *Brain*, 119, 1991–2000.

Aniskiewicz AS (1979). Autonomic components of vicarious conditioning and psychopathy. *J Clin Psychol*, 35, 60–7.

Arsenio WF and Fleiss K (1996). Typical and behaviourally disruptive children's understanding of the emotion consequences of socio-moral events. *Br J Dev Psychol*, 14, 173–86.

Bachevalier J (1994). Medial temporal lobe structures and autism: a review of clinical and experimental findings. *Neuropsychologia*, 32, 627–48.

Baddeley A and Della Sala S (1998). Working memory and executive controls. In *The Prefrontal Cortex*, ed. AC Roberts, TW Robbins and L Weiskrantz, pp. 9–21. New York: Oxford University Press.

Barratt ES (1994). Impulsiveness and aggression. In *Violence and Mental Disorders: Developments in Risk Assessment*, ed. J Monahan and H Steadman, pp. 61–79. Chicago: University of Chicago Press.

Baumrind D (1971). Current patterns of parental authority. *Dev Psychol Monogr*, 94, 132–42.

Baumrind D (1983). Rejoinder to Lewis's interpretation of parental firm control effects: are authoritative families really harmonious? *Psychol Bull*, 94, 132–42.

Bechara A, Tranel D, Damasio H, Adolphs R, Rockland C and Damasio AR (1995). Double dissociation of conditioning and declarative knowledge relative to the amygdala and hippocampus in humans. *Science*, 269, 1115–18.

Bechara A, Damasio H, Damasio AR and Lee GP (1999). Different contributions of the human amygdala and ventromedial prefrontal cortex to decision-making. *J Neurosci*, 19, 5473–81.

Berkowitz L (1993). *Aggression: Its Causes, Consequences, and Control.* Philadelphia: Temple University Press.

Blackburn R (1988). Psychopathy and personality disorder. In *Adult Abnormal Psychology*, ed. E Miller and PJ Cooper, pp. 218–44. Edinburgh: Churchill Livingstone.

Blair RJR (1995). A cognitive developmental approach to morality: investigating the psychopath. *Cognition*, 57, 1–29.

Blair RJR (1997). Moral reasoning in the child with psychopathic tendencies. *Pers Ind Diff*, 22, 731–9.

Blair RJR (1999). Responsiveness to distress cues in the child with psychopathic tendencies. *Pers Ind Diff*, 27, 135–45.

Blair RJR (2001). Neuro-cognitive models of aggression, the antisocial personality disorders, and psychopathy. *J Neurol Neurosurg Psychiatry*, 71, 727–31.

Blair RJR and Cipolotti L (2000). Impaired social response reversal: a case of "acquired sociopathy". *Brain*, 123, 1122–41.

Blair RJR and Coles M (2001). Expression recognition and behavioral problems in early adolescence. *Cognit Dev*, 15, 421–34.

Blair RJR and Morton J (1995). Putting cognition into sociopathy. *Brain Behav Sci*, 18, 548.

Blair RJR, Jones L, Clark F and Smith M (1995*a*). Is the psychopath "morally insane"? *Pers Ind Diff*, 19, 741–52.

Blair RJR, Sellars C, Strickland I et al. (1995*b*). Emotion attributions in the psychopath. *Pers Ind Diff*, 19, 431–7.

Blair RJR, Jones L, Clark F and Smith M (1997). The psychopathic individual: a lack of responsiveness to distress cues? *Psychophysiology*, 34, 192–8.

Blair RJR, Morris JS, Frith CD, Perrett DI and Dolan R (1999). Dissociable neural responses to facial expressions of sadness and anger. *Brain*, 122, 883–93.

Blair RJR, Colledge E, Murray L and Mitchell DG (2001*a*). A selective impairment in the processing of sad and fearful expressions in children with psychopathic tendencies. *J Abnorm Child Psychol*, 29, 491–8.

Blair RJR, Colledge E and Mitchell DG (2001*b*). Somatic markers and response reversal: is there orbitofrontal cortex dysfunction in boys with psychopathic tendencies? *J Abnorm Child Psychol*, 29, 499–511.

Brody GH and Shaffer DR (1982). Contributions of parents and peers to children's moral socialization. *Dev Rev*, 2, 31–75.

Burgess PW, Alderman N, Evans J, Emslie H and Wilson BA (1998). The ecological validity of tests of executive function. *J Int Neuropsychol Soc*, 4, 547–58.

Camras LA (1977). Facial expressions used by children in a conflict situation. *Child Dev*, 48, 1431–5.

Chaplin TC, Rice ME and Harris GT (1995). Salient victim suffering and the sexual responses of child molesters. *J Consult Clin Psychol*, 63, 249–55.

Cleckley H (1976). *The Mask of Sanity*. St Louis, MO: Mosby.

Cornell DG, Warren J, Hawk G, Stafford E, Oram G and Pine D (1996). Psychopathy in instrumental and reactive violent offenders. *J Consult Clin Psychol*, 64, 783–90.

Damasio AR (1994). *Descartes' Error: Emotion, Rationality and the Human Brain*. New York: Putnam (Grosset Books).

Damasio AR, Tranel D and Damasio HC (1991). Somatic markers and the guidance of behavior: theory and preliminary testing. In *Frontal Lobe Function and Dysfunction*, ed. HS Levin, HM Eisenberg and AL Benton, pp. 217–29. New York: Oxford University Press.

Davis M (2000). The role of the amygdala in conditioned and unconditioned fear and anxiety. In *The Amygdala: A Functional Analysis*, ed. JP Aggleton, pp. 289–310. Oxford: Oxford University Press.

Duncan J (1986). Disorganisation of behavior after frontal lobe damage. *Cognit Neuropsychol*, 3, 271–90.

Eibl-Eibesfeldt I (1970). *Ethology: The Biology of Behavior*. New York: Holt, Rinehart and Winston.

Ekman P and Friesen WV (1976). *Pictures of Facial Affect*. Palo Alto: Consulting Psychologists Press.

Elliot FA (1978). Neurological aspects of antisocial behavior. In *The Psychopath*, ed. WH Reid. New York: Bruner/Mazel.

Eslinger PJ and Damasio AR (1985). Severe disturbance of higher cognition after bilateral frontal lobe ablation: patient EVR. *Neurology*, 35, 1731–41.

Everitt BJ, Cardinal RN, Hall J, Parkinson JA and Robbins TW (2000). Differential involvement of amygdala subsystems in appetitive conditioning and drug addiction. In *The Amygdala: A Functional Analysis*, ed. JP Aggleton, pp. 289–310. Oxford: Oxford University Press.

Eysenck HJ (1964). *Crime and Personality*. London: Routledge and Kegan Paul.

Fine C (2000). *Expectation Violations and Emotional Learning*. London: University College London.

Fine C and Blair RJR (2000). Mini review: the cognitive and emotional effects of amygdala damage. *Neurocase*, 6, 435–50.

Fisher L and Blair RJR (1998). Cognitive impairment and its relationship to psychopathic tendencies in children with emotional and behavioural difficulties. *J Abnorm Child Psychol*, 26, 511–19.

Fowles DC (1988). Psychophysiology and psychopathy: a motivational approach. *Psychophysiology*, 25, 373–91.

Frick PJ and Hare RD (in press). *The Psychopathy Screening Device*. Toronto: Multi-Health Systems.

Frick PJ, O'Brien BS, Wootton JM and McBurnett K (1994). Psychopathy and conduct problems in children. *J Abnorm Psychol*, 103, 700–7.

Fuster JM (1980). *The Prefrontal Cortex*. New York: Raven Press.

Gallagher M, McMahan RW and Schoenbaum G (1999). Orbitofrontal cortex and representation of incentive value in associative learning. *J Neurosci*, 19, 6610–14.

Gernsbacher MA and Faust ME (1991). The mechanism of suppression: a component of general comprehension skill. *J Exp Psychol Learn Memory Cognit*, 17, 245–62.

Gorenstein EE (1982). Frontal lobe functions in psychopaths. *J Abnorm Psychol*, 91, 368–79.

Gorenstein EE and Newman JP (1980). Disinhibitory psychopathology: a new perspective and a model for research. *Psychol Rev*, 37, 301–15.

Grafman J, Schwab K, Warden D, Pridgen BS and Brown HR (1996). Frontal lobe injuries, violence, and aggression: a report of the Vietnam head injury study. *Neurology*, 46, 1231–8.

Graves R, Landis T and Goodglass H (1981). Laterality and sex differences for visual recognition of emotional and non-emotional words. *Neuropsychologia*, 19, 95–102.

Gray JA (1971). *The Psychology of Fear and Stress*. London: Weidenfeld and Nicolson.

Gray JA (1987). *The Psychology of Fear and Stress*, 2nd edn. Cambridge: University of Cambridge Press.

Hare RD (1965). Temporal gradient of fear arousal in psychopaths. *J Abnorm Psychol*, 70, 442–5.

Hare RD (1978). Electrodermal and cardiovascular correlates of psychopathy. In *Psychopathic Behavior: Approaches to Research*, ed. RD Hare and D Schalling, pp. 107–43. Chichester: John Wiley and Sons.

Hare RD (1982). Psychopathy and physiological activity during anticipation of an aversive stimulus in a distraction paradigm. *Psychophysiology*, 19, 266–71.

Hare RD (1991). *The Hare Psychopathy Checklist–Revised*. Toronto, Ontario: Multi-Health Systems.

Hare RD (1998). Psychopathy, affect and behavior. In *Psychopathy: Theory, Research and Implications for Society*, ed. DJ Cooke, AE Forth and RD Hare, pp. 81–105. Dordrecht: Kluwer Academic Publishers.

Hare RD, Frazelle J and Cox DN (1978). Psychopathy and physiological responses to threat of an aversive stimulus. *Psychophysiology*, 15, 165–72.

Hare RD, Hart SD and Harpur TJ (1991). Psychopathy and the DSM–IV criteria for antisocial personality disorder. *J Abnorm Psychol*, 100, 391–8.

Harpur TJ and Hare RD (1994). Assessment of psychopathy as a function of age. *J Abnorm Psychol*, 103, 604–9.

Harpur TJ, Hare RD and Hakstian AR (1989). Two-factor conceptualization of psychopathy: construct validity and assessment implications. *Psychol Assess J Consult Clin Psychol*, 1, 6–17.

Hart SD, Forth AE and Hare RD (1990). Performance of criminal psychopaths on selected neuropsychological tests. *J Abnorm Psychol*, 99, 374–9.

Hatfield T, Han JS, Conley M, Gallagher M and Holland P (1996). Neurotoxic lesions of basolateral, but not central, amygdala interfere with Pavlovian second-order conditioning and reinforcer devaluation effects. *J Neurosci*, 16, 5256–65.

Hoffman ML (1988). Moral development. In *Developmental Psychology: An Advanced Textbook*, ed. M Bornstein and M Lamb, pp. 497–548. Hillsdale, NJ: Lawrence Erlbaum Associates.

Hoffman ML (1994). Discipline and internalisation. *Dev Psychol*, 30, 26–8.

Hoffman ML and Saltzstein HD (1967). Parent discipline and the child's moral development. *J Pers Social Psychol*, 5, 45–57.

House TH and Milligan WL (1976). Autonomic responses to modeled distress in prison psychopaths. *J Pers Social Psychol*, 34, 556–60.

Johns JH and Quay HC (1962). The effect of social reward on verbal conditioning in psychopathic and neurotic military offenders. *J Consult Clin Psychol*, 26, 217–20.

Kandel E and Freed D (1989). Frontal lobe dysfunction and antisocial behavior: a review. *J Clin Psychol*, 45, 404–13.

Killcross S, Robbins TW and Everitt BJ (1997). Different types of fear-conditioned behavior mediated by separate nuclei within amygdala. *Nature*, 388, 377–80.

Krakowski M, Czobor P, Carpenter MD et al. (1997). Community violence and inpatient assaults: neurobiological deficits. *J Neuropsychiatry Clin Neurosci*, 9, 549–55.

LaBar KS, LeDoux JE, Spencer DD and Phelps EA (1995). Impaired fear conditioning following unilateral temporal lobectomy in humans. *J Neurosci*, 15, 6846–55.

LaPierre D, Braun CMJ and Hodgins S (1995). Ventral frontal deficits in psychopathy: neuropsychological test findings. *Neuropsychologia*, 33, 139–51.

LeDoux J (2000). The amygdala and emotion: a view through fear. In *The Amygdala: A Functional Analysis*, ed. JP Aggleton, pp. 289–310. Oxford: Oxford University Press.

Levenston GK, Patrick CJ, Bradley MM and Lang PJ (2000). The psychopath as observer: emotion and attention in picture processing. *J Abnorm Psychol*, 109, 373–86.

Lorenz K (1966). *On Aggression*. New York: Harcourt Brace Jovanovich.

Luria A (1966). *Higher Cortical Functions in Man*. New York: Basic Books.

Lykken DT (1957). A study of anxiety in the sociopathic personality. *J Abnorm Social Psychol*, 55, 6–10.

Mealey L (1995). The sociobiology of sociopathy: an integrated evolutionary model. *Behav Brain Sci*, 18, 523–99.

Moffitt TE (1993*a*). Adolescence-limited and life-course-persistent antisocial behavior: a developmental taxonomy. *Psychol Rev*, 100, 674–701.

Moffitt TE (1993*b*). The neuropsychology of conduct disorder. *Dev Psychopathol*, 5, 135–52.

Morgan AB and Lilienfeld SO (2000). A meta-analytic review of the relation between antisocial behavior and neuropsychological measures of executive function. *Clin Psychol Rev*, 20, 113–36.

Morris JS, Frith CD, Perrett DI et al. (1996). A differential response in the human amygdala to fearful and happy facial expressions. *Nature*, 383, 812–15.

Morris JS, Scott SK and Dolan RJ (1999). Saying it with feeling: neural responses to emotional vocalizations. *Neuropsychologia*, 37, 1155–63.

Newman JP (1998). Psychopathic behaviour: an information processing perspective. In *Psychopathy: Theory, Research and Implications for Society*, ed. DJ Cooke, AE Forth and RD Hare, pp. 81–105. Dordrecht: Kluwer Academic Publishers.

Newman JP and Kosson DS (1986). Passive avoidance learning in psychopathic and nonpsychopathic offenders. *J Abnorm Psychol*, 95, 252–6.

Newman JP and Schmitt WA (1998). Passive avoidance in psychopathic offenders: a replication and extension. *J Abnorm Psychol*, 107, 527–32.

Newman JP, Patterson CM and Kosson DS (1987). Response perseveration in psychopaths. *J Abnorm Psychol*, 96, 145–8.

Newman JP, Schmitt WA and Voss WD (1997). The impact of motivationally neutral cues on psychopathic individuals: assessing the generality of the response modulation hypothesis. *J Abnorm Psychol*, 106, 563–75.

Nucci LP and Herman S (1982). Behavioral disordered children's conceptions of moral, conventional, and personal issues. *J Abnorm Child Psychol*, 10, 411–25.

O'Brien BS and Frick PJ (1996). Reward dominance: associations with anxiety, conduct problems, and psychopathy in children. *J Abnorm Child Psychol*, 24, 223–40.

Ogloff JR and Wong S (1990). Electrodermal and cardiovascular evidence of a coping response in psychopaths. *Crimin Justice Behav*, 17, 231–45.

Patrick CJ (1994). Emotion and psychopathy: startling new insights. *Psychophysiology*, 31, 319–30.

Patrick CJ, Bradley MM and Lang PJ (1993). Emotion in the criminal psychopath: startle reflex modulation. *J Abnorm Psychol*, 102, 82–92.

Patrick CJ, Cuthbert BN and Lang PJ (1994). Emotion in the criminal psychopath: fear image processing. *J Abnorm Psychol*, 103, 523–34.

Patterson CM and Newman JP (1993). Reflectivity and learning from aversive events: toward a psychological mechanism for the syndromes of disinhibition. *Psychol Rev*, 100, 716–36.

Perry DG and Perry LC (1974). Denial of suffering in the victim as a stimulus to violence in aggressive boys. *Child Dev*, 45, 55–62.

Phelps EA, O'Connor KJ, Gatenby JC, Gore JC, Grillon C and Davis M (2001). Activation of the left amygdala to a cognitive representation of fear. *Nat Neurosci*, 4, 437–41.

Phillips ML, Young AW, Senior C et al. (1997). A specified neural substrate for perceiving facial expressions of disgust. *Nature*, 389, 495–8.

Phillips ML, Young AW, Scott SK et al. (1998). Neural responses to facial and vocal expressions of fear and disgust. *Proc R Soc Lond Biol Sci* 265, 1809–17.

Prather MD, Lavenex P, Mauldin-Jourdain ML et al. (2001). Increased social fear and decreased fear of objects in monkeys with neonatal amygdala lesions. *Neuroscience*, 106, 653–8.

Raine A, Buchsbaum MS, Stanley J, Lottenberg S, Abel L and Stoddard J (1994). Selective reductions in prefrontal glucose metabolism in murderers. *Biol Psychiatry*, 15, 365–73.

Raine A, Lencz T, Bihrle S, LaCasse L and Colletti P (2000). Reduced prefrontal gray matter volume and reduced autonomic activity in antisocial personality disorder. *Arch Gen Psychiatry*, 57, 119–27.

Rapcsak SZ, Galper SR, Comer JF et al. (2000). Fear recognition deficits after focal brain damage: a cautionary note. *Neurology*, 54, 575–81.

Roberts AC, Robbins TW and Weiskrantz L (1998). *The Prefrontal Cortex: Executive and Cognitive Functions.* Oxford: Oxford University Press.

Rogers RD and Robbins TW (2001). Investigating the neurocognitive deficits associated with chronic drug misuse. *Curr Opin Neurobiol*, 11, 250–7.

Rolls ET (1997). The orbitofrontal cortex. *Philos Trans R Soc, B* 351, 1433–43.

Schalling D (1978). Psychopathy-related personality variables and the psychophysiology of socialization. In *Psychopathic Behavior: Approaches to Research*, ed. RD Hare and D Schalling, pp. 85–106. Chichester: John Wiley and Sons.

Schmitt WA, Brinkley CA and Newman JP (1999). Testing Damasio's somatic marker hypothesis with psychopathic individuals: risk takers or risk averse? *J Abnorm Psychol*, 108, 538–43.

Schneider F, Gur RE, Mozley LH et al. (1995). Mood effects on limbic blood flow correlate with emotional self-rating: a PET study of oxygen-15 labeled water. *Psychiatry Res: Neuroimag*, 61, 265–83.

Schoenbaum G, Chiba AA and Gallagher M (1998). Orbitofrontal cortex and basolateral amygdala encode expected outcomes during learning. *Nat Neurosci*, 1, 155–9.

Schoenbaum G, Chiba AA and Gallagher M (2000). Changes in functional connectivity in orbitofrontal cortex and basolateral amygdala during learning and reversal training. *J Neurosci*, 20, 5179–89.

Scott SK, Young AW, Calder AJ, Hellawell DH, Aggleton JP and Johnson M (1997). Impaired auditory recognition of fear and anger following bilateral amygdala lesions. *Nature*, 385, 254–7.

Seguin JR, Boulerice B, Harden PW, Tremblay RE and Pihl RO (1999). Executive functions and physical aggression after controlling for attention deficit hyperactivity disorder, general memory, and IQ. *J Child Psychol Psychiatry*, 40, 1197–208.

Shallice T (1988). *From Neuropsychology to Mental Structure.* Cambridge: Cambridge University Press.

Shapiro SK, Quay HC, Hogan AE and Schwartz KP (1988). Response perseveration and delayed responding in undersocialised aggressive conduct disorder. *J Abnorm Psychol*, 97, 371–3.

Smetana JG (1993). Understanding of social rules. In *The Child as Psychologist: An Introduction to the Development of Social Cognition*, ed. M Bennett, pp. 111–41. New York: Harvester Wheatsheaf.

Sprengelmeyer R, Rausch M, Eysel UT and Przuntek H (1998). Neural structures associated with the recognition of facial basic emotions. *Proc R Soc Lond B*, 265, 1927–31.

Stevens D, Charman T and Blair RJR (in press). Recognition of emotion in facial expressions and vocal tones in children with psychopathic tendencies. *J Genet Psychol*.

Strauss E (1983). Perception of emotional words. *Neuropsychologia*, 21, 99–103.

Thorpe SJ, Rolls ET and Maddison S (1983). The orbitofrontal cortex: neuronal activity in the behaving monkey. *Exp Brain Res*, 49, 93–115.

Tranel D and Damasio H (1994). Neuroanatomical correlates of electrodermal skin conductance responses. *Psychophysiology*, 31, 427–38.

Trasler G (1978). In *Psychopathic Behavior: Approaches to Research*, ed. RD Hare and D Schalling. Chichester: John Wiley and Sons.

Volkow ND and Tancredi L (1987). Neural substrates of violent behavior. A preliminary study with positron emission tomography. *Br J Psychiatry*, 151, 668–73.

Whalen PJ, Shin LM, McInerney SC and Rauch SL (1998). Greater fMRI activation to fearful vs. angry expressions in the amygdaloid region. *Neurosci Abstr*, 24, 692.

Williamson S, Hare RD and Wong S (1987). Violence: criminal psychopaths and their victims. *Can J Behav Sci*, 19, 454–62.

Williamson S, Harpur TJ and Hare RD (1991). Abnormal processing of affective words by psychopaths. *Psychophysiology*, 28, 260–73.

Part IX

Drug use and abuse

19

The contribution of genetically manipulated animals to the study of stimulant and alcohol addiction

David N Stephens, Andy N Mead and Tamzin L Ripley

University of Sussex, Falmer, UK

Introduction

As in other areas of biology, behavioural neuroscience has been revolutionized in the past decade by advances in genomics. The sequencing of the human genome, as well as those of the mouse and of invertebrate species, has opened the prospect of understanding the extent to which psychiatric conditions depend upon variations in genetic makeup. At the same time, advances in genetic technology have made studies of functional genomics possible. The ability to manipulate the genetic makeup of organisms, such as the mouse, by specific targeting of mutations in selected genes has provided an impetus for behavioural scientists to match technical advances in genomics with technical developments of their own. The area of drug abuse and dependence has been among the beneficiaries of these developments. However, even after such a short period of experience, it has become clear that the new science of behavioural genomics not only offers opportunities, but also raises questions that are peculiar to the new field.

Knockouts and transgenics

Two basic techniques are used to generate mice with 'targeted mutations', either by deletion of the gene of interest (knockouts, 'null mutants' or -/-), or by inserting a novel gene or multiple copies of the gene of interest into the genome (transgenics). While the terms 'knockout' and 'transgenic' are sometimes used interchangeably when referring to genetically engineered organisms, they do represent two distinctly different procedures, as illustrated in Figure 19.1, with separate problems resulting from the method used for their generation.

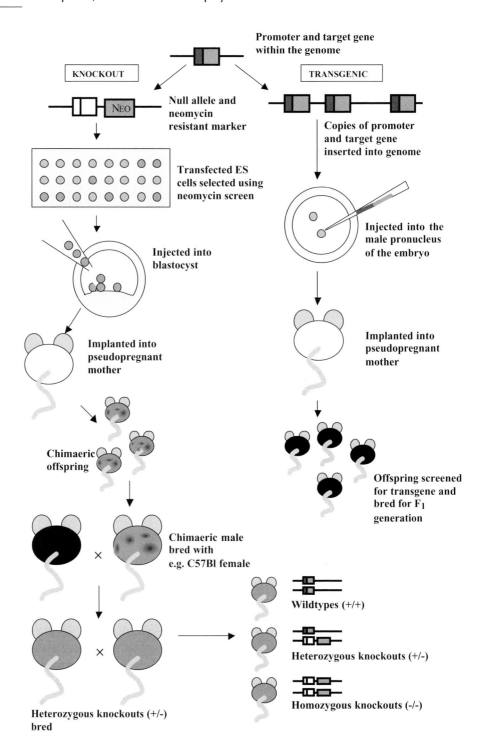

Transgenic mice are created by the insertion of foreign DNA into the host genome by a process of nonhomologous recombination. It is important to note that the foreign DNA sequence is inserted at random locations within the host genome, a process that may disrupt other genes. Thus, to be confident that any differences observed in the transgenic mice are due to the introduced DNA sequence, mice derived from a number of transgenic lines using the same construct should be tested. In addition, it is not possible to know how many copies of the gene have been inserted in the case of transgenic mice, and the number of copies can influence the level of expression of the gene product (Friend et al. 1992). Since the insertion of the transgene sequence into the mouse genome is not under the control of the experimenter, and in different replications of an experiment the transgene may be inserted at different loci within the genome, it may come under the control of different regulatory genes. Although this appears to be an unwelcome feature, it can be exploited in that in different progenitor lines, a particular transgene may be under the control of different promotors, and may thus be expressed in different cells and tissues, giving rise, potentially, to different behavioural effects.

Figure 19.1 Two basic techniques are used to generate mice with 'targeted mutations', either by deletion of the gene of interest (knockouts, 'null mutants' or -/-), or by inserting a novel gene or multiple copies of the gene of interest into the genome (transgenics).

Transgenic mice are created by the insertion of foreign DNA into the host genome by a process of nonhomologous recombination. The foreign DNA sequence is inserted at random locations, and in multiple copies within the host genome, a process that may disrupt other genes. Since the insertion of the transgene sequence into the mouse genome is not under the control of the experimenter, and in different replications of an experiment the transgene may be inserted at different loci within the genome, it may come under the control of different regulatory genes. The generation of knockout mice involves targeted insertion of foreign DNA into embryonic stem (ES) cells. DNA sequences of interest are then incorporated into the host genome by a process of homologous recombination, replacing the wildtype sequence. Since the foreign DNA sequence will not be incorporated into all blastocysts, the vector carrying the gene of interest also contains the genes for markers. The neo^r gene encodes an enzyme that provides resistance against the antibiotic neomycin. Thus, if ES cells that have been exposed to the vector are subsequently exposed to neomycin, only cells that have incorporated the neo^r gene (and thus, also the targeted gene to which it is linked) will survive. Using this technique, those ES cells in which homologous recombination of the foreign DNA has occurred can be selected, and subsequently injected into the blastocysts, before implantation into the uterus. In some cases, the mutated stem cells will develop into germ cells, and the resultant offspring can then be identified, and used to breed lines of knockout mice. The fact that the gene insertion is targeted to a specific location allows greater confidence in the specificity of the mutation, concerning both location and number of gene copies.

The generation of knockout mice involves targeted insertion of foreign DNA into embryonic stem (ES) cells. DNA sequences of interest are then incorporated into the host genome by a process of homologous recombination, replacing the wildtype sequence. Since the foreign DNA sequence will not be incorporated into all blastocysts, the vector carrying the gene of interest also contains the genes for markers, such as the *neo*[r] gene, and the *tk* gene. The *neo*[r] gene encodes an enzyme that provides resistance against the antibiotic neomycin, while the *tk* gene encodes thymidine kinase, which phosphorylates gancyclovir. Thus, if ES cells that have been exposed to the vector are subsequently exposed to neomycin, only cells that have incorporated the *neo*[r] gene (and thus, also the targeted gene to which it is linked) will survive. Similarly, if the *tk* gene is placed outside of the homologous regions of the endogenous and foreign DNA, only cells in which homologous recombination has occurred (therefore splicing out the *tk* gene) will survive exposure to gancyclovir. Using this technique, those ES cells in which homologous recombination of the foreign DNA has occurred can be selected, and subsequently injected into the blastocysts, before implantation into the uterus.

The term 'knockout' refers to a particular method of targeted mutation, whereby the endogenous gene is replaced or disrupted. Using a similar technique, it is also possible to insert multiple copies of the target gene, resulting in overexpression, or to introduce subtle disruptions (mutations) of the target gene (knock-ins). While both the transgenic and the knock-in methods will introduce foreign DNA into the genome, the knock-in method holds distinct advantages. The fact that the gene insertion is targeted to a specific location allows greater confidence in the specificity of the mutation, concerning both location and number of gene copies.

Nevertheless, the insertion of the neomycin cassette, essential for selecting stem cells, into the genome is not without effect, and may alter the expression of neighbouring genes. Frequently, families of functionally related genes are clustered at the chromosomal level (Homanics et al. 2000) and under the control of common transcription processes. Deletion of one member of the family, together with the associated insertion of the neomycin-resistant gene, may therefore disrupt the control of several genes with related functions, in addition to deleting the gene of interest (see discussion below on GABA$_A$ receptor α6 subunit function).

Opportunities offered by genetically manipulated animals

The ability to manipulate single genes offers a potentially powerful tool to neuroscientists. Although the technology required to produce such knockout animals is novel, the approach is not dissimilar to traditional behavioural pharmacological approaches to studying function. In behavioural pharmacology, a particular aspect of neuronal function is postulated to contribute to a behaviour of interest – for instance that the action of a neurotransmitter at a particular receptor is important in the ability of an animal to perform a behaviour. A drug is then chosen which is thought to interact specifically with the receptor to block the action of the neurotransmitter; the drug is administered, and its effects on the behaviour observed. Clearly, in order to test the function of a particular protein, an appropriate drug must be available. The first obvious advantage of the availability of knockout technology is that even if no such drug is available, the target can still be studied. A second advantage is that genetic manipulations of this sort are extremely specific; only the targeted protein is affected, whereas even so-called selective drugs are very likely indeed to interact with far more targets than the protein of interest, even if those other targets are not always known. Furthermore, since many of the hypotheses with which behavioural pharmacology interests itself derive from the use of drugs (which may have multiple targets), it is extremely useful to have a nondrug approach to testing the hypothesis. To the extent that knockout mice behave in the same way as mice treated with a drug acting as an antagonist or inhibitor of the protein do, then they provide independent support for a drug-derived hypothesis.

Problems of work with genetically manipulated animals

On the other hand, as with any type of manipulation, transgenic technology brings with it problems of interpretation. Some of these are addressed below. A more extensive account is provided by recent books by Crawley (2000) and by Crusio and Gerlai (1999).

Developmental

Since gene mutations are typically introduced at the single-cell or blastocyst stage of development, consideration must also be given to the consequences of development in the presence of the mutation. If the mutation affects a gene that normally plays a role in the development of the mouse, then there are likely to be consequences of the mutation on the subsequent behaviour and physiology of the adult mouse. It then becomes difficult to decide whether any behavioural consequences of the gene deletion are attributable to abnormal development, or to the absence of the gene product at the time the experimental manipulation is performed. Many neurotransmitter systems are involved not only in neuronal communication in the adult, but also in determining neuronal connectivity during development, so that mice in which neuronal signalling has been impaired may be wired differently from their wildtype controls. For instance, mice in which the gene for dopamine D2 receptors has been deleted show developmental changes in maturation of excitatory synapses in striatum, resulting in altered glutamatergic transmission in adulthood (Tang et al. 2001). Morphologically, a subpopulation of medium-sized spiny neurons from D2 receptor-deficient mice displays a decreased number of dendritic spines (on to which glutamatergic neurons synapse), compared with cells from wildtype mice (Cepeda et al. 2001). Such results provide evidence that D2 receptors not only are involved in dopaminergic synaptic transmission, but also play an important role in the regulation of glutamate receptor-mediated activity in the corticostriatal or thalamostriatal pathways.

Thus, if the administration of a drug to a D2 knockout mouse has different effects from its effect in the wildtype strain, it is not clear whether this is because dopaminergic transmission is impaired, or because the differences reflect the developmental effects of the gene deletion on glutamatergic transmission. If the behavioural phenotype of a neurotransmitter receptor knockout differs from the behaviour of a wildtype mouse administered a specific antagonist of the receptor, it is possible that the difference reflects differences in development of the knockout.

In the case of gene knockout mutations, there is also the possibility of other mechanisms compensating for the lack of the targeted gene. If protein A is deleted by genetic engineering, it is possible that protein B, which serves a similar function in the wildtype, may be overexpressed to compensate for the absence of protein A. Deletion of the dopamine transporter (DAT), which is responsible for clearing dopamine from the synapse, is thought to result in overexpression of the noradrenaline transporter (NAT) by dopamine neurons. Since NAT is also capable of transporting dopamine, some consequences of deleting DAT may be ameliorated by the compensatory overexpression of NAT (Carboni et al. 2001).

Genetic background

The genetic background of mutant mice is another factor that must be given careful consideration when planning studies. There are distinct behavioural and neurochemical differences between different inbred mouse strains and those in which mutations have been induced (Phillips et al. 1999), and the effect of a mutation can differ depending on which strain is used (see Gerlai 1996 for a review). For this reason, it is recommended that any mutation should be compared across several genetic backgrounds. While this is good advice, it is frequently impractical for a behavioural scientist to cross the mutation of interest into several background strains, so most studies are carried out using a single background strain.

In both knockout and transgenic mice, following the implantation of the fertilized egg (transgenic mice) or blastocyst (knockout mice), the resultant offspring are examined to detect the presence or absence of the gene of interest. Those that do possess the targeted gene construct will be heterozygous (containing one copy of the mutant gene and one copy of the wildtype gene). By mating of heterozygotes, mice homozygous for the mutation (containing two copies of the mutant gene) will be produced. In order to produce sufficient mice for experimental purposes, further breeding will be necessary. Breeding from heterozygote mice requires genotyping of the offspring since each litter will contain a mixture of homozygous mutants, homozygous wildtypes and heterozygous offspring. Discussion of genotyping is beyond the scope of this chapter, but is not trivial, or inexpensive, when considering the number of animals required for well-controlled behavioural experiments. Breeding from homozygous knockouts or transgenic animals is sometimes simpler, but raises several major issues. Sometimes the homozygous knockouts show poor reproductive success, ruling out this strategy. However, even if this is not an issue, repeated breeding of 'pure lines' of genetically manipulated and wildtype mice from a small population of progenitor animals can easily result in accidental incorporation of other genetic changes in one line but not the other (genetic drift), so that eventually the knockout and wildtype populations may differ in ways other than the targeted gene manipulation. Some experimenters avoid this issue by breeding only one generation from homozygous animals derived from F_1 breeding of heterozygote pairs, using the F_2 generation of knockouts and wildtypes for experiments. While this is very likely to avoid genetic drift, it must be considered that the genetic manipulation may give rise to alterations in mothering, so that any differences arising in the offspring may result from mutation-induced changes in the behaviour of the mother, rather than from direct effects of the gene on the behaviour of the offspring being studied. Since changes in mothering can have long-term effects on the adult behaviour of the offspring, this is as much an issue for those who use F_2 offspring for the experimental work as those who breed from homozygous lines.

In order to minimize the possibility of such confounds, homozygous mutant mice from the breeding of heterozygous mutants are best compared with wildtype mice from the same litter. However, particularly in behavioural studies, this is frequently not practical because of the large numbers of mice required to carry out systematic and well-controlled experiments. Breeding strategies have been suggested (Silva et al. 1997) to reduce the problems associated with background strains.

Inducible transgenic mice

Many of the problems of abnormal development resulting from genetic manipulation can be overcome using inducible transgenes. This technology utilizes the ability of the antibiotic, doxycycline, to inhibit the activity of a tetracycline transactivator (tTA) gene which drives the activity of a second transgene which encodes the protein of interest. By maintaining the genetically manipulated mice on a water supply containing low levels of doxycycline, production of the target protein is inhibited until a stage of development of interest, at which point the doxycycline is removed from the drinking water, allowing the second transgene to be expressed (see Self 1999). This is a particularly powerful tool, especially since it is possible to include a specific neuronal gene promotor, such as that for tyrosine hydroxylase (Min et al. 1996), in the cassette which is inserted into the mouse genome, so that activation of the target transgene can be made both tissue- and stage-of-development-specific.

Transgenic mice in addiction research

The availability of genetically manipulated mice has allowed behavioural neuro-scientists to test hypotheses on the molecular basis of drug action, frequently by deleting the gene for the molecular target at which the drug of abuse is thought to act. Sometimes, these studies have simply confirmed hypotheses derived from more conventional pharmacological techniques, though some interesting anomalies have been discovered. Foremost among these was the observation that mice in which the gene encoding the DAT had been deleted nevertheless continued to self-administer cocaine (Rocha et al. 1998*a*), and to show cocaine-conditioned place preference (Sora et al. 1998). These anomalies are discussed in more detail below.

A second approach has been the exploitation of genetically manipulated mice to study processes involved in receptor regulation. This approach has been particularly used in alcohol research (see below). Third, drug abuse depends on adaptive processes in the brain related on the one hand to learning, but also to the development of drug dependence. In this context, mutant mice have been exploited in research into the mechanisms of synaptic plasticity and learning in the context of drug abuse (Ripley et al. 1999).

Transgenic mice in psychostimulant research

A surprisingly limited number of studies have been carried out using genetically manipulated mice to study the neurobiological substrates of drug abuse. One of the most intensively studied is the DAT knockout (Giros et al. 1996), which Rocha et al. (1998*a*) reported to maintain cocaine self-administration, despite deletion of the presumed site of action of cocaine. This mouse provides an excellent example of many of the issues which complicate the interpretation of behavioural data from genetically manipulated mice.

DAT -/- mice display hyperactivity in both the home cage and a testing environment, accompanied by a greatly reduced rate of habituation (Giros et al. 1996; Sora et al. 1998; Gainetdinov et al. 1999). As a result, comparisons of psychostimulant effects on activity in wildtypes and knockouts have necessarily been from different baseline levels. The results of these studies have provided contrasting conclusions. Giros et al. (1996) and Sora et al. (1998) report a lack of effect of psychostimulants, consistent with the idea that DAT is an important site of action of these drugs.

However, others have reported a suppressant effect of psychostimulant treatment (Gainetdinov et al. 1999). At least in the first two of these studies, it is not clear whether the DAT knockout is actually insensitive to the stimulant properties of psychostimulants, or whether the hyperactivity of this mouse masks the stimulant effects. Similar problems of interpretation associated with a hyperactive behavioural phenotype have been encountered with deletions of the D1 and D3 dopamine receptor genes (Xu M et al. 1997, 2000; Carta et al. 2000), as well as with mice lacking the gene for the glutamatergic AMPA receptor subunit GluR1 (Vekovischeva et al. 2001; AN Mead and DN Stephens, unpublished manuscript). In some cases, given sufficient exposure to the testing apparatus, it has been possible to equalize baselines prior to drug administration, offering a partial solution to the problem. The occurrence of a basally hypoactive phenotype has also been reported. For example, mice lacking D2 or D4 dopamine receptors display a reduced activity response in a novel environment (Chen et al. 2001; Rubinstein et al. 1997), as do mice lacking the noradrenaline transporter (Xu F et al. 2000). One further important consideration when assessing the stimulant properties of psychostimulants is the reaction of knockout mice to the injection procedure itself. Not only is there the possibility of the injection procedure reinstating basal differences in activity in animals whose activity levels have been equalized by habituation, but also the possibility that the mutants will respond differently to the stress of the injection. In an attempt to remove these potential problems, AN Mead et al. (unpublished manuscript) administered the drug intravenously, thus allowing mice to be fully habituated to the environment, and removing effects of the handling associated with an injection procedure. The results of this study demonstrated that the stress of the injection procedure might be an important factor in the apparent enhanced sensitivity of NAT knockout mice to cocaine, since, in contrast to experiments requiring handling of the animals for drug administration, cocaine was actually less potent in stimulating activity in the knockout when administered intravenously.

The activity levels of mutant mice, both basal and following psychostimulant administration, can also have important consequences on other behaviours maintained by psychostimulants. For example, much of the work into the reinforcing properties of psychostimulants has employed the self-administration (Rocha 1999) and conditioned place-preference paradigms (Mead and Stephens 1999). Much effort has gone into developing techniques of intravenous self-administration of drugs of abuse in the mouse, since the value of this technique for assessing reinforcement in other species is generally recognized. Often, mice are trained to self-administer drug through an indwelling intravenous catheter, using operant techniques, though the acute insertion of an intravenous line into the tail vein has also been used for short-term experiments (Kuzmin et al. 2000). A change in the vigour with which mutant mice perform the operant response to activate the drug infusion (increased rates, or higher breakpoints on progressive ratio schedules) is taken as evidence for alterations in the reinforcing properties of the drugs in the mutants. As with other species, the dose–response curve describing rates of operant performance of different drug doses usually has an inverted-U form. Since both small increases or decreases from the optimal drug dose will result in a decrease in rates of operant output, it is difficult to draw conclusions regarding the direction of change in reinforcing efficacy of a drug in genetically manipulated mice from studies using a limited range of doses. Nevertheless, the practicalities of obtaining sufficient genetically manipulated mice often prevent rigorous testing over a wide dose range. Furthermore, it needs to be recognized that rates of self-administration reflect not only the reinforcing, but also other, properties of the drugs. Operant behaviour may be affected by gene manipulations that influence aspects of learning and memory, activity and sensory perception as well as those that alter positive or negative reinforcement, and the gene of interest may interact with these functions. For this reason, a thorough behavioural characterization of a knockout mouse is a prerequisite before attempts to understand more complex behaviours can proceed. Several workers in the field have proposed batteries of tests with which to obtain an initial evaluation of sensory, motor and motivational competence in knockout mice, important before proceeding to more complex analyses (Gold 1999; Crawley 2000).

Since catheter patency is relatively short in mice, it is common to use training procedures whose limitations are well recognized in other species. Among these are pretraining the mice to lever press for food prior to self-administration training, and providing 'priming' (a free dose) with drug at the start of the session. Psychostimulants facilitate responding for conditioned reinforcers associated with the food (Robbins et al. 1983), and increase rates of lever pressing as a result of their stimulant properties. The initial priming dose may thus act to facilitate responding for stimuli previously conditioned adventitiously to food delivery, or may increase the probability of lever-pressing as a result of enhanced activity, thereby engendering further cocaine infusions. Unequivocal interpretation of the consequences of the genetic manipulation in terms of reward may therefore be inappropriate. These behavioural issues can interact with the abnormal behavioural phenotype of the genetically manipulated animal. If the mouse is spontaneously hyperactive, or shows a changed response to the drug, then this will result in an apparent change in the reinforcing qualities of cocaine.

We have already pointed to the possibility that gene deletion early in development may lead to compensatory changes in the organism during development. Again, the DAT knockout provides an excellent example. Initial studies suggested that this mouse was still sensitive to the reinforcing properties of cocaine in both self-administration (Rocha et al. 1998*a*) and conditioned-place-preference para-digms (Sora et al. 1998), despite cocaine failing to increase extracellular dopamine in the caudate putamen of these mice (Fauchey et al. 2000). These studies questioned the importance of the DAT and dopamine in the reinforcing actions of cocaine, one of the fundamental tenets of behavioural pharmacology of abused drugs. It has subsequently been suggested, however, that cocaine does increase extracellular dopamine in the nucleus accumbens (Carboni et al. 2001), and these workers postu-lated that in the case of the DAT knockout, cocaine increased extracellular dopamine through blockade of NATs. An alternative possibility is that serotonin transporters (SETs) substitute for DAT in the DAT knockout animals since mice in which both DAT and SET are deleted do not show place preference to cocaine (Sora et al. 2001). Thus, it appears that, although the DAT knockout mouse is sensitive to the reinforc-ing properties of cocaine, this may be due to compensatory mechanisms (expression or involvement of the NAT or SET in place of DAT in dopamine neurons), and not due to a lack of involvement of the DAT in cocaine's effects in the 'normal' wildtype mouse. Interestingly, NAT knockout mice are supersensitive to psychostimulants (Xu F et al. 2000). Although AN Mead et al. (unpublished manuscript) question whether the heightened sensitivity may be a heightened response to stress, it is worth considering whether the heightened effects of psychostimulants in NAT knockouts may reflect a compensatory increase in DAT expression.

The necessity of thorough behavioural analysis in interpreting changes in self-administration behaviour is also illustrated by our own work on the tPA -/- mouse. tPA is a serine protease involved in synaptic plasticity, and as such, was postulated to play a role in behavioural sensitization mechanisms which may lead to facili-tation of drug self-administration. In keeping with this general idea, tPA -/- mice showed facilitated sensitization to cocaine. However, in a cocaine self-administration paradigm, they did not show changed rates of cocaine self-administration in an operant task in which a short time-out period, when drug was not available, was programmed following each cocaine delivery (Ripley et al. 1999). Nevertheless, the pattern of operant behaviour was changed, so that tPA -/- mice showed over-responding during time-out periods. In the absence of time-out periods, the tPA -/- mice rapidly obtained repeated doses of cocaine, sufficient to be lethal (unpublished). Although overresponding was not seen with a conventional reinforcer (milk), further behavioural analysis (Ripley et al. 2001) suggested that early in operant training, tPA -/- mice may be impulsive, overresponding even on schedules under which such overresponding leads to loss of reinforcer. Differences between tPA -/- and wildtype mice in responding for cocaine thus appear to reflect a more general behavioural deficit in these animals. Whether the apparent changes in the drug-related behavioural phenotype of other genetically manipulated mice also reflect more general behavioural alterations has seldom been approached.

Many workers in the area of behavioural phenotyping argue for the establishment of standard methodologies in which all genetically manipulated mice should be characterized. Our experience with tPA -/- mice illustrates the danger of this approach; each genetic manipulation will throw up its own idiosyncratic behaviour which needs thorough characterization, which should not be limited to a prescribed series of tests.

Transgenic mice in nicotine research

The subunit composition of the neuronal nicotinic acetylcholinergic receptors (nAChrs) is crucial to the understanding of the reinforcing effects of nicotine. The members of this heterogeneous receptor family, consisting of a pentameric ligand-gated ion channel, composed of α and β subunits ($\alpha2$–$\alpha9$, $\beta2$–$\beta4$), differ in their pharmacology and distribution in the central nervous system (Changeux et al. 1998; for review see Lloyd and Williams 2000). To examine the effect of different subunit composition on nicotine-mediated behaviours, knockout mice lacking the genes that encode specific subunits have been generated (Picciotto et al. 1995).

The most widespread subunit is $\beta2$, which is found throughout the central nervous system and has been implicated in Parkinson's disease, cognition, neurodegeneration, pain, anxiety and depression. It has also been shown to be important in the nicotine-induced activation of the ventrotegmental area dopamine neurons, thought to be the mechanism of the stimulant, and rewarding properties of nicotine in rats. Mice that lack $\beta2$ possess high-affinity binding sites for nicotine (Picciotto et al. 1995) and do not show nicotine-induced increases in dopaminergic neuronal firing (Lena and Changeux 1999), nor do they show a nicotine-induced dopamine release in the ventral striatum (Picciotto et al. 1998). In keeping with these observations, Picciotto et al. (1998) reported the inability of mice lacking the $\beta2$-subunit to self-administer nicotine. The animals were initially trained to self-administer cocaine, in which task their performance was equivalent to that of wildtype controls. When switched to nicotine the wildtype mice continued to nose-poke for the drug. However, $\beta2$ null mutants extinguished this behaviour in a similar pattern to wildtype mice when switched to saline treatment. As the $\beta2$ mutants will respond for both cocaine and natural reinforcers (food) it seems unlikely that this effect was due to an inability to perform or learn the task. However, it has been shown that antagonism of the nicotinic receptor with mecamylamine disrupted place-preference conditioning to cocaine whilst nicotine itself potentiated this effect. $\beta2$ null mutant mice also showed decreased placed preference to low doses of cocaine (5 mg/kg; Zachariou et al. 2001). These results may suggest that extinction of nicotine self-administration in the $\beta2$ mutants may also reflect a weaker conditioning during the initial training with cocaine.

As the β2-subunit is often found in combination with the α4-subunit it is important to also investigate the role of this subunit in the reinforcing effects of nicotine. Both the α4 knockout and α4 knock-in mice display increased anxiety, poor motor learning, excessive ambulation and reduced nigrostriatal dopamine function on ageing (Ross et al. 2000; Labarca et al. 2001). The α4-subunit plays a major role in the neuroprotective effects of nicotine upon parkinsonian-like damage in vivo (Ryan et al. 2001) and is also responsible for the antinociceptive actions of nicotine (Marubio et al. 1999). However, no work to date has investigated the role of this subunit in the reinforcing properties of nicotine.

Transgenic mice in alcohol research

Alcohol is known to exert its pharmacological effects through a number of mechanisms, many of them the result of interactions with both ligand-gated and voltage-gated ion channels. The function of many of these channels is so fundamental to neurotransmission that genetic manipulations are often so deleterious that the mutant animals are grossly abnormal, or not viable. Thus, the most likely contributors to alcohol's effects are precisely those genes which are most difficult to study using targeted gene manipulations.

Monoamine systems

The reinforcing properties of alcohol, like those of most other drugs of abuse, are thought to be mediated in part by its ability to facilitate transmission in dopamine neurons, leading to increased dopamine release in nucleus accumbens (Di Chiara and Imperato 1988). Both D1 (El-Ghundi et al. 1998) and D2 (Phillips et al. 1998) dopamine receptor knockout mice consume less alcohol, the D2 -/- mice showing an apparent aversion to ethanol, relative to the high preference and consumption exhibited by wildtype littermates. Sensitivity to ethanol-induced locomotor impairment is also reduced in these mutant mice and D2 -/- mice also show a deficit in alcohol-conditioned place preference (Cunningham et al. 2000). D2 -/- mice have reduced sensitivity to the locomotor stimulant properties of alcohol (Phillips et al. 1998) and are impaired in the operant self-administration of ethanol (Risinger et al. 2000). However, the D2 -/- mice also showed a lower rate of lever pressing for water, saccharin and food. While largely consistent, the significance of these observations as evidence for an important role of D2 receptors in mediating alcohol's effects is questionable, since D2 -/- mice show lower spontaneous activity (Kelly et al. 1998) and their behaviour has analogies with parkinsonian symptomatology (Baik et al. 1995). The D2 -/- mouse may thus simply be more sensitive than wildtypes to the work requirement necessary to obtain reinforcers in operant tasks. Some strains of rat bred selectively to prefer ethanol in choice procedures show decreased D2 receptor binding (Stefanini et al. 1992; McBride et al. 1993), which would seem to be in disagreement with the findings from the genetically manipulated mice. Given the evidence of developmental changes in glutamatergic transmission seen in D2 knockout mice (Tang et al. 2001), one might also speculate that any behavioural differences in response to alcohol seen in D2 -/- mice could reflect the developmental changes, and a change in alcohol's interaction with the glutamate system. These studies thus provide only limited evidence of a role for D2 receptors in mediating ethanol's effects.

Similar arguments may be relevant in considering genetic manipulations of other dopamine receptor subtypes. Although D4 receptor knockouts are more sensitive to the stimulant effects of alcohol, as well as to cocaine and methamphetamine (Rubinstein et al. 1997), they also show a reduced baseline level of locomotor activity, and show compensations for the deletion during development (Drago et al. 1998). Unfortunately, further information on the consequences of deletions of this dopamine receptor subtype for ethanol-related behaviours is not available. This is a criticism which can be made of many studies employing gene manipulation; following an initial pioneering publication in a prominent journal, often using methods which, though rapid and convenient, do not provide much insight into behavioural mechanisms, further characterization is not carried out.

Serotonin systems have long been implicated in certain forms of alcoholism, and in alcohol-motivated behaviour. A possible means by which serotonergic transmission affects ethanol reward is through the regulation of the activity of dopamine neurons by serotonin inputs. 5HT1b receptor knockouts have been extensively studied, and have been reported to show altered dopamine, as well as 5HT, metabolism (Ase et al. 2000), and enhancement of both basal and cocaine-evoked dopamine release (Shippenberg et al. 2000). These mice have been reported to show enhanced self-administration of cocaine (Rocha et al. 1998b), and to consume twice as much alcohol as their wildtype controls (Crabbe et al. 1996). It should be noted, however, that this latter observation has not been replicated in subsequent studies (Crabbe et al. 1999; Bouwknecht et al. 2000), and Risinger et al. (1999) reported that 5HT1b knockout mice did not respond for ethanol in operant experiments. Crabbe et al. (1999) attribute the loss of the alcohol hyperdipsia over several generations of breeding of the manipulated strains to a subtle change in the genetic background of the 5HT1b -/- mice. While this remains speculation, it emphasizes the insecurity of drawing negative conclusions regarding the contribution of a particular gene to behaviour if the genetic manipulation is not tested on a very wide variety of genetic backgrounds.

A second 5HT receptor subtype, 5HT3, has also been suggested to modulate dopamine activity. 5HT3 receptor antagonists decrease ethanol-induced dopamine release in nucleus accumbens (Wozniac et al. 1990), so that reduction of 5HT receptor expression might be expected to decrease the rewarding properties of ethanol. In fact, overexpression of the receptor in mice resulted in decreased preference for ethanol in a two-bottle choice test (Engel et al. 1998). Engel and colleagues ascribe the unexpected result to an increased sensitivity of the mice to the stimulant properties of ethanol (Engel and Allan 1999). Again, the apparent contradiction between conclusions from pharmacological and gene-knockout experiments may suggest developmental changes in the 5HT3 knockouts.

Opioids

The reinforcing properties of ethanol have been ascribed to effects mediated by opioid peptides, particularly β-endorphin (Ulm et al. 1995). Nevertheless, mice deficient in β-endorphin acquired an operant hole-poke task to obtain intravenously administered ethanol (Grahame et al. 1998), and did not differ from wildtype littermates in their preference for ethanol in a two-bottle free-choice paradigm (though, curiously, the heterozygotes drank more; Grisel et al. 1999). Work with μ-receptor knockout mice is more consistent with the pharmacologically derived hypotheses, alcohol-preferring strains of rats (Soini et al. 1999; McBride et al. 1998) and mice (de Waele and Gianoulakis 1997) expressing higher densities of μ-receptors. Pharmacological antagonism of opiate receptors decreases ethanol consumption in both humans (O'Malley 1995) and monkeys (Rodefer et al. 1999). In keeping with these earlier findings, Roberts et al. (2000) found μ-receptor knockout mice to take fewer ethanol reinforcers when required to nose-poke, or to lever press, as the operant response to obtain ethanol, though the knockouts responded more than wildtype mice when the reinforcer was food or sucrose. Knockout mice also consumed less 10% ethanol in a two-bottle choice test, but not when ethanol was the sole available fluid. The mice in this study were male, but in another two-bottle choice experiment, employing a wide range of ethanol concentrations, Hall et al. (2001) found no differences across knockout, heterozygotes and wildtype male mice. Nevertheless, female knockout mice did show increased ethanol preference. It may be significant that although both groups employed mice bred on a mixed C57Bl/129sv background, the mice originated from two separate attempts at creating the knockout. Furthermore, the Roberts mice were bred in Strasbourg, France, and imported into the USA for the behavioural testing, whereas the Hall mice were bred in the institute in which they were tested. The stress associated with international travel might have been expected to contribute to the behavioural phenotype of Roberts' mice, and it is therefore satisfying that despite different origins, and different life histories, rather similar consequences of the mutation were observed. Hall et al. (2001) also found deficits in both knockout and heterozygous female mice in the ability of ethanol both to support a conditioned place preference, and to enhance locomotor activity, again consistent with a broad pharmacological literature suggesting a role for μ-opioid receptors in the rewarding effects of ethanol.

Amino acid transmitters

Primary among alcohol's effects is its action at γ-aminobutyric acid A (GABA$_A$) receptor-gated chloride channels to facilitate inhibition of neuronal activity. The GABA$_A$ family of receptors is complex, and the functional role of its many subtypes is only beginning to be discovered. GABA is the brain's most important inhibitory transmitter, and deletion of genes encoding GABA$_A$ receptor subunits and leading to disruption of receptor function is frequently lethal early in development, or gives rise to grossly impaired animals. Recent attempts to understand the contribution of individual subunits to brain function have exploited the ability of benzodiazepine drugs to facilitate GABA's action at GABA$_A$ receptors. Single-point mutations of the α-subunit of GABA receptors (which result in the substitution of the amino acid arginine for histidine at position 101 of the protein) result in receptors that are insensitive to benzodiazepines, though they retain apparently unchanged responses to the neurotransmitter GABA itself. Since responsivity to the natural transmitter remains unchanged, these animals show no developmental deficits, but do show changed behavioural responses to benzodiazepines (Rudolph et al. 1999; Low et al. 2000; McKernan et al. 2000). Using such 'knock-in' methods, it has been suggested that α1-containing GABA$_A$ receptors are involved in the sedative properties of benzodiazepines, while α2-containing receptors may contribute to their anxiolytic effects. These are subtle and exciting approaches, but the conclusions reached remain controversial (Wisden and Stephens 1999) since the behavioural analyses used to characterize the mutant mice are frequently considerably less sophisticated than the molecular genetic techniques used to generate the animals.

Benzodiazepines are abused by certain populations, and an insight into the contribution of the receptor subtypes for benzodiazepine abuse and dependence is also likely to provide insight into the importance of these receptors for ethanol abuse and dependence. α1-subunit mutants do not show a normal sedative effect of benzodiazepines, but a locomotor stimulant response instead. Since locomotor stimulation is a common feature of many abused drugs, α1(H101R) mutants may be a useful model for studying benzodiazepine abuse. However, despite the stimulant effects of midazolam in these mutants, they did not show behavioural sensitization to repeated administration of midazolam nor facilitated conditioned place preference to the benzodiazepine (Reid et al. 2001), confirming differences between the mechanisms underlying abuse of benzodiazepines and psychostimulant drugs.

Such sophisticated molecular approaches do not yet lend themselves directly to the study of alcohol, since there does not appear to be a similar binding site for alcohol on the GABA$_A$ receptor. Nevertheless, some evidence has been adduced on the contribution of GABA$_A$ subunits to alcohol's behavioural effects. Studies using conventional pharmacological methods had suggested important roles of α6 subunit-containing GABA$_A$ receptors (found exclusively in cerebellar granule cells) in mediating alcohol's effects, and the ability of a benzodiazepine receptor inverse agonist to antagonize some of those behavioural effects. A spontaneous point mutation (from Arg to Glu at position 100) in the gene encoding α6 subunits, conferring loss of inverse agonist binding, has been reported in an alcohol-nontolerant rat line, suggesting that this subunit is important in behavioural sensitivity to alcohol. It is thus of some interest that α6 knockout mice do not show changed sensitivity to the behavioural effects of alcohol, or in development of tolerance or withdrawal sensitivity (Homanics et al. 1997, 1998). However, there appear to be compensatory changes in response to the mutation (e.g. loss of δ subunits, an increase in the number of receptors containing the β subunit of the GABA$_A$ receptor), and an increase in expression of a potassium channel (Nusser et al. 1999). These changes may be regarded as compensatory for the loss of α6-containing receptors, and may account for the failure to observe an altered response to alcohol. Furthermore, the gene encoding α6 subunits is located on the chromosome in a cluster with other subunits of the GABA$_A$ receptor, including α1- and β2-subunits. Disruption of α6 expression also decreases expression of these genes (Uusi-Oukari et al. 2000), which contribute to GABA$_A$ receptor function throughout the brain. The behavioural consequences of changes in the expression of these subunits is difficult to predict, so that the complexity of the effects resulting from α6 deletion makes interpretation of the behavioural consequences of this knockout impossible.

Early evidence from in vitro studies suggested that another subunit, γ2, an essential constituent of many GABA$_A$ receptors throughout the CNS, is an absolute requirement for alcohol's ability to potentiate the action of GABA at the receptor (Wafford et al. 1991; Wafford and Whiting 1992; but see Mehta et al. 1999). This subunit exists in two forms produced by alternative splicing of the mRNA. The γ2-long (γ2L) variant differs from the γ2-short (γ2S) variant in possessing a 24-base-pair sequence that encodes an eight-amino-acid part of an intracellular loop of the subunit protein, that contains a phosphorylation site amenable to modification by intracellular events. Although mice engineered to lack the 24 base-pairs do not differ from wildtypes in their behavioural phenotype, or in their behavioural or electrophysiological response to alcohol (perhaps because they show increased expression of γ2S), mice carrying either the γ2L or γ2S transgene developed significantly less tolerance to the ataxic effects of ethanol (but not less severe withdrawal following chronic treatment; Wick et al. 2000). These observations point to the sometimes subtle consequences of genetic manipulation for the action of abused drugs, allowing insights not readily obtained from conventional approaches.

Genetically manipulated mice are particularly valuable in studying mechanisms underlying modification of receptor function by drugs of abuse. A common mechanism by which receptor function is modified rapidly is by phosphorylation – the attachment of phosphate groups to specific amino acids making up the receptor to change their signalling properties. A number of enzymes which phosphorylate (thereby desensitizing) $GABA_A$ receptors are known to be affected by ethanol, among them members of the protein kinase C (PKC) family (Stubbs and Slater 1999). PKCγ null mutants are less sensitive to the sedating effects of alcohol than wildtype mice (Harris et al. 1995), and the development of tolerance was also decreased, at least in some background strains (Bowers et al. 1999, 2000).

In contrast to PKCγ-mutant mice lacking PKCε showed *increased* sensitivity to alcohol's sedative effects, as well as to the effects of other $GABA_A$ receptor allosteric ligands (Hodge et al. 1999). $GABA_A$ receptors in membranes isolated from the frontal cortex of PKCε null mice were also supersensitive to allosteric activation by ethanol and a benzodiazepine. Despite increased sensitivity to the effects of ethanol, following withdrawal of chronic ethanol, convulsant sensitivity was reduced in ethanol-fed PKCε null mutant mice compared to ethanol-fed wildtype mice. These data demonstrate that deletion of PKCε results in diminished progression of ethanol withdrawal-associated seizure severity (Olive et al. 2001). Behaviourally, PKCε -/- mice show reduced operant ethanol self-administration and an absence of ethanol-induced increases in extracellular dopamine levels in the nucleus accumbens, while mesolimbic dopamine responses to cocaine (20 mg/kg i.p.) or high potassium concentrations (100 mM) in these mice were comparable with those of wildtypes (Olive et al. 2000). This pattern of results is curious. There is no reason to think that the three aspects of the ethanol behavioural phenotype mentioned (increased sensitivity to sedative effects of ethanol, reduced sensitivity to its withdrawal, and reduced effects of ethanol on dopamine release and impaired self-administration) are related.

A further kinase, cyclic AMP-dependent PKA, has also been implicated in mediating certain of the acute and chronic cellular responses to alcohol (Diamond and Gordon 1997) and chronic ethanol has been reported to increase cAMP levels and PKA activity in the nucleus accumbens of rats (Ortiz et al. 1995). PKA consists of regulatory subunits RI and RII and catalytic (C) subunits (Brandon et al. 1997), the regulatory subunits being responsible for the activation of PKA by cAMP. The regulatory (R) and catalytic subunits are encoded by separate genes (Brandon et al. 1997), and deletion of the regulatory RIIβ gene results in increased consumption of ethanol in two-bottle choice drinking experiments, over a wide range of ethanol concentrations (6–20%). Increases in drug-related behaviours are generally more impressive than decreases, which may be due to nonspecific effects of the gene manipulation, but it should be noted that these mice were less sensitive to the sedative effects of ethanol. In contrast, RIβ knockouts showed normal ethanol consumption (Thiele et al. 2000). The changed behavioural effects of ethanol were associated with a reduction in cAMP-stimulated PKA activity in accumbens, amygdala and hippocampus. Although it is not yet understood how downregulation of PKA activity contributes to changes in alcohol-related behaviour, high levels of ethanol drinking in both rodents (Kurtz et al. 1996) and humans (Schuckit 1994) are often associated with tolerance to ethanol, and may lead to alcoholism (Schuckit 1994). These insights into the importance of receptor phosphorylation in determining responsiveness to ethanol would not have been achievable without transgenic technology.

If the contribution of genetically manipulated mice to understanding ethanol's interaction with GABA$_A$ receptors is still at an early stage, their contribution to understanding the interaction of ethanol with excitatory receptors has been even more limited. Ethanol acts as a functional antagonist of glutamatergic NMDA receptors (Woodward 2000), possibly by enhancing phosphorylation of a tyrosine-containing intracellular element of the receptor. Mice lacking Fyn, a nonreceptor type tyrosine kinase, were hypersensitive to the hypnotic effect of ethanol and insensitive to ethanol-induced phosphorylation of the receptor. An acute tolerance to ethanol inhibition of NMDA (N-methyl-D-aspartate) receptor-mediated excitatory postsynaptic potentials in hippocampal slices developed in control mice but not in Fyn-deficient mice (Miyakawa et al. 1997). This observation currently stands alone in the area of addiction in analyses of NMDA receptor function using genetic manipulation.

Conclusions

The benefits of transgenic and knockout technology for understanding processes underlying drug addiction have been equivocal. While single gene deletions can tell us much about protein interactions at the cellular level, at the behavioural level, much caution must be exercised. It must be remembered that in an animal with a particular gene deleted, just as in an animal with a lesion in a discrete brain area, one is not studying the function of the deleted element, but how the animal functions in the absence of the gene or neuronal system. The extent to which one can deduce the role of the deleted element in intact animals from such studies will vary.

It is clear that the kinds of question being asked in ethanol research are rather different from those being asked in psychostimulant research. Genetically manipulated animals are being used in psychostimulant research to test hypotheses relating to known sites of action of abused drugs. Thus, research using mutations of dopamine transporters and dopamine receptors predominates. It has become clear that simple answers are not readily forthcoming, partly because of the problems of compensatory and developmental changes inherent in research with mutant animals, but also because the rigour of behavioural analysis of mutant animals has not yet reached the level in the rest of behavioural neuroscience. Behavioural analysis of targeted mutants is still in its infancy, and as more behaviourally trained scientists enter the field, we can expect an improvement in this area, just as the development of inducible knockouts will help avoid issues of developmental changes. In the alcohol area, studies using receptor knockouts have suffered from similar problems, but also from the fact that genetic manipulations of some of the main targets of ethanol result in death early in development, or severely altered behaviour. Nevertheless, use of genetically manipulated mice has provided insights into the regulation of receptors at which ethanol acts, some of which would not have been possible without the new technology.

Use of genetically manipulated animals in behavioural research is still at an early stage, and, like many innovations, will require time before it matures and takes its place alongside better-established approaches for studying the neurobiology of drug abuse and dependence. The availability of knock-in techniques allowing point mutations in genes to modify, but not completely disrupt, their function, and the growth in the availability of inducible knockouts will no doubt contribute to more sophisticated approaches and more consistent agreement between pharmacological and genomic approaches. At the same time, it is to be hoped that more sophistication develops in behavioural analysis, and that the limitations of animal models are both recognized and accepted by molecular biologist colleagues, understandably impatient to discover the importance of their expensively created knockout mouse. Hopefully, behavioural genomics has already passed the point of attempting to identify the gene 'for' a particular behaviour, and is moving towards an understanding of the panoply of processes which contribute to drug abuse and dependence.

REFERENCES

Ase AR, Reader TA, Hen R, Riad M and Descarries L (2000). Altered serotonin and dopamine metabolism in the CNS of serotonin 5-HT(1A) or 5-HT(1B) receptor knockout mice. *J Neurochem*, 75, 2415–26.

Baik JH, Picetti R, Saiardi A et al. (1995). Parkinsonian-like locomotor impairment in mice lacking dopamine D2 receptors. *Nature*, 377, 424–8.

Bouwknecht JA, Hijzen TH, van der Gugten J, Maes RA, Hen R and Olivier B (2000). Ethanol intake is not elevated in male 5-HT(1B) receptor knockout mice. *Eur J Pharmacol*, 403, 95–8.

Bowers BJ (2000) Applications of transgenic and knockout mice in alcohol research. *Alcohol Res Health*, 24, 175–84.

Bowers BJ, Owen EH, Collins AC, Abeliovich A, Tonegawa S and Wehner JM (1999). Decreased ethanol sensitivity and tolerance development in gamma-PKC null mutant mice is dependent on genetic background. *Alcohol Clin Exp Res*, 23, 387–97.

Bowers BJ, Collins AC and Wehner JM (2000). Background genotype modulates the effect of γ-PKC on the development of rapid tolerance to ethanol-induced hypothermia. *Addict Biol*, 5, 47–58.

Brandon EP, Idzerda RL and McKnight GS (1997). PKA isoforms, neural pathways, and behaviour: making the connection. *Curr Opin Neurobiol*, 7, 1397–403.

Carboni E, Spielewoy C, Vacca C, Nosten-Bertrand M, Giros B and Di Chiara G. (2001). Cocaine and amphetamine increase extracellular dopamine in the nucleus accumbens of mice lacking the dopamine transporter gene. *J Neurosci*, 21, 1–4.

Carta AR, Gerfen CR and Steiner H (2000). Cocaine effects on gene regulation in the striatum and behavior: increased sensitivity in D3 receptor-deficient mice. *Neuroreport*, 11, 2395–9.

Cepeda C, Hurst RS, Altemus KL et al. (2001). Facilitated glutamatergic transmission in the striatum of D2 dopamine receptor-deficient mice. *J Neurophysiol*, 85, 659–70.

Changeux JP, Bertrand D, Corringer PJ et al. (1998). Brain nicotinic receptors: structure and regulation, role in learning and reinforcement. *Brain Res Rev*, 26, 198–216.

Chen J-F, Moratella R, Impagnatiello F et al. (2001). The role of the D2 dopamine receptor (D2R) in A2A adenosine receptor (A2AR)-mediated behavioral and cellular responses as revealed by A2A and D2 receptor knockout mice. *Proc Natl Acad Sci USA*, 98, 1970–5.

Crabbe JC, Phillips TJ, Feller DJ et al. (1996). Elevated alcohol consumption in null mutant mice lacking 5HT1b receptors. *Nat Genet*, 14, 98–101.

Crabbe JC, Wahlsten D and Dudek BC (1999). Genetics of mouse behavior, interactions with laboratory environment. *Science*, 284, 1670–2.

Crawley JN (2000). *What's Wrong with My Mouse? Behavioural Phenotyping of Transgenic and Knockout Mice.* New York: John Wiley and Sons.

Crusio WE and Gerlai RT (1999). *Handbook of Molecular Genetic Techniques for Brain and Behavioral Research.* London: Elsevier.

Cunningham CL, Howard MA, Gill SJ, Rubinstein M, Low MJ and Grandy DK (2000). Ethanol-conditioned place preference is reduced in dopamine D2 receptor-deficient mice. *Pharmacol Biochem Behav*, 67, 693–9.

Diamond I and Gordon AS (1997). Cellular and molecular neuroscience of alcoholism. *Physiol Rev*, 77, 1–20.

Di Chiara G and Imperato A (1988). Drugs abused by humans preferentially increase synaptic dopamine concentrations in the mesolimbic system of freely moving rats. *Proc Natl Acad Sci USA*, 85, 5274–8.

Drago J, Padungchaichot P, Accili D and Fuchs S (1998). Dopamine receptors and dopamine transporter in brain function and addictive behaviors: insight from targeted mouse mutants. *Dev Neurosci*, 20, 188–203.

El-Ghundi M, George SR, Drago J et al. (1998). Disruption of dopamine D1 receptor gene expression attenuates alcohol seeking behaviour. *Eur J Pharmacol*, 353, 149–58.

Engel SR and Allen AM (1999). 5-HT3 receptor overexpression enhances ethanol sensitivity in mice. *Psychopharmacology*, 144, 411–15.

Engel SR, Lyons CR and Allan AM (1998). 5-HT3 receptor overexpression decreases ethanol self-administration in transgenic mice. *Psychopharmacology*, 140, 243–8.

Fauchey V, Jaber M, Bloch B and Le Moine C (2000). Dopamine control of striatal gene expression during development: relevance to knockout mice for the dopamine transporter. *Eur J Neurosci*, 12, 3415–25.

Friend WC, Clapoff S, Landry C et al. (1992). Cell-specific expression of high-levels of human S100-Beta in transgenic mouse-brain is dependent on gene dosage. *J Neurosci*, 12, 4337–46.

Gainetdinov RR, Wetsel WC, Jones SR, Levin ED, Jaber M and Caron MG (1999). Role of serotonin in the paradoxical calming effect of psychostimulants on hyperactivity. *Science*, 283, 397–401.

Gerlai R (1996). Gene-targeting studies of mammalian behavior: is it the mutation or the background phenotype? *Trends Neurosci*, 19, 177–81.

Giros B, Jaber M, Jones SR, Wightman RM and Caron MG (1996). Hyperlocomotion and indifference to cocaine and amphetamine in mice lacking the dopamine transporter. *Nature*, 379, 606–12.

Gold LH (1999). Hierarchical strategy for phenotypic analysis in mice. *Psychopharmacology*, 147, 2–4.

Grahame NJ, Low MJ and Cunningham CL (1998). Intravenous self-administration of ethanol in beta-endotrophin-deficient mice. *Alcohol Clin Exp Res*, 22, 1093–8.

Grisel JE, Mogil JS, Grahame NJ et al. (1999). Ethanol oral self-administration is increased in mutant mice with decreased beta-endorphin expression. *Brain Res*, 835, 62–7.

Hall FS, Sora I and Uhl GR (2001). Ethanol consumption and reward are decreased in mopiate receptor knockout mice. *Psychopharmacology*, 154, 43–9.

Harris RA, McQuilkin SJ, Paylor R, Abeliovich A, Tonegawa S and Wehner JM (1995). Mutant mice lacking the g isoform of protein kinase C show decreased behavioral actions of ethanol and altered function of g-aminobutyrate type A receptors. *Proc Natl Acad Sci USA*, 92, 3658–62.

Hodge CW, Mehmert KK, Kelley SP et al. (1999). Supersensitivity to allosteric GABA(A) receptor modulators and alcohol in mice lacking PKCepsilon. *Nat Neurosci*, 2, 997–1002.

Homanics GE, Ferguson C, Quinlan JJ et al. (1997). Gene knockout of the alpha 6 subunit of the gamma-aminobutyric acid type A receptor: lack of effect on responses to ethanol, pentobarbital, and general anaesthetics. *Mol Pharmacol*, 51, 588–96.

Homanics GE, Le N, Kist R, Mihalek A, Hart A and Quinlan J (1998). Ethanol tolerance and withdrawal responses in GABAA receptor alpha6 subunit null allele mice and in inbred C% and BL/6J and Strain 129/svJ mice. *Alcohol Clin Exp Res*, 22, 259–65.

Homanics GE, Harrison NL, Quinlan JJ et al. (2000). Role of the GABA(A)beta2, GABA(A)alpha6, GABA(A)alpha1 and GABA(A)gamma2 receptor subunit genes cluster in drug responses and the development of alcohol dependence. *Neurochem Int*, 37, 413–23.

Kelly M, Rubinstein M, Phillips TJ et al. (1998). Locomotor activity in D2 dopamine receptor-deficient mice is determined by gene dosage, genetic background and developmental adaptations. *J Neurosci*, 18, 3470–9.

Kurtz DL, Stewart RB, Zweifel M, Li TK and Froehlich JC (1996). Genetic differences in tolerance and sensitization to the sedative/hypnotic effects of alcohol. *Pharmacol Biochem Behav*, 53, 585–91.

Kuzmin AV, Gerrits MA, Zvartau EE and van Ree JM (2000). Influence of buprenorphine, butorphanol and nalbuphine on the initiation of intravenous cocaine self-administration in drug naive mice. *Eur Neuropsychopharmacol*, 10, 447–54.

Labarca C, Schwarz J, Deshpande P et al. (2001). Point mutant mice with hypersensitive α4 nicotinic receptors show dopaminergic deficits and increased anxiety. *Proc Natl Acad Sci USA*, 98, 2786–91.

Lena C and Changeux JP (1999). The role of beta 2-subunit-containing nicotinic acetylcholine receptors in the brain explored with a mutant mouse. *Ann NY Acad Sci*, 868, 611–16.

Lloyd GK and Williams M (2000). Neuronal nicotinic acetylcholine receptors as novel drug targets. *J Pharm Exp Ther*, 292, 461–7.

Low K, Crestani F, Keist R et al. (2000). Molecular and neuronal substrate for the selective attenuation of anxiety. *Science*, 290, 131–4.

Marubio LM, del Mar Arroyo-Jimenez M et al. (1999). Reduced antinociception in mice lacking neuronal nicotinic receptor subunits. *Nature*, 398, 805–10.

McBride WJ, Murphy JM, Gatto GJ et al. (1993). CNS mechanisms of alcohol self-administration. *Alcohol Alcohol Suppl*, 2, 463–7.

McBride WJ, Chernet E, McKinzie DL, Lumeng L and Li TK (1998). Quantitative autoradiography of mu-opioid receptors in the CNS of alcohol-naive alcohol-preferring P and -nonpreferring NP rats. *Alcohol*, 16, 317–23.

McKernan RM, Rosahl TW, Reynolds DS et al. (2000). Sedative but not anxiolytic properties of benzodiazepines are mediated by the GABA$_A$ receptor α1 subtype. *Nat Neurosci*, 3, 587–92.

Mead AN and Stephens DN (1999). Blockade of the expression of a place preference conditioned to amphetamine, by an antagonist of the strychnine-insensitive glycine site of the NMDA receptor, but not by an AMPA receptor antagonist. *J Pharmacol Exp Ther*, 290, 9–15.

Mehta AK, Kist F, Mihalek RM, Aul JJ and Firestone LL (1999). Normal electrophysiological and behavioral responses to ethanol in mice lacking the long splice variant of the gamma2 subunit of the gamma-aminobutyrate type A receptor. *Neuropharmacology*, 38, 253–65.

Min N, Joh TH, Corp ES, Baker H, Cubells JF and Son JH (1996). A transgenic mouse model to study transsynaptic regulation of tyrosine hydroxylase gene expression. *J Neurochem*, 67, 11–18.

Miyakawa T, Yagi T, Kitazawa H et al. (1997). Fyn-kinase as a determinant of ethanol sensitivity: relation to NMDA-receptor function. *Science*, 278, 573.

Nusser Z, Ahmad Z, Tretter V et al. (1999). Alterations in the expression of GABAA receptor subunits in cerebellar granule cells after the disruption of the alpha6 subunit gene. *Eur J Neurosci*, 11, 1685–97.

Olive MF, Mehmert KK, Messing RO and Hodge CW (2000). Reduced operant self-administration and in vivo dopamine responses to ethanol I PKC epsilon-deficient mice. *Eur J Neurosci*, 1, 4131–40.

Olive MF, Mehmert KK, Nannini MA, Camarini R, Messing RO and Hodge CW (2001). Reduced ethanol withdrawal severity and altered withdrawal-induced c-fos expression in various brain regions of mice lacking protein kinase C-epsilon. *Neuroscience*, 103, 171–9.

O'Malley SS et al. (1995). Integration of opioid antagonists and psychosocial therapy in the treatment of narcotic and alcohol dependence. *J Clin Psychiatry*, 56 (Suppl. 7), 30–8.

Ortiz J, Fitzgerald LW, Charlton M et al. (1995). Biochemical actions of chronic ethanol exposure in the mesolimbic dopamine system. *Synapse*, 21, 289–98.

Phillips TJ, Brown KJ, Burkhart-Kasch S et al. (1998). Alcohol preference and sensitivity are markedly reduced in mice lacking dopamine D2 receptors. *Nat Neurosci*, 1, 610–15.

Phillips TJ, Hen R and Crabbe JC (1999). Complications associated with genetic background effects in research using knockout mice. *Psychopharmacology*, 147, 5–7.

Picciotto MR, Zoli M, Lena C et al. (1995). Abnormal avoidance learning in mice lacking functional high-affinity nicotine receptor in the brain. *Nature*, 374, 65–7.

Picciotto MR, Zoli M, Rimondini R et al. (1998). Acetylcholine receptors containing the beta2 subunit are involved in the reinforcing properties of nicotine. *Nature*, 391, 173–7.

Reid L, McKernan RM and Stephens DN (2001). Does the α_1 GABA$_A$ receptor subtype play a role in mediating the dependence and abuse potential of benzodiazepines? *Behav Pharmacol*, 12 (Suppl. 1), S82.

Ripley TL, Rocha BA, Oglesby MW and Stephens DN (1999). Increased sensitivity to cocaine, and over-responding during cocaine self-administration in tPA knockout mice. *Brain Res*, 826, 117–27.

Ripley TL, Horwood JM and Stephens DN (2001). Evidence for impairment of behavioural inhibition in performance of operant tasks in tPA-/- mice. *Behav Brain Res*, 125, 215–27.

Risinger FO, Doan AM and Vickrey AC (1999). Oral operant ethanol self-administration in 5-HT1b knockout mice. *Behav Brain Res*, 102, 211–15.

Risinger FO, Freeman PA, Rubinstein M, Low MJ and Grandy DK (2000). Lack of operant ethanol self-administration in dopamine D2 receptor knockout mice. *Psychopharmacology*, 152, 343–50.

Robbins TW, Watson BA, Gaskin M and Ennis C (1983). Contrasting interactions of pipradrol, d-amphetamine, cocaine, cocaine analogues, apomorphine and other drugs with conditioned reinforcement. *Psychopharmacology*, 80, 113–19.

Roberts AJ, McDonald JS, Heyser CJ et al. (2000). μ-opioid receptor knockout mice do not self-administer alcohol. *J Pharmacol Exp Ther*, 293, 1002–8.

Rocha BA (1999). Methodology for analyzing the parallel between cocaine psychomotor stimulant and reinforcing effects in mice. *Psychopharmacology*, 147, 27–9.

Rocha BA, Fumagalli F, Gainetdinov RR et al. (1998a). Cocaine self-administration in dopamine-transporter knockout mice. *Nat Neurosci*, 1, 132–7.

Rocha BA, Scearce-Levie K, Lucas JJ et al. (1998b). Increased vulnerability to cocaine in mice lacking the serotonin-1B receptor. *Nature*, 393, 175–8.

Rodefer JS, Campbell UC, Cosgrove KP and Carroll ME (1999). Naltrexone pretreatment decreases the reinforcing effectiveness of ethanol and saccharin but not PCP or food under concurrent progressive-ratio schedules in rhesus monkeys. *Psychopharmacology*, 141, 436–46.

Ross SA, Wong JY, Clifford JJ et al. (2000). Phenotypic characterization of an alpha 4 neuronal nicotinic acetylcholine receptor subunit knock-out mouse. *J Neurosci*, 20, 6431–41.

Rubinstein M, Phillips TJ, Bunzow JR et al. (1997). Mice lacking dopamine D4 receptors are supersensitive to ethanol, cocaine and methamphetamine. *Cell*, 90, 991–1001.

Rudolph U, Crestani F, Benke D et al. (1999). Benzodiazepine actions mediated by specific γ-aminobutyric acidA receptor subtypes. *Nature*, 401, 796–800.

Ryan RE, Ross SA, Drago J and Loiacono RE (2001). Dose-related neuroprotective effects of chronic nicotine in 6-hydroxydopamine treated rats, and loss of neuroprotection in alpha4 nicotinic receptor subunit knockout mice. *Br J Pharmacol*, 132, 1650–6.

Schuckit MA (1994). Low level of response to alcohol as a predictor of future alcoholism. *Am J Psychiatry*, 151, 184–9.

Self DW (1999). Comparison of transgenic strategies for behavioral neuroscience in rodents. *Psychopharmacology*, 147, 35–7.

Shippenberg TS, Hen R and He M (2000). Region-specific enhancement of basal extracellular and cocaine-evoked dopamine levels following constitutive deletion of the serotonin (1B) receptor. *J Neurochem*, 75, 258–65.

Silva AJ, Simpson EM, Takahashi JS et al. (1997). Mutant mice and neuroscience: recommendations concerning genetic background. *Neuron*, 19, 755–9.

Soini SL, Honkanen A, Hyytia P and Korpi ER (1999). [3H]ethylketocyclazocine binding to brain opioid receptor subtypes in alcohol-preferring AA and alcohol-avoiding ANA rats. *Alcohol*, 18, 27–34.

Sora I, Wichems C, Takahashi N et al. (1998). Cocaine reward models: conditioned place preference can be established in dopamine- and in serotonin-transporter knockout mice. *Proc Natl Acad Sci USA*, 95, 7699–704.

Sora I, Hall FS, Andrews AM et al. (2001). Molecular mechanisms of cocaine reward: combined dopamine and serotonin transporter knockouts eliminate cocaine place preference. *Proc Natl Acad Sci USA*, 98, 5300–5.

Stefanini E, Frau M, Garau MG, Garau B, Fadda F and Gessa GL (1992). Alcohol-preferring rats have fewer dopamine D2 receptors in the limbic system. *Alcohol Alcohol*, 27, 127–30.

Stubbs CD and Slater SJ (1999). Ethanol and protein kinase C. *Alcohol Clin Exp Res*, 23, 1552–60.

Tang K-C, Low MJ, Grandy DK and Lovinger DM (2001). Dopamine-dependent synaptic plasticity in striatum during in vivo development. *Proc Natl Acad Sci USA*, 98, 1255–60.

Thiele TE, Willis B, Stadler J, Reynolds JG, Bernstein IL and McKnight GS (2000). High ethanol consumption and low sensitivity to ethanol-induced sedation in protein kinase A-mutant mice. *J Neurosci*, 20, RC75 (1–6).

Ulm RR, Volpicelli JR and Volpicelli LA (1995). Opiates and alcohol self-administration in animals. *J Clin Psychiatry*, 56 (Suppl. 7), 5–14.

Uusi-Oukari M, Heikkila J, Sinkkonen ST et al. (2000). Long-range interactions in neuronal gene expression: evidence from gene targeting in the GABA(A) receptor beta2-alpha6-alpha1-gamma2 subunit gene cluster. *Mol Cell Neurosci*, 16, 34–41.

Vekovischeva OY, Zamanillo D, Echenko O et al. (2001). Morphine-induced dependence and sensitization are altered in mice deficient in AMPA-type glutamate receptor-A subunits. *J Neurosci*, 21, 4451–9.

de Waele JP and Gianoulakis C (1997). Characterization of the mu and delta opioid receptors in the brain of the C57BL/6 and DBA/2 mice, selected for their differences in voluntary ethanol consumption. *Alcohol Clin Exp Res*, 21, 754–62.

Wafford KA and Whiting PJ (1992). Ethanol potentiation of GABA-A receptors requires phosphorylation of the alternatively-spliced variant of the gamma 2 subunit. *FEBS Lett*, 313, 113–17.

Wafford KA, Burnett DM, Leidenheimer HJ et al. (1991). Ethanol sensitivity of the GABA-A receptor expressed in *Xenopus* oocytes requires 8 amino acids contained in the gamma 2L subunit. *Neuron*, 7, 27–33.

Wick MJ, Radcliffe RA, Bowers BJ et al. (2000). Behavioural changes produced by transgenic overexpression of gamma2L and gamma2S subunits of the GABA-A receptor. *Eur J Neurosci*, 12, 2634–8.

Wisden W and Stephens DN (1999). Towards better benzodiazepines. *Nature*, 401, 751–2.

Woodward JJ (2000). Ethanol and NMDA receptor signaling. *Crit Rev Neurobiol*, 14, 69–89.

Wozniac KM, Pert A and Linnoila M (1990). Antagonism of 5-HT3 receptors attenuates the effects of ethanol on extracellular dopamine and serotonin in nucleus accumbens. *Eur J Pharmacol*, 187, 287–9.

Xu F, Gainetdinov RR, Wetsel WC et al. (2000). Mice lacking the norepinephrine transporter are supersensitive to psychostimulants. *Nat Neurosci*, 3, 465–71.

Xu M, Koeltzow TE, Santiago GT et al. (1997). Dopamine D3 receptor mutant mice exhibit increased behavioral sensitivity to concurrent stimulation of D1 and D2 receptors. *Neuron*, 19, 837–48.

Xu M, Guo Y, Vorhees CV and Zhang J (2000). Behavioral responses to cocaine and amphetamine administration in mice lacking the dopamine D1 receptor. *Brain Res*, 852, 198–207.

Zachariou V, Caldarone BJ, Weathers-Lowin A et al. (2001). Nicotine receptor inactivation decreases sensitivity to cocaine. *Neuropsychopharmacology*, 24, 576–89.

20

The neuropsychology of chronic drug abuse

Robert D Rogers[1] and Trevor W Robbins[2]

[1] University of Oxford, Oxford, UK; [2] University of Cambridge, Cambridge, UK

Introduction

There are at least two ways in which cognitive impairments might contribute to drug misuse and drug dependence or addiction. Cognitive impairments, perhaps involving heightened impulsivity, may facilitate drug-seeking behaviour but also undermine the extent to which drug users are able to assimilate and benefit from treatment programmes that often have strong educational and cognitive components (McCrady and Smith 1986; Majewska 1996).

Recent research has seen a rapid expansion of the investigation of neurocognitive deficits in drug abusers and on the relationship between these deficits and neurochemical, morphological and functional pathologies associated with chronic drug use. This research is now able to call upon advances from several areas of cognitive neuroscience, encompassing neuroanatomy and molecular pharmacology (Gurevich and Joyce 1999; Ongur and Price 2000), psychological theory concerning the nature of motivated action and reinforcement mechanisms as they relate to drugs of abuse (see Altman et al. 1996; Everitt et al. 2001 for reviews), and imaging methodologies (Breiter et al. 1997; Volkow et al. 1997; Gollub et al. 1998; Liu et al. 1998) and event-based electroencephalography (McKetin and Solowij 1999) that allow investigation of the physiological correlates of cognitive and emotional activity in the brain. Moreover, the scope of this research is expanding with the preliminary investigation of neurocognitive deficits associated with drugs, such as ketamine, whose potential for abuse is only recently becoming apparent (Curran and Morgan 2001).

Notwithstanding the impact of these technical and theoretical resources, it is important to acknowledge at the outset that gaining an understanding of the neuropsychological correlates of human drug abuse presents a set of difficult clinical, methodological and theoretical problems, which we shall first describe briefly. In subsequent sections, we consider the neurocognitive deficits that have been associated with the 'illicit' use of cannabis, stimulants and opiates. We do not discuss the well-documented neurocognitive correlates of prolonged use of alcohol or nicotine, or the more commonly prescribed drugs liable to abuse, such as the benzodiazepines. Comprehensive reviews are already available elsewhere (Allen et al. 1997; Rusted et al. 1998). However, we shall refer to studies of the neuropsychology of alcohol abuse where this is pointedly relevant, i.e. in studies into cognitive deficits in stimulant-abusers, as discussed below.

Theoretical and methodological issues

Drugs of abuse affect neurotransmitter pathways with relatively diffuse patterns of innervation over wide cortical areas and, particularly, in the forebrain (Altman et al. 1996; Cooper et al. 1996; Feldman et al. 1997). Partly for this reason, there have been few, if any, convincing demonstrations that the prolonged abuse of different classes of drug (e.g. stimulants vs. hypnotics/opiates) is associated with discriminable neuropsychological deficits (e.g. memory vs. attention).

We now understand the molecular and neuronal basis of action of many drugs of abuse, as well as the neural loci at which they exert their reinforcing actions – mainly from research in experimental animals (Altman et al. 1996; Feldman et al. 1997). There is much focus, for example, on the hypothesis that a final common pathway of effects of many drugs of abuse, including opiates, stimulants, cannabinoids, alcohol and nicotine, is upon dopamine-dependent functions of the nucleus accumbens, a structure in the basal forebrain that forms an interface between the limbic and motor systems (see Altman et al. 1996 or Robbins and Everitt 1999 for a brief review). This is the case even though only stimulant drugs, such as amphetamine or cocaine, have their initial site of action at dopamine neurons within the nucleus accumbens. However, ancillary effects of drugs of abuse at other receptors and other loci may contribute to the overall pattern of behavioural and cognitive effects observed. This will especially be the case following chronic administration. Moreover, the nucleus accumbens itself forms a node within a number of neural networks that include both limbic and cortical connections (see Figure 20.1). Thus, it is likely that both acute as well as chronic effects of drugs will disrupt the functioning of circuitry with functions in both cognitive and emotional processing. Indeed, later in this chapter we shall be reviewing evidence of pathological effects of drugs of abuse that affect several of the structures shown in Figure 20.1.

Although the chronic use of illicit drugs may be associated with a rather generalized profile of neuropsychological deficits, it is important to note that there are marked differences in the patterns of innervation associated with distinct neurotransmitter systems. For example, the noradrenergic innervation of the dorsal striatum is quite sparse relative to that of the dopamine systems, whereas the innervation

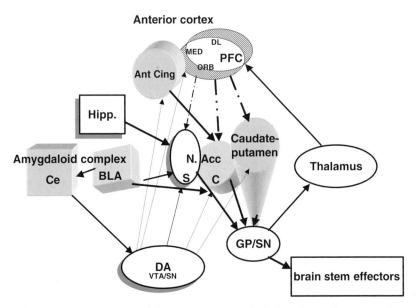

Figure 20.1   Schematic representation of the neural network including the nucleus accumbens
(N. Acc. – note the shell (S) and core (C) subregions) and other structures of the striatum
(e.g. caudate–putamen) and their relationships with the amygdala (Ce, central nucleus;
BLA, basolateral region), the hippocampus (Hipp), prefrontal cortex (PFC) and its
dorsolateral (DL), orbitofrontal (ORB) and medial (MED) divisions, and the anterior
cingulate (Ant Cing) cortex. Note also the feedback loops to the cortex via the thalamus
and the output to brain stem structures via the globus pallidus (GP) and substantia nigra,
pars reticulata (SN). The mesocorticolimbic dopamine (DA) pathways originating from the
ventral tegmental area (VTA) are important sites of action of many drugs of abuse,
especially stimulants such as amphetamine and cocaine. They run parallel to the DA
innervation of the dorsal striatum (caudate–putamen) from the substantia nigra, pars
compacta (affected in Parkinson's disease). Many of the structures and systems shown in
this figure are targets for disruptive and even toxic effects following chronic exposure to
drugs of abuse that may affect cognitive functioning (see text).

of the cerebral cortex by the ascending dopamine systems is primarily to anterior
portions of the cerebral cortex, for example, the prefrontal cortex. There are differences in distribution across cortical laminae or layers in different cortical regions
(Lewis 2001). Substantial differences also exist between the distributions and functions of various receptor subtypes (Feldman et al. 1997). Thus, dopamine D1 type
receptors are most densely distributed in the anterior cortical regions, whereas D2
receptors are found in greater numbers in subcortical areas (Gurevich and Joyce
1999). The receptors of the cannabinoid system are most concentrated in the hippocampal cortical fields and relatively sparse in the brain stem (see Herkenham et al.

1990). Consequently, in addition to a general pattern of cognitive deficits commonly associated with chronic misuse of all or most illicit drugs, there may be subtle differences between these patterns of deficit reflecting underlying differences in modes of actions of different drugs.

Resolving such differences in neurocognitive deficits on the basis of the existing literature is problematic. First, published studies of the neuropsychological performance of samples of illicit drug abusers have employed traditional neuropsychological tests with variable psychometric reliability and sensitivity for neural dysfunction. Second, while studies of the acute effects of different kinds of drugs of abuse conducted by experimental psychologists have tended to pursue particular cognitive paradigms (e.g. vigilance tests in the case of stimulants; Koelega 1993), studies of the chronic effects conducted by neuropsychologists have used broader batteries of tasks (e.g. the Halstead–Reitan battery), making comparisons difficult. However, recent developments of standardized neuropsychological batteries such as the Cambridge Neuropsychological Test Automated Battery (CANTAB), that have been validated in studies encompassing neurological (Sahakian and Owen 1992), imaging (Lee et al. 2000) and pharmacological (Elliott et al. 1997) research offer the opportunity to relate deficits in drug-abusing groups to underlying pathology.

In this context, the results of neuropsychological investigations – and for that matter, brain-imaging studies – have to be bolstered by converging evidence from other methodologies that do not rely on correlational information. Specifically, research with animal models is needed to establish that prolonged administration of such drugs produces the same kind of cognitive and behavioural changes demonstrated in the kind of studies discussed below. These additional animal models will provide the means to distinguish cognitive deficits reflecting cumulative change to neurotransmitter function resulting from prolonged abuse and preexisting neurodevelopmental abnormality.

Finally, research into neurocognitive deficits associated with drug abuse also needs to allow for a complicated set of clinical variables. The two most prominent confounding factors are the duration of time between last use of drug and neuropsychological assessment, and the need to control for polydrug abuse. However, there are other clinical factors associated with chronic drug abuse that complicate interpretation of results in the absence of carefully controlled positive control groups. These include elevated rates of comorbid psychiatric disorders, and variable levels of concurrent medication for psychiatric disorders and for substance abuse itself (e.g. methadone medication). Additionally, drug abuse can itself represent an independent pathway to major physical illnesses, such as HIV infection, that can then further compromise neurocognitive functioning (Bassoa and Bornstein 2000). Addressing these difficulties simultaneously has not been possible in any of the published studies to date. So the best research in this area has necessarily been concerned with narrowly defined issues, and reflects the clinical diversity of drug abuse. The studies have utilized many different methodological designs, including cross-sectional and prospective longitudinal studies.

Cannabis

In general, the evidence that cannabis use is associated with neurocognitive deficits persisting beyond the residual effects of the drug has been summarized as relatively weak (Pope et al. 1995, 2001). However, Block and Ghoneim (1993) reported that heavy marijuana users show small but significant impairments in memory retrieval, verbal expression and mathematical reasoning compared with a matched group of healthy, non-drug-using controls. The marijuana users actually showed small improvements in concept formation (i.e. abstraction). The hypothesis that prolonged cannabis use is associated with persisting, albeit subtle, cognitive changes was also strengthened by a large prospective study involving both younger and older cohorts of Costa Rican cannabis users and appropriately matched nonusing control groups (Fletcher et al. 1996). In this study, appropriate comparisons of differences between cannabis user groups and their respective controls (matched for age and ability) suggested that prolonged use of cannabis is associated with problems in the recall of items from list-learning tasks, and impairments in the performance of selective and divided attention tests. However, a recent large-scale study that compared the performance of a sample of current heavy cannabis users, a sample of former heavy cannabis users and a sample of control subjects with only very limited cannabis experience on a comprehensive battery of tests of attention and memory found only subtle deficits in the former users up to 7 days after the last dose of cannabis but no deficits 28 days later. Thus, it may be safest to conclude that impairments associated with prolonged cannabis are not reliably detected with traditional neuropsychological instruments (Pope et al. 2001).

Using EEG methodologies as a means of identifying changes in attentional processing that might not be detectable with traditional neuropsychological tests, and employing closely matched groups of light and heavy cannabis users, Solowij et al. (1995) and Solowij (1995) reported that heavy, chronic use of cannabis may be associated with subtle changes in attentional processing, as indicated by altered 'processing negativity' and attenuated P300 amplitudes within an event-related potential (ERP)-related paradigm. The weight of evidence available from these studies tends to suggest problems in the efficient selection of relevant stimulus information and in filtering out irrelevant material, which appear to persist following many years of abuse (Solowij et al. 1995).

Some of the more recent studies have suggested that cannabis may also be associated with developmental changes at a functional and neural level. A small number of studies have suggested that, when all the identifiable confounding factors have been controlled for, prenatal use of cannabis may have deleterious effects on the cognitive function of offspring; there is a specific suggestion that these effects have their greatest impact on 'executive function' mediated by the frontal lobes (Fried and Smith 2001). There have also been reports that deficits in visual scanning function (which undergoes maturation between 12 and 15 years of age) are best predicted by an earlier onset age of cannabis use (<16 vs. >16 years) (Ehrenreich et al. 1999). In general, these results are consistent with claims (Fletcher et al. 1996) that attentional processing may be particularly affected by cannabis abuse (Solowij 1998). Despite these data, the available research suggests that chronic cannabis use is associated with only subtle neurocognitive changes compared, for example, with those seen in neurological illness (Fletcher et al. 1996). Such deficits also appear to depend on prolonged, heavy consumption of the drug (Solowij 1998).

Evidence for actual neural disruption associated with chronic use of cannabis is currently even less substantive. There is some evidence that repeated treatment with 9-tetrahydrocannabinol (THC) and synthetic cannabinoid-receptor agonists, such as WIN 55,212-2, may produce morphological changes within the hippocampus, more closely resembling ischaemic or toxic damage than the effects of stress, and which might explain some of the learning and memory changes associated with cannabis use (Lawston et al. 2000). Only a few studies have examined structural or functional changes in human cannabis users. Volkow et al. (1996) reported lower baseline cerebellar metabolism in chronic cannabis users than in control volunteers, but greater increases in orbitofrontal areas and the basal ganglia after THC treatment. The finding that frontal functioning associated with the acute effects of THC was differentially changed in the chronic users suggests that alterations in the processing of frontostriatal circuitry may mediate some of the clinical manifestations of cannabis use. Consistent with this possibility, repeated administration of THC in rats has also been found to reduce prefrontal dopamine metabolism (Jentsch et al. 1998b).

Finally, while, altered cerebellar activity in chronic cannabis users has continued to accumulate (Block et al. 2000a), structural and functional changes in humans may depend critically on length of use. Thus, Wilson et al. (2000) reported that relatively early onset of cannabis use (<17 years) is associated with structural abnormalities including reduced whole brain volume and percentage of grey matter, but higher global cerebral blood flow. By contrast, Block et al. (2000b) have reported magnetic resonance findings that frequent use of marijuana in younger subjects is associated only with lower ventricular cerebrospinal fluid volume.

In summary, the chronic and heavy use of cannabis may be associated with quite subtle changes in cognitive function. Many of the existing data suggest problems with attention as well as memory. However, whether such changes are permanent remains unconfirmed while the nature of their relationship with underlying functional and structural abnormalities and the impact of cannabis use on subsequent neurodevelopment are attracting greater study.

Stimulants

Following the dramatic upsurge in cocaine use, the early 1980s saw a significant increase in research into the cognitive effects of prolonged stimulant abuse. In general, this work has tended to focus on problems in visuomotor performance, attention and verbal memory (Berry et al. 1993; Beatty et al. 1995; Roselli and Ardila 1996). Several studies have examined the question of whether the neuropsychological deficits associated with cocaine use diminish with prolonged abstinence, with some evidence that cocaine use is associated with residual cognitive deficits persisting for at least several months (O'Malley et al. 1992; Strickland et al. 1993). Convergent evidence to strengthen this possibility was provided by the findings that regional cerebral blood flow is reduced in the frontal lobes of abstinent cocaine abusers (Volkow et al. 1992, 1993). In particular, Volkow et al. (1993) used positron emission tomography (PET) 2-deoxy-2 [18 F] fluoro-D-glucose (FDG) as well as dopamine D2 ligand-binding methodology to demonstrate reduced D2 receptor availability in 20 male chronic cocaine abusers, compared with 38 male control subjects, that correlated with reduced metabolism in the orbital prefrontal cortex. These reductions in D2 receptor availability remained evident for 3–4 months of detoxification, suggesting that cocaine abuse is associated with persisting changes in corticostriatal functioning.

In the context of hypotheses about the neural basis of neuropsychological deficits in cocaine users, it is important to note that cocaine is also associated with a variety of pathologies that could be expected to impair cognition directly. These include cerebral vasculitis, stroke, seizures and intracranial haemorrhage. Moreover, there have been suggestions that the simultaneous use of cocaine and alcohol impairs cognitive abilities through the neurotoxic effects of cocaethylene (Jatlow 1995). As against this, there is only mixed evidence that joint abuse of cocaine and alcohol is associated with larger deficits than abuse of cocaine alone (Carroll et al. 1993; Robinson et al. 1999).

Studies focusing on the impact of clinical factors have adopted the approach of regressing standardized performance measures, encompassing many different traditional indices of verbal memory, visual memory, executive functioning, visuoconstruction and visuoperception, psychomotor speed and manual dexterity, against drug-related variables such as frequency of use, intensity of use and duration of use, while controlling for the effects of demographic and psychometric measures such as age, gender, level of attained education and ethnicity. For example, Bolla et al. (1999) examined 30 abstinent chronic cocaine abusers and 21 non-drug-using control subjects matched for age, education and intelligence. Regression analysis

Table 20.1. Distinct cognitive profiles in chronic drug abuser groups

	Amphetamine	Heroin
Decision-making variable		
Decision quality	X	O
Deliberation time	X	X
Per cent bets	X	O
Other cognitive tests		
ED shift	X	x
ID shift	O	X
Visual pattern recognition	X	X

X, highly significant deficit; x, significant deficit; O, No significant deficit.
ED, extradimensional; ID, intradimensional. See text for explanation of
other variables.
Source: Summary of some of the main results from Rogers et al.
(1999*b*) and Ornstein et al. (2000).

indicated that greater intensity and earlier cocaine use in abstinent users is associated with more marked deficits in executive control, visuospatial abilities, psychomotor speed and manual dexterity (see also Strickland et al. 1997). Follow-up work suggested that dose-related deficits in verbal learning and memory persist over 4 weeks of abstinence (Bolla et al. 2000).

While most research has utilized traditional neuropsychological instruments as indices of functioning of particular cortical regions (e.g. anterior frontal, temporal or parietal lobes), recent research has employed tools validated with both neurological and brain-imaging studies. Ornstein et al. (2000) compared 23 chronic amphetamine abusers, 22 chronic opiate abusers and groups of non-drug-using controls on a selection of tests including those selected from the CANTAB battery, each test being validated against a background of studies with neurological patients with focal lesions of the frontal or temporal lobes or neurodegenerative diseases such as Parkinson's, Huntington's or Alzheimer's diseases. Importantly, further validation was provided by studies with brain-imaging techniques in normal volunteers (Lee et al. 2000) and also psychopharmacological studies of effects of acute doses in normal volunteers (Elliott et al. 1997: Rogers et al. 1999*a*). The neuropsychological tests employed included recognition memory, spatial working memory, planning, sequence-generation and learning, visual discrimination learning and attentional-set-shifting. In general, deficits were more marked in the amphetamine than in the opiate abusers. However, there were differences in the profile of deficits of the amphetamine abusers compared with that of the opiate abusers (see Table 20.1 for summary). Thus, while both groups were impaired at tasks involving short-term spatial memory, the amphetamine abusers were worse than the opiate abusers and control volunteers at shifting an attentional set. The opiate abusers were worse at generalizing an already acquired attentional set to new learning and were also impaired in acquiring a strategy in a sequence learning procedure. These results suggest that there are cognitive deficits in amphetamine and opiate abusers, perhaps relating to underlying frontal lobe pathology (Liu et al. 1998), but with some evidence of more specific deficits in each case (Table 20.1). Recent work has extended the ERP methodology previously used in chronic cannabis users (Solowij 1995) to demonstrate problems in attentional mechanisms of amphetamine abusers, as measured by processing negativity and reduced P300 amplitude anomalies (McKetin and Solowij 1999).

Other work has explored more advanced proposals about the clinical significance of neurocognitive deficits in stimulant abusers. This work has focused on the role of the frontal lobes. Specifically, chronic drug abusers exhibit several of the behavioural changes associated with focal lesions of the frontal lobes – lack of behavioural regulation, altered decision-making and a lack of concern for the consequences of actions. Therefore, Rogers et al. (1999b) tested the hypothesis that drug abusers should also show deficits on neuropsychological measures of functions that depend on the frontal lobes. Independent samples of 18 chronic amphetamine-dependent individuals, 13 opiate-dependent individuals, 10 patients with focal lesions of the dorsolateral prefrontal cortex (PFC), 10 patients with lesions of the orbital PFC and 26 non-drug-using controls completed a computerized decision-making task. Consistent with recent reports of deficient decision-making in neurological samples (see Bechara et al. 1994; Rahman et al. 2001 for review), patients with orbital prefrontal lesions took significantly longer to make their decisions than both the patients with dorsolateral prefrontal lesions and the normal controls, and were more likely to choose the response option that was least likely to lead to reward. Both drug-dependent groups showed the same increase in the time taken to make decisions as the patients with the orbital lesions but, critically, only the chronic amphetamine abusers exhibited the same tendency to choose the least optimal choices. Moreover, reduced optimal choices were also associated with number of years of abuse, suggesting an association between prolonged use and decision-making impairment.

These data suggest that chronic amphetamine abuse is associated with altered functioning of the circuitry, involving the ventral PFC, ventral striatum and amygdala, that mediates decision-making, and are consistent with results indicating that prolonged stimulant use is associated with altered metabolism in the orbital cortex (Volkow et al. 1993). Moreover, comparable deficits in decision-making in non-drug-using control volunteers who underwent rapid dietary tryptophan depletion, leading to reduced central serotonin function (Young et al. 1985), suggest that altered neuromodulation of this circuitry underpins the deficits in the abuser groups.

Recent autopsy data have further strengthened this hypothesis by providing evidence of reduced serotonin in the orbital prefrontal cortex and reduced dopamine in the striatum of methamphetamine abusers (Wilson et al. 1996a, b).

Widespread deficits in frontal lobe functioning of chronic amphetamine and opiate abusers may be related to altered monoamine activity that, through relatively diffuse patterns of innervation across the forebrain and frontal cortex, mediate changes in behavioural control. Grant et al. (2000) conducted a well-designed study to test the specificity of frontal lobe deficits in a group of 30 polydrug abusers and 24 healthy controls. Both groups completed a 'gambling task' with established sensitivity to orbital cortical damage (Bechara et al. 1994, 2001), and the Wisconsin Card Sorting Test (WCST; Anderson et al. 1991) that previous imaging studies have suggested is associated with dorsolateral prefrontal cortical function. Deficits were evident in decision-making but not on the WCST. Concurrently, Bechara et al. (2001) have demonstrated that polydrug abusers, with histories of both stimulant and alcohol abuse, also show impaired performance on the same decision-making measure as used by Grant et al. (2000). Since three separate studies (Rogers et al. 1999b; Grant et al. 2000; Bechara et al. 2001) have now shown deficits in the decision-making of groups of chronic drug abusers, there is a strong case for the 'working hypothesis' that chronic abuse of drugs is associated with altered orbital prefrontal cortex functioning (Robbins and Everitt 1999; London et al. 2000).

Supporting the growing evidence (see Box 20.1 for summary) for frontal lobe deficits in chronic drug abusers, recent work with animal models has extended the now well-known demonstrations that repeated administrations of methamphetamine produces reduced levels of monoamines in the frontal cortex (Ricaurte et al. 1984) by examining behavioural, as well as neurochemical, sequelae. Thus, repeated phencyclidine treatment has been found to reduce both prefrontal dopamine (Jentsch et al. 1998a) and performance in an object-retrieval memory task (Jentsch et al. 1999, 2000), and to impair inhibition of conditioned responding (Jentsch and Taylor 2001). The same group (Jentsch et al. 2002) has also recently found that acute or repeated, intermittent administrations of doses (2 or 4 mg/kg) of cocaine for up to 30 days impaired the reversal, but not the acquisition, of object discriminations. The significance of this finding is that reversal learning is known to depend particularly on circuitry incorporating the orbitofrontal cortex, amygdala and nucleus accumbens in monkeys (Dias et al. 1996) and humans (Rahman et al. 1999). Thus, this type of deficit may be a particularly good 'marker' for abnormalities in this network. In an analogous way, administering escalating doses of amphetamine to rhesus monkeys has been found to alter, for up to 28 days, behavioural responses to later amphetamine challenge on spatial delayed-response tasks associated particularly with the circuitry of the dorsolateral prefrontal cortex (Castner and Goldman-Rakic 1999). In a study that is in many ways complementary

---

Box 20.1 Milestones in determining neurotoxic effects of stimulant drugs: experimental, postmortem neuropathological and neuroimaging approaches

Long-term effects of repeated methamphetamine on dopamine (DA) and 5-hydroxy-tryptamine (5HT) neurons in experimental animals (Ricaurte et al. 1984; Woolverton et al. 1989).

Striatal DA terminal markers reduced in brain tissue of chronic methamphetamine abusers

Serotonin (5HT) metabolites reduced in orbitofrontal cortex of chronic methamphetamine abusers (Wilson et al. 1996*a*, *b*).

Striatal dopamine D2 receptors reduced in chronic cocaine abusers (positron emission tomography; PET) (Volkow et al. 1993).

Reduced metabolism/blood flow in cingulate and frontal cortex (PET) (Volkow and Fowler 2000).

Chronic amphetamine and morphine in rats induce structural changes in neurons in frontostriatal circuitry (Robinson and Kolb 1999*a*, *b*).

---

to these findings, analysis using PET methodology of effects of repeated doses of amphetamine comparable with those used recreationally by humans have demonstrated depleted monoamines in monkeys (Villemagne et al. 1998), further supporting the hypothesis that neuropsychological deficits in chronic stimulant abusers may reflect cumulative effects to ascending chemical pathways modulating the information processing of the frontal lobes.

Using a micro-anatomical approach, Robinson and Kolb (1999*a*) have extended earlier work investigating the way in which repeated administration of stimulant drugs can produce structural, as well as functional, changes in the frontostriatal circuitry proposed to mediate some of the cognitive disturbances seen in drug abusers (see Rogers et al. 1999*b*; London et al. 2000). Specifically, rats were treated with either amphetamine or cocaine and then left for between 24–25 days before killing and Golgi–Cox staining. Stimulant treatment increased the number of dendritic branches and the density of dendritic spines on medium spiny neurons in the shell of the nucleus accumbens, and on apical dendrites of layer V pyramidal cells in the prefrontal cortex. Cocaine also increased branching and spine density on the basilar dendrites of pyramidal cells. These changes are interesting in that they resemble in some ways classical effects of environmental enrichment in rats (Rosenzweig and

Bennett 1996); thus the extent to which the changes produce pathological cognitive or behavioural effects is not yet clear. In future studies, the concurrent use of behavioural paradigms, tapping such relevant functions as impulse control (see also Cardinal et al. 2001), offers the opportunity to investigate underlying changes in neural function consequent to prolonged administration of stimulant drugs, which may underpin observable cognitive failures in chronic drug abusers.

There has been recent emphasis on the potential neurobiological underpinnings of neuropsychological deficits associated with repeated exposure to 3,4-dioxyethylenemethamphetamine (MDMA; 'ecstasy'). This interest follows several demonstrations that even moderate doses of MDMA produce reductions in markers of serotonergic function and persisting morphological changes in several animal models (e.g. Commins et al. 1987; Ricaurte et al. 1992). Such evidence converges with that of reduced serotonin receptor binding in MDMA users with appropriate ligand-imaging methodologies (McCann et al. 1998; Semple et al. 1999). To go with these findings, several studies have now shown that MDMA users are impaired on tests of memory, and, sometimes, more complex tests of attention compared with non-drug-using controls and other drug-abusing groups (Krystal et al. 1992; Parrott et al. 1998; Bolla et al. 1999; McCann et al. 1999; Gouzoulis-Mayfrank et al. 2000).

The neural basis for these deficits is unclear at the current time, with some recent studies suggesting that concomitant use of cannabis accounts for at least some of the deficits observed in MDMA users (Rodgers 2000; Croft et al. 2001). However, at least two studies that controlled for clinical confounding variables such as use of other illicit drugs and personality variables associated with drug use suggest that MDMA use may not lead to generalized deficits on, for example, tests of frontal lobe function, but may be associated with problems in various forms of memory function and impulse control mechanisms (Morgan 1998, 1999, 2000). Additionally, further research is needed to investigate the relationship between these cognitive impairments and the lowered mood consequent to MDMA use (Curran and Travill 1997), and also the possibility of deficits in affective learning, which have been shown recently to be sensitive to serotonergic manipulation in healthy volunteers (Rogers et al. 1999*a*). Finally, work with animal models suggests that neuromodulatory changes may persist for between 5 and 7 years following MDMA treatment; however, there has been little work to discover whether the cognitive deficits seen in MDMA users persist in the abstinent state. Reneman et al. (2001) report that both current MDMA users and MDMA users that have abstained from use for at least 1 year show impairments on several indices of memory compared with non-drug-using controls, but that only the current MDMA users show reductions in the density of the serotonin transporter as measured by single photon emission computed tomography (SPECT). The authors suggest that some MDMA-related neurochemical changes may be reversible, while cognitive changes may persist.

McCann and Molliver (2001) caution that changes in radioligand binding may underestimate underlying neurochemical change consequent to MDMA use, and that further work with animal models is needed to clarify the causal relationship between MDMA use and cognitive deficits in clinical samples. It is worth noting that MDMA use may also be too recent a phenomenon for well-designed studies to address the persistence of cognitive deficits over the periods of time over which serotonergic changes have been observed in animal studies up to 5–7 years (Woolverton et al. 1987).

Opiates

There has been much less research into the neuropsychological deficits associated with chronic opiate abuse in comparison with that of cannabis and stimulants. A few relatively early studies reported impairments in groups of opiate abusers on traditional batteries of neuropsychological tests such as the Halstead–Reitan battery, the Wechsler Adult Intelligence Scale (WAIS) and aphasia tests (Grant et al. 1978). Hill and Mikhael (1979) found some evidence of impairment in several measures of memory but less impairment in the capacity for abstraction and reasoning (e.g. the Category tests). Marked impairment in memory function in opiate abusers is broadly consistent with recent data indicating that chronic administration of opiates interferes with neurogenesis within the hippocampus under conditions of forced administration and self-administration in rats (Eisch et al. 2000).

Partly because of the lack of deficits on tasks of abstraction, some investigators have concluded that opiate abuse does not involve deficient frontal lobe functioning (Bruhn and Maage 1975; Rounsaville 1982). However, recent work utilizing more sensitive measures that have been validated with both neurological and functional-imaging studies has shown that opiate abusers are impaired in the completion of tasks sensitive to frontal lobe damage (Ornstein et al. 2000), although these deficits do not appear to include problems with altered attentional control or altered decision-making (Rogers et al. 1999b; Ornstein et al. 2000). The finding that opiate abusers were not as impaired as stimulant abusers on the decision-making task should be interpreted with caution and does not preclude that opiate abusers do not have deficits in choices involving different rewards and punishment. Thus, Madden et al. (1997) report that, in choices between hypothetical monetary rewards, opiate abusers tend to choose the smaller rewards rather more frequently than did non-drug-using controls. Moreover, this tendency was enhanced when the reward was heroin compared with money. Further research with such procedures may clarify whether such patterns of choices reflect increased trait impulsivity as measured by personality inventories previously seen in other populations of drug abusers (Rosenthal et al. 1990). Procedures that probe clinically relevant behavioural patterns, or traits, offer the prospect of establishing links between hypotheses about underlying psychological and neural dysfunction and drug abuse as it presents in the clinic.

A particular difficulty in the interpretation of neuropsychological deficits in opiate abusers is the high incidence of methadone treatment. Methadone treatment may itself induce cognitive deficits through its own pharmacological actions. To date, published studies have not attempted to address this issue. There is much less evidence for persisting structural or functional changes in brain function following repeated administration of opiates than is the case for stimulants and even cannabis. However, Robinson and Kolb (1999*b*) have reported that repeated administration of morphine can lead to morphological change in the frontal cortex of rats that might underpin the kinds of deficits reported by Ornstein et al. (2000). Combining research with animal models, perhaps involving delay-discounting paradigms (Madden et al. 1997; Cardinal et al. 2001) and regimes of opiate treatment, are needed to establish whether morphological changes can induce cognitive changes analogous to those seen in humans after opiate abuse.

Conclusions

The development of improved preventative and treatment programmes for drug misuse will benefit from improved knowledge about any possible role of cognitive dysfunction in the onset and maintenance of drug-seeking behaviour. Simultaneously, diagnostic systems need to be refined to characterize more precisely the nature of substance abuse disorders at various stages in their pathology so that the clinical impact of (neuro)cognitive dysfunction can be more fully appreciated. It seems likely that drug abuse is associated with deficits involving attentional, mnemonic and response-based cognitive mechanisms. These deficits are often relatively subtle and, while apparent across drug preferences, do have an uncertain relationship with the abstinent state. For these reasons, the next stage of research will need to identify groups of abusers with more consistent and homogeneous patterns of drug use, and to employ methodologies that characterize acute cognitive effects of drugs of abuse and of concurrent medication.

Future research needs to link the neurocognitive deficits in chronic drug abusers to patterns of brain physiology demonstrated by the major imaging modalities. The growing evidence that substance abuse involves dysfunction across several levels of the cognitive system, including the limbic–striatal circuitry mediating incentive/motivational processes in respect of the drugs of abuse, and the frontostriatal circuitry mediating attentional, decisional and output mechanisms (Jentsch and Taylor 1999) points to valid areas of inquiry.

One example of such an approach relates to the recent suggestion that decreased D2 receptor activity in the striatum disturbs the functioning of circuitry of the orbitofrontal and cingulate cortices, possibly mediating cognitive deficits associated with drug abuse (Volkow and Fowler 2000). The demonstration that D2 receptor availability correlated with craving in the case of the right orbital prefrontal cortex and right striatum, and with mood in the case of prefrontal cortical metabolism, indicates the relevance of future studies that can establish the relationship between underlying neural pathology, cognitive dysfunction and measurable features of drug dependence (e.g. craving). Such studies also provide a pointer to the conjoint use of monoaminergic (and other) agents as a means of correcting these disturbances. Finally, these developments need to be linked to the developing work on genetically mediated individual differences in receptor function (see Chapter 19 by Stephens et al.) and cognitive and behavioural paradigms with proven construct validity, to establish whether these neurocognitive deficits are the result of long-term drug use and represent an important precursor of compulsive patterns of drug-seeking and drug-taking behaviour characteristic of addiction itself.

Acknowledgements

Supported by a Programme grant from the Wellcome Trust and completed within the MRC Co-operative in Brain, Behaviour and Psychiatry. We should like to thank A Bechara and S Grant for helpful discussions.

REFERENCES

Allen DN, Goldstein G and Seaton BE (1997). Cognitive rehabilitation of chronic alcohol abusers. *Neuropsychol Rev*, 7, 21–39.

Altman J, Everitt BJ, Glautier S et al. (1996). The biological, social and clinical bases of drug addiction: commentary and debate. *Psychopharmacology*, 125, 285–345.

Anderson SW, Damasio H, Jones RD and Tranel D (1991). Wisconsin Card Sorting Test performance as a measure of frontal lobe damage. *J Clin Exp Neuropsychol*, 13, 909–22.

Bassoa MR and Bornstein RA (2000). Neurobehavioral consequences of substance and HIV infection. *J Psychopharmacol*, 14, 228–37.

Beatty WW, Katzung VM, Moreland VJ and Nixon SJ (1995). Neuropsychological performance of recently abstinent alcoholics and cocaine abusers. *Drug Alcohol Depend*, 37, 247–53.

Bechara A, Damasio AR, Damasio H and Anderson SW (1994). Insensitivity to future consequences following damage to human prefrontal cortex. *Cognition*, 50, 7–15.

Bechara A, Dolan S, Denburg N, Hindes A, Anderson SW and Nathan PE (2001). Decision-making deficits, linked to dysfunctional ventromedial prefrontal cortex, revealed in alcohol and stimulant abusers. *Neuropsychologia*, 39, 376–89.

Berry J, van Gorp W, Herzberg DS et al. (1993). Neuropsychological deficits in abstinent cocaine abusers: preliminary findings after two weeks of abstinence. *Drug Alcohol Depend*, 32, 231–7.

Block RI and Ghoneim MM (1993). Effects of chronic marijuana use on human cognition. *Psychopharmacology*, 110, 219–28.

Block RI, O'Leary DS, Ehrhardt JC et al. (2000*a*). Effects of frequent marijuana use on brain tissue volume and composition. *Neuroreport*, 11, 491–6.

Block RI, O'Leary DS, Hichwa RD et al. (2000*b*). Cerebellar hypoactivity in frequent marijuana users. *NeuroReport*, 11, 749–53.

Bolla KI, McCann UD and Ricaurte GA (1998). Impaired memory function in (±) 3, 4-methylenedioxymethamphetamine (MDMA, 'ecstasy') users. *Neurology*, 51, 1532–7.

Bolla KI, Rothman R and Cadet JL (1999). Dose-related neurobehavioral effects of chronic cocaine use. *J Neuropsychiatry Clin Neurosci*, 11, 361–9.

Bolla KI, Funderburk FR and Cadet JL (2000). Differential effects of cocaine and cocaine alcohol on neurocognitive performance. *Neurology*, 54, 2285–92.

Breiter HC, Gollub RL, Weisskoff RM et al. (1997). Acute effects of cocaine on human brain activity and emotion. *Neuron*, 19, 591–611.

Bruhn P and Maage N (1975). Intellectual and neuropsychological functions in young men with heavy and long-term patterns of drug abuse. *Am J Psychiatry*, 132, 397–401.

Cardinal RN, Pennicott DR, Sugathapala CL, Robbins TW and Everitt BJ (2001). Impulsive choice induced in rats by lesions of the nucleus accumbens core. *Science*, 292, 2499–501.

Carroll KM, Rounsaville BJ and Bryant KJ (1993). Alcoholism in treatment-seeking cocaine abusers: clinical and prognostic significance. *J Stud Alcohol*, 54, 199–208.

Castner SA and Goldman-Rakic PS (1999). Long-lasting psychotomimetic consequences of repeated low-dose amphetamine exposure in rhesus monkeys. *Neuropsychopharmacology*, 20, 10–28.

Commins DL, Vosmer G, Virus GM, Woolverton WL, Schuster CR and Seiden LS (1987). Biochemical and histological evidence methylenedioxymethamphetamine (MDMA) is toxic to neurons in the rat brain. *J Pharmacol Exp Ther*, 241, 338–45.

Cooper JR, Bloom FE and Roth RH (1996). *The Biochemical Basis of Neuropharmacology*, 7th edn. New York: Oxford University Press.

Croft RJ, Mackay AJ, Mills AT and Gruzelier JG (2001). The relative contributions of ecstasy and cannabis to cognitive impairment. *Psychopharmacology*, 153, 373–9.

Curran HV and Morgan C (2001). Cognitive, dissociative and psychotogenic effects of ketamine in recreational users on the night of drug use and 3 days later. *Addiction*, 95, 575–90.

Curran HV and Travill RA (1997). Mood and cognitive effects of +/-3,4-methylenedioxyamphetamine (MDMA, 'ecstasy'): week-end 'high' followed by mid-week low. *Addiction*, 92, 821–31.

Dias R, Robbins TW and Roberts AC (1996). Dissociation in prefrontal cortex of affective and attentional shifts. *Nature*, 380, 69–72.

Ehrenreich H, Rinn T, Kunert HJ et al. (1999). Specific attentional dysfunction in adults following early start of cannabis use. *Psychopharmacology*, 142, 295–301.

Eisch AJ, Barrot M, Schad CA, Self DW and Nestler EJ (2000). Opiates inhibit neurogenesis in the adult rat hippocampus. *Neurotoxicol Teratol*, 97, 7579–84.

Elliott R, Sahakian BJ, Matthews K, Bannerjea A, Rimmer J and Robbins TW (1997). Effects of methylphenidate on spatial working memory and planning in healthy young adults. *Psychopharmacology*, 131, 196–206.

Everitt BJ, Dickinson A and Robbins TW (2001). The neuropsychological basis of addictive behaviour. *Brain Res Rev*, 36, 129–38.

Feldman RS, Meyer JS and Quenzer L (1997). *Principles of Neuropsychopharmacology.* Sunderland, MA: Sinauer Associates.

Fletcher JM, Page B, Francis DJ et al. (1996). Cognitive correlates of long-term cannabis use in Costa Rica men. *Arch Gen Psychiatry*, 53, 1051–7.

Fried PA and Smith AM (2001). A literature review of the consequences of prenatal marijuana exposure: an emerging theme of a deficiency in aspects of executive function. *Neurotoxicol Teratol*, 23, 1–11.

Gollub RL, Breiter HC, Kantor H et al. (1998). Cocaine decreases cortical cerebral blood flow but does not obscure regional activation in functional magnetic resonance imaging in human subjects. *J Cereb Blood Flow Metab*, 18, 724–724.

Gouzoulis-Mayfrank E, Daumann J, Tuchtenhagen F et al. (2000). Impaired cognitive performance in drug free users of recreational ecstasy (MDMA). *J Neurol Neurosurg Psychiatry*, 68, 719–25.

Grant I, Adams KM, Carlin AS, Rennick PM, Judd LL and Schoof K (1978). Collaborative neuropsychological study of polydrug users. *Arch Gen Psychiatry*, 35, 1063–74.

Grant S, Contoreggi C and London ED (2000). Drug abusers show impaired performance in a laboratory test of decision-making. *Neuropsychologia*, 38, 1180–7.

Gurevich EV and Joyce JN (1999). Distribution of dopamine D3 receptor expressing neurons in the human forebrain: comparison with D2 receptor expressing neurons. *Neuropsychopharmacology*, 20, 60–80.

Herkenham M, Lynn AB, Little MD et al. (1990). Cannabinoid receptor localization in brain. *Proc Natl Acad Sci USA*, 87, 1932–6.

Hill SY and Mikhael MA (1979). Computerised transaxial tomographic and neuropsychological evaluations in chronic alcohol and heroin abusers. *Am J Psychiatry*, 136, 598–602.

Janowsky DS and Risch C (1979). Amphetamine psychosis and psychotic symptoms. *Psychopharmacology*, 65, 73–7.

Jatlow P (1995). Cocaethylene. What is it? *Am J Clin Pathol*, 104, 120–1.

Jentsch JD and Taylor JR (1999). Impulsivity resulting from frontostriatal dysfunction in drug abuse: implications for the control of behavior by reward-related stimuli. *Psychopharmacology*, 146, 373–90.

Jentsch JD and Taylor JR (2001). Impaired inhibition of conditioned responses produced by sub-chronic administration of phencyclidine to rats. *Neuropsychopharmacology*, 24, 66–74.

Jentsch JD, Dazzi L, Chhatwal JP, Verrico CD and Roth RH (1998a). Reduced prefrontal cortical dopamine, but not acetylcholine, release in vivo after repeated, intermittent phencyclidine administration to rats. *Neurosci Lett*, 258, 175–8.

Jentsch JD, Verrico CD, Dung L and Roth RH (1998b). Repeated exposure to 9-tetrahydrocannabinol reduces prefrontal cortical dopamine in the rat. *Neurosci Lett*, 246, 169–72.

Jentsch JD, Taylor JR, Redmond DE Jr, Elsworth JD, Youngren KD and Roth RH (1999). Dopamine D4 receptor antagonist reversal of subchronic phencyclidine-induced object retrieval/detour deficits in monkeys. *Psychopharmacology*, 142, 78–84.

Jentsch JD, Roth RH and Taylor JR (2000). Object retrieval/detour deficits in monkeys produced by prior subchronic phencyclidine administration: evidence for cognitive impulsivity. *Biol Psychiatry*, 48, 415–24.

Jentsch JD, Olausson P, De La Garza R and Taylor JR (2002). Impairments of learning reversal and response perseveration after repeated, intermittent cocaine administration in monkeys. *Neuropsychopharmacology*, 26, 183–90.

Koelega HS (1993). Stimulant drugs and vigilance performance: a review. *Psychopharmacology*, 111, 1–16.

Krystal JH, Price LH, Opsahl C, Ricaurte GA and Heninger GR (1992). Chronic 3,4-methylenedioxymethamphetamine (MDMA) use: effects on mood and neuropsychological function. *Am J Drug Alcohol Abuse*, 18, 331–41.

Lawston J, Borella A, Robinson JK and Whitaker-Azmitia PM (2000). Changes in hippocampal morphology following chronic treatment with the synthetic cannabinoid WIN 55,212-2. *Brain Res*, 877, 407–10.

Lee ACH, Owen AM, Rogers RD, Sahakian BJ and Robbins TW (2000). Utility of CANTAB in functional neuroimaging. In *Functional Neuroimaging in Child Psychiatry*, ed. M Ernst and JM Rumsey, pp. 366–78. Cambridge: Cambridge University Press.

Lewis DA (2001). The catecholamine innervation of the primate cerebral cortex. In *Stimulant Drugs and ADHD: Basic and Clinical Neuroscience*, ed. MV Solanto, AFT Arnsten and FX Castellanos, pp. 77–103. New York: Oxford University Press.

Liu X, Matochik JA, Cadet JL and London ED (1998). Smaller volume of prefrontal lobe in polysubstance abusers: a magnetic resonance imaging study. *Neuropsychopharmacology*, 18, 243–52.

London ED, Ernst M, Grant S, Bonson K and Weinstein A (2000). Orbitofrontal cortex and human drug abuse: functional imaging. *Cereb Cortex*, 10, 334–42.

Madden GJ, Petry NM, Badger GJ and Bickel WK (1997). Impulsive and self-control choices in opioid-dependent patients and non-drug-using control participants: drug and monetary rewards. *Exp Clin Psychopharmacol*, 5, 256–62.

Majewska MD (1996). Cocaine addiction as a neurological disorder: implication for treatment. *NIDA Res Monogr*, 1631–2.

McCann UD and Molliver ME (2001). 'Ecstasy' and serotonin neurotoxicity. New findings raise more questions. *Arch Gen Psychiatry*, 58, 901–6.

McCann UD, Szabo Z, Scheffel U et al. (1998). Positron emission tomographic evidence of toxic effect of MDMA ('ecstasy') on brain serotonin in human beings. *Lancet*, 352, 1433–7.

McCann UD, Mertl M, Eligulahvilli and Ricaurte GA (1999). Cognitive performance in (±) 3,4-methylenedioxymethamphetamine (MDMA, 'ecstasy') users: a controlled study. *Psychopharmacology*, 143, 417–25.

McCrady BS and Smith DE (1986). Implications of cognitive impairment for the treatment of alcoholism. *Alcohol Clin Exp Res*, 10, 145–59.

McKetin R and Solowij N (1999). Event-related potential indices of auditory selective attention in dependent amphetamine users. *Biol Psychiatry*, 45, 1488–97.

Morgan MJ (1998). Recreational use of ecstasy (MDMA) is associated with elevated impulsivity. *Neuropsychopharmacology*, 19, 253–64.

Morgan MJ (1999). Memory deficits associated with recreational use of 'ecstasy' (MDMA). *Psychopharmacology*, 141, 30–6.

Morgan MJ (2000). Ecstasy (MDMA): a review of its possible persistent psychological effects. *Psychopharmacology*, 152, 230–48.

O'Malley S, Adamse M, Heaton RK and Gawin FH (1992). Neuropsychological impairment in chronic cocaine abusers. *Am J Drug Alcohol Abuse*, 18, 131–44.

Ongur D and Price JL (2000). The organization of networks within the orbital and medial prefrontal cortex of rats, monkeys and humans. *Cereb Cortex*, 10, 206–19.

Ornstein TJ, Iddon JL, Baldacchino AM et al. (2000). Profiles of cognitive dysfunction in chronic amphetamine and heroin abusers. *Neuropsychopharmacology*, 23, 113–26.

Parrott AC, Lees A, Garnham NJ, Jones M and Wesnes K (1998). Cognitive performance in recreational users of MDMA or ecstasy. *J Psychopharmacol*, 12, 79–83.

Pope HG, Gruber AJ and Yurgelun-Todd D (1995). The residual neuropsychological effects of cannabis: the current status of research. *Drug Alcohol Depend*, 38, 25–34.

Pope HG, Gruber AJ, Hudson JI, Huesis MA and Yurgelun-Todd D (2001). Neuropsychological performance of long-term cannabis users. *Archiv Gen Psychiatry*, 58, 909–15.

Rahman S, Sahakian BJ, Hodges JR, Rogers RD and Robbins TW (1999). Specific cognitive deficits in mild frontal variant frontotemporal dementia. *Brain*, 122, 1469–93.

Rahman S, Sahakian BJ, Cardinal R, Rogers RD and Robbins TW (2001). Decision-making and neuropsychiatry. *Trends Cognit Sci*, 5, 271–7.

Reneman L, Lavalaye J, Schmand B et al. (2001). *Archiv Gen Psychiatry*, 58, 901–6.

Ricaurte GA, Schuster CR and Seiden LS (1984). Long-term effects of repeated methamphetamine administration on dopamine and serotonin neurons in the rat brain: a regional study. *Brain*, 193, 153–63.

Ricaurte GA, Martello A, Katz JL and Martello MB (1992). Lasting effects of (±)-3,4-methylenedioxymethamphetamine (MDMA) on central serotonergic neurons in nonhuman primates: neurochemical observations. *J Pharmacol Exp Ther*, 261, 616–22.

Robbins TW and Everitt BJ (1999). Drug addiction: bad habits add up. *Nature*, 398, 567–70.

Robinson JE, Heaton RK and O'Malley S (1999). Neuropsychological functioning in cocaine abusers with and without alcohol dependence. *J Int Neuropsychol Soc*, 5, 10–19.

Robinson TE and Kolb B (1999*a*). Alterations in the morphology of dendrites and dendritic spines in the nucleus accumbens and prefrontal cortex following repeated treatment with amphetamine or cocaine. *Eur J Neurosci*, 11, 1598–604.

Robinson TE and Kolb B (1999*b*). Morphine alters the structure of neurons in the nucleus accumbens and neocortex of rats. *Synapse*, 33, 160–2.

Rodgers J (2000). Cognitive performance amongst recreational users of 'ecstasy'. *Psychopharmacology*, 151, 19–24.

Rogers RD, Blackshaw AJ, Middleton HC et al. (1999*a*). Tryptophan depletion impairs stimulus–reward learning while methylphenidate disrupts attentional control in healthy young adults: implications for the monoaminergic basis of impulsive behaviour. *Psychopharmacology*, 146, 482–91.

Rogers RD, Everitt BJ, Baldacchino A et al. (1999*b*). Dissociating deficits in the decision-making cognition of chronic amphetamine abusers, opiate abusers, patients with focal damage to prefrontal cortex, and tryptophan-depleted normal volunteers: evidence for monoaminergic mechanisms. *Neuropsychopharmacology*, 20, 322–9.

Roselli M and Ardila A (1996). Cognitive effects of cocaine and polydrug abuse. *J Clin Exp Neuropsychol*, 18, 122–35.

Rosenthal TL, Edwards NB, Ackerman BJ, Knott DH and Rosenthal RH (1990). Substance abuse patterns reveal contrasting personality traits. *J Subst Abuse*, 2, 255–63.

Rosenzweig MR and Bennett EL (1996). Psychobiology of plasticity: effects of training and experience on brain and behavior. *Behav Brain Res*, 78, 57–65.

Rounsaville BJ (1982). Neuropsychological functioning in opiate addicts. *J Nerv Ment Dis*, 170, 209–16.

Rusted JM, Mackee A, Williams R and Willner P (1998). Deprivation state but not nicotine content of the cigarette affects responding by smokers on a progressive ratio task. *Psychopharmacology*, 140, 411–17.

Sahakian BJ and Owen AM (1992). Computerised assessment in psychiatry using CANTAB: discussion paper. *J R Soc Med*, 85, 399–402.

Semple DM, Ebmeier KP, Glabus MF, O'Carroll RE and Johnstone EC (1999). Reduced in vivo binding to the serotonin transporter in the cerebral cortex of MDMA ('ecstasy') users. *Br J Psychiatry*, 175, 63–9.

Solowij N (1995). Do cognitive impairments recover following cessation of cannabis use? *Life Sci*, 56, 2119–26.

Solowij N (1998). *Cannabis and Cognitive Functioning*. Cambridge: Cambridge University Press.

Solowij N, Michie PT and Fox AM (1995). Differential impairments of selective attention due to frequency and duration of cannabis use. *Biol Psychiatry*, 37, 731–9.

Strickland TL, Mena I, Villanueva-Meyer J et al. (1993). Cerebral perfusion and neuropsychological consequences of chronic cocaine use. *J Neuropsychiatry Clin Neurosci*, 5, 419–27.

Strickland TL, Stein RA, Khalsa H and Andre K (1997). Gender differences in neuropsychological test performance among cocaine abusers. *Arch Clin Neuropsychol*, 12, 410–11.

Villemagne V, Yuan J, Wong DF et al. (1998). Brain dopamine in baboons treated with doses of methamphetamine comparable to those recreationally abused by humans: evidence from [11C]WIN-35,428 positron emission tomography studies and direct in vitro determinations. *J Neurosci*, 18, 419–27.

Volkow ND and Fowler JS (2000). Addiction, a disease of compulsion and drive: involvement of the orbitofrontal cortex. *Cereb Cortex*, 10, 318–25.

Volkow ND, Hitzemann R, Wang G-J et al. (1992). Long-term frontal brain metabolic changes in cocaine abusers. *Synapse*, 11, 184–90.

Volkow ND, Fowler JS, Wang GJ et al. (1993). Decreased dopamine D2 receptor availability is associated with reduced frontal metabolism in cocaine abusers. *Synapse*, 14, 169–77.

Volkow ND, Gillespie H, Mullani N et al. (1996). Brain glucose metabolism in chronic marijuana users at baseline and during marijuana intoxication. *Psychiatry Res*, 67, 29–38.

Volkow ND, Wang G-J, Fischman MW et al. (1997). Relationship between subjective effects of cocaine and dopamine transporter occupancy. *Nature*, 386, 827–30.

Wilson JM, Kalasinsky KS, Levey AI et al. (1996*a*). Striatal dopamine nerve terminal markers in human, chronic methamphetamine users. *Nat Med*, 2, 699–703.

Wilson JM, Levey AI, Bergeron C et al. (1996*b*). Striatal dopamine, dopamine transporter, and vesicular monoamine transporter in chronic cocaine users. *Ann Neurol*, 40, 428–39.

Wilson W, Mathew R, Turkington T, Hawk T, Coleman RE and Provenzale J (2000). Brain morphological changes and early marijuana use: a magnetic resonance and positron emission tomography study. *J Addict Dis*, 19, 1–22.

Woolverton WL, Ricaurte GA, Forno LS and Seiden LS (1987). Long-term effects of chronic methamphetamine administration in rhesus monkeys. *Brain Res*, 486, 73–8.

Young SN, Smith SE, Pihl RO and Ervin FR (1985). Tryptophan depletion causes a rapid lowering of mood in normal males. *Psychopharmacology*, 87, 173–7.

Index

Note: page numbers in bold denote illustrations or tables